Disability Rights Handbook

22nd edition
April 1997–April 1998

by Judith Paterson

Address list compiled by Lorna Reith,
Pauline Day, Vincent Luttman

Acknowledgements

With thanks to contributors to this edition of the Handbook: David Brodie, Mike Ellison, Geoffrey Ferres, Harry Harmer, Simon Osborne, Earl Piggott-Smith, Lorna Reith, Sylvia Saxton, Pauline Thompson, Peter Turville, Sally West and John Zebedee.

I would also like to thank those who contributed comments or helped with the checking of this year's Handbook: Dave Allsop (Ferret Information Systems), Stephen Cragg, Nadya Kassam, Duncan Lane (London Advice Services Alliance), Vincent Luttman, Dominic Milne, Iain Murray, Nick Robinson, Alun Thomas, Pauline A Thompson MBE.

Thanks also to colleagues at Disability Alliance for their work on sales administration, distribution and for their practical support: Henry Conway, Terry DeBrou, Abi Franses, Kathryn Hindley, Marilyn Howard, Sharon Kelly, Sue Kenney, Philomena Murphy, Michael Stavri, Damon Willcox and Pam Wright. For their support and encouragement, thanks to Emily Paterson and Hugh Paterson.

This year once again, I am very grateful for the invaluable assistance of staff at the DSS for checking and commenting on drafts at short notice – and to Lorna Dacres at the Information Division for co-ordinating this. I would also like to acknowledge the helpful comments from staff at the Department for Education and Employment, the Department of Health, Department of the Environment and the Independent Review Service for the Social Fund.

I am ever grateful to Richard Bates at Discript for his fast and accurate artwork. Many thanks also to Anderson Fraser for print and print management, in particular to Debbie Kamofsky.

Disability Alliance wishes to gratefully acknowledge the financial support of London Boroughs Grants Committee and the Department of Health towards our rights service.

Special acknowledgement goes to Sally Robertson who wrote the Disability Rights Handbook from the 6th edition through to the 18th edition.

We do our best to ensure the information in the Handbook is correct. However, changes in the law after April 1997 might affect the accuracy of some of the information. Where this could be important to you, you should check the details with a local advice centre or your local DSS office. If you think anything in the Handbook is incorrect, please write and tell us. Thanks to all those who wrote in to us this year with comments and suggestions on the Handbook. Your contributions are always welcome.

Contents

Benefits Checklist **4**

Section A **Overview**
Chapters
1 Introduction **7**
2 Disability Discrimination Act **10**

Section B **Income support**
Chapter
3 Income support **14**

Section C **Housing and council tax benefits**
Chapters
4 Housing benefit and council tax benefit **39**
5 Council tax **55**

Section D **Social fund**
Chapters
6 Regulated social fund **59**
7 Discretionary social fund **60**

Section E **Unable to work?**
Chapters
8 Incapacity for work **67**
9 Contributions and credits **76**
10 Statutory sick pay **80**
11 Incapacity benefit **85**
12 Transitional rules **89**
13 Severe disablement allowance **91**

Section F **Unemployment to employment**
Chapters
14 Jobseeker's allowance **98**
15 Employment and training **108**
16 Disability working allowance **111**

Section G **Care and mobility**
Chapters
17 Disability living allowance **119**
18 Attendance allowance **140**
19 Invalid care allowance **142**
20 Help with mobility needs **145**

Section H **Special compensation schemes**
Chapters
21 Industrial injuries scheme **148**
22 War disablement pension **156**
23 Criminal injuries compensation **159**
24 Vaccine damage payments **161**
25 Compensation recovery **162**

Section I **Children and young people**
Chapters
26 Maternity rights **163**
27 Child benefit **165**
28 Family credit **167**
29 Children with disabilities **169**
30 Young people with disabilities **171**
31 Financing studies **172**

Section J **Practical help at home**
Chapters
32 Care services **177**
33 Help with equipment **182**
34 Help with buying your own care **184**

Section K **Residential care**
Chapters
35 Help with residential care **187**
36 Benefits in care – since April 1993 **190**
37 Charging for residential care **193**
38 Benefits in care – before April 1993 **198**

Section L **Hospital and abroad**
Chapters
39 Going into hospital **203**
40 Hospital – one year on **208**
41 Going abroad **209**

Section M **Retirement**
Chapters
42 Early retirement **213**
43 Benefits in retirement **213**
44 Retirement pensions **216**
45 Home responsibilities protection **220**

Section N **Other money matters**
Chapters
46 Widows **222**
47 Christmas bonus **224**
48 Health benefits **224**
49 Housing grants **226**
50 Child support **231**
51 Income tax **233**

Section O **Appeals and information**
Chapters
52 Claims and appeals **236**
53 Free legal help **251**
54 Complaining to the Ombudsman **252**

Useful Publications **254**

Disability Alliance Publications List **255**

Blue pages   Address List **257**

Index **271**

Benefits checklist

This checklist is intended as a quick guide to help you see which benefits you might be entitled to, so that you can look up the relevant chapter. It is not a guide to the benefits themselves – you still need to read the information in the chapters. More than one of the circumstances below may apply to you and you may well qualify for more than one benefit, especially if you have low savings and income. Box A.2 in Chapter 1 tells you which benefits depend on your National Insurance record and which are affected by other income.

Circumstance	Benefit
Incapable of work	
■ employed	**statutory sick pay (SSP)**
■ after 28 weeks SSP, or not employed	**incapacity benefit**
■ not enough NI contributions for incapacity benefit, and you're 80% disabled or incapable of work since before age 20	**severe disablement allowance**
■ if you can't get any of these, or can but still do not have enough to live on	**income support**
Unemployed or working less than 16 hours a week	
■ payable for 26 weeks if you've paid enough NI contributions	**contribution-based jobseeker's allowance (JSA)**
■ if you've not paid enough NI contributions, or your contribution-based JSA has run out or is not enough to live on	**income-based jobseeker's allowance**
■ if you don't have to sign on for work (eg you're incapable of work, disabled, a carer, single parent or 60 or over) and any income or savings are low	**income support**
Working at least 16 hours a week	
■ you have a child	**family credit**
■ you have a disability and get a qualifying incapacity or disability benefit	**disability working allowance**
Injured or contracted disease in work	
■ you are disabled through an industrial accident or prescribed disease	**industrial injuries disablement benefit**
■ the industrial accident or disease occurred before 1.10.90 and your earnings capacity is reduced	**reduced earnings allowance**
■ replaces reduced earnings allowance when you give up regular employment after pension age	**retirement allowance**
Disabled due to vaccine damage	**vaccine damage payment**
Injured due to violent crime	**criminal injuries compensation**
War disablement	
■ injured because of service in the Armed Forces, or a civilian disabled due to the 1939–45 war	**war disablement pension**
■ your husband died because of the war, or because of service in the Armed Forces	**war widow's pension**
Retirement	
■ from age 60 for women, or 65 for men	**retirement pension**
■ to top up your pension	**income support**
Need help with NHS costs, glasses, hospital fares	**health benefits**
Caring	
■ you care for a disabled person for at least 35 hours a week	**invalid care allowance**

Problems with walking

■ aged under 65 when you claim (under 66 if you claim before 6.10.97)	**disability living allowance mobility component**
■ hire or buy a car using the mobility component	**Motability**
■ if you get higher rate mobility component	**road tax exemption**
■ parking concessions	**orange badge scheme**

Practical help at home

■ practical help if you are disabled	**care services, eg home help, meals on wheels**
■ equipment and adaptations	**help from Social Services, or the NHS**

Need help with personal care

■ aged under 65 when you claim (under 66 if you claim before 6.10.97)	**disability living allowance care component**
■ aged 65 or over when you claim	**attendance allowance**
■ severely disabled and need help with personal care or household assistance	**Independent Living Funds**

Housing problems

■ repairs, adaptations, improvements	**housing grants (renovation and disabled facilities grants)**
■ help with the mortgage	**income support, income-based jobseeker's allowance**
■ help with the rent	**housing benefit**
■ help with the council tax	**council tax benefit, disability reduction or discount scheme**

Pregnancy

■ employed	**statutory maternity pay (SMP)**
■ recently employed or self-employed, but not entitled to SMP	**maternity allowance**
■ not entitled to SMP or maternity allowance	**incapacity benefit**
■ help with maternity expenses	**social fund maternity payment**
■ for free milk and vitamins	**health benefits**

Responsibility for children

■ responsible for a child under 16, or 16–19 in full-time, non-advanced education	**child benefit**
■ looking after a child whose parents are dead; or one is dead and other untraceable or in prison	**guardian's allowance**
■ working 16 hours a week or more	**family credit**
■ disabled child	**disability living allowance, Family Fund**
■ for free milk and vitamins	**health benefits**

Death

■ widow under 60 or whose husband did not get retirement pension	**widow's payment**
■ widow with a dependent child	**widowed mother's allowance**
■ widow aged over 45 when husband dies or widowed mother's allowance ended	**widow's pension**
■ help with the cost of a funeral	**social fund funeral payment**

If you do not have enough to live on

■ not working, or working less than 16 hours a week – if you have to sign on for work	**income support** **income-based jobseeker's allowance**
■ working at least 16 hours a week and have a child	**family credit**
■ disabled and working 16 hours or more a week	**disability working allowance**
■ paying rent for your home	**housing benefit**
■ paying council tax	**council tax benefit**

If you have needs difficult to meet out of regular income

■ if you get income support or income-based jobseeker's allowance	**social fund community care grant**
■ if you've had income support or income-based jobseeker's allowance for at least 26 weeks	**social fund budgeting loan**
■ following emergency or disaster	**social fund crisis loan**

This section of the Handbook looks at the following:

Introduction	Chapter **1**
Disability Discrimination Act	Chapter **2**

Overview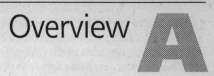

1 Introduction

1. What does the Handbook include?

This Handbook is intended as a comprehensive guide to social security benefits for disabled people, their families, carers and the many professionals who work with them. You may find it helpful to start by looking at the benefits checklist at the front of the Handbook. In addition to social security benefits, the Handbook covers practical help and services and other essential matters such as income tax, council tax and housing grants.

Much of the Handbook applies to disabled and non-disabled people alike. But it is specifically aimed at disabled people, whatever their impairment – physical, mental or sensory, whatever the degree of severity, and however they became disabled, from birth or acquired, contracted in war, at work or at home.

2. Disability Rights Bulletins

Besides the Handbook, we publish regular *Disability Rights Bulletins*. These update the Handbook and deal with changes in the law or administrative practices, government proposals for future changes and also look at some topics in greater depth than is possible in the Handbook.

We will publish three *Disability Rights Bulletins* to update this 22nd edition of the Handbook. The 23rd edition of the Handbook will be published in May 1998.

PLEASE REMEMBER TO ORDER YOUR 23RD EDITION OF THIS HANDBOOK BEFORE MAY 1998.

3. Disability and benefits

What is disability?
Few of your rights depend on what your condition is called. In most cases, your right to a benefit or service depends on the effect of your disability on your life. Within the social security system there are four main tests of disability:
- **incapacity for work** – used for statutory sick pay, incapacity benefit and severe disablement allowance; also for industrial injuries benefits and war pensioners' unemployability allowance and for income support. There are different tests of incapacity depending on the benefit you claim;
- **needing care, supervision or watching over by another person** – used for disability living allowance (DLA) care component and attendance allowance. A similar test is used for the constant attendance allowance under the industrial and war disablement schemes;
- **unable or virtually unable to walk** – used for DLA mobility component and for war pensioners' mobility supplement;
- **degree of disablement** – used for severe disablement allowance, industrial disablement benefit, war disablement pension and vaccine damage payments.

In addition there are two other definitions in use:
- **substantially and permanently handicapped** – used for registering as disabled with a local authority Social Services Department;
- **physical or mental impairment which has a substantial and long-term adverse effect on a person's ability to carry out**

A.1 The costs of disability

Disability inevitably leads to extra costs. It is far more difficult for a disabled person to manage on the same income as someone of the same age who is not disabled. Yet the average disabled person has a much lower income than the average non-disabled person. And, despite the range of benefits and other help available to people with disabilities, not all people manage to work their way through the jungle and claim their full legal entitlements. The weekly loss can be substantial.

Even among people who have claimed all they are entitled to there are still anomalies. People who are equally severely disabled can be entitled to different amounts of non-means-tested income. How old you were when you became disabled; how you became disabled; the effects of your disability; how long you have lived in the UK; and whether you worked and paid the right National Insurance contributions at the right time: all can make a difference to the total amount you may be entitled to.

The disability gap
Without going through any means test, different people who are equally and extremely severely disabled, could be entitled to:
- a maximum of £386.15 from the war disablement scheme;
- a maximum of £373.24 from the industrial injuries scheme and disability living allowance (DLA);
- a maximum of £159.70 from incapacity benefit and DLA;
- a maximum of £135.00 from severe disablement allowance (SDA) and DLA.

The gap between the maximum and minimum help available without going through a means-test now stands at £251.15 a week. But including possible entitlement to means-tested income support only cuts the disability gap to £231.95. Income support means an extra £19.20 for the SDA claimant; (or if the person is now aged over 60, an extra £24.80). Maximum incapacity benefit is £5.50 higher than income support rates (10p lower if you are now aged over 60).
NB These figures assume the person became disabled before age 35. They don't include allowances for adult or child dependants, or for housing costs. The income support figure includes the allowance for a person aged over 25, and a disability premium. Including a severe disability premium cuts the disability gap to £194.80 (£189.20, if you are now aged over 60). The war pension figure includes the age allowance payable at the age of 65.

normal day-to-day activities – used to define who is covered by the Disability Discrimination Act 1995.

Besides these main tests of disability, you may find that there are other criteria you must satisfy in order to get a particular benefit or service. The individual chapters give details of these.

The different types of benefits

Broadly speaking benefits can be divided into three categories: those which are intended to replace earnings; those which compensate for extra costs; and those which help alleviate poverty. The first category includes those benefits which are to compensate you if you are unable to work through sickness, disability, unemployment, pregnancy, retirement or caring responsibilities. In general these benefits are not subject to a means-test but some will depend on your National Insurance contribution record – see Box A.2. Benefits available to contribute towards the extra costs of disability or of caring for children are not means tested nor do they depend on National Insurance contributions. Those benefits intended to alleviate poverty by providing a basic income or topping up a low income are subject to a means-test.

4. The law

Every decision on any claim for benefit depends on something in the law. Primary legislation, in Acts of Parliament, sets out the framework and gives the Secretary of State specific powers to make regulations giving detailed provisions. The Acts of Parliament most commonly referred to in the Handbook are the Social Security Contributions and Benefits Act 1992 (SSCBA) and the Social Security Administration Act 1992 (SSAA). These consolidated and replaced almost all the previous social security Acts.

Case law

Besides the Acts and regulations, you may also need to consider case law. Social Security Commissioners hear appeals from Social Security Appeal Tribunals, Disability Appeal Tribunals and Medical Appeal Tribunals. The decisions they make, as well as decisions of the courts, make up social security case law. This clarifies any doubt about the meaning of the law, or its application to individual cases. Where case law sets up a general principal, that also sets a precedent which should be followed in similar cases. For more details, see Box O.6 in Chapter 52.

Practice – getting answers

If in doubt, check the actual law rather than guidebooks. Always check to see if a word or phrase is being used in a technical way. It may be defined in an Act, or in regulations. Or it may have been considered in case law. If a word or phrase has not been defined in law or case law, check a good dictionary: it has its ordinary English meaning.

If you are not sure about something, contact your local DSS office – see Box A.3. Ask for an explanation and outline of the exact basis (with references) for what has been, or is, happening.

It is always worth contacting an advice agency who may have copies of the law and relevant text books. Your local library may also be able to assist. Remember, if you feel a decision about your benefit is wrong you may be able to appeal, see Chapter 52.

5. Department of Social Security

The Department of Social Security (DSS) is responsible for most of the help available for people with disabilities. Almost all social security benefits are now administered by the Benefits Agency, an Executive Agency of the DSS.

Responsibility for making policy stays with the DSS. This includes setting the framework of policy objectives and resources for the delivery and administration of social security benefits.

The Secretary of State still has a decision-making role. However, some Secretary of State decisions have been formally delegated to the Benefits Agency's Chief Executive, while others remain with the policy sections of the DSS. Of course ultimately the Secretary of State for Social Security remains legally responsible for all decisions made on his behalf.

The DSS is currently engaged in a huge exercise known as the Change Programme to achieve massive savings in administration.

The day-to-day running of the social security system is the responsibility of the Benefits Agency whose Chief Executive is

---

A.2 Which benefits are affected by other income or NI contributions?

The following benefits, known as **means-tested benefits**, *are* affected by most other types of income and savings. However your National Insurance contribution record does not matter.

Means-tested benefits
- income support
- income-based jobseeker's allowance
- family credit
- disability working allowance
- housing benefit
- council tax benefit
- social fund

The following benefits, known as **non-means-tested benefits**, *are not* usually affected by other money that you have. For some of these benefits, your National Insurance record does not matter: they are listed here as **non-contributory benefits**. However for the others you must have sufficient contributions, and they are listed here as **contributory benefits**.

Non-contributory
- attendance allowance
- child benefit
- disability living allowance
- guardian's allowance
- industrial injuries benefits
- invalid care allowance
- retirement pension: category C or D
- severe disablement allowance
- statutory maternity pay
- statutory sick pay
- war disablement pensions

Contributory
- contribution-based jobseeker's allowance
- incapacity benefit
- maternity allowance
- retirement pension: category A or B
- widowed mother's allowance
- widow's payment
- widow's pension

accountable to the Secretary of State for Social Security. The Benefits Agency's headquarters is in Leeds.

The Benefits Agency has in turn contracted out some of its functions to private companies. For example, Benefits Agency leaflets are now distributed by The Stationery Office Ltd which before privatisation was Her Majesty's Stationery Office.

In this Handbook we continue to refer to the system as a DSS system, eg 'contact your local DSS office', 'write to the DSS', etc. This reflects the legal reality.

Besides the Benefits Agency, four other Executive Agencies deal with aspects of DSS operations: Child Support Agency, Contributions Agency, Information Technology Agency, War Pensions Agency.

The administration of benefits for unemployed people through Jobcentres is a joint activity which involves Benefits Agency staff and staff employed in the Employment Service, an Executive Agency of the Department for Education and Employment.

Local offices

Most benefits are dealt with by local offices. Your local phone book should make it clear which office you should contact – see Box A.3.

Small numbers of local offices, usually three, make up a Benefits Agency district. One of these offices is usually a district headquarters known as the District Office.

Each district is managed by a District Manager who has some freedom in how the district is run – so long as s/he stays within the agreed budget, overall guidelines, and specific performance targets (for example, on the accuracy of decisions and clearance times for benefit claims). Each District Manager answers to an Area Director.

In some parts of London, you may just have a branch office, with the work being done at one of three Benefits Centres in Glasgow, Belfast or Makerfield: your local office will give you full details.

Central offices

Some benefits are dealt with not by local offices but by one or more remote centres: for example disability living allowance and attendance allowance have a network of 11 Disability Benefits Centres as well as the central Unit at Fylde.

If you want to claim a benefit which is dealt with by a central office rather than by your local DSS office, the claim form for that benefit will tell you where you should send the form.

6. Northern Ireland

In Northern Ireland the Department of Health and Social Services is responsible for all social security matters, but benefits are administered by the Social Security Agency whose Chief Executive is accountable to the Secretary of State for Northern Ireland.

Northern Ireland has its own legislation, and the structure and organisation of the system is different from Great Britain. However, the rates of social security benefits and the qualifying conditions are similar to those in Great Britain – apart from the survival of rate rebates.

7. Who's who in the benefit system?

Different DSS offices are likely to be organised in slightly different ways. What follows is a rough sketch – you'll find more details in the chapters on the individual benefits. The main rules about claims, decision-making and appeals are also covered in Chapter 52. However, in all cases, you have a right to expect a good standard of service. The overall standards are set out in the Benefits Agency's Customer Charter – you can get a copy from your local office.

Each District, as well as every other management unit within the Agency, must publish its annual business plan to show how it intends to work. Your District may also provide a more user-friendly guide to its services, or its own Customer Charter.

If you want to know how your local office is organised, ask to speak to Customer Services. A Customer Services Officer can explain things and send you any relevant information.

Administrative staff – The people you see or talk to when you visit or phone a DSS office are not usually legally responsible for making a decision on your claim. Although they will do the support and maintenance work for claims, and may handle many routine claims, particularly for the means-tested benefits, these must in law be decided by an Adjudication Officer. So, if you think a decision is wrong, ask to speak to the section supervisor. S/he will usually be an *Adjudication Officer* (AO). If you think someone has just made a mistake, it might also be worth involving the Assistant Manager who is responsible for the benefit you are claiming.

Secretary of State – Note that some decisions are taken by the Secretary of State (usually by someone specially appointed to act on his behalf), not by an Adjudication Officer. There is no right of appeal to a tribunal against Secretary of State decisions – but you can ask for them to be looked at again. Many of these decisions are about procedures, rather than how much benefit you are entitled to. For example, the Secretary of State decides whether to replace a missing giro; or to pay two benefits in a combined order book. Chapter 52 has more detail about the Secretary of State's role.

Adjudication Officer (AO) – The AO is legally responsible for decisions on your entitlement to almost all benefits but won't always be based in your local office. So it may be best to write rather than phone. If you don't like a decision, ask for an explanation, in writing if possible. If you are not satisfied, appeal to an independent tribunal. The letter giving you the decision must always explain what you can do next. Before you get to a tribunal a different AO will look at your case, and may even change the decision in your favour.

Adjudicating medical authority – Industrial disablement benefit and severe disablement allowance have a different decision-making system. An adjudicating medical authority, either a single doctor, or two doctors sitting as a medical board, is responsible for a medical decision on percentage disablement. The AO then makes a decision on other aspects of your claim. If you disagree with the medical decision, you can appeal to an independent Medical Appeal Tribunal – see Chapter 52 for details.

Social Security Appeal Tribunal (SSAT) – The SSAT hears appeals against decisions of Adjudication Officers: except where that appeal concerns a disability question for disability living allowance (DLA), disability working allowance (DWA) or attendance allowance. The SSATs are run by the Independent Tribunal Service. Their role and powers are explained in Chapter 52.

Disability Appeal Tribunal (DAT) – The DAT hears appeals against decisions of Adjudication Officers which involve a disability question for DLA, DWA or attendance allowance. Like the SSAT, it is run by the Independent Tribunal Service. Chapter 52 explains its role and powers.

Social Security Commissioner – If an appeal tribunal refuses your appeal, you can apply for permission to appeal (on a point of law) to the Social Security Commissioners. They are lawyers of at least 10 years standing. They have the same status as High Court Judges. Their decisions set precedents and form 'case law'. We quote a few useful decisions in this

Handbook: eg R(S)6/85 and CM/60/86. Box O.6 in Chapter 52 explains what each reference means. Chapter 52 explains more about appealing to the Commissioners.

Social fund – For the discretionary social fund there is a different decision-making system. Initial decisions are taken by a *social fund officer*, with an ultimate right of review by a *social fund inspector* – see Chapter 7.

8. Complaints and suggestions

If you want to complain about something, or have suggestions for how Benefits Agency services could be improved, start by contacting the office dealing with the matter. It may be possible to sort things out easily. It is always best to complain as soon as something goes wrong. Don't wait until you get a decision on your claim – a complaint should not prejudice your chances of success.

If you have a complaint about a DSS doctor, you can write directly to the Director of the Benefits Agency Medical Services – see the Address List at the back of the Handbook.

In most other cases, ask the DSS for leaflet BAL 1. This outlines the sort of steps you can take if you want to complain or suggest something.

If you feel you have been treated unfairly or discriminated against or if you have special needs that are not being met, you should ask the DSS for leaflet LBF 1 – *Let's be Fair*.

If your concern is about the way in which things are, or have been done, or about practical matters such as access problems, contact the Customer Service Manager. S/he will respond in 7 days. If you're not satisfied with the response, contact the Manager of that DSS office; then the Chief Executive of the Benefits Agency. If a problem continues for some time, it can be helpful to involve your MP. If you think there is a case of maladministration, you can complain to the Ombudsman – see Chapter 54.

Compensation
In some cases you might be entitled to a special payment if the DSS has made a mistake and you've lost out financially, or your benefit payment has been interrupted or delayed – see Chapter 52. Information about special payments is in the leaflet BAL 1 – *Tell us about it* – which you can get from the DSS.

2 Disability Discrimination Act

1. Introduction

After many years of campaigning by disabled people and their supporters the Government finally introduced the Disability Discrimination Act (DDA) 1995. The DDA makes it unlawful to discriminate against disabled people in connection with employment, the provision of goods, facilities and services or the disposal or management of premises. The Act also places obligations on educational establishments, sets up a National Disability Council and allows the Government to set standards and targets for accessible public transport.

Disability Alliance, together with many other disability organisations, is strongly critical of the Act. We believe it falls far short of the comprehensive civil rights legislation which the disability movement had campaigned for. For example, under the Act employers with less than 20 staff are exempt from the employment provisions; there is no Commission, like the Equal Opportunities Commission or the Commission for Racial Equality, with enforcement powers or the ability to take up individual cases; the Act does not give disabled children equal rights of access to school; and, some of the provisions of the Act will not come into force until the next century.

However, the DDA does provide new rights for many disabled people and we believe it is important that people are aware of their rights. Disability Alliance does not have the resources to offer expert advice on the DDA, but we give suggestions of places to go for further information and help in Box A.4.

2. How is disability defined?

The DDA defines disability as *'a physical or mental impairment which has a substantial and long-term adverse effect on [your] ability to carry out normal day-to-day activities'.*

'Impairment' includes sensory impairments (for example, blindness or deafness), learning disabilities and mental illness. *'Substantial'* is defined as meaning more than minor. *'Long-term'* means effects which have lasted at least 12 months, or are likely to last at least 12 months, or are likely to last for the rest of your life. The definition also includes you if you have had a disability in the past, even if you no longer have that disability. In addition, you are covered by the Act if you have a severe disfigurement, even though it may not have any effect on your ability to carry out normal activities.

Further information about the definitions of *substantial*

A.3 Contacting the DSS

The address of your nearest social security office is in the phone book under 'Benefits Agency'. If you are in any doubt, just phone up and ask which is the right office for you. The addresses of the central units are listed in our Address List at the back of the Handbook.

Benefit Enquiry Line (BEL)
This specialises in benefits for people with disabilities. Call 0800 882200. If you have a textphone, call 0800 243355. The lines are open 8.30am – 6.30pm Monday to Friday and 9am – 1pm Saturday. Your call is free. BEL can provide general benefits advice or information. They cannot deal with your particular problems themselves, but this means your call is confidential and nothing you ask or say will go onto your file.

Forms Completion Service
Staff will fill in your claim form for you over the phone and send it to you to check and sign (can be in braille or large print). The service covers ICA, SDA, DWA, DLA, AA, industrial injuries benefit for bronchitis and emphysema. Call 0800 441144.

Incapacity Benefit Line
Staff can send information and leaflets on incapacity benefit, but do not give advice. Call 0800 868868.

Northern Ireland
To find your local social security office, look in the phone book under 'Social Security'.
NI Freeline Social Security – call 0800 616757
NI Benefit Enquiry Line (BEL) – call 0800 220674
If you have a textphone, call 0800 243787.
All three lines are open 9am – 5pm Monday to Friday.

and *long-term* are to be found in guidance issued by the Government – see Box A.4

'Day-to-day activities' involve the following: moving from place to place, manual dexterity, physical co-ordination, continence, the ability to lift, carry or move ordinary objects, speech, hearing or eyesight, memory or the ability to concentrate, learn or understand and being able to recognise physical danger.

If you have a progressive condition, such as cancer or multiple sclerosis, you will not be covered just because your condition has been diagnosed. You will only come under the definition used in the DDA from the time that you first develop symptoms that affect your ability to carry out day-to-day activities. Similarly, you will not be covered by the Act just because you have a genetic predisposition to a particular condition, such as Huntington's chorea or thalassaemia.

If your disability is helped by medication or by equipment such as a hearing aid or artificial limb, this will not be taken into account when considering whether your impairment has a substantial effect on your day-to-day activities. Note, however, that an exception is made if you wear glasses or contact lenses in that it is the effect on your vision **with** the lenses that is considered.

Registered disabled people – If you were registered as a disabled person under the Disabled Persons (Employment) Act 1944, or the Disabled Persons (Employment) Act (Northern Ireland) 1945 on both 12.1.95 and 2.12.96 then you will automatically be covered by the DDA for three years from 2.12.96.

3. Your employment rights

From 2.12.96 it is unlawful for an employer to treat you less favourably than someone else because of your disability, unless they can show that such treatment is 'justified'. The DDA covers temporary staff and contract workers, as well as permanent employees. The Act covers all employment matters, including recruitment, training, access to a company pension scheme, promotion and dismissal. Employers will also be liable for the actions of their agents. So, for example, companies which use recruitment agencies will be responsible for ensuring that their agency is acting lawfully. The government has published a Code of Practice on the employment provisions of the Act – see Box A.4.

Reasonable adjustments

The DDA requires employers to make 'reasonable adjustments' (changes) to the workplace and to employment arrangements so that a disabled employee, or disabled job applicant, is not at any substantial disadvantage. Reasonable adjustments include changes to the physical environment, such as widening a doorway to allow for wheelchair access or allocating a specific parking space for a disabled person. The term also includes changes to arrangements in the workplace, such as flexible working hours, purchasing specialised equipment, providing additional training or allowing time off for treatment.

If your employer does not own premises but rents on a lease then the landlord cannot unreasonably refuse permission for the premises to be altered to accommodate you. If a landlord does unreasonably refuse your employer permission to alter your workplace then you can take the landlord to an Industrial Tribunal – see below.

What can you do if you are discriminated against?

If you think you have been discriminated against you can take your complaint to an Industrial Tribunal. You can ask ACAS (the Advisory Conciliation and Arbitration Service) for help. In Northern Ireland the relevant body is the Labour Relations Agency. If you are a trade union member you should seek assistance from your union.

Exemptions – The DDA does not apply to employers with fewer than 20 employees. Nor does it apply to people serving in the armed forces, police officers, firefighters, prison officers, those working on board ship, aircraft or hovercraft or anyone whose work is mainly outside the UK. Small employers are however encouraged to follow the guidance in the Code of Practice.

Trade organisations, including trade unions, professional associations and Chambers of Commerce also have a duty under the DDA not to discriminate against you as a member or potential member. In the future the Government will introduce regulations which will impose a duty on trade organisations to make 'reasonable adjustments' for their potential and existing members.

From 2.12.96, the schemes for registering as disabled run by the Employment Service and the Quota Designated Employment scheme ended. You can no longer register as a disabled person for employment purposes. Note that this is different from registers of disabled people kept by local authority Social Services Departments.

A.4 For more information

You can get a Disability Discrimination Act Information Pack (DL50) from the DDA Information Line. There is also a range of Government booklets available covering different aspects of the DDA. Call 0345 622 633 or 0345 622 644 (textphone). Information is also available in Welsh, braille, audio cassette and as a special pack for people with learning disabilities.

Transport

Information about the Transport provisions of the Act can be obtained from *Department of Transport Mobility Unit, Zone 1/11, Great Minster House, 76 Marsham Street, London SW1P 4DR* (0171 271 5259; minicom 0171 271 5252).

Guidance and Codes of Practice

- *Disability Discrimination Act 1995: Guidance on matters to be taken into account in determining questions relating to the definition of disability* (£7.50)
- *Disability Discrimination Act 1995: Code of Practice – Rights of Access. Goods, Facilities, Services and Premises* (£6)
- *Disability Discrimination Act 1995: Code of Practice for the elimination of discrimination in the field of employment against disabled persons or persons who have had a disability* (£9.95)

Available in print, braille, audio-cassette and Welsh from *The Stationery Office Ltd (formerly HMSO), Publications Centre, PO Box 276, London SW8 5DT*.

Further information

You may find it helpful to contact: the RNIB; RADAR; the Disability Law Service; or your local law centre (see our Address List).

Useful books include *Disability Discrimination – the New Law (2nd Edition)* by Brian J Doyle and *Disability Discrimination Act* by Caroline Gooding.

Local authorities may find publications produced by the Local Government Information Unit (0171 608 1051) helpful.

4. Access to goods and services

Since 2.12.96 it has been unlawful for agencies (service providers) who provide goods, facilities or services directly to the general public to discriminate against disabled people. Service providers include commercial businesses such as shops, hotels, banks, cinemas, restaurants and telecommunications companies. The term also includes those providing public services such as hospitals, railway stations, libraries, swimming pools and government offices. The size of the company makes no difference, nor does it matter whether or not you pay for the service. Insurance companies are also covered but special rules apply. Note, however, that private clubs and associations are exempt from the Act in relation to serving their members.

You will have been discriminated against if a service provider treats you less favourably than someone else for a reason relating to your disability, and this treatment cannot be 'justified'. Examples of discrimination would include refusing to serve you, offering you a lower standard of service or less favourable terms. There are some grounds under which treating a disabled person less favourably can be justified, for example, health and safety where a risk can be proven. Further information can be found in the Code of Practice – see Box A.4.

Reasonable adjustments

In the future, service providers will also be required to make 'reasonable adjustments' to ensure that you have access to their service. The Act mentions three types of adjustments: to make reasonable changes to policies, practices or procedures that make it unreasonably difficult for disabled people to use their service; to take reasonable steps to obtain aids, such as induction loops, that will help disabled people use their service; and to take reasonable steps to remove or alter a feature of their premises that makes it unreasonably difficult or impossible for a disabled person to use the service. If the feature cannot be changed the service provider will be expected to find an alternative way of providing the service. These duties will be phased in over the period 1998-2005 but the Government is yet to confirm the implementation timetable or explain in detail what these new duties will entail in practice.

The Government has published a Code of Practice which contains practical advice for service providers – see Box A.4.

5. Housing

From 2.12.96 it has been unlawful for anyone letting or selling land or property to discriminate against disabled people. Most types of premises are included in the provisions – houses, flats, hostels and business premises – though hotels and guest houses are covered by the Access to Goods and Services section of the Act, as is the provision of general housing information – see 4 above.

The DDA applies to almost any agency involved in letting or selling property including: councils, housing associations, private landlords, estate agencies, accommodation agencies, banks and building societies, property developers and owner occupiers.

You will have been discriminated against if you are treated less favourably than someone else for a reason relating to your disability and this treatment cannot be 'justified'. For example, if you were charged a higher rent or a higher deposit than other tenants, for a reason related to your disability, then your landlord would be guilty of discrimination.

Note though, that the Act exempts landlords who let rooms to six or fewer people in their own homes and there is no legal obligation on anyone selling or letting property to alter the premises in order to make them accessible for you.

6. Education

This section of the DDA came into force in September 1996. Although the education provisions of the DDA do not give you any enforceable rights as an individual, it is worth noting that if an education building is being used for non-educational purposes then the other provisions (eg Access to Goods and Services) of the Act still apply, other than when a school is used as a polling station since voting is not covered under the Act.

Schools

The Act places a duty on schools in England and Wales to include in their annual reports; details of their arrangements for admitting disabled pupils, how they will ensure that those pupils receive the same treatment as other pupils and what facilities they will provide to enable disabled pupils to access the education being offered.

The DDA does not apply to schools in Scotland or Northern Ireland. The relevant legislation in Scotland is the Education (Scotland) Act 1980 and in Northern Ireland it is Article 8(3) of the Education (Northern Ireland) Order 1996.

Further education

The DDA places a duty on Further Education Funding Councils in England and Wales to ensure that further education colleges publish disability statements with information about their facilities for disabled students. The Act also requires the Funding Councils to report back to Government on their progress. Statutes are already in force covering development plans in further education colleges in Scotland. Further education colleges in Northern Ireland are not currently covered but may be in future.

Higher education

The DDA places a duty on Higher Education Funding Councils in England, Wales and Scotland to take account of the needs of disabled students and to require institutions which they fund to provide disability statements. The DDA does not apply to higher education institutions in Northern Ireland.

7. Transport

The Public Transport Vehicles section of the Act covers taxis, buses, coaches, trains and trams. Transport termini (airports, bus and rail stations, etc) are covered under the Access to Goods and Services section of the Act – see 4 above. The Act gives the Government the power to require all new public transport vehicles and newly licensed taxis to be accessible to disabled people. However, the Act also gives the Government a fairly wide power to grant exemptions.

Taxis will also be required to carry service animals (guide dogs) without charging extra. Mini-cabs are not covered by the Act.

This section of the Act has not yet been implemented but regulations are expected that will require all trains and trams brought into use after the end of December 1998 to be accessible.

The Department of Transport Mobility Unit produces information bulletins on the transport provisions of the Act – see Box A.4.

8. The National Disability Council (NDC)

The NDC is an independent body, set up under the Act to advise the Government. It covers England, Wales and Scotland; there is a separate Northern Ireland Disability Council. Members of the NDC are appointed by the Secretary of State for

Social Security or by the Department of Health and Social Services for Northern Ireland. The Government has stated that at least half the members of the NDC will be either disabled people or parents of disabled children.

The NDC has to produce an annual report which is laid before Parliament (or the Northern Ireland Assembly). Its role is to advise Government about eliminating and reducing discrimination and all aspects of the operation of the Act except employment. The National Advisory Council on Employment of People with Disabilities is responsible for advising the Government on issues relating to employment and training.

The NDC is **not** able to take up individual complaints of discrimination. The NDC can be contacted at *6th Floor, The Adelphi, 1-11 John Adam Street, London WC2N 6HT*.

9. Enforcing your rights

If you have a complaint under the employment provisions of the DDA you can seek redress through an Industrial Tribunal. A questionnaire procedure will assist you in determining whether you have a strong case. Rights under the other provisions of the Act are enforceable through the County Court (the Sheriff Court in Scotland). You can make a complaint to the Pensions Ombudsman if you think that the managers of a pension scheme have discriminated against you – see Box M.2 in Chapter 44.

Under the Act it is unlawful to victimise you if you try to enforce your rights. Anyone who helps you make a complaint about discrimination is also protected, this includes people who provide information or give evidence for you in a court or tribunal. The Act also makes it unlawful for a person to knowingly help another person to discriminate against you.

If you are successful in a Tribunal or Court you can obtain damages for financial loss or hurt feelings. Courts can also impose injunctions on the service provider.

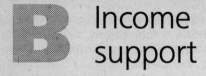

B Income support

This section of the Handbook looks at the following:

Who can get income support?	Chapter **3A**
Income support amounts	Chapter **3B**
Income and capital	Chapter **3C**
Claims, payments and appeals	Chapter **3D**

3 Income support

In this chapter we look at:

A. Who can get income support?
What is income support?	see 1
The starting conditions	see 2
Who is eligible for income support?	see Box B.1
Presence in Great Britain	see 3
Aged 16 or over	see 4
Full-time education	see 5
Full-time or part-time work	see 6
People from abroad	see 7

B. Income support amounts
How do you work out your entitlement?	see 8
What is your applicable amount?	see 9
Transitional protection	see Box B.2
The personal allowances	see 10
The premiums	see 11
The disability premium	see 12
The severe disability premium	see 13
The family premium	see 14
The disabled child premium	see 15
The carer premium	see 16
The pensioner premium	see 17
The enhanced pensioner premium	see 18
The higher pensioner premium	see 19
Housing costs	see 20
Which mortgages and loans are covered?	see 21
The assessment of mortgage and loan interest	see 22
When entitlement to housing costs begins	see 23

C. Income and capital
What are your resources?	see 24
Earnings from work	see 25
Income from benefits and pensions	see 26
Charitable and voluntary payments	see 27
Other kinds of income	see 28
Capital limits	see 29
How is capital valued?	see 30
Benefit weeks and paydays	see Box B.3
What capital is disregarded?	see 31

D. Claims, payments and appeals
How do you claim?	see 32
How is your IS paid?	see 33
Supplementary benefit	see Box B.4
Reviews and appeals	see 34
For more information	see Box B.5

A. WHO CAN GET INCOME SUPPORT?

1. What is income support?

Income support (IS) is a means-tested benefit which does not depend on your National Insurance contributions. It is intended to provide for basic living expenses for yourself and for your family. It can be paid on its own if you have no other income, or topping up other benefits or earnings from part-time work, up to the basic amount the law says you need to live on. If you don't have much money coming in, it is always worth checking to see if you might qualify for income support.

Income support is for people who are not required to sign on for work, for example those who are incapable of work through ill health or disability, carers, lone parents and people aged 60 or over. Box B.1 lists the groups of people who are eligible for income support. If you are not in one of these groups, you are not eligible for income support and should claim income-based jobseeker's allowance (JSA) instead. This replaced income support in October 1996 for those required to sign on for work.

Income support can help towards mortgage interest payments and certain other housing costs.

If you get income support, you may also get housing benefit and council tax benefit to help with your rent and council tax. You won't have to go through a separate means test (see Chapter 4).

Getting income support may also entitle you to other types of help, such as free prescriptions and dental treatment (Chapter 48), housing grants (Chapter 49) and help from the social fund (Chapters 6 and 7).

2. The starting conditions

To qualify for IS there are 7 key starting conditions. If you pass these tests, you are generally eligible for IS. However, for each key rule there is at least one exception, sometimes more;
- you must be in Great Britain – see 3; and
- you must be aged 16 or older – see 4; and
- you must not be in full-time, non-advanced education – see 5; and
- you must not be working 16 or more hours a week – see 6; and
- if you have a partner, s/he must not be working 24 or more hours a week – see 6; and
- your capital (and any capital belonging to a partner, but not to a dependent child) must be no more than £8,000 (if you live permanently in residential care the limit is £16,000) – see 29; and
- you must be in one of the specified categories of people eligible for income support (eg incapable of work, over 60, carer, etc) – see Box B.1.

If you pass these tests, you'll be entitled to IS if your income, worked out under the IS rules, is less than your 'applicable amount' (the amount the law says you need to live on).

If you have no income at all, you'll be paid the full amount of your IS 'applicable amount'.

If you have some income, but it is less than your IS 'applicable amount', IS is payable to bridge the gap between that income and your IS 'applicable amount'.

If your income is higher than your IS 'applicable amount', you won't be entitled to IS. But you may be entitled to housing and/or council tax benefit.

For some groups of people there are special rules. The IS rules for people in residential care or nursing homes are explained in Chapters 36 and 38.

If you are classed as a 'person from abroad', you are not entitled to ordinary IS, but you may be able to get an urgent cases payment – see 7.

Entitled to jobseeker's allowance? – If you are entitled to either income-based or contribution-based jobseeker's allowance, or your partner is entitled to income-based jobseeker's allowance, you cannot get income support at the same time. You can switch claims if you find you've made the wrong choice – see 32.

3. Presence in Great Britain

IS can be paid for the first 4, or 8 weeks of a temporary absence from Britain. Chapter 41 explains the conditions. There are no other exceptions to this rule.

As well as being present in Great Britain, you must also be 'habitually resident' in the UK, Channel Islands, the Isle of Man or the Republic of Ireland – see 7.

4. Aged 16 or over

If you are aged under 16 you cannot get IS in your own right in any circumstances.

If you are under 19 and still at school or doing a non-advanced course at college, you are usually excluded from IS – your parents can claim child benefit for you and include you in their IS claim. But in some circumstances you can claim IS in your own right while you are at school– see 5. If you are a student, ie you are under 19 and on an advanced course, or you are 19 or over and in full-time education (advanced or non-advanced), see Chapter 31 for details of IS entitlement.

Once you've left school, from the first Monday after the end of the school holiday following your school leaving date, you are eligible for IS in the same way as anyone else. So long as you fit into one of the situations outlined in Box B.1 which exempt you from signing on for work, you are eligible to claim. If you don't fit into one of these groups, you should claim jobseeker's allowance instead. But there are extra tests for 16 and 17 year olds claiming jobseeker's allowance – see Chapter 14(19).

5. Full-time education

You are excluded from IS if you are aged 16, 17 or 18 and are treated as a child for Child Benefit Act purposes – see Chapter 27: ie you are at school, or doing a non-advanced course at college, for 12 or more hours a week. But even if you are at school, you won't be excluded from IS if:
- you are severely mentally or physically disabled and your disability means that you would be unlikely to find work within a year if you were to leave school now and sign on for work; or
- you get child benefit for a child living with you (provided no-one also gets child benefit for you); or
- you have no parent, and no-one is legally responsible for you or acting in place of your parents; or
- you are living away from your parents (and anyone acting in their place) and they cannot support you as they are chronically sick or disabled, in custody, or prohibited from coming in to Britain: seek advice; or
- you have to live away from your parents (and anyone acting in their place) because:
  – you are estranged from them; or
  – you are in physical or moral danger; or
  – there is a serious risk to your physical or mental health; or
- you are a refugee on an English course – see Box B.1; or
- you have left care and are living independently.

Reg 13, IS (General) Regs

If you are aged 19 or over and on a full-time course, you will be treated as a student whether your course is advanced or non-advanced. Chapter 31 explains which students are entitled to IS.

6. Full-time or part-time work

You are excluded from IS if you, or your partner, are in *'remunerative work'*. This means that you are not entitled to IS if you, the claimant, work for 16 hours or more a week, or if your partner works for 24 hours or more a week.

To count as 'remunerative' it must be work *'for which payment is made or which is done in expectation of payment'*. Lunch breaks, if you are paid for them, count towards the 16 hours. Some people may be treated as still being in full-time work: eg if you are off work because of a holiday, or during a period covered by pay in lieu of notice. But if you are off work because you are ill or on maternity leave, you are not treated as being in remunerative work, even if you are getting sick pay or maternity pay from your employer. Once you have stopped working, you are not excluded from IS if you continue to get disability working allowance or family credit, nor during a period covered by your last normal earnings.

If you or your partner are working part-time while on IS, you can build up entitlement to a lump sum Back to Work Bonus – see Box F.2 in Chapter 14.

If you come within one of the exceptions listed below, you can qualify for IS even if you are working for 16 or more hours a week. If your partner is working 24 or more hours a week, s/he must come within one of these exceptions. Although you are not excluded from IS on account of the number of hours you work in these cases, any earnings you may have are taken into account in the usual way. If you have an additional occupation which is not in one of these exceptions, the hours you work in that occupation do count towards the 16 hour or 24 hour remunerative work limit – but see the note below if you are a carer.

You are not treated as being in remunerative work if:
- because of your disability, physical or mental, either:
  – your earnings are reduced to 75% or less of what someone without your disability would reasonably be expected to earn if they worked the same number of hours in your type of job, or in a comparable job in the area; or
  – your hours of work are 75% or less of what someone without your disability would reasonably be expected to undertake in your type of job, or in a comparable job in the area;

    DSS guidance advises that your own evidence of reduced earnings or hours should normally be accepted. But the Adjudication Officer may get more evidence from the Employment Service, employment agencies, Social Services Departments or disability charities if they need this to make a comparison;
- you are eligible for IS because you are caring for a person

who gets attendance allowance, or the middle or higher rate of DLA care component, or you get ICA – see Box B.1; note that DSS guidance advises that if this exception applies then you are not excluded from IS even if you have another job (AOG 25216). For example, if you care for your mother during the day and she gets attendance allowance, and you also work 20 hours a week in a supermarket in the evenings, because you are a carer none of your hours count, not even the 20 hours evening work; (for JSA only the hours you spend caring are disregarded and you must not be employed as a paid carer);
- you are working as a childminder in your home; (note that for JSA childminding does count as remunerative work);
- you are working as a local authority councillor, a part-time fire fighter, a member of the Territorial Army or reserve forces, a lifeboat crew member, or running or launching a lifeboat, or as an auxiliary coastguard involved in coast rescue duties;
- you are getting a state training allowance;
- you are a volunteer, or working for a charity or voluntary organisation, but only if the only payment you receive, or expect to receive, is a payment to cover your actual expenses. If the AO is not *'satisfied that it is reasonable for [you] to provide [your] services free of charge'*, s/he may treat you as having 'notional' earnings – see 24. If you are paid (or notionally paid) anything else, even if that is below your earnings disregard, all your hours of 'work' go into the melting pot. If your average hours are 16 or more a week, you'll be excluded from IS;
- you are held to be involved in a trade dispute (but not during the first 7 days after the day you stopped work);
- you are *'in employment'* and live in, or are temporarily away from, a residential care or nursing home, if either you, or your partner, are receiving a care home rate or residential allowance;
- you are a foster parent or you are paid by a health authority, local authority or voluntary organisation to provide respite care in your own home for someone who does not normally live with you;
- you are working 16 or more hours a week, but under 24 hours and are still covered by the transitional protection set out in regs 22 to 24 of the Income Support (General) Amendment (No 4) Regulations 1991. Your right to IS is protected until you cease to be entitled to IS (on the basis of working under 24 hours) for over 8 consecutive weeks (12 weeks, if you lose IS but are covered by the work 'trial period' provisions – seek advice).

Reg 6, IS (General) Regs

7. People from abroad

If you are defined as a 'person from abroad', you are not entitled to ordinary IS, although you might be able to get an

---

B.1 Who is eligible for income support?

The categories of people who are eligible for IS are set out in Schedule 1B of the IS (General) Regulations 1987. You are eligible for IS if you meet any one of the conditions below. You must also pass the means-test and other IS conditions described in this chapter to be entitled to IS – see 2. Income support is only for people who are not expected to sign on as available for work. If none of the categories below apply to you, you cannot get IS and should claim jobseeker's allowance instead. From October 1996, jobseeker's allowance replaced unemployment benefit and income support for those required to sign on as available for work.

Age
- ❑ You are 60 or older.
- ❑ On 6.10.96 or at any time in the 8 weeks before 6.10.96, you were receiving IS and were between age 50 and 59 and in the past 10 years had not worked for 16 or more hours in any week and had no prospect of getting work, and would not have been made to sign on if you had claimed IS or SB. This category is transitionally protected for those who satisfied it before jobseeker's allowance was introduced on 7.10.96. You lose this protection if you stop claiming IS for more than 8 weeks. If you reclaim within 8 weeks you are still covered unless you worked for 16 hours or more in any week.

Sickness or disability
- ❑ You are entitled to statutory sick pay.
- ❑ You are incapable of work.
  This is assessed under the 'own occupation' or 'all work' tests (see Chapter 8). You must send in medical certificates until you are assessed under (or exempted from) the all work test. You can be treated as incapable of work in some circumstances (see Chapter 8(4)). You are still eligible for IS under this category if you are treated as capable of work because of 'misconduct', failure without good cause to accept medical treatment or failure to observe certain rules of behaviour (see Chapter 8(6)).
- ❑ You have appealed against a decision that you are capable of work. This category continues to apply until the final decision on your appeal (eg by the Commissioner if you further appeal the SSAT decision). This category depends on which test of incapacity was applied:
- if the decision is under the 'own occupation' test you must continue to send in medical certificates. IS is paid at the normal rate;
- if the decision is under the 'all work' test, you don't need to send in medical certificates. IS will be reduced by 20% of the single person's personal allowance for your age group (unless you are eligible for IS under one of the other categories in this box, eg you are a carer). But if you were getting invalidity benefit or SDA on 12.4.95, or you were continuously incapable of work for 28 weeks before 13.4.95, and this is the first time the all work test has been applied, this reduction does not apply. If you win your appeal the reduction will be repaid. See Chapter 14(8) – you may be better off claiming JSA;
- you are not eligible for IS under this category while you are appealing against a decision treating you as capable of work because you failed without good cause to return the all work test questionnaire or attend a medical examination, or you were doing work that was not permitted. You should claim JSA instead, unless any of the other categories in this box applies.

para 24, Sch 1B and reg 22A IS (General) Regs

- ❑ You are registered as blind (in Scotland, certified as blind). If you regain your sight, you don't have to sign on during the 28 weeks after you are taken off the register.
- ❑ You are mentally or physically disabled, working 16 or more hours a week, and are not treated as being in remunerative work because your hours or earnings are 75% or less than that of a person without your disability in the same job (see 6).

urgent cases payment – see below. You count as a 'person from abroad' if:
- you have limited leave to enter or remain in the UK subject to having no recourse to public funds; or
- you have overstayed your limited leave; or
- you are subject to a deportation order; or
- you are alleged to be an illegal entrant by the Home Office; or
- you have temporary admission; or
- you have never had a decision on your immigration status; or
- you are an EC national and have been required to leave the UK by the Secretary of State; or
- you are a sponsored person whose sponsor has signed an undertaking and less than 5 years have elapsed since you entered the UK or since the undertaking was signed (whichever is the later); or
- you are in any of the above categories and you have applied to the Home Office for asylum; or
- you are not 'habitually resident' in the UK, Channel Islands, the Isle of Man or the Republic of Ireland – see below.

If you are treated as a 'person from abroad', it is important to seek advice. If you are refused benefit because you are a 'person from abroad' you may be able to get help from your local Social Services Department. If you have children, they may be able to provide a payment for food under Section 17 of the Children Act 1989, and accommodation under Section 20. If you don't have children your local Social Services Department should provide you with accommodation and food if you have no other source of assistance available to you (*R v London Borough of Hammersmith*, TLR 19.2.97).

Habitual residence
Anyone who claims IS (or income-based JSA, housing or council tax benefit) from 1.8.94 has to show they are 'habitually resident' to be eligible for benefit. However, the test should not be applied if:
- you are an EC national with 'worker status', or the 'right to reside' (under EC worker Directives); or
- you have refugee status; or
- you have exceptional leave to remain.

'Worker status' and 'right to reside' are defined in EC law. Generally, EC nationals who are in employment will have both worker status and the right to reside in the UK. But once that employment ends, this status may be lost. If you or your partner have never worked in the UK, you will not have the right to reside. This does not mean you lose the right to be in the UK, but you do have to show you are habitually resident to get IS, HB or CTB. If you are a 'person from abroad' who qualifies for urgent cases payments (eg you are an asylum seeker) you should still get benefits despite the test.

❑ You are in employment while living in (or temporarily absent from) a residential care or nursing home, and you or your partner receive either a residential allowance or care home rate.

Education and training
❑ You are entitled to IS while at school, or in full-time non-advanced education, eg if your severe disability means you would be unlikely to get a job within the next 12 months (see 5).
❑ You are a student and your applicable amount includes the disability premium or severe disability premium; or you have been incapable of work (or entitled to SSP) for 28 weeks (two or more periods of incapacity can be added together provided they are no more than 8 weeks apart).
❑ You are a student who gets a disabled student's allowance because of your deafness: see Chapter 31.
❑ You are a student and have either been getting IS as a disabled student since immediately before 1.9.90; or in the 18 months before your current claim began you were either getting IS as a disabled student under the pre-1.9.90 rules, or were getting IS when at school because of your disability.
❑ You are on a Youth Training Scheme (or equivalent).
❑ You are a refugee and start attending an English course for over 15 hours a week during your first year in Great Britain: you are eligible under this category only for up to 9 months.

Caring
❑ You are *'regularly and substantially engaged in caring for another person'* and either you are getting ICA, or the person you are looking after gets attendance allowance (or constant attendance allowance), or the middle or higher rate of DLA care component.
  If s/he has claimed DLA or AA, you'll be eligible for up to 26 weeks, unless a decision is made sooner. You are eligible if s/he has an advance award of DLA middle or higher rate care component or AA but is still in the qualifying period. If ICA stops, or the person you are looking after stops getting AA or the middle or higher rate of DLA care component, you continue to be eligible for 8 weeks.
❑ If you would have been eligible for IS as a carer had you made a claim for IS, then you are eligible for IS for 8 weeks from the date your ICA and/or the disabled person's qualifying benefit stops.
❑ You are looking after a member of your IS family who is *'temporarily ill'*.

Childcare responsibility
❑ You are a lone parent and responsible for a child under 16 who is a member of your household.
❑ You are single or a lone parent and are fostering a child under 16 through a local authority or voluntary organisation.
❑ You are looking after a child under 16 because the child's parent, or the person who usually looks after the child, is ill, or is temporarily away from his or her home.
❑ Your partner is temporarily outside the UK and you are responsible for a child under 16 who is a member of your household.

Pregnancy
❑ You are pregnant and incapable of work because of your pregnancy.
❑ If you are, or have been pregnant, you are eligible for IS during the period starting with the 11th week before your expected week of confinement and ending 7 weeks after the date on which your pregnancy ended.

Other
❑ You are getting IS as a 'person from abroad'.
❑ You are required to attend court as a JP, juror, witness, defendant or plaintiff.
❑ You are remanded or committed in custody for trial or sentencing.
❑ You are held to be involved in a trade dispute.

If you are not exempted from the habitual residence test, the AO will decide whether you are habitually resident or not. The regulations do not define 'habitual residence', but there is guidance and case law that applies.

The rules are complicated, so seek advice if you are caught by this test. It is very important to appeal if you are refused benefit and to get good advice and representation. A high proportion of appeals against the habitual residence test are being won.

'Urgent cases'

If you count as a 'person from abroad' (see above), you may be entitled to IS under the 'urgent cases' provisions if:

- you are on limited leave and are dependent on funds from abroad which are temporarily disrupted (payment will last for a maximum of 6 weeks); or
- you have a sponsor who signed an undertaking and less than 5 years have passed since you entered the UK (or since the undertaking was signed) and your sponsor has died (payment can continue indefinitely); once the 5 years have passed you can go on to 'normal' IS; or
- you have applied for asylum 'on arrival' in the UK. The DSS take this to mean before clearing immigration control. But the words 'on arrival' are not defined and should therefore be given their ordinary everyday meaning. There have been successful appeals by people who have applied for asylum immediately after clearing immigration control; or
- you have applied for asylum or appealed against a refusal of asylum and were entitled to IS before 5.2.96.

'Urgent cases' payments of IS are worked out under different rules from ordinary IS. We don't cover assessments of urgent cases payments here – seek advice.

If you are entitled to IS 'urgent cases' as an asylum-seeker, entitlement will stop if you receive a negative decision on your application or appeal after 5.2.96.

If you are not entitled to IS 'urgent cases' as an asylum-seeker and are subsequently granted refugee status you are entitled to 'urgent cases' payments backdated to the date of your asylum application or to the date that benefit stopped because of a negative decision on your application, but you must claim within 28 days of receiving the letter notifying you of your refugee status. The payment is disregarded as capital for 52 weeks.

B. INCOME SUPPORT AMOUNTS

8. How do you work out your entitlement?

- ❏ Add up your total capital resources. If your (and your partner's) capital is more than £8,000 (or £16,000 if you live in residential care), you won't be entitled to IS – but it is worth double checking that you've applied the law correctly (see 24 and 31).
- ❏ Work out your IS family's 'applicable amount' (see 9).
- Add up your personal allowances (see 10).
- Add up your entitlement to the premiums (see 11–19). Maximum entitlement to the premiums would be:
  - one (at the single or couple rate) out of the disability premium, pensioner premium, enhanced pensioner premium or higher pensioner premium; **plus**
  - one family premium (ordinary rate); **plus**
  - disabled child premium(s); **plus**
  - severe disability premium; **plus**
  - a carer premium for each eligible person.
- Add up any IS housing costs (see 20).
- Add up any residential allowance (see Chapter 36).

The sum total of all these is your IS applicable amount.
❏ Now add up your total income resources (see 24).
If you have capital over £3,000 (or £10,000 if you are in residential care), don't forget the 'tariff income' (see 29).
❏ Deduct your income from your applicable amount.
If your income is less than your applicable amount, IS makes up the difference in full – provided you pass the other tests. Even if your income is more than your applicable amount, it may be worth claiming IS to make sure that you haven't made a mistake with the figures, or in applying the law.

If you get confused, remember the golden rule – if in doubt, claim or ask for a written explanation! Remember the second rule – keep a copy of your letter and follow it up if you don't get a reply!

9. What is your applicable amount?

The applicable amounts are set by Parliament. They can be seen as the amount the law says you need to live on. The applicable amount consists of:

- a personal allowance – for a single claimant, or for a couple, and for each dependent child in your IS family;
- a premium – a flat-rate extra amount if you satisfy certain conditions;
- certain housing costs.

Your entitlement to all of these is taken into account when your IS claim is assessed. The Adjudication Officer (AO) will add up your total applicable amount. S/he will also assess your income under the IS rules. If your income is lower than your applicable amount, the difference is payable as IS, if you've passed all the other tests.

If you want to check that your IS has been correctly worked out, ask for a detailed notice of assessment, on form A124. This form gives more detail than the shorter form, A14N. If there is some part of the assessment which you don't understand, or are doubtful about, ask the AO for a written explanation: including references to the exact legal basis for that decision.

Your family

If you are a single person, with no partner or dependent children living with you, the AO will look only at your own needs and resources. If you are one of a couple (married or living together as husband and wife), the AO will normally take into account both of your needs and resources. If you have dependent children living with you, their needs and income will be added to your own. But a child's capital is not added to your own capital.

If you are a lone parent, with a dependent child living with you, your child's needs and income are added to your own.

Children – In a few cases a child who is living with you won't count as a dependant (eg s/he is in advanced education: above A level and OND standard). In others, a child will still count as a dependant even though s/he is not living with you. If a child is in local authority care, or detained in custody, but is at home with you for part of a week, you'll get a reduced-rate allowance for him or her. Generally you are treated as responsible for a child if you get child benefit for them. But if you are 'responsible' for a young person who has a child of their own for whom they get child benefit, you are treated as responsible for both of them.

If you are not sure how or why a child has been excluded from (or included in) the IS assessment, ask the AO for a written explanation. If a child becomes a claimant in his or her own right, s/he is excluded from your IS family – see Chapter 30.

Special groups

Residential care – If you are living in local authority residential accommodation, your applicable amount is worked out differently – see Chapter 36. If you are in an independent residential care or nursing home, your position depends on whether or not you have a 'preserved right' to IS under special rules. Chapters 36 and 38 explain both assessments, as well as the benefit implications of staying in residential care. In general, if you enter an independent residential care or nursing home on or after 1.4.93, your 'applicable amount' is worked out in the normal way, but with an extra residential allowance – see Chapter 36(5). If you live permanently in a residential care or nursing home, the capital limits are higher – see 29 below.

Hospital – If you, or a member of your family, are in hospital, your applicable amount may be reduced – see Chapter 39.

Urgent cases – If you are in one of the 2 groups of people who can claim IS on an 'urgent need' basis, it is worked out under different rules. Urgent cases payments only apply if you are waiting for income which you are due to be paid, or if you count as a 'person from abroad' (see 7 above) – seek advice.

10. The personal allowances

Under IS, the AO just has to take into account your age, whether you are one of a married or unmarried couple, and whether you are responsible for a dependent child.

If you have a child, the AO normally just has to check the child's age, whether s/he lives with you, whether you get child benefit for him or her, and whether s/he has capital of over £3,000. If a child has capital of over £3,000, you won't get an allowance, or the disabled child premium, for that child; but even if s/he is your only child, you still qualify for the family premium.

Rates of personal allowances

If you are aged under 18 – The rate you get depends on meeting other conditions.

❑ **Couple** – In the table of weekly rates below, the stars mean:
  * includes couples where one is under 18 but is eligible for IS or would be eligible for income-based JSA if s/he had been registered for work or YT, or is subject to a Secretary of State's direction for discretionary JSA;
  ** only if one is responsible for a child; or each would be eligible for IS if they were single; or the claimant's partner would be eligible for income-based JSA if they had been registered for work or YT, or is subject to a Secretary of State's direction for discretionary JSA. If only one of the couple is eligible for IS, etc, the personal allowance is £29.60. However, the personal allowance would be £38.90 if the person who is eligible for IS would, if s/he had been registered for work or YT, have fallen into one of the groups of people who can get income-based JSA during the child benefit extension period (see Chapter 14(19));
  *** only if the other is under 18 and not eligible for IS, income-based JSA or subject to a Secretary of State's direction for discretionary JSA.

❑ **Single person or lone parent** – You get the higher rate of £38.90 if you qualify for a disability premium, or you would be eligible for income-based JSA during the child benefit extension period if you had been registered for work or YT (see Chapter 14(19)).

para 1, Sch 2, IS (General) Regs

Personal allowances

		Weekly rates
Couple	both aged 18+*	£77.15
	both under 18**	£58.70
	one aged 25+***	£49.15
	one aged 18–24***	£38.90
Lone parent	aged 18+	£49.15
	aged under 18 (higher rate)	£38.90
	aged under 18 (lower rate)	£29.60
Single person	aged 25 or older	£49.15
	aged 18–24	£38.90
	aged under 18 (higher rate)	£38.90
	aged under 18 (lower rate)	£29.60
Dependent child (see below)	aged 16–18	£29.60
	aged 11–16	£24.75
	aged 0–11	£16.90

Amounts for dependent children

The amount for a child goes up to that for the next age band from the first Monday in September following the child's 11th or 16th birthday. For 18 year olds the allowance ends on the day before the dependent child's 19th birthday.

For example, if your child's 11th birthday is on 31 October 1997, you will continue to get the age 0–11 personal allowance for her/him until 6 September 1998, increasing to the age 11–16 band from 7 September 1998.

Before this rule was changed on 7.4.97, the amount for a child increased from the actual date of the child's 11th or 16th birthday, and a higher rate was payable for 18 year olds. There is transitional protection.

If your child is already aged 11, 16 or 18 before 7.4.97 – You do not have to wait until September for the increase. You will get £24.75 for your child aged 11, and £29.60 for your child aged 16. You will get the higher rate of £38.90 for your dependent child aged 18. This applies to claims made both before and after 7.4.97.

B.2 Transitional protection

Transitional protection allows for additional payments for people who would otherwise have lost money at the point of the changeover from supplementary benefit to income support in April 1988.

Once a transitional addition has been properly worked out, it cannot be increased. It can only be reduced, withdrawn and/or restored following certain changes in circumstances. Generally, an increase in IS applicable amounts, leads to an equivalent cut in your transitional addition, so the amount of money you get stays the same. The overall idea is to transfer former SB claimants to normal IS as quickly as possible.

Chapter 4 in the 15th edition of our Disability Rights Handbook describes the system of transitional protection, and Chapter 4 in our 18th edition outlines the rules for cutting, withdrawing and restoring transitional additions. Send us a large, stamped self-addressed envelope for copies.

A special transitional addition is also payable to some of the 1000 claimants who were getting a domestic help addition of £10 or more in the last week of supplementary benefit. Unlike the ordinary transitional addition, the special transitional addition increases when other benefits are uprated. More details are in Chapter 4 of our 15th edition.

11. The premiums

There are eight different weekly premiums. Each one has specific qualifying conditions, which are detailed in 12 to 19 below. Some premiums you can get in addition to any other premium. Others overlap with each other and you can only get one of these at a time – you get the one that is worth the most.

❏ *You may qualify for any or all of the following premiums.*

- family premium – ordinary rate £10.80
- or – lone parent rate £15.75
- disabled child premium £20.95
- carer premium £13.35
- severe disability premium £37.15

❏ *Plus you may qualify for one of the following premiums. If you qualify for more than one, you'll only get the larger amount. If you are a lone parent and you are entitled to one of these premiums, your family premium switches to the ordinary rate.*

	Single	Couple
disability premium	£20.95	£29.90
pensioner premium	£19.65	£29.65
enhanced pensioner premium	£21.85	£32.75
higher pensioner premium	£26.55	£38.00

12. The disability premium

The disability premium is payable only while the person who qualifies is aged under 60. Once s/he reaches 60, the higher pensioner premium will normally be payable instead.

The disability premium for a single claimant aged from 16 to 60 is £20.95. For a couple, the disability premium is £29.90 – whether one or both of the couple count as disabled.

The disability premium can be awarded on top of a family premium, disabled child premium, carer premium and severe disability premium. But if you are a lone parent, you'll get the ordinary rate instead of the lone parent rate of the family premium.

There are three ways of qualifying for the disability premium:
- you must be aged under 60 and pass at least one of the disability conditions; or
- your partner is aged under 60 and s/he passes at least one of the disability conditions; or
- the person who is, or becomes, the IS claimant is aged under 60 and passes the incapacity condition.

The disability conditions (claimant or partner)
You (or your partner) must be:
- registered as blind, or taken off that register in the past 28 weeks; or
- getting one of the following qualifying benefits:
  - attendance allowance
    (or constant attendance allowance)
  - disability living allowance
  - disability working allowance
  - long-term incapacity benefit
  - mobility supplement
  - severe disablement allowance

(but you, or your partner, must satisfy the conditions for getting that benefit yourself. It doesn't count if you are paid someone else's benefit as an appointee; nor if you just get your partner's benefit because s/he has been in hospital for 52 or more weeks); or
- still getting help under the pre-1976 vehicle scheme – eg an invalid trike.

You also qualify if you are paid incapacity benefit at the long-term rate because you are terminally ill.

If you get one of these qualifying benefits backdated, write and ask the AO for a review and to award the disability premium from either the start of your IS claim or the start of your award of the qualifying benefit – whichever is the later. For entitlement to a disability premium before 13.4.95, invalidity benefit is also a qualifying benefit.

If you have been getting long-term incapacity benefit or SDA, and have already qualified for the disability premium, the premium won't be withdrawn if you go on a course, such as YT, for which a state training allowance is payable, or if the course counts as provided or approved by the Secretary of State for Employment under s.2, Employment and Training Act 73. Nor will the premium be withdrawn if the overlapping benefit rules mean that you cannot be paid your long-term incapacity benefit or SDA: eg because you start to receive widowed mother's allowance or a widow's pension.

If your DLA stops when you are in hospital, you won't also lose the disability premium until your personal allowance is reduced – see Chapter 39.

The incapacity condition (claimant only)
You must be the IS claimant. If you are one of a couple, you must become the IS claimant – see 32 below. But you don't have to have been the IS claimant during the qualifying period for a disability premium under this incapacity condition.

To qualify under the incapacity condition, you must:
- have been incapable of work or entitled to statutory sick pay during the qualifying period of 52 weeks (or 28 weeks if you are terminally ill); and
- still be incapable of work.

Incapable of work – For the first 28 weeks of your incapacity the DSS may check to see if you can carry out your normal job, based on medical certificates provided by your doctor. This is the 'own occupation' test. It applies if you have worked for at least 16 hours a week for more than 8 weeks out of the last 21 weeks before you became incapable of work.

After 28 weeks, you will be tested on your ability to carry out a range of activities, such as walking, sitting and standing; this is based on a questionnaire and a statement from your doctor, but may also include a medical examination. This is the 'all work' test. The 'all work' test is applied from the beginning of the qualifying period if you have not had enough recent employment for the own occupation test to apply. Some people are exempt from the all work test – see Chapter 8(9). We look at the assessment of incapacity for work in more detail in Chapter 8.

In practice, it may take some time for the actual assessment under the all work test to be completed. Until you are assessed, you must continue to send in medical certificates.

These tests of incapacity were introduced in April 1995. If you already qualified for a disability premium under the incapacity condition before then, you will still have to be assessed under the new all work test to continue to qualify, unless you fall into an exempt group. There is an extra exempt group for some people aged 58 or over on 13.4.95 – see Chapter 12(7).

Qualifying period – During the 52 week qualifying period, if you stop being incapable of work for an interval of no more than 8 weeks, you won't have to start at the beginning again. The two spells of incapacity are linked together. For example, you fall sick on 1.6.97, then on 1.9.97 you decide to look for work and sign on as unemployed, but on 1.10.97 you fall sick again. You were capable of work for 30 days. This is less than 8 weeks, so the days of sickness from June to August are added to days of sickness from October onwards. You would have served the 52 week qualifying period by 30.6.98.

You don't have to be in receipt of IS during the qualifying period, so if you have already been incapable of work for 52 weeks before you claim, the disability premium will be included immediately.

The qualifying period is 28 weeks if you are 'terminally ill'. You count as terminally ill if you *suffer from a progressive disease and [your] death can reasonably be expected within 6 months'*.

Before 13.4.95, the qualifying period under the incapacity condition for the disability premium was 28 weeks (196 days) in all cases. If you were incapable of work before then but had not yet reached the 197th day of incapacity, you had to serve the full 52 week qualifying period. Your days of incapacity before 13.4.95 count towards the 52 weeks, providing you were incapable of work on 12.4.95. The linking rule outlined above does not apply before 13.4.95; for the part of the qualifying period before then, your incapacity must be continuous.

After you have qualified – If you stop being incapable of work, you will lose the disability premium unless you can pass the 'disability condition' (eg you get one of the qualifying benefits) – see above. But if you fall sick again no later than 8 weeks afterwards, you will go straight back on to the disability premium. You won't have to serve the 52 week qualifying period again.

If you go on a training course such as YT, you will not lose the disability premium.

Applying for the premium – Send in the claim pack, SC1, which you can get from your doctor's surgery, and a sicknote from your doctor on form Med 3. If you have been incapable of work but not sending in medical certificates, ask your doctor for a backdated sicknote on form Med 5. Send a separate letter to the income support section of your local DSS, if possible with a photocopy of the medical certificate. You should be able to get free stamped addressed envelopes at the Post Office.

If you are refused backdated incapacity benefit because you claimed late, this does not prevent days of incapacity in that past period counting towards the disability premium.

Note that the rules on assessing incapacity for work outlined here and described in Chapter 8 only apply to days of incapacity on or after 13.4.95. So decisions on incapacity for periods before then must be made under the old rules (see the 19th edition of this Handbook).

13. The severe disability premium

The severe disability premium (SDP) can be awarded on top of the ordinary disability premium, or the higher pensioner premium. It is £37.15 for each person who qualifies.

To qualify, you must be:
- an IS claimant;
- who gets DLA care component at the middle or higher rate, or attendance allowance (or constant attendance allowance); and
- no-one gets invalid care allowance for looking after you; and
- you technically count as 'living alone'.

Couples – If you are one of a couple, you can also qualify for the SDP if:
- both you and your partner get DLA care component at the middle or higher rate, or attendance allowance (or constant attendance allowance); and
- you technically count as 'living alone'; and
- someone gets invalid care allowance for looking after just one of you; or
- no-one gets invalid care allowance for looking after either

you, or your partner.

If your partner is registered blind you can still qualify for the SDP even though s/he does not get DLA or attendance allowance. You are treated as if you were a single person.

If you both get middle or higher rate care component or attendance allowance, and no-one gets invalid care allowance (ICA) for looking after either you or your partner, your SDP will be £74.30.

If you both get middle or higher rate care component or attendance allowance, and one person gets ICA for looking after you (or your partner), your SDP will be £37.15. If two people are getting ICA for looking after you and your partner, you won't get the SDP. Note that it is quite possible for you to get ICA for looking after your partner (as well as your own care component or attendance allowance). If you, or your partner, or both of you, get ICA for looking after the other, that excludes you from the single (or double) SDP. But since 1.10.90, you can get the carer premium(s).

Getting ICA?

If someone gets ICA for looking after you, that excludes you from the SDP. If ICA is not payable to your carer, for whatever reason, you can get the SDP. For example, if ICA cannot be paid to your carer because s/he gets another non-means-tested benefit (such as incapacity benefit) which cancels out ICA under the overlapping benefit rules, you'll nevertheless be entitled to the SDP. In this example, your carer also qualifies for a carer premium – see 16 below.

Neither you, nor your carer, can be forced to claim ICA. Although the DSS will ask you if anyone is caring for you, and will send you the ICA claim form to give to your carer, nothing should happen if a non-resident carer decides not to claim ICA. By the same token, you cannot stop your carer claiming ICA – so long as s/he meets, or is able to meet, the qualifying conditions for getting ICA. If s/he spends less than 35 hours from Sunday through to Saturday looking after you, s/he won't normally be eligible for ICA.

However, do note that the deprivation of income and notional income rules apply also to ICA – see 24 below. Seek expert advice if you, or your carer, fall foul of these rules. If your carer is not part of your IS family, and is not also getting IS, income-based JSA, housing benefit, DWA, or family credit, these rules cannot affect either of you.

Remember that you are only excluded from the SDP if your carer is actually paid an amount of ICA. If s/he already receives a non-means-tested benefit of £37.35 or more, a claim for ICA won't affect your SDP for, even if s/he is entitled to ICA, the overlapping benefit rules mean that s/he cannot be paid ICA.

Your premium is only affected once ICA is actually awarded. Arrears of ICA for the period before the date of the award will not affect your severe disability premium.

'Living alone'?

You are ruled out of the SDP if you have a partner who is not also getting the middle or higher rate of DLA care component, or attendance allowance, unless your partner is registered blind, or if you have any people who are classed as *'non-dependants'* who live with you. A 'non-dependant' is someone who lives in your home (unless they are in the list below) usually an adult son or daughter, friend or relative.

The presence of the following people in your home is ignored:
- anyone aged under 18;
- a dependent child aged 18 who is part of your IS family;
- someone who gets the middle or higher rate of DLA care component, or attendance allowance (or constant

attendance allowance);
- anyone who is registered blind;
- someone who does not *'normally'* reside with you – because they normally live elsewhere, they cannot count as a non-dependant; (there is no definition of 'normally resides' in terms of time, frequency or anything else – see CSIS/100/93);
- someone who is not a *'close relative'* and *'jointly occupies'* your dwelling as a co-owner or who is sharing legal liability to make 'rent' payments – a joint occupier, such as a joint tenant, cannot count as a non-dependant. If a co-owner or joint tenant is a close relative of you (or your partner), s/he will count as a 'non-dependant' (and so exclude you from the SDP) unless:
  – the co-ownership or joint liability began before 11.4.88; or
  – the co-ownership or joint liability began after 11.4.88 but began *'on or before the date upon which [you or your] partner first occupied the dwelling in question'* – reg 3(2C) IS (General) Regulations;
- someone who is not a close relative and who is your resident *'landlord'*, sharing living accommodation with you – to whom you, or your partner, are *'liable to make payments on a commercial basis in respect of [your] occupation of [his or her] dwelling'*;
- someone who is not a close relative and who shares living accommodation with you and is *'liable to make payments on a commercial basis to [you or your partner] in respect of [his or her] occupation of [your] dwelling'* – a licensee, tenant or sub-tenant cannot count as a non-dependant;
- a live-in helper who has been placed with you by a 'charitable or voluntary body' (not by a public or local authority), where the organisation (not the helper) charges you for that help – the charge need only be nominal.

If you are already getting the SDP and someone else joins your household *'for the first time in order to care for you'*, the SDP continues for up to 12 weeks after the date s/he joins your household. This is to give him or her time to claim ICA. Once ICA is paid, the SDP stops. This rule applies only where the carer would otherwise count as a non-dependant – because s/he intends to make his or her home with you for long enough so that s/he can be said to reside with you.

Close relatives and living arrangements
A 'close relative' means only a parent, parent-in-law, son, daughter, son/daughter-in-law, step-parent, step-son/daughter, brother, sister, or the (married or unmarried) partner of any of those. If you have a licence or tenancy agreement with a relative, who is not a close relative, you (or they) would only be excluded from the SDP while you are residing with them if your occupancy agreement was not on a 'commercial basis'.
Living independently? – If you have entirely separate living accommodation, you cannot be said to *'normally reside'* with other people living under the same roof. For example, if you live in a separate 'Granny flat', your right to the SDP is not affected – even if a close relative lives under the same roof.

If you are living under the same roof as other people, with a separate bedroom, kitchen and living room, you won't count as 'residing' with those other people – so you can qualify for the SDP. It makes no difference if you share a bathroom, lavatory or any communal area (which does not include any communal rooms unless you are living in sheltered accommodation).
Separate liability – If you share a living room or kitchen with other people but are *'separately liable to make payments in respect of [your] occupation of the dwelling to the landlord'*, you won't count as 'residing with' those other people – even if they are close relatives. The DSS see this as typically covering someone in supported lodgings.

Protecting pre-21.10.91 SDPs
If you are a co-owner or joint tenant with a 'close relative' and had an award of IS, including an SDP, in the week before 21.10.91, your position is protected. This also applies if you had a claim or request for a review lodged before 21.10.91. That claim or review must result in an award of SDP under the old pre-11.11.91, rules. If an SDP was not included in the assessment of your IS in respect of the week before 21.10.91, you may still be protected. If you had a break from IS which straddled 21.10.91 and, under the old rules, were entitled to an SDP both before and after the break, you will be protected if:
- the break was no more than 8 weeks or less (for any reason); or
- the break was no more than 12 weeks (covered by the work 'trial period' provisions); or
- you have just finished employment training or an employment rehabilitation course and re-claim IS immediately.

If your SDP is protected, that protection will survive changes in the type of agreement, in the parties to the agreement, and will even survive a move of home – see reg 4(9) IS (General) Amendment (No.6) Regs 1991. It cannot survive a carer getting ICA, or a non-dependant joining your home. If you have a break off income support after 21.10.91, you can regain your protected SDP on a similar basis to that outlined above.

Hospital
If you enter hospital, the SDP will be withdrawn once your care component or attendance allowance is withdrawn – usually once you've been in hospital for 4 weeks.

For couples, if both of you get the care component or attendance allowance, and one or both of you enters hospital, you will still get the SDP even after the care component or attendance allowance is withdrawn but the SDP will only be paid at the rate of £37.15. But if both of you are in hospital, the SDP is withdrawn in any case after 6 weeks.

If your carer enters hospital and loses ICA, you may qualify for the SDP while s/he is in hospital. By the same token, you may lose the SDP for a period if your carer's ICA becomes payable once his or her usual overlapping benefit is reduced after 6 weeks in hospital.

14. The family premium
This is awarded if you have a dependent child aged under 19. There are two different rates of the family premium. You will get either:
- the *ordinary rate* of £10.80 – if you are one of a couple; or you are a lone parent who is entitled to a disability premium or any of the pensioner premiums; or
- the *lone parent rate* of £15.75 – if you are a lone parent (and you're not entitled to a disability premium or any of the pensioner premiums).

The ordinary rate can be awarded in addition to any of the other premiums covered in this chapter. The lone parent rate can be awarded in addition to a disabled child premium, carer premium and severe disability premium. But if you get a disability premium or any pensioner premium, you get the ordinary rate instead of the lone parent rate. This replaced the lone parent premium from 7.4.97.

To qualify for the family premium, your IS family must include a child aged under 19. The family premium is fixed at £10.80 or £15.75 regardless of the number of children you have.

If you have just one child, and get the full personal

allowance for that child, you will also be entitled to the family premium.

If you have just one child, and get a reduced-rate allowance for that child, your family premium will be reduced pro-rata – see 9 above.

If you have just one child and s/he does not count as a member of your family, you won't get the child's personal allowance, nor will you get the family premium or disabled child premium. For example, this would happen where your former partner gets child benefit in respect of that child.

If you have just one child living with you and s/he has capital of over £3,000, you will get the family premium even though you cannot get an allowance for the child (or the disabled child premium).

If you are normally one of a couple but your partner is temporarily living apart from you, you may count as a lone parent. For example, you'll count as a lone parent if your partner is now 'permanently' in a residential care or nursing home; or where s/he has been in hospital for 52 weeks; or where s/he is in prison or is detained in a special hospital (eg Broadmoor). You'll also count as a lone parent where your partner is living apart from you and doesn't intend to return.

15. The disabled child premium

The disabled child premium (DCP) can be awarded in addition to any of the other premiums covered in this chapter. The disabled child premium is £20.95 for each child who lives with you and counts as disabled.

Your child counts as disabled if s/he:
- is registered as blind, or was taken off that register within the past 28 weeks; or
- gets disability living allowance; or
- no longer gets DLA because s/he is a patient – so long as s/he is still treated as being a member of your IS family.

However, the DCP won't be paid for a child if that child has capital of over £3,000. Apart from this point, the rules for paying, or not paying, or paying a reduced-rate of DCP are the same as the rules for the family premium – see above.

There is no lower age-limit in law for registering a child as blind. Apply (in writing) to your Social Services (or Social Work) Department for registration as soon as you are given a diagnosis, or you think one likely. Contact the RNIB if you experience difficulty. If a delay in registration is unreasonable, consider complaining to the Local Ombudsman – see Chapter 54.

If a child is not registered as blind, and is not terminally ill, the earliest age at which you can get the DCP for him or her is 3 months (when DLA care component normally first becomes payable). If s/he qualifies for DLA mobility component, the DCP would be paid from his or her 5th birthday at the earliest. If none of these apply, no DCP is payable.

16. The carer premium

The carer premium was introduced from 1.10.90. It can be awarded in addition to any of the other premiums covered in this chapter. It is £13.35 a week for each person who qualifies.

You'll qualify for a carer premium if you or your partner:
- are actually paid an amount of invalid care allowance (ICA); or
- have an underlying entitlement to ICA: you are entitled to ICA but it cannot be paid because of the overlapping benefit rules.

Paid ICA
If you are actually paid ICA, there are no extra rules for getting a carer premium. However, do note that the person you are caring for will be excluded from the SDP.

Overlapped ICA
If you only have an underlying entitlement to ICA, there are some extra rules:
- you must have claimed (or re-claimed) ICA on or after 1.10.90; and
- you are entitled to ICA but the overlapping benefit rules mean that you cannot be paid ICA because you receive another non-means-tested benefit of £37.35 or more a week; and
- the person you are caring for must continue to receive attendance allowance or the middle or higher rate of DLA care component.

Note that if you have overlapped ICA, you can qualify for a carer premium and the person you are caring for will still be entitled to the severe disability premium.

Overlapping benefits – You must be entitled to ICA, so that some ICA would be paid but for the overlapping benefit rules. These rules mean that you cannot be paid the full amount of ICA at the same time as receiving the full amount of your entitlement to: incapacity benefit, severe disablement allowance, unemployability supplement, maternity allowance, widowed mother's allowance, widow's pension, industrial death benefit, contribution-based JSA and retirement pension. In general ICA is reduced by the amount of the other listed benefit payable for the same period. Unless you receive less than £37.35 a week from a listed benefit, your ICA will be cancelled out.

Although you can get the carer premium whether or not your ICA is overlapped, the person you are caring for will lose their SDP if you are paid ICA. The person you are caring for can only qualify for the SDP if you can't be paid ICA (either because ICA is completely overlapped, or you haven't claimed it).

8 week extension
The carer premium continues for 8 weeks after you would otherwise have ceased to be entitled to it. Your caring role can have ended temporarily or permanently and for any reason at all. For example, you are entitled to the carer premium for 8 weeks after you lose ICA, or after the disabled person loses attendance allowance, or for 8 weeks after s/he dies. During this 8 week extension of the carer premium you continue to be eligible for IS as a carer. After this you will be expected to sign on and claim JSA instead, unless you are eligible for IS in another way – see Box B.1.

Age
Chapter 43(4) looks at the position for people over 65.

17. The pensioner premium

To qualify for the pensioner premium (PP), you (or your partner) must be aged from 60 to 74 (inclusive). For a single claimant, the PP is £19.65. For a couple, where one or both of you are within the PP age band, the pensioner premium is £29.65.

If you (or your partner) are disabled, check to see if you can get the higher pensioner premium instead.

18. The enhanced pensioner premium

To qualify for the enhanced pensioner premium (EPP), you (or your partner) must be aged 75-79 (inclusive). For a single claimant, the EPP is £21.85. For a couple, where one or both of you are within the EPP age band, the premium is £32.75.

If you (or your partner) are disabled, check to see if you can get the higher pensioner premium instead.

19. The higher pensioner premium

The higher pensioner premium (HPP) is £26.55 for a single claimant; £38.00 for a couple.

The severe disability premium, the family premium, the carer premium(s) and the disabled child premium can all be awarded on top of the HPP. But if you get the HPP and you are a lone parent, your family premium will be at the ordinary rate, not the lone parent rate.

If you, or your partner, are 60 or over, you can't keep the disability premium – you'll get the HPP instead – but this gives you a better deal.

There are four ways of qualifying for the HPP. The first way is easy. The second method has a few snags, which may tip you into methods 3 or 4. Methods 3 and 4 may well cause difficulty.

1. You (or your partner) are aged 80 or older. OR
2. You (or your partner) satisfy the 'disability condition' used for the ordinary disability premium – see 12 above. If you no longer get a qualifying benefit (and cannot pass the disability condition in any other way), you may be able to keep your HPP – see below (under 'Method 2: the snags'). OR
3. You were getting the disability premium under the 'incapacity condition' within 8 weeks of your 60th birthday – see 12 above for details of the incapacity condition; see below for more details of this 8 week linking rule. OR
4. You were the IS claimant and were getting the disability premium within 8 weeks of your 60th birthday only because your partner alone satisfied the disability condition – see below for more about this 8 week linking rule.

Method 2: the snags

One of the ways of passing the disability condition depends on receiving one of the qualifying benefits.

SDA – If your SDA is overlapped by retirement pension, your HPP continues. However, if the HPP wasn't paid before you claimed retirement pension, claiming SDA afterwards can only get you the HPP if SDA is more than your retirement pension.

Incapacity benefit – If your long-term incapacity benefit ends because you move to retirement pension instead, you won't lose your right to the HPP if you remain continuously entitled to IS (apart from breaks of 8 weeks or less). If the incapacity benefit was paid to your partner, s/he must still be alive.

Invalidity benefit – If your invalidity benefit stopped because you moved to retirement pension, you keep your right to the HPP provided you were getting HPP under this rule on 12.4.95 or at any time in the 8 weeks beforehand. You must remain continuously entitled to IS (apart from breaks of 8 weeks or less).

The 8 week linking rule

If the only way you can qualify for the HPP is under method 3 or 4 above, there is an extra condition. Since reaching 60, you must have continued to get IS, apart from any breaks of 8 weeks or less. If you cease to get IS for 8 weeks and 1 day, you'll no longer qualify for the HPP but will get the lower PP or EPP, depending on your age.

If you stop getting IS for a period of 8 weeks or less which includes your 60th birthday, you'll be treated as having been continuously entitled to IS. Thereafter, the normal 8 week linking rule will apply.

If you qualified for the HPP only because of your partner's situation, you won't lose the HPP altogether if your partner dies or you are separated. Method 4 can apply so long as you were the IS claimant and getting a disability premium within the 8 weeks surrounding your 60th birthday. The rate at which you get IS makes no difference.

20. Housing costs

If you have rent to pay you may get help from housing benefit – see Chapter 4. For help with the cost of residential care, see Chapters 36 and 38. Mortgage interest payments and certain other housing costs are covered by income support. DSS leaflet, IS8, outlines the help available for home owners.

The basic rules

Housing costs may be included in your IS applicable amount if:
- you or your partner are liable for the housing costs at the home you live in – see below; and
- the type of housing costs are covered by IS – see below; and
- your mortgage was not taken out while you or your partner were on IS or income-based JSA or between claims (there are some exceptions) – see 21.

The amount of housing costs met by IS is worked out taking into account the following factors:
- the ceiling on loans of £100,000 (there are some exceptions) – see 22;
- the standard rate of interest applied to loans – see 22;
- the waiting period (ie the number of weeks you must be entitled to IS before housing costs are included in your applicable amount) – see 23;
- whether your housing costs are 'excessive' – see 22;
- deductions for any 'non-dependants' living with you (eg adult son or daughter, friend or relative: see 13) – the law assumes they are contributing towards your housing costs, whether they are paying anything or not. Unless your circumstances, or your non-dependant's, exempt you from the deduction, an amount is deducted from your assessed housing costs. IS rules are the same as for housing benefit (see Chapter 4(22)) unless your non-dependant has weekly gross income of £152 or more, in which case the maximum IS deduction is £33. No deduction is made from your IS housing costs if a deduction for that non-dependant is already being made from your housing benefit.

There were substantial changes to the rules on housing costs which came into effect on 2.10.95. The transitional protection for existing claimants is described in 22 below.

Liability for housing costs

You (or a member of your IS family) must be liable for housing costs for the home you live in. You are treated as liable if it is considered reasonable to do so and you have to meet the costs in order to carry on living in your home because the liable person is not meeting them.

Absence from home – Generally you can only get help on one home at a time and this must be the home that you occupy. In some situations you are treated as occupying your home when you are not actually present there, eg during a temporary absence of up to 13 weeks (or 52 weeks in some cases), or for up to 4 weeks when moving home. Chapter 4(6) and (7) cover the extra conditions – the housing benefit rules are almost the same as the IS rules.

Housing costs covered by IS

The following housing costs can be included as part of your IS applicable amount:
- mortgage interest payments – see 21;
- interest on loans for certain repairs and improvements – see 21;

- service charges – these are charges payable as a condition of your occupancy (eg under a lease) which relate to the provision of adequate accommodation. House insurance can be included if payments are made under the terms of the lease (rather than as a condition of the mortgage). Service charges for repairs and improvements listed in 21 below are not met by IS, although you can get help to pay interest on a loan taken out to pay these charges. Service charges are not met where these would be ineligible under the housing benefit rules – see Chapter 4(8);
- ground rent, feu duty, or other rent payable under a long lease of over 21 years;
- payments under a co-ownership scheme;
- rent if you are a Crown tenant;
- payments on a tent;
- rentcharges – this is a nominal rent that may be charged to a freeholder.

Paragraphs 15–17, Schedule 3, IS (General) Regs

Housing costs not covered by IS
IS does not include the cost of:
- water charges;
- housing costs covered by housing benefit;
- fuel charges and other ineligible service charges – see Chapter 4(8);
- charges for emptying a cesspit or septic tank;
- endowment premiums or capital repayments payable on a mortgage;
- mortgage interest on a new or additional loan taken out while you were on IS or income-based JSA or between claims (but there are exceptions) – see 21.

Following the changes to the rules on 2.10.95, some previously eligible housings costs are no longer covered by IS: arrears of mortgage interest payments; loans for repairs and improvements which do not fit the new criteria; extra help to separated couples with loans secured on the home which were not for house purchase. If, in the benefit week including 1.10.95, your applicable amount included interest for such a loan, it will continue to be covered so long as you or your partner remain on IS, disregarding any breaks in IS entitlement of 12 weeks or less. If you separate from your partner, you keep this protection.

21. Which mortgages and loans are covered?
IS only covers interest on mortgages (or higher purchase agreements or other loans) used:
- to buy your home – this includes buying your home jointly with others, a leaseholder buying the freehold, or buying out a joint owner;
- to pay off an earlier loan, but only to the extent that the earlier loan would have been covered by IS. For example, if your outstanding mortgage was £10,000 and you borrow, say, £12,000 to repay that first mortgage, IS can only cover the interest on £10,000 of the second loan;
- for certain repairs and improvements – see below.

Where a loan is taken out partly for a different purpose (eg a business loan), IS will not cover that part of the loan.

If your loan is covered by IS, an amount is added to your applicable amount, worked out according to the rules in 22 below. (See 23 below for when entitlement to housing costs can begin.) This amount is not paid to you but is deducted from your benefit and paid 4-weekly in arrears directly to your lender if they are part of the mortgage direct scheme.

Mortgages taken out while on IS or income-based JSA or between claims
The general rule is that IS does not meet mortgage interest on a loan taken out to buy a home while you or your partner were on IS or income-based JSA or within a break in entitlement of 26 weeks or less. The intention is to restrict your entitlement to the level of help (if any) you were already entitled to, either from IS, JSA or from housing benefit. Once a restriction is made, it continues to apply until you have a break in entitlement to IS or income-based JSA of over 26 weeks. Some loans are exempt from the restrictions – see below.

These restrictions do not apply to loans for repairs and improvements. Before the rules changed on 2.10.95, help with interest payments on repairs and improvement loans taken out while on IS could, in some cases, be restricted. If you had interest on a loan refused or restricted under the old rules (Schedule 3, para 5A, IS (General) Regs), you should ask for a review. Provided your loan is for eligible repairs and improvements, IS should include the interest payments assessed under the normal rules.

Replacement or additional loans – If you already have a mortgage and you increase it or take out an additional loan while on IS or between claims (eg if you take on a bigger mortgage to move home or buy out a joint owner), IS does not meet the additional amount. You can replace one mortgage with another provided the new mortgage is for the same amount or less. Where your new mortgage has been used to buy a home, and you pay off all or part of an earlier eligible loan in respect of another property from the sale of that property, then IS on the new mortgage is restricted to the amount of the earlier loan. This allows separated couples who sell their home to each have IS paid for mortgage interest on a new home at the full amount of the previous mortgage.

If you were previously getting housing benefit – If you take on a mortgage while on IS, income-based JSA, or between claims, the amount of IS for mortgage interest and for other housing costs (such as service charges and ground rent) is restricted to the level of housing benefit payable to you or your partner in the week before the week you buy the home. If you were getting both housing benefit and IS/JSA housing costs in that week, perhaps because you were on a shared ownership scheme, the restriction is to the total of the housing benefit payable plus the IS/JSA housing costs included in your applicable amount. The restricted amount can only subsequently go up to take account of increases in the standard rate of mortgage interest (see 22 below) or increases in other housing costs (service charges, etc).

If in the week before you buy the home you were not getting any housing benefit, for example you lived in your parents' home, then none of the mortgage interest is met by IS.

If your applicable amount previously included only housing costs other than for loan interest (eg service charges or ground rent) – If you take on a mortgage while on IS, income-based JSA or between claims, IS is restricted to the level of housing costs included in your applicable amount in the week before the week you buy a home. The restricted amount can only then increase if the standard rate of mortgage interest goes up or there is an increase in service charges or ground rent, etc.

Loans exempt from restrictions – In the following cases, loans are exempt from the restrictions described above, and IS for housing costs is worked out under the usual rules:
- any loan taken out before 3.5.94;
- a loan taken out, or an existing loan increased, to buy *'alternative accommodation more suited to the special needs of a disabled person'* than your previous home. This could include moving home to be nearer a carer. A person is treated

as disabled if they satisfy the conditions for a disability premium, disabled child premium, enhanced or higher pensioner premium at the date the loan is taken out, but they don't actually have to be getting any of these premiums or be entitled to IS;
- an additional or increased loan taken out because you've sold your home to buy another solely in order to provide separate bedrooms for children of different sexes aged 10 or over who are part of your family.

Paragraph 4, Schedule 3, IS (General) Regs

Loans for repairs and improvements

IS covers the interest on loans taken out and used within 6 months to pay for repairs and improvements to your home. These must be *'undertaken with a view to maintaining the fitness of the dwelling for human habitation'* and come within the following categories:
- adapting your home for *'the special needs of a disabled person'*; this could include adapting the home to house a carer; the disabled person must satisfy the conditions for a disability premium, disabled child premium, enhanced or higher pensioner premium, but need not actually get any of these premiums;
- provision of a bath, shower, sink, lavatory, ventilation, natural lighting, electric lighting and sockets, insulation of the home;
- provision of facilities for preparing and cooking food, storing fuel or refuse, or for drainage;
- provision of separate bedrooms for children of different sexes aged 10 or over who are part of your family;
- repairs to existing heating systems or of unsafe structural defects;
- damp proof measures.

Loans to pay service charges for any of these works are covered, as are loans used to pay off an existing loan for repairs but only to the extent that the existing loan would have qualified.

Paragraph 16, Schedule 3, IS (General) Regs

If your loan is covered by IS, an amount is added to your applicable amount, worked out according to the rules in 22 below.

The rules covering loans for repairs and improvements were changed on 2.10.95. If, in the benefit week which included 1.10.95, you were entitled to IS for a loan which qualified under the old rules but not the new, that loan continues to be covered until you or your partner have a break in your IS entitlement of over 12 weeks. If you separate from your partner, you keep this protection.

22. The assessment of mortgage and loan interest

There is a limit of £100,000 on the amount of eligible loans on which interest payments are met by IS. Provided the total amount of outstanding capital on your mortgage(s) and/or loan(s) is no more than £100,000 and your housing costs are not 'excessive', the interest to be met by IS is worked out on the whole of the eligible capital, using the standard rate of interest. In most cases there is a waiting period before the loan interest is included in your applicable amount – see 23 below. Once interest is included, reductions to the amount of eligible capital owing (eg if you reduce it with capital repayments) are only taken into account after a year and then annually.

The ceiling

If your loan (or the total of your loans) is above the ceiling of £100,000, the interest to be met by IS is worked out only on the first £100,000. Loans taken out to adapt the home *'for the special needs of a disabled person'* are exempt and do not count towards this limit – see 'Loans for repairs and improvements' above. If you are eligible for IS for housing costs on two homes, the ceiling is applied separately to each home. Any payments from a mortgage protection insurance policy to cover the interest on the part of a loan above the ceiling are disregarded as income for IS – see 28.

The £100,000 ceiling applies to IS claims made from 9.4.95. If you have been on IS continuously since before this, loans will be met up to the level of the ceiling that applied at the time you made your claim: £125,000 between 11.4.94 and 8.4.95; £150,000 between 2.8.93 and 10.4.94; no limit prior to 2.8.93. A break off IS of just one day is enough to end this protection. Loans which you take out or increase while on IS are subject to whichever ceiling applies at the time you do so.

Excessive housing costs

The amount of housing costs met by IS may be restricted if they are regarded as 'excessive', ie your home is larger than you need for your household, or the immediate area is more expensive than other areas in which there is suitable alternative accommodation, or your housing costs are higher than those for suitable alternative accommodation in the area.

But no restriction is made if it is not reasonable to expect you to move taking into account the availability of suitable alternative accommodation and the level of housing costs in the area, and the circumstances of you and your family. In particular, the age and health of yourself and your family must be considered, your employment prospects, and the effect of a move on the children's education. But other factors could also be relevant, eg you provide care, or rely on the care or support of someone nearby.

No restriction is made for the first 26 weeks of your claim, or following a review, if you could afford the costs when you took them on; nor for a further 26 weeks if you're doing your best to find cheaper accommodation. The 26 weeks continues to run during a break in IS of 12 weeks or less.

Where a restriction is applied, the amount of loan to be met is restricted to the amount you need to obtain suitable alternative accommodation.

Calculating the interest

Once the amount of capital outstanding on your eligible loan/s has been established, the interest to be included in your IS applicable amount is calculated on that capital (less any MIRAS due) using, in most cases, a standard interest rate. The rate is linked to an average of the interest rates charged by the top building societies.

Standard interest rates

from 2.10.95	**8.39%**	from 1.9.96	**7.16%**
from 28.1.96	**8.00%**	from 22.12.96	**6.89%**
from 28.4.96	**7.74%**	from 20.4.97	**7.20%**
from 30.6.96	**7.48%**		

The standard interest rate is applied in all cases, with one exception. Where your actual interest rate is less than 5% on the day your housing costs are first included in your IS applicable amount (ie after any relevant waiting period), it is your actual interest rate on that day that is applied. Changes in actual interest rate are ignored until it increases to at least 5%. The standard interest rate will be applied in the following benefit week and any further increases or reductions in the actual interest rate are ignored. Thus you may end up getting more from IS, or less, than the mortgage interest you are due to pay.

Arrears of interest cannot be met.

This method of calculating the interest was introduced on 2.10.95. Before this IS was worked out using actual interest rates. There is transitional protection for those who would otherwise lose out at the time the rules changed.

Transitional protection
This is worked out by comparing the amount of eligible housing costs met by IS before and after the introduction of the standard interest rate on 2.10.95. If you had housing costs included in your IS applicable amount in the benefit week which included 1.10.95, these are reassessed the following week under the new rules. If the new assessment is lower, the difference is added back on, so there is no change in the amount you receive for mortgage/loan interest.

The amount of transitional protection (called the '*add back*') cannot increase, but it can be reduced. If you have more than one loan, the 'add back' is calculated separately for each loan. Reduction in 'add back' on one loan does not affect the other.

The 'add back' is reduced by the amount of any later increase in housing costs, eg because of an increase in the standard interest rate. For example, say your weekly mortgage interest on 1.10.95 was £70 and when reassessed using the standard interest rate this went down to £65. The 'add back' is £5. A later increase in the standard interest rate puts the mortgage interest payable up £2 to £67. The 'add back' goes down to £3. You still get £70 in total (£67 mortgage interest plus £3 'add back'). But then the standard interest rate goes down putting the mortgage interest payable down to £64. The 'add back' stays at £3 and your total housing costs including the 'add back' is now £67.

You lose this transitional protection if you or your partner have a break in IS entitlement of over 12 weeks, or there is a spell when your applicable amount does not include housing costs (eg you are no longer responsible for the loan). But you can transfer the 'add back' to your partner if s/he becomes the IS claimant.

If you were only getting 50% mortgage interest paid on 1.10.95 because of the 16-week waiting period, you continue to get the same amount regardless of changes in mortgage interest rates until the end of the 16-week waiting period. The standard interest rate is then applied, the 'add back' is calculated and included in your entitlement.

23. When entitlement to housing costs begins
In most cases there is a waiting period from the start of your IS entitlement before housing costs are included in your applicable amount. Generally, the length of the waiting period depends on whether you took out your mortgage or other housing costs before or after 2.10.95.

Note that the waiting period begins from the start of your IS entitlement even if you have no housing costs at the time. So if you take out a loan while on IS and you are eligible for help with the costs (see 21 above), your IS is reviewed and housing costs can be included immediately; the waiting period does not start from the time you take out the loan.

If you are not entitled to IS because your income or capital is over the limit, or there is a break in your claim, see below. In some cases the waiting period can run even though you are not getting IS.

No waiting period
If you or your partner are aged 60 or over – Eligible housing costs are included in your applicable amount from the beginning of your IS entitlement, or from the day you reach 60 if you are part-way through the waiting period.
Certain housing costs – There is no waiting period for payments under a co-ownership scheme, rent for a Crown tenant or payments on a tent. These are included from the start of your IS entitlement.

'8 to 26-week' waiting period
Housing costs agreements made before 2.10.95 – If your loan or other housing costs arose under an agreement made before 2.10.95, your housing costs are included in your IS applicable amount as follows. If you've been continuously entitled to IS (or treated as entitled to IS – see below if you're not entitled to IS during the waiting period) for:
- less than 8 weeks – no housing costs are met;
- at least 8 weeks but less than 26 weeks – 50% of assessed housing costs are included;
- 26 weeks or more – 100% of assessed housing costs are included.

Replacement loans – If, on or after 2.10.95, you replace one mortgage or loan with another, the '8 to 26-week' waiting period applies only where the new loan is between the same parties, for the same property and for the same amount or less and replaces a loan that was taken out before 2.10.95. Otherwise the 39-week waiting period applies.

Special circumstances – If your loan or housing costs agreement was made on or after 2.10.95, the '8 to 26-week' waiting period applies nevertheless if you yourself are in one of the following groups at the time you make your IS claim:
- you are eligible for IS as a carer – see Box B.1;
- you have been refused payments under a mortgage protection insurance policy because you are suffering from a pre-existing medical condition, or because you have HIV; or
- you are a prisoner on remand; or
- you have a child and are claiming IS because your partner has died or your partner has 'abandoned' you. If you become one of a couple and you have not yet been on IS for 39 weeks, you lose this protection and the 39-week waiting period applies instead.

39 week waiting period
Housing costs agreement made on or after 2.10.95 – If your loan or other housing costs arose under an agreement made on or after 2.10.95, 100% of assessed housing costs are included in your applicable amount after you have been continuously entitled to IS (or treated as entitled – see below) for 39 weeks. You get no help with housing costs for the first 39 weeks of your claim. But if you come under one of the 'special circumstances' above at the time you claim IS, the '8 to 26-week' waiting period applies instead.

If you're not entitled to IS during the waiting period
Throughout the waiting period, you must be entitled to IS, although breaks in entitlement of 12 weeks or less are ignored. A break in IS entitlement of more than 12 weeks puts you back to the start. But there are linking rules that, in some situations, allow the period in between the end of one IS claim and the beginning of another to count towards the waiting period as though you had been entitled to IS throughout, and allow a period when your partner was the claimant to count.

If you have other income or your capital is over £8,000, you might find that you're not entitled to IS until your applicable amount goes up after the waiting period when the housing costs are included. In this case, the waiting period can run while you are entitled to certain benefits or National Insurance credits, or if you are a carer or single parent – see below.

During a break in IS claims, or a change of claimant – You are treated as entitled to IS:
- during a gap between claims for IS or income-based JSA of 12 weeks or less;
- for any period that it is decided on review or appeal that you were entitled to IS or income-based JSA;
- for the same period your ex-partner was getting IS or income-based JSA for both of you, if you claim within 12 weeks of separating;
- for the same period that your new partner was getting IS or income-based JSA as a single person or lone parent, if you claim within 12 weeks of becoming a couple;
- during the time your partner was getting IS or income-based JSA for both of you if you swap to become the claimant yourself;
- during the time someone was claiming IS or income-based JSA for you as their dependent child, if you claim within 12 weeks of the end of the claim and your claim includes a child who was also their dependant;
- during a gap between claims of 26 weeks or less where your last claim included housing costs after the waiting period, your IS or income-based JSA stopped because of child support payments and you reclaim because the payments are reduced either due to a change in the law or because an interim assessment has been replaced;
- during a gap between claims while you or your partner are on a government training scheme or employment rehabilitation scheme.

If your income or capital is over the IS limit – If you cannot get IS only because your income is higher than your applicable amount and/or your capital is over £8,000, you are treated as entitled to IS for up to 39 weeks if you satisfy one of the following conditions on each day (but gaps of up to 12 weeks are allowed):
- you are entitled to unemployment benefit, contribution-based jobseeker's allowance, statutory sick pay or incapacity benefit; or
- you are entitled to National Insurance credits for incapacity for work or unemployment (see Chapter 9(2)); or
- you are treated as entitled to IS during a break in IS claims, or because of a change in claimant (see the rules above); or
- you are eligible for IS as a carer (see Box B.1) or you are a lone parent, (provided you are not working 16 hours or more a week, your partner is not working 24 hours or more a week, you are not a student who is excluded from IS (see Chapter 31(5)) and you're not absent from the UK other than in circumstances described in Chapter 41(4)); the 39 weeks runs from when your IS claim is refused, so don't delay putting in your claim.

If you also have a mortgage protection policy, the 39 weeks is extended to cover the period that payments are made under the policy, provided your capital is within the limit (£8,000 or less) throughout.

Once you have qualified for housing costs – You will not have to serve the waiting period again if you have a break in your claim of 12 weeks or less, or your claims can be linked under one of the other linking rules described above.

If you have a break in claim of 26 weeks or less and you have been getting payments from an insurance policy for unemployment which have run out, your two claims are linked and the period in between ignored, so housing costs will resume from the start of your linked claim.

C. INCOME AND CAPITAL

24. What are your resources?

The IS assessment takes into account any income and capital you may have. All income is considered, including earnings, benefits and pensions. But your income or capital may be either ignored completely, ignored partly or fully taken into account.

If you have earnings, the amount that is disregarded generally depends on which premiums you are entitled to. We outline the assessment of earnings and how much is disregarded in 25 below. If you have income other than earnings, such as other benefits or pensions, see 26 to 28 below to check whether any (or all) of your income may be disregarded.

Capital includes savings, investments, some lump-sum payments, the value of property and land. If you borrow money, that will almost always count as money which you possess (generally as capital if it is a one-off loan or, in some cases, as income where it is part of a series of payments). If you intend to borrow a sum to use for a specific purpose, wait until you actually need to spend that money – don't borrow in advance of your need. Seek expert advice if credit or loans are taken into account. If capital which you possess outside the UK is taken into account, seek expert advice.

If you have capital of over the lower limit of £3,000, look at 31 below to see if any can be disregarded, and 29 below for the way in which capital affects the amount of benefit you get.

Generally it is clear whether a particular resource is income or whether it is capital. But in some cases, capital is treated as income and vice versa – see below.

In some cases you can be treated as possessing income or capital that you don't actually have – see below under 'notional income' or 'notional capital'.

There are specific rules for liable relative payments, child support maintenance, students and urgent cases payments. We don't cover these rules here, so seek advice if any of these apply. If you are a student, see Chapter 31 for more information.

Whose income and capital is included?
If you are one of a couple (married or living together as husband and wife), your partner's income and capital are added to your own. Otherwise only your own income and capital are taken into account. Children's income may be partly taken into account.

Dependent children – Unless the payment is maintenance, part of a dependent child's income may be ignored. If the child's own income is greater than the amount of their personal allowance (and the disabled child premium if s/he qualifies), the excess is disregarded. A dependent child's earnings are ignored unless s/he gets a job of at least 16 hours a week during the holiday after leaving school for good. In this case earnings will count (less the disregarded amount – see 25 below under 'Dependent child's earnings') against the child's personal allowance and the disabled child premium; any earnings above this are ignored.

Capital belonging to a dependent child is not treated as yours. It is ignored when working out your savings for the capital limits. But if s/he has capital of over £3,000 (not including disregarded capital), your IS assessment won't include the personal allowance or disabled child premium for that child. But neither will it include any of that child's income (other than maintenance payments). Your IS will still include the family premium.

Income or capital?

There is usually no problem deciding whether a particular resource is income or capital. But the distinction is not defined in the regulations. Where it is unclear the general principle (developed in case law) is that payments of income recur periodically and do not include ad hoc payments, whereas capital payments are one-off and not linked to a particular period (although capital may be paid in instalments).

In some cases the rules treat capital as income and vice versa – see below.

Income generated from capital – Income derived from capital is ignored as income but is treated as capital from the date it is normally due to be credited to you, *except* for income derived from the following items of disregarded capital (see 31 below):
- your home;
- premises you've acquired to live in, but have not yet been able to move in to;
- premises occupied by a partner, or ex-partner (but not estranged or divorced) or relative who is aged 60 or more or is incapacitated;
- your former home if you are estranged or divorced;
- premises you are taking reasonable steps to sell;
- premises you intend to occupy and are taking legal steps to obtain possession;
- premises you intend to occupy but which need essential repairs;
- business assets;
- trust fund from compensation for personal injury.

Reg 48(4) IS (General) Regs

Any mortgage payments, council tax or water charges paid in respect of the premises (other than the home you live in) during the period in which you receive income from those premises can be set off against that income. The amount above this is taken into account as income.

Para 22(2), Schedule 9, IS (General) Regs

If you let out your property and it is not covered under one of the exceptions above, rent is treated as capital, not as income. The full amount is taken into account as capital without any deductions for mortgage payments, etc.

Income treated as capital – The following payments of income are treated as capital:
- income derived from capital (but see above);
- income tax refunds, except for those involved in a trade dispute;
- irregular charitable or voluntary payments;
- holiday pay which is payable more than 4 weeks after the employment ends;
- advance of earnings or a loan from an employer;
- compensation for loss of full-time employment if it is less than a week's legal maximum;
- payment for a discharged prisoner;
- arrears of local authority residence order or custody payments;
- a bounty paid no more than once a year for a part-time fire fighter, or coast rescue duties, running a lifeboat, or to a member of the Territorial Army.

Reg 48, IS (General) Regs

Capital treated as income – If any capital is payable by instalments, each instalment outstanding when your claim is decided (or on the first day for which IS is paid if this is earlier) or at a later review, is treated as income if the total of all your capital, including the outstanding instalments, adds up to over £8,000. If your total capital adds up to £8,000 or less, each instalment is treated as a payment of capital. For people living permanently in residential care, the capital limit is £16,000. If the instalments aren't made by a liable relative, and are made to a dependent child, they will be treated as income if the outstanding instalments together with his or her other capital would take him or her over the £3,000 capital limit for a child.

Any payment under an annuity is treated as income.

If you or your partner have been involved in a trade dispute, any tax refund is treated as income, as are certain payments made by Social Services Departments under the Children Act, or under the Social Work (Scotland) Act.

Student loans (administered by the Student Loan Company) and Career Development Loans are treated as income.

Any capital treated as income is disregarded as capital.

Reg 41, reg 44(1), reg 66A IS (General) Regs

Notional income

Income that you do not actually possess may be taken into account in some circumstances.
- You are treated as possessing any income of which you have deprived yourself in order to get IS or increase your IS.
- You are treated as possessing any income that would be available to you on application. This also applies to social security benefits (but only up until the time you put in a claim) except jobseeker's allowance, family credit and disability working allowance, and the extra child benefit payable to lone parents (equivalent to the old one parent benefit).

The rule does not apply to payments from a discretionary trust, or from a personal injury compensation trust. Nor does it apply to income from a personal pension scheme, or retirement annuity contract as long as you are aged under 60. If you are 60 or over and you fail to purchase an annuity with the money available from the pension fund, and you've deferred or not taken all the necessary steps to draw an income from the pension (or the scheme does not allow for income withdrawal), you are assumed to have a notional income of the maximum amount of pension available to you.
- If you are a volunteer, or engaged by a charitable or voluntary organisation, notional earnings cannot be assumed if it is reasonable for you to provide your services free of charge. If it is reasonable to expect you to charge for your services, or you are performing a service for someone else in some other capacity, you are treated as having *'such earnings (if any) as is reasonable for that employment unless [you] satisfy [the AO] that the means of that person are insufficient for him to pay or to pay more for the service'*. If notional earnings are assumed, seek expert help with your appeal. A carer may count as a 'volunteer'- see CIS/93/91 – but see CIS/701/94 for exemptions.
- You are treated as possessing any income owing to you. There are exceptions, eg income from a discretionary or personal injury trust, or delays in social security benefits.
- Any payment made towards the cost of your residential care or nursing home is treated as your income, but some of this may be ignored (see 28 below).

Reg 42, IS (General) Regs

Notional capital

If you are held to have 'deprived' yourself of some capital in order to get IS, or to get extra benefit, the law says that that capital must be treated as if you still had it. It is called 'notional' capital. In some cases, the amount of notional capital along with your actual capital will exclude you from benefit. Or you may still be entitled to benefit, but because of your notional capital, the assessment is based on a higher tariff income than your actual capital warrants – see 29.

If there were good and sensible reasons for spending your capital, and getting IS (or more IS) wasn't a significant motive for spending part of your savings, you should be OK. It is worth appealing if capital you no longer have is taken into account, but do seek expert advice and check Commissioners' decisions R(IS)1/91, R(SB)11/82, R(SB)38/85, R(SB)40/85, R(SB)9/91 and CIS/242/93.

If you are held to have 'notional' capital on this basis, you won't be excluded from IS permanently, nor will a tariff income be based permanently on the higher amount of 'notional' capital. The AO will apply the 'diminishing capital rule' which reduces the amount of notional capital over time – see below. Ask the AO to explain, in writing, how this will apply to you. Chapter 52(7) covers the separate diminishing capital rule for overpayments. It is not possible to deprive yourself of 'notional' capital, only 'actual' capital is subject to this rule.

Reducing 'notional' capital – Your notional capital is treated as having been reduced by the amount of benefit 'lost' over a set period.

If you are held to have deprived yourself of an amount of capital, the AO will work out:
- how much benefit you would have been entitled to in the normal way if you had no notional capital – (A)
- how much benefit, if any, you are entitled to on the basis of your notional capital (as well as any actual capital) – (B)
- (A) minus (B) = the benefit you have lost – (LB 1).

If you have also 'lost' any of the other income-related benefits, the AO (or local authority) will add on those amounts of 'lost' benefit, eg LB 1 (income support) + LB2 (housing benefit) + LB 3 council tax benefit) = total lost benefit (TLB).

Your notional capital is treated as being reduced each week by your total lost benefit – (TLB).

When you claim an income-related benefit, the decision on your claim will include the amount of that particular benefit which you have 'lost' because of notional capital. Keep that decision letter – you may need to produce it when you claim any of the other income-related benefits. You only need to produce it if you are also held to have deprived yourself of some capital in order to get the other benefit(s): eg if you are excluded from IS because of notional capital, and you are also held to have deprived yourself of some capital to get HB and/or council tax benefit (CTB), you will need to show the IS decision letter to the local authority sections dealing with your HB/CTB claims. Note that it is quite possible to have completely different decisions on deprivation of capital, and different amounts of notional capital, for each benefit.

If you still get benefit – Each time your notional capital goes below another tariff income step, you will be entitled to some more benefit. Or a change of circumstances may increase or reduce your benefit. Both (A) and (B) will be re-calculated, giving you a new amount of 'lost' benefit (LB 1.2 . . .;). For the other benefits, the amount of 'lost' benefit may also change – so you add on (LB 2.2 etc). Your notional capital will now be treated as being reduced by your current total lost benefit – (TLB 2 . . .;). Note that a family credit or DWA award cannot be varied until your next claim.

If you don't get benefit – Once your total lost benefit is worked out, it cannot be reduced. It can only be increased so as to enable your notional capital to diminish faster. Unless you have a change of circumstances, your total lost benefit can only be re-calculated after 26 weeks (20 weeks for DWA, 22 weeks for family credit, but to take effect from after 26 weeks). The onus is on you to make a fresh claim for each benefit affected by the deprivation of capital rule and to produce the decision letters showing the amount(s) of the other 'lost' benefit(s). If there is only a small amount of 'notional' capital, you might well become entitled to some benefit within a matter of weeks.

You do not have to wait the full 26 weeks before making a fresh claim. That time limit is only relevant for re-calculating your total lost benefit if there have been no changes of circumstances affecting your entitlement beforehand.
Reg 51A, IS (General) Regs

More deprivation? – If you have actual capital as well as notional capital, you should still be careful about how you spend your actual capital. Obviously you will have to draw on actual capital to help supplement your income and to cover expenses that cannot be met by benefit. But the deprivation of capital rule can be re-applied.

Before 1.10.90 – Since 1.10.90, regulations have established a specific 'diminishing notional capital' rule described above. However, in R(IS)1/91 a Tribunal of Commissioners decided that income support law already included a more generous diminishing notional capital principle – based on reasonable expenses, rather than being tied to benefit rates. Therefore notional capital before 1.10.90 should be dealt with under this more favourable principle, rather than under the current rules.

25. Earnings from work

How earnings from employment are assessed
The IS assessment is normally based on your actual earnings in respect of a particular week. If you are paid monthly, that month's pay is multiplied by 12 and then divided by 52 to arrive at the weekly amount. However, if the amount of your income varies from week to week, there is discretion to take a more representative period and work out your average earnings over that period. If you have a regular pattern, or cycle, of working some weeks on, some weeks off, your average weekly earnings may be worked out over your working cycle: that average is then also taken into account in your 'off' weeks.
Reg 32(1) and 32(6), IS (General) Regs

If you have just retired, or your job has ended, or you are off sick, or your job has been interrupted for some other reason (but not if you have been suspended from work), your last normal earnings as an employee will usually be disregarded. You cannot be excluded from IS during the period covered by normal last earnings: only during a period covered by pay in lieu of notice, holiday pay within a set period, a retainer fee, or pay in lieu of remuneration (but not a periodic redundancy payment).

Earnings not clear? – If it is not clear exactly how much you earn a week, the AO will estimate how much it is reasonable to take into account. If this is not possible, a payment 'on account' may be made. If you are not being paid, or are underpaid for a service, 'notional' earnings may be taken into account – see 24.
Reg 42(5) and 42(6), IS (General) Regs

Working out net earnings
Do not count the following as earnings: any payment in kind, meal vouchers, sickness or maternity pay, or occupational pension (see 26 below for how benefits and pensions are treated). Don't count *'any payment in respect of expenses wholly, exclusively and necessarily incurred in the performance of the duties of the employment'*.

An advance of earnings, or a loan, counts as capital. Count any other payment from your employer as earnings – eg bonuses; commission; payments towards travel expenses between your home and workplace, or towards childminding fees; retainers (from your employer or from a boarder); pay in lieu of notice; and holiday pay (unless you get it more than 4 weeks after you last worked).

Reg 35, IS (General) Regs

Deduct from your earnings – income tax; National Insurance contributions; half of any contribution towards an occupational or personal pension scheme.

Earnings disregards

Once you have worked out your total earnings as above, you now deduct the appropriate 'earnings disregard'.

This is limited to an overall maximum of £15 per week of a single person's earnings, or of the joint earnings of a couple. But you have to qualify for the £15 overall maximum earnings disregard. If you cannot qualify for the £15 earnings disregard, you are limited to an earnings disregard of £5 if you are single, or £10 for a couple.

The £15 earnings disregard – Deduct £15 a week from joint earnings if any of the following apply.

❑ You qualify for an adult disability premium (or would qualify for it if you weren't in hospital, or in a residential care or nursing home).

❑ You qualify for a carer premium – the disregard applies to the earnings of the carer; if your earnings are less than £15, up to £5 can be disregarded from your partner's earnings subject to the overall £15 maximum.

❑ You qualify for the lone parent rate of the family premium (or would qualify for it if you weren't in a residential care or nursing home, or also entitled to the pensioner premium; but not if you are also entitled to the higher pensioner premium).

❑ You qualify for the higher pensioner premium (or would qualify for it if you weren't in hospital etc) – but only where you, or your partner, were working immediately before reaching 60. You must also have been entitled to the £15 disability premium earnings disregard at that time. Since then, you must have continued in part-time employment, apart from breaks of 8 weeks or less.

❑ You are one of a couple and your IS would include a disability premium but for the fact that the higher pensioner premium or enhanced pensioner premium are applicable (or you would meet this condition if you weren't in hospital etc). Either you or your partner must be under 60 with either one of you in part-time employment.

❑ You are one of a couple, with one of you aged 60 or over and the other aged 75–79 (inclusive), if immediately before the younger person reached 60 either one of you were in part-time employment and the claimant qualified for the enhanced pensioner premium and was getting the £15 earnings disregard outlined immediately above. Since that time you must have continued in part-time work apart from breaks of 8 weeks or less.

❑ You are working in one of the jobs listed below, up to £15 of those earnings are disregarded:
- a part-time fire fighter;
- an auxiliary coastguard on coast rescue activities;
- helping operate or launch a life boat;
- a member of any territorial or reserve force.

If both of a couple are doing this type of work, you are still restricted to the joint earnings disregard of £15. If one of you is doing an ordinary part-time job, up to £5 of his/her earnings can be ignored, so long as that doesn't take you over the £15 joint disregard.

If you cannot qualify for the £15 earnings disregard – Deduct £5 from earnings if you are single. Deduct £10 from joint earnings if you are in a couple, whether one or both of you are working.

If you qualify for the higher pensioner premium after reaching 60, or requalify after a break of 8 weeks and 1 day or longer, you are restricted to the £5 earnings disregard (or £10 for couples) – unless the 8-week linking rule can be extended: see below.

Dependent child's earnings – If a dependent child gets a job, working for 16 or more hours a week, during the holiday after leaving school for good, deduct the following from his or her earnings:

- £15, plus any earnings above the amount of the child's personal allowance and the disabled child premium – but only if s/he qualifies for the disabled child premium (or would if s/he was not in a residential care or nursing home). If disability reduces his or her earning capacity to less than 75% of what a non-disabled person would 'normally be expected to earn', s/he doesn't count as being in remunerative work, so all those earnings are ignored. OR
- £5, plus any balance above the child's personal allowance.

The 8-week linking rule – If your break from IS is covered by the work 'trial period', the linking period is extended to 12 weeks.

If your break from IS is because you (or your partner) are on an employment rehabilitation course, or taking part in training arranged under s.2, Employment and Training Act 1973, the whole of that break is ignored. However, if you get a 'disability' earnings disregard, a break of no more than 8 weeks coming after a spell of training, is also ignored.

How self-employed earnings are assessed

IS has specific rules to work out income from self-employment. It is based on the net cash flow of your business, or of your share of the business. If you get royalties or copyright payments, seek advice.

Take full gross receipts of the business – This is all the money you receive in respect of and generated by the business over a specific trading period, normally one year; but if you've recently started self-employment, or there has been a change which is likely to affect the normal pattern of business, the AO can pick a different period which is more representative of your average weekly earnings.

Work out net profit – deduct:

- if you work as a childminder, two thirds of those earnings; OTHERWISE
- *'any expenses wholly and exclusively defrayed [ie actually paid] in that period for the purposes of that employment'*: this is subject to some exceptions and extra rules in reg 38(5) to (7) IS General Regs, eg the expenses must be *'reasonably incurred'*, and business entertainment is specifically excluded. Note that expenses can be apportioned between business and personal use – see R(FC)1/91 and R(IS)13/91;
- a repayment of capital on any loan used for replacing equipment or machinery, or for repairing existing business assets (less any insurance payments);
- the excess of any VAT paid, over VAT received;
- expenditure out of income to repair an existing business asset (less any insurance payment);
- interest (but not capital) payments on a loan taken out for the purposes of the employment.

The sum you are left with after these deductions is your net profit.

From your net profit, deduct:

- income tax – this is just your appropriate personal tax allowances, on a pro rata basis if necessary: see Chapter 51;

- Class 2 and Class 4 contributions – see Chapter 9(1);
- half of any contribution to a personal pension scheme.

Now check above to see which of the £15, £10 or £5 earnings disregards applies.

26. Income from benefits and pensions

Most benefits are taken into account in full in the IS assessment (less any income tax payable). For example, retirement pension and incapacity benefit are both taken into account in full. But some benefits are either wholly or partly disregarded.

The following benefits are ignored completely
- housing benefit;
- council tax benefit;
- war pensioners mobility supplement;
- disability living allowance (DLA), attendance allowance, constant attendance allowance, mobility allowance, exceptionally severe disablement allowance (payable under the war or industrial disablement schemes only). But if you are in a residential care or nursing home and have preserved rights, DLA care component, or attendance allowance, etc of up to £49.50 a week is taken into account as income. If the RCH/NH rates would not apply because of Sch 4, Part II IS General Regs, attendance allowance etc is ignored – see Chapter 38;
- any ex-gratia payment made to compensate for the non-payment of DLA, mobility or attendance allowance (as above), or of a war disablement or war widow's pension, or of income support;
- any social fund payment;
- any payment(s) of the £10 Christmas bonus;
- any resettlement benefit paid on discharge from hospital;
- any special war widow's payment or supplementary pension;
- any payment or repayment of health benefits and any payment made instead of milk tokens or vitamins – see Chapter 48;
- dependants' additions to non-means-tested benefits if the dependant is not a member of your family.

The following benefits are partly ignored
Deduct up to £10 of:
- a war disablement pension; or
- war widow's pension; or
- comparable pensions paid under non-UK social security legislation, or to victims of Nazi persecution.

If £10 of a war pension is ignored, you can also have £10 of a regular charitable payment ignored – see 27. The mobility supplement, constant attendance allowance, severe disablement occupational allowance and exceptionally severe disablement allowance paid with a war pension are completely disregarded.

Statutory sick pay and statutory maternity pay
Statutory sick pay and statutory maternity pay are taken into account in full, less any Class 1 NI contributions, tax, and half of any contributions towards an occupational or personal pension scheme.

Occupational and personal pensions
Occupational and personal pensions are normally taken into account in full, less any tax payable. State retirement pensions are also taken into account in full, less tax. Income from a personal pension that would be available to you on application, may be taken into account as 'notional income' – see 24 above.

If you live in a residential care or nursing home and have preserved rights (see Chapter 38), half of any occupational or personal pension or income from a retirement annuity contract is disregarded if you pay at least this amount to your husband or wife for their maintenance. The disregard continues during a temporary absence from the care home.

27. Charitable and voluntary payments

Some types of charitable and voluntary payments (except maintenance or liable relative payments, or payments made to a striker) are completely disregarded as income.

If the payment is towards the cost of residential care, see also 28 below.

Disregarded regular payments
The following payments made to you, or to any member of your IS family, should be ignored as income: any charitable or voluntary payment made or due to be made at regular intervals which is intended and used for an item *other than* food, ordinary clothing or footwear, household fuel, rent or rates for which housing benefit is payable, any housing costs which are met by IS, or any residential care or nursing home charges met by IS if you have preserved rights (see 28), or is used for any council tax, or water charges for which you are liable. Ordinary clothing or footwear is defined as items for *'normal daily use, but does not include school uniforms, or clothing or footwear used solely for sporting activities'*.

Examples of allowable items include payments intended and used for: annual veterinary checkups and inoculations for a pet, annual service charges for electrical and gas equipment and appliances, hire purchase or other regular payments for a car, wheelchair, electrical and gas equipment and appliances, furniture and furnishings. However, paying for adaptations to your car is almost certainly a one-off payment. It would be treated as capital and taken into account (but would only affect benefit if it takes existing capital above £3,000); unless it was paid to a third party when it would be disregarded (see 28 below).
Para 15, Schedule 9, IS (General) Regs

Note that you must use the whole of the payment for the allowable item or need: any cash left over after you have paid for the item would be taken into account as income, subject to the £20 disregard – see below.

Regular payments partly disregarded – If it cannot be completely disregarded under the rules above, then up to £20 a week of any regular charitable or voluntary payment is ignored as income. £20 is the maximum that can be disregarded in any week no matter how many payments are made.

If you get £10 disregarded from a war disablement pension or war widow's pension, or from a student loan, or £5 disregarded from student's covenant income, there is an overriding limit of £20 on the total weekly disregards, so you could not also get the full £20 disregard on charitable or voluntary payments.

Payments made to a third party (rather than to yourself) are dealt with under the 'third party' rules – see 28 below.

Irregular payments
If the cash payments from any charity or voluntary payments are not made, or due to be made to you (rather than to a third party – see 28) at regular intervals, those payments are treated as capital. Gifts of money from liable relatives are treated as capital. Irregular gifts in kind from a charity are disregarded.

Payments from specific trusts
Any payments, in kind or cash, made by the Macfarlane

Trusts, the Fund, the Eileen Trust or the Independent Living Funds are ignored completely.

Any payment made by, or on behalf of a person with haemophilia who received money from the Macfarlane Trust, or a person who received money from the Fund or the Eileen Trust, or their partner, is disregarded in full if it originates from the trust money. To qualify for the disregard the payment must be made to (or for the benefit of) the partner or former partner of the person who is making the payment (unless you are estranged or divorced), or to dependent children (if they are a member of the donor's family, or were, but are now a member of the claimant's family). If the person making the payment has no partner or dependent children, a payment (including a payment from their estate if they are now dead) to their parent, step-parent, or guardian is disregarded until the end of 2 years after his/her death; so long as the payment originates from any of these trusts.

28. Other kinds of income

Payments to third parties
A payment of income made to a third party in respect of a member of your IS family, can be taken into account only to the extent that it is used for the food, ordinary clothing or footwear, household fuel, rent or rates for which housing benefit is payable, or any housing costs which are covered by IS of any member of your IS family, or is used for any council tax or water charges for which you or your partner are liable. Ordinary clothing or footwear does not include school uniforms or sportswear.
Regulation 42(4), IS (General) Regs

Any payment made to a third party towards the cost of your residential care or nursing home is treated as your income. But some of this income may be ignored under other rules – see below.

If someone pays a third party to do or provide something which is not in the list above, its value will be ignored. For example, paying for your car to be repaired or adapted; or paying someone else to supply you with cat food; or paying your TV rental.

If a payment would have been ignored had it been paid to a third party, rather than to you, that payment will be ignored. It must be intended for and used to buy or pay for an item not in the list above.

Payments in kind
Any income in kind is ignored, eg things like a free bus pass, tins of cat food, food, cigarettes, petrol etc (even where a liable relative is giving you the items). But these payments are taken into account if you are involved in a trade dispute.

Payments for residential care and nursing homes
Some payments towards the cost of your care can be disregarded as income for IS. See also Chapters 36 and 38.
If the local authority arranged your care – If the local authority has arranged your preferred choice of residential care or nursing home which is more expensive than the local authority would usually expect to pay, any charitable or voluntary payment made or due to be made at regular intervals to meet the difference is ignored as income. See Chapter 35(4).
para 15A, Sch 9, IS (General) Regs
If the local authority did not arrange your care – Any payment intended for and used to meet the residential care or nursing home charge is partly ignored. The amount ignored is the weekly accommodation charge less your IS applicable amount less an amount for personal expenses (£14.10 for an adult).

The payment need not be from a charity, or a voluntary payment.
para 30A, Sch 9, IS (General) Regs
If you have preserved rights – Any payment to you is ignored which is *'intended and used as a contribution towards'* – the part of a residential care or nursing home charge which is not met by IS, ie is above the appropriate limit for the type of accommodation you are in.

A regular charitable or voluntary payment intended and used towards charges that are met by IS has the first £20 a week disregarded – see 27.
para 30(1)(e) and para 15(1), Sch 9, IS (General) Regs

Miscellaneous income
The following types of income are ignored:
- Victoria Cross/George Cross annuities and analogous payments;
- any educational maintenance allowance for a dependent child at school or college;
- any expenses paid to a volunteer – but only if you are paid nothing else by the charity or organisation, and aren't treated as having 'notional' earnings;
- any contribution towards living and accommodation costs made to you by someone living as a member of your household (but not if they are a commercial boarder, or a sub-tenant);
- if the child has capital of over £3,000, disregard the whole of an adoption or custodianship allowance; otherwise ignore any amount above the child's personal allowance and disabled child premium;
- any fostering allowance;
- any payment made *'by a health authority, local authority or voluntary organisation to the claimant in respect of a person who is not normally a member of the claimant's household but is temporarily in his care'*. Generally this covers respite care payments, for overnight (or longer) stays, or for just a few hours in the day. But the payment cannot be made by the person you are looking after;
- any payment under the Community Care (Direct Payments) Act 1996 or s.12B Social Work (Scotland) Act 1968;
- any discretionary payment from a Social Services or Social Work Department made under s.17 or 24, Children Act, or s.12, 24 or 26, Social Work (Scotland) Act (but not to a striker's family);
- any payment made to a juror or a witness in respect of attendance at court (but not if it was to compensate for loss of earnings or for loss of benefit);
- any payment under the Assisted Prison Visits scheme;
- any payment to help a disabled person get, or keep, work which is made under the Disabled Persons (Employment) Act 1944 (or the equivalent for training) – but not if it is a state training allowance;
- up to £10 pw of the maximum student loan given your situation – whether or not you have applied for the maximum student loan – see Chapter 31;
- up to £5 pw of any excess of a student's covenant income above the assessed parental contribution, or above the standard maintenance grant – see Chapter 31;
- if you are eligible for IS as a student, certain parts of your grant are disregarded – see Chapter 31;
- a Career Development Loan except for any part applied for and used for specified living expenses;
- any student grant or loan after you have completed your course;
- if you are doing Youth Training, Training for Work, or an

employment rehabilitation course:
- payments made to reimburse your travel expenses;
- a 'living away from home' allowance if housing benefit does not cover your extra housing costs;
- a training premium;
■ if you have a sub-tenant or tenant (but not if that person lives as a member of your household, nor if you provide them with meals):
  - £4 from the 'rent' they pay you; plus
  - £9.25 if that 'rent' includes an amount for heating;
■ if you provide board and lodging in your own home, £20 and half of the remainder of the weekly charge paid by each person provided with such accommodation (even if that person lodges with you for just one night). If your boarder is disabled, nothing extra is disregarded;
■ payments under a mortgage protection policy used to meet repayments on a mortgage or on a loan for repairs and improvements that are covered by IS (see 21 above) up to the amount of loan interest not met in your applicable amount, plus the amount due in capital repayments or endowment premiums, and either the premiums on the mortgage protection policy or premiums on a buildings insurance policy;
■ payment (from any source) made to you which is intended and used as a contribution towards: the payments due on a loan secured on your home which is not covered by IS (see 21 above); housing costs covered by IS but not met in your applicable amount; capital repayments or endowment premiums on loans covered by IS; premiums on a policy taken out to meet any of the above costs or for buildings insurance; any rent not met by housing benefit;
■ deduct the part of a home income plan annuity which covers the net interest payable on the loan used to buy the annuity. Income from any other type of annuity counts in full. (The full qualifying conditions are listed in p.17, Sch 9, IS General Regs);
■ income abroad while transfer to the UK is prohibited;
■ charges for currency conversion if income is not paid in sterling.

29. Capital limits

The upper limit is £8,000. While the value of all your capital resources (or notional capital resources) is £8,000.01 or more, you are excluded from benefit. If a child's own capital adds up to over £3,000, no personal allowance or disabled child premium can be paid for that child. But some types of capital are disregarded, or ignored, for these capital limits and for the lower limit at which a tariff income begins to be assumed (see below).

Tariff Income – If your capital is £3,000 or less, your benefit is not affected. While the value of your capital is from £3,000.01 to £8,000 (inclusive), a deduction is made from benefit which is known as 'tariff income'. £1 pw is taken into account for each £250 or part of £250 from £3,000.01 to £8,000. Thus if capital is from £3,250.01 to £3,500, £2 is taken into account. Each time your capital gets into the next block of £250 (even by as little as one penny), an additional £1 is deducted. If your capital is from £7,750.01 to £8,000, the tariff income is £20 pw.

If tariff income is included in your assessment, do notify the DSS if the amount of your capital changes. If your savings drop to the next lower tariff income band and you haven't told the DSS, you'll be getting too little IS. If your savings have increased to the next higher tariff income band and you haven't told the DSS, you'll have been overpaid benefit. Watch out for the 'notional capital rule' – see 24 above. It is sensible to keep records, and all receipts, to show how and why you spent your savings.

If you go into residential care – From 8.4.96, the capital limits are higher if you move permanently into a residential care or nursing home. The upper limit is £16,000. If you have capital above £16,000, you are excluded from IS. The lower limit at which a tariff income begins to be assumed is £10,000. Tariff income is calculated in the same way as outlined above. If your stay is only temporary, the capital limit remains at £8,000. See Chapters 36 and 38.

30. How is capital valued?

Capital is calculated at it's current market or surrender value, less 10% if there would be costs involved in selling, and less

---

B.3 Benefit weeks and paydays

The IS benefit week and payday rules depend on whether your IS is paid in advance or in arrears. Your IS is normally paid on the same day and at the same intervals as any other benefit you get. If you are incapable of work, your IS is paid fortnightly in arrears.

Payment in advance

IS is paid in advance only where you (the IS claimant – not your partner) are:
■ getting retirement pension; or
■ over pension age and not getting severe disablement allowance or incapacity benefit and neither you or your partner are involved in a trade dispute (unless you were getting IS immediately before the dispute started); or
■ getting widowed mother's allowance or a widow's pension (but not if you are signing on for work, or providing medical evidence of incapacity, whether you are doing this voluntarily or because you have to); or
■ returning to work after a trade dispute.

Benefit week – If you are paid IS in advance, your IS benefit week is the 7 days starting with your payday. For example, the retirement pension pay day is a Monday. Your IS pay day will also be on that Monday. Your IS benefit week will end on the following Sunday.

First payment of IS – For IS in advance, the first payment won't begin until your IS payday. If your IS claim is received by the DSS on your payday, payment of IS will begin from that day. If your claim isn't received (or treated as having been received) on an IS payday, you won't get benefit until the next IS payday. You could lose up to 6 days benefit. However, if IS is awarded for a definite period which is not a complete benefit week (or weeks), entitlement begins on your date of claim.

Payment in arrears

Benefit week – Your IS benefit week is the period of 7 days ending with your IS payday.
First payment of IS – For IS in arrears, you can be paid from the date your claim was received (or treated as received) in a DSS office.

Changes of circumstances

The date from which a change of circumstances can be put into

any mortgage or debt secured on the property.
Jointly owned capital – If you own property jointly with one or more others, you are treated as though you own an equal share. Thus if 4 people jointly possess an item of capital in an actual split of 80%, 10%, 5% and 5%, each of you will be treated as possessing 25% of that capital. The market value of your share is worked out assuming that you are the sole owner, and assuming that none of the joint owners lives in the property, and then dividing the resulting value by the number of joint owners. The valuation must take account of anyone else who lives there who is not a joint owner.

If you can split up a joint holding into something you own outright (equal to your real actual share), that does not count as 'deprivation'; eg you might split a joint account into separate accounts. It can be argued that you should only be treated as owning an equal share of a capital asset under this rule (reg 52 IS General Regs) if you have a joint beneficial ownership of the whole capital asset (see CIS/7097/95). If the capital is not jointly owned but rather is held in undivided shares, the rule should not apply. Instead, the amount of the share to which you are beneficially entitled, equal or unequal, is the actual capital possessed by you.

31. What capital is disregarded?

Your home
The following items are disregarded:
- the value of your own home;
- the value of any premises occupied wholly or partly by your partner or by a 'relative', if they are aged 60 or more, or incapacitated; or former partner if you are not 'estranged or divorced';
- the value of your former home for 26 weeks after you left it because of divorce or estrangement from your former partner;
- the value of premises you've acquired if you intend to move in within 26 weeks of the date of purchase (longer is allowed if that is reasonable in the circumstances to enable you to get possession and move in);
- any sum 'directly attributable' to the proceeds of the sale of your former home, which you intend to use to buy another home within 26 weeks of that sale, or *'such longer period as is reasonable in the circumstances to enable [you] to complete the purchase'*;
- any sum paid to you because of damage to, or loss of the home or any personal possession and intended for its repair or replacement, or any sum given or loaned to you expressly for essential repairs or improvements to the home, will be ignored for 26 weeks if you are going to use that sum for its intended purpose: longer if that is reasonable in the circumstances;
- any sum deposited with a housing association as a condition of occupying the home is ignored. If you've removed that deposit and intend to use it to buy another home it can be ignored on the same basis as the proceeds of the sale of a former home;
- the value of premises which you are taking reasonable steps to dispose of for 26 weeks from *'the date on which [you] first took such steps, or such longer period as is reasonable in the circumstances to enable [you] to dispose of those premises'*;
- the value of premises which you intend to occupy as your home if you are taking steps to obtain possession and have either sought legal advice or commenced legal proceedings in order to obtain possession. The value is ignored for 26 weeks from the date on which you first sought such advice, or started proceedings (whichever is earlier); but it may be ignored for a longer period if that is reasonable in the circumstances;
- the value of premises which you intend to occupy as your home once *'essential repairs or alterations'* make the premises *'fit for such occupation'* for 26 weeks from the date on which you first took steps to get the premises repaired or altered, or such longer period as is reasonable in the circumstances to enable the works to be carried out and for you to move in. This can help if you need to make adaptations because of a disability, eg install a ground floor bathroom;
- any grant under S.129, Housing Act 1988, or S.66, Housing (Scotland) Act 1988 to be used to buy premises you intend to live in as your home, or to do repairs or alterations needed to make the premises fit for you to live in. The grant

---

effect varies depending on whether you are paid IS in arrears or in advance. An award can also be reviewed in advance of an expected change. These standard rules are subject to the exceptions listed below: unless you are covered by an exception, or reg 17(3), Claims and Payments Regs is used to make an award for a definite period, you might find that a change is cancelled out by another change in the same benefit week if both have to be put into effect from the same day. In addition, if you are away from the residential care or nursing home in which you usually live for 6 days, or less, that won't be treated as a change of circumstances.

IS in advance – In this case, a change can have effect only from a payday. If the date your circumstances actually changed is a payday, the cash effect of that change is implemented from that date. If your circumstances change on any other day, the cash effect of that change can only be implemented from the next payday. You could lose up to 6 days benefit.

IS in arrears – If you are paid IS in arrears, the cash effect of any change is implemented from the first day of the benefit week in which the change happened. In some cases you will gain (eg for a child born in the middle of your benefit week, you'll get the full rate). In others you lose (eg death in the middle of a benefit week).

Exceptions – If you are affected by any of the changes listed below, your IS will be altered with effect from the date of that change, and then again from the day after the date on which that change ended. All but the first change applies whether IS is paid in arrears or advance. (Note that any income is taken into account from the first day of the benefit week in which it is due to be paid.)

❑ Your IS is paid in arrears and your entitlement ends for a reason other than that your income exceeds your applicable amount.
❑ A child who is normally in care or detained in custody lives with you for part only of the benefit week.
❑ You or your partner enter a nursing home or a residential care home for a period of not more than 8 weeks.
❑ You or a member of your family cease to be a patient for less than a week.
❑ A striker becomes incapable of work, or enters the maternity pay period.
❑ During your IS award you claim another social security benefit and, as a result, your benefit week changes.
❑ You become, or cease to be, a prisoner.

is ignored for 26 weeks, or such longer period as is reasonable in the circumstances to enable you to complete buying, repairing, or altering the premises.

Benefits
Arrears (or an ex-gratia payment) of the following benefits are ignored for 52 weeks after you get them: disability living allowance, attendance allowance (or equivalent under the industrial injuries or war pensions schemes), mobility allowance, housing benefit, council tax benefit, community charge benefit, transitional relief payments, special war widow's payment, IS, income-based JSA, earnings top-up, supplementary benefit, disability working allowance, family credit or family income supplement.

Any payment or repayment of a health benefit in respect of NHS prescription charges, dental charges or hospital travelling expenses is ignored for 52 weeks after you receive the money. Any payment made instead of milk tokens or free vitamins is ignored for 52 weeks after you receive the payment.

Any social fund payment is completely ignored.

Personal possessions
The value of any personal possessions is ignored except those bought to reduce your capital in order to get more benefit. A compensation payment for loss or damage of personal possessions which is to be used for repair or replacements is ignored for 26 weeks, or longer if that is reasonable.

Trust funds
A trust fund created from payments for a personal or criminal injury is completely ignored. 'Personal injury' includes a disease and injury suffered as a result of a disease – R(SB)2/89. Trusts created from compensation and Vaccine Damage Payments are clearly covered; so too may a trust of funds collected for a person because of their personal injuries. Actual payments received count in full as income or capital, depending on the nature of the payment.

For under 18s, damages awarded for personal injury, or compensation for the loss of a parent, where capital is administered by the Courts ('infant funds in court') are ignored. Actual payments received count in full as income or capital, depending on the nature of the payment.

The value of the right to receive any income under a life interest or from a liferent (this is a type of trust in Scotland) is ignored. Actual income received counts in full as income.

Any payment made under the Macfarlane Trusts, the Fund, the Eileen Trust or the Independent Living (Extension) or (1993) Funds is ignored. Any payment which derives from a payment made under the Macfarlane Trusts, the Fund or the Eileen Trust may also be ignored (see 27 above).

Other capital
The following types of capital are disregarded:
- any future interest in property other than land or premises on which you have granted a lease or tenancy;
- the capital value of the 'right to receive' any income under an annuity, and the 'surrender value' of an annuity;
- the capital value of the right to receive any income which is disregarded because it is frozen abroad: seek advice;
- the full surrender value of any life insurance policy;
- any payment from social services made under s.17 or 24, Children Act, or Ss.12, 24 or 26, Social Work (Scotland) Act, – unless made to a striker's family;
- a refund of tax which was deducted on loan interest if that loan was taken out in order to buy the home, or to carry out repairs or improvements to the home;
- the value of the right to receive an occupational or personal pension; and the value of any funds held under a personal pension scheme or retirement annuity contract;
- the value of the right to receive any rent except where you have a future interest in the property;
- any payment in kind made by a charity;
- business assets while you are 'engaged as a self-employed earner' are ignored. If you've ceased that self-employment, the assets will be ignored for as long as is reasonable in the circumstances to allow you to dispose of them. However, if sickness or disability mean that you cannot work as a self-employed earner, your business assets will be disregarded for 26 weeks from your date of claim: longer if that is reasonable in the circumstances. You must intend to start or resume work in that business as soon as you are able to, or as soon as you recover;
- any 'training bonus' of £200 or less;
- any payment made to a juror or witness in respect of attendance at a court (but not if it was to compensate for loss of earnings or for loss of benefit);
- any payment made under the Assisted Prison Visits scheme: for 52 weeks after you receive the payment;
- any payment (but not a state training allowance, or a training bonus) to help a disabled person get, or keep, work, which is made under the Disabled Persons (Employment) Act 1944 (or the equivalent for training);
- a start-up capital programme under the Blind Homeworkers' scheme;
- where any payment of capital 'falls to be made by instalments, the value of the right to receive any outstanding instalments' – see also 24 above, 'Capital treated as income';
- payment to you as holder of the Victoria Cross or George Cross.

Sch 10, IS (General) Regs

D. CLAIMS, PAYMENTS AND APPEALS

32. How do you claim?
You can start off your claim by phoning your local DSS office or by using the coupon in leaflet IS1. Say that you wish to claim IS. The DSS will send you a claim form, SP1 for pensioners, A1 for others. You can also get a claim form from a post office or advice centre. If you do this, phone the DSS to tell them that you intend to claim IS. That way your benefit can be backdated to the date of your call. You can fill in the form yourself, but don't hesitate to ask the DSS or an advice centre for help as soon as you need it. If you would prefer an interview, tell the DSS. You can be seen in your own home, or at the DSS office.

So long as you send in the form (properly completed) within one month of the date you phoned or wrote to the DSS asking for a claim form (or otherwise notified them of your intention to claim), your claim is treated as made on the date of that first contact.
Reg 6(1)(aa) Claims & Payments Regs

Supporting evidence – From 6.10.97 there are new strict rules requiring you to give all the information and send in all the supporting documents specified in the claim form, for your claim to be accepted as properly made. So long as you do this within a month of the date you first notified the DSS of your intention to claim, your date of claim will be the date of that first contact.

If you have problems getting the necessary information or evidence within the month, tell the DSS straightaway and send in your claim form anyway. If your difficulty is for one of the reasons specified in the regulations as acceptable (eg you have a physical, mental, learning or communication difficulty and it is not reasonably practicable for you to get help) then your claim will still be treated as made on the date you notified the DSS of your intention to claim. There is space on the claim form for you to tell the DSS what these problems are. The Secretary of State decides whether your reasons will be accepted so there is no right of appeal if you disagree. See Chapter 52(2) for more details.

Reg 4(1A), (1B), Reg 6(1A) Claims & Payments Regs

Late claims – If you think you were entitled to IS before you put in your claim, ask, in writing, for your claim to be backdated. IS can be backdated for up to 3 months if you have 'special reasons' why you couldn't reasonably have been expected to claim earlier – see Chapter 52(4).

Waiting for a decision on another benefit? – Sometimes entitlement to another benefit, can mean that you become entitled to IS because your 'applicable amount' goes up. For example if you get ICA, that qualifies you for a carer premium, or if you get DLA that qualifies you for a disability premium. Don't wait for a decision on the benefit you've claimed. Put in a claim for IS straightaway, otherwise you could lose out. For example, if you've claimed DLA and think you might also become entitled to IS, put in your IS claim straightaway. Although your IS claim may be refused to begin with, once you get the DLA decision, ask for a review of the decision on the IS claim. Your IS can then be fully backdated to the date of the original IS claim or to the date from which the DLA is awarded.

Who should make the claim?

You can make the claim yourself, or if necessary, someone can make the claim on your behalf. If you are unable to act for yourself, the Secretary of State can appoint someone else (a parent or carer) to take over management of your claim.

Couples

Only married couples, or a man and woman living together as husband and wife can count as a couple for IS.

If one is eligible for IS – If you are eligible for IS but your partner would be required to sign on for benefit, you can choose which of you should make a claim for your family – either you claim IS or your partner claims jobseeker's allowance (JSA). You can't get both at the same time unless your partner is only claiming contribution-based JSA. In this case you can claim IS to top up the JSA.

Whether you claim IS or JSA, the amount of benefit is usually the same but:

- IS is tax free whereas JSA is taxable;
- JSA is not payable for the first 3 'waiting days' at the start of the claim;
- you avoid the risk of JSA 'sanctions' if you claim IS instead.

If you claim IS, your partner can sign on voluntarily at the Jobcentre to secure National Insurance credits. If you find you've made the wrong choice, simply put in a claim for IS. The AO will stop the JSA award if your IS claim is successful.

If both are eligible for IS – You can choose which of you should make the claim for your family. There are some points to consider in deciding which of you should be the IS claimant.

- If the only way you can qualify for a disability premium is because you are incapable of work (but not receiving a qualifying benefit), you have to be the claimant – see 12.
- If you are appealing against an 'all work' test incapacity decision and are subject to a reduction in IS, your partner should be the claimant so that full-rate IS can be paid – see Box B.1.
- To qualify for a Christmas bonus, the claimant must be over pension age.
- If the current IS claimant is getting a transitional addition, this ends if you switch roles.

You can switch roles at any time. Your partner just has to put in a claim for IS with your agreement that s/he should make the claim. If your IS has been, or now will be, paid in advance, write *'please treat this claim as though it were made on the appropriate pay day so that IS for our family can continue without any break in payment'*.

33. How is your IS paid?

Payment is usually by means of an order book which can be cashed at the post office of your choice. You can also opt to have your IS paid directly into a bank or building society. If you are also entitled to incapacity benefit, SDA, or attendance allowance, or DLA, the payments will normally be made together. Over the next 3 years order books are to be replaced gradually by benefit payment cards which you take to the post office to get your benefit.

If you need money urgently at the start of your claim, the DSS should make the first payment by giro.

Payment is usually made in arrears, but if you're getting certain other benefits, it may be paid in advance – see Box B.3.

Small payments – If you are entitled to less than £1 a week in IS, it will be paid to you weekly only if it can be paid along with another benefit. Otherwise, it will usually be paid in one sum every 13 weeks (but never more slowly).

The minimum payment of IS is 10p per week. If you are entitled to IS of 9p or less a week, that can only be paid to you if it can be paid along with another benefit. If you cannot be paid IS because of this minimum payment rule, you don't count as being 'on IS' for housing or council tax benefit purposes – you have to go through the separate benefit assessments – see Chapter 4.

Direct payments from benefit – Income support for mortgage

B.4 Supplementary benefit

Income support replaced supplementary benefit in April 1988. Since 16.11.92, it is no longer possible to make a wholly new claim to supplementary benefit (SB). Reg 49, Claims and Payments Regulations, was abolished from 16.11.92. Reg 49 had 'saved' the Supplementary Benefits Act 1976 and regulations made under it. It allowed new claims to be made in respect of entitlement up to April 1988. The end of reg 49 means that the AO has no jurisdiction to deal with SB claims which are made on or after 16.11.92.

However, if you had claimed SB at the time, or made a backdated SB claim before 16.11.92, including where you were wrongly refused benefit, you can still get an AO decision on that claim, or make an appeal, or late appeal, or pursue a review under reg 57, SS (Adjudication) Regs 1995 of the past decision on your entitlement to SB. This is because reg 13, SS (Adjudication) Amendment (No 2) Regulations 1987, is still in force. Reg 13 saves the original 1986 Adjudication Regulations so that they *'shall continue to apply to the adjudication of claims and questions relating to any benefit payable under the SBA 76'*.

B.5 For more information

All the abbreviations, and what they mean, are listed at the back of the Handbook.

Box O.4 in Chapter 52 and the list of Useful Publications at the back of the Handbook list a number of other guides which might help you. You can see copies of the law relating to social security, reported decisions of the Social Security Commissioners, and the official guidance manuals at your local DSS office. See also DSS leaflet, IS 20 – *A Guide to Income Support*.

The law on income support

The Acts
The Social Security Contributions and Benefits Act 1992 (SSCBA)
The Social Security Administration Act 1992 (SSAA)

The Regulations
Income Support (General) Regulations 1987, as amended
Social Security (Claims and Payments) Regulations 1987 as amended
IS (Transitional) Regulations 1987 as amended
IS (Transitional) Regulations 1988
Social Security (Adjudication) Regulations 1995 as amended

Case law
There may be reported or unreported Commissioners' decisions that would help if you are appealing, or you may find that one is used against you in an appeal. *CPAG's Income Related Benefits: The Legislation* (Sweet & Maxwell) contains detailed footnotes to the law and references to relevant decisions. If this is not enough detail, you can buy reported decisions from The Stationery Office (you should also be able to see copies at your local DSS office) and unreported decisions directly from the Office of the Social Security Commissioners.

interest is paid direct when a lender is a member of the Mortgage Interest Direct Scheme. For other costs part of your benefit (up to a ceiling) may be deducted and paid direct to a third party if you have enough benefit, and usually where you have built up a debt. The order of priority for direct payment deductions is: housing costs, fuel costs, water charges, community charge and council tax, court fines and compensation orders, and maintenance payments.

The rules on direct payments are in Sch 9 and 9A, SS (Claims and Payments) Regs 1987. The Fines (Deductions from IS) Regs 1992 also enable fines or compensation orders to be deducted from your benefit. Deductions for community charge and council tax are covered under the Community Charge (Deductions from IS) Regs 1990, and the Council Tax (Deductions from IS) Regs 1993.

34. Reviews and appeals

When you first claim, or when there is a major change in your applicable amount or resources, and thus a change in the amount of benefit you get, you will be sent a short notice of assessment (form A14N). You can ask for a more detailed notice of assessment (on form A124) at any time.

If your IS claim is turned down, or you don't think you've been awarded the right amount, ask for an A124 to show you how the AO worked things out. You can also ask for a written statement of reasons for any decision within 3 months of the date that decision was sent to you.

The time limit for appealing to a Social Security Appeal Tribunal is also 3 months. If you want to appeal, it is important to keep to that time limit even if you are still waiting for a written statement of reasons. If you delay, you can ask for a review of the past decision. If the AO refuses to review, or refuses to revise the decision on review, you will be able to appeal against that new decision. You can only get up to one month's arrears unless:
- the review is because of a delay in a decision on another benefit – see 32; or
- reg 57 of the Adjudication Regs 1995 applies (full backdating on review) – see Chapter 52(10)(e); or
- your request for the review was made before 7.4.97 – in this case you can get up to 52 weeks arrears.

See Chapter 52 for more about reviews and appeals.

Housing and council tax benefits

This section of the Handbook looks at the following:

Housing benefit and council tax benefit	Chapter **4**
Council tax	Chapter **5**

4 Housing benefit and council tax benefit

In this chapter we look at:

What is housing benefit?	see 1
Who can get HB?	see 2
What is rent?	see 3
Why housing benefit may not cover all your rent	see Box C.1
Housing costs HB cannot meet	see 4
Liability for rent on your normal home	see 5
Temporary absence	see 6
Moving home and getting HB on two homes	see 7
How much of your rent is taken into account?	see 8
Rent restrictions	see 9
What is council tax benefit?	see 10
Who can get CTB?	see 11
Liability for council tax on your normal home	see 12
Why CTB may not cover all your council tax	see Box C.2
How much of your council tax is taken into account?	see 13
For more information	see Box C.3
How to claim HB and CTB	see 14
When your HB/CTB starts, changes and ends	see 15
How your HB/CTB is paid	see 16
Getting more benefit	see 17
Underpayments	see 18
Overpayments	see 19
Decisions and appeals	see 20
How much benefit?	see 21
Non-dependants	see 22
Capital	see 23
Income	see 24
Applicable amounts	see 25
Second adult rebate	see 26
HB for rates in Northern Ireland	see 27

1. What is housing benefit?

Housing benefit (HB) helps people pay their rent. It is also known as a rent rebate or rent allowance. (In Northern Ireland it also helps people pay their rates – see 27.)

In nearly all cases, local authorities run the HB scheme. But in a few cases, other organisations run the scheme for their tenants, and in some areas local authorities have contracted out part of the administration to private firms. Local authorities are paid central government subsidy for much of the HB they award and for some of their administration costs.

Rules and regulations – In England, Wales and Scotland, the framework for the scheme is in the Social Security Contributions and Benefits Act 1992 and the Social Security Administration Act 1992. The details are in the Housing Benefit (General) Regulations 1987, as amended. Local authorities have a duty to allow members of the public to inspect the Acts and regulations.

2. Who can get housing benefit?

You can get HB if you satisfy all the following conditions:
- you are not excluded from getting HB – see below;
- you are liable to pay rent on your normal home – see 5;
- your capital is no more than £16,000 – see 23;
- you are on income support (IS) or income-based job-seeker's allowance (JSA) or have fairly low income – see 21;
- you claim and provide the information requested – see 14.

People who cannot get housing benefit
If you are in any of the following groups, you are excluded altogether from getting HB.

People in residential care or nursing homes – There are some exceptions – see Chapter 36.

'Persons from abroad' – This does not cover every non-UK national, but it does cover some UK nationals who do not habitually reside in the UK. The details are in Chapter 3(7). If you are in a couple, and only one of you is a 'person from abroad', the other one can get HB for you both.

Many full-time students – Full-time students cannot get HB unless they fall within certain groups. Many students with disabilities do, however, fall within one of those groups. The details are in Chapter 31(5). If you are in a couple and only one of you is a full-time student, the other one can get HB for you both.

Members of religious orders – If you are maintained by the order.

People who live with a landlord who is a close relative – If you live with your landlord and your landlord is a close relative, you cannot get HB. Sharing just a bathroom, toilet, hallway, stairs or passageways does not count as living with your landlord. A 'close relative' means only a parent, parent-in-law, step-parent, son, daughter, son/daughter-in-law, step-son/daughter, sister, brother or the (married or unmarried) partner of any of those.

People who live with a landlord on a non-commercial basis – If you live with your landlord on a non-commercial basis, you cannot get HB. Sharing just a bathroom, toilet, hallway, stairs or passageways does not count as living with your landlord. An example would be someone who just pays something towards their food, but does not pay a commercial rent.

People with contrived lettings – If your or your landlord's primary or dominant purpose in creating your letting agreement was to take advantage of the HB scheme, you cannot get HB unless you were liable for rent there on some other basis during the 8 weeks before the letting agreement was created.

People with contrived joint lettings – If you jointly rent your home, but during the 8 weeks before your joint letting agreement was created you were a non-dependant of the other joint occupier(s), you cannot get HB. The other joint occupier(s) can get HB as though you were still a non-dependant rather than a joint occupier. But this rule does not apply if the joint letting agreement was created for a genuine reason (rather than to take advantage of the HB scheme).

3. What is rent?

You can get HB towards almost any kind of rent, whether you pay it to a local authority (including a health authority), a New Town, the Development Board for Rural Wales, Scottish Homes, a housing association, a co-op, a hostel, a bed and breakfast hotel, a private company, or a private individual (including a resident landlord – but see 2). This is true whether your letting is a 'tenancy' or 'licence'; whether your payments are for 'rent' or for 'use and occupation' or for 'mesne profits' or 'violent profits'; and whether you have a written letting agreement or an agreement entered into by word of mouth. If you are buying a share of your council or housing association home, but still pay rent, you can get HB towards the rent (and you may be able to get IS or income-based JSA towards your mortgage interest). You can also get HB towards the following, which all count as 'rent' for HB purposes:
- mooring charges and/or berthing fees for a houseboat (as well as your rent, if you do not own it);
- site fees for a caravan or mobile home (as well as your rent, if you do not own it);
- payments to a charitable almshouse;
- payments under a 'rental purchase' agreement;
- payments (in Scotland) on a croft or croft land.

4. Housing costs that housing benefit cannot meet

You cannot get HB towards any of the following (though some of them may be met by IS or income-based JSA – see Chapter 3(20) and Chapter 14(20):
- payments on residential care or nursing homes (there are some exceptions – see Chapters 36 and 38);
- any payments you make on your home if you own it or have a long lease (over 21 years);
- any payments you make in a 'co-ownership scheme' where, if you left, you would be entitled to a sum based on the value of your home;
- rent if you are a Crown tenant (there is a separate scheme for Crown tenants). But tenants of the Crown Estate Commissioners and the Duchies of Cornwall and Lancaster can get HB;
- hire purchase or credit sale agreements;
- conditional sale agreements (unless for land);
- payments on a tent.

C.1 Why housing benefit may not cover all your rent

If you are eligible for HB, your HB may not cover all of your rent.
This could be because:
- your rent includes service charges or other things which have to be deducted in the calculation of HB – see 8;
- the rent officer fixes a 'maximum rent' on your home – see 9;
- you have one or more non-dependant(s) in your home and a deduction has to be made because of this – see 22;
- the level of your income means that you do not qualify for the whole of your rent to be met – see 21.

---

5. Liability for rent on your normal home

The general rule is that, to get HB, you must be personally liable to pay the rent on your home. And you can only get HB on one home at a time, which is the home *'normally occupied'* by yourself and any members of your family. However, there are exceptions to these points as described in the next few paragraphs.

Couples – If you are in a couple, either one of you can get HB towards the rent on your normal home, even if the letting agreement is in one name only.

Joint occupiers – We use 'joint occupiers' to mean two or more people (other than a couple) who are jointly liable to pay the rent on their home. If you are a joint occupier, you can get HB towards a share of the rent on your normal home. This 'share' is assessed by taking into account the number of joint occupiers and how much each of you pays.

Large families – If your family is so large that your local authority has allocated you two council homes, you can get HB on both.

Students – Some students who have to maintain two homes can get HB on both (if they are eligible for HB in the first place) – see Chapter 31(5).

Repairs to your home

If your landlord agrees not to collect rent while you do repairs to your home, you can carry on getting HB for the first 8 weeks. After that, you cannot get HB until you start paying rent again.

If you have to move into temporary accommodation while your normal home is being repaired, you can get HB on the temporary accommodation – but only if you are not liable for rent or mortgage interest on your normal home.

If you take over paying someone else's rent

If the person who is liable for the rent on your home stops paying it, and you take over the payments in order to continue living there, you can get HB towards the rent – even though you are not legally liable for it. This applies if your partner has left you, and in any other reasonable case.

6. Temporary absence

There are three different rules – described below – which relate to different circumstances.

The 13-week rule

You can get HB for up to 13 weeks during a temporary absence from your normal home if:
- you intend to return to occupy it as your home; and
- the part you normally occupy has not been let or sub-let; and
- your absence is unlikely to exceed 13 continuous weeks.

If your absence is *'likely'* to exceed 13 continuous weeks, you cannot get HB for any time you are away (unless you qualify under the 52-week rule below). If you cannot make an estimate of the length of your absence, you are unlikely to get HB during any of it. So if possible always give your local authority an estimate.

This rule applies to all absences (including absences outside the UK) apart from those mentioned below. In calculating the length of a prison sentence, the length of the sentence includes periods of temporary release, but should be reduced by any remission allowable for good behaviour.

The 52-week rule

You can get HB for up to 52 weeks during a temporary

absence from your normal home if:
- you intend to return to occupy it as your home; and
- the part you normally occupy has not been let or sub-let; and
- your absence is unlikely to exceed 52 weeks or, in exceptional circumstances, is unlikely to substantially exceed 52 weeks; and
- your absence is for any of the reasons listed below.

Who the rule applies to – You can get HB under this rule if you are:
- a patient in a hospital or similar institution in the UK or abroad;
- receiving medical treatment or medically approved care or convalescence (other than in a residential care or nursing home) in the UK or abroad;
- accompanying your child or partner who is receiving the above (but not convalescence);
- providing care to a child whose parent or guardian is receiving the above (but not convalescence);
- providing medically approved care to anyone in the UK or abroad;
- receiving care in a residential care or nursing home (but not for a trial period: see below);
- on an approved training course in the UK or abroad;
- on remand awaiting trial or awaiting sentencing;
- a vulnerable student (in certain circumstances);
- in fear of violence (the conditions are the same as in the rule about getting HB on two homes in such cases – see 7).

If you cannot make an estimate of the length of your absence, you are unlikely to get HB during any of it. So if possible always give your local authority an estimate.

Trial periods in residential care or nursing homes
You can get HB for up to 13 weeks during an absence from your normal home if:
- you are trying out a residential care or nursing home to see whether it suits your needs; and
- you intend to return to your normal home if it does not; and
- the part you normally occupy has not been let or sub-let.

7. Moving home and getting housing benefit on two homes

The general rule
When you move from one rented home to another, you can get HB on both homes for up to 4 weeks if you have actually moved into the new home but cannot avoid liability for rent on the old home (eg because you have had to move unexpectedly and have to give notice on your old home). This general rule applies only if you have actually moved into the new home. Exactly what it means to 'move in' can be interpreted in different ways, so it is often worth getting advice. However, different rules – some more generous – apply if you move for one of the following reasons.

Fear of violence – This rule applies if you move because of fear that violence may occur:
- in your old home – in this case the rule applies regardless of who might cause the violence; or
- in the locality – in this case only if the violence would be caused by a (former) partner or member of your family.

In either case, you can get HB on both homes for up to 52 weeks – so long as you intend to return to your old home at some point and your local authority agrees it is reasonable to pay HB on both. You do not have to say exactly when you intend to return: it should be sufficient if you intend to return when it becomes safe to do so. If you do not intend to return, you can only get HB for both for up to 4 weeks – under the general rule above.

Waiting for your new home to be adapted – If you do not move into a new rented home straight away because you have to wait for it to be adapted to meet your disablement needs or those of any member of your family, and your local authority agrees the delay is reasonable, you can get HB for up to 4 weeks before you actually move in. And if you are liable for rent on your old home, you can get HB on both during those 4 weeks.

Waiting for a social fund payment before moving home – If you do not move into a new rented home straight away because you have asked for a social fund payment to help with the move or with setting up home, and your local authority agrees the delay is reasonable, you can get HB for up to 4 weeks before you actually move in. But this rule only applies if there is a child under the age of 6 in your family, or you or your partner are aged 60 or more, or you qualify for one of the HB disability or pensioner premiums – see 25 (look at 'Your premiums'). And under this rule you cannot get HB on your old home at the same time.

When you leave hospital or a residential care or nursing home – If you do not move into a new rented home straight away because you are waiting to leave hospital or a residential care or nursing home, and your local authority agrees the delay is reasonable, you can get HB for up to 4 weeks before you actually move in.

Claiming on time – In the last three cases, you must make your claim straight away: it is not enough to wait until you have actually moved in (unless your local authority backdates your claim – see 17). If your local authority rejects that claim, but you reapply within 4 weeks of actually moving in, the rejected claim must be reconsidered.

8. How much of your rent is taken into account?

Your rent may include things like water charges, fuel, meals or other services; or you may rent a garage with your home. As detailed below, HB cannot be awarded towards all of these things. The HB calculation is based on your *'eligible rent'*. This means:
- the actual rent on your home,
- plus in some cases the rent on a garage,
- minus amounts for water, fuel, meals and certain other services.

Exceptions – In certain cases, the HB calculation is based instead on a 'maximum rent' fixed by the rent officer – see 9.

Converting rent to a weekly figure
HB is worked out on a weekly basis, so your rent has to be converted as follows.
- For rent due fortnightly, divide the amount by 2.
- For rent due four-weekly, divide the amount by 4.
- For rent due daily (eg in a hostel), multiply the amount by 7.
- For rent due calendar-monthly, the law allows two methods. The more common is to multiply the amount by 12 (giving an annual figure), then divide by 365 (giving a daily figure), then multiply by 7. The alternative is to divide a particular month's rent by the number of days in that month (28, 29, 30 or 31) and then multiply by 7. The two methods give different results.

Garages
If you rent a garage, this is included as part of the rent on your home only if you were obliged to rent the garage from the

beginning of your letting agreement, or you are making (or have made) all reasonable efforts to stop renting it.

Water charges and council tax included in your rent
If your rent includes water or sewerage charges, the actual amount of the charge for your home (or if your water is metered, an estimate) is deducted. If your rent includes a contribution towards the council tax because your landlord pays it, not you, this is included as part of your eligible rent.

Other charges: general conditions
The rules for several service charges are given below, saying whether they can be taken into account as part of your eligible rent. But even when they can, there are two further conditions.
- The amount of the charge must be reasonable for the service provided. If it is not reasonable, the unreasonable part is deducted.
- Payment of the charge must be a condition of occupying your home – whether from the beginning of your letting agreement or from later on. If it is not a condition of occupying the home, the whole charge is deducted.

Exceptions – If the rent officer has fixed a 'maximum rent' for your home, s/he also fixes a value for some of the services – see 9.

Fuel and related charges
If your rent includes fuel of any kind, the actual amount of the fuel charge is deducted if there is evidence of how much it is (eg in your rent book or letting agreement). If there is no evidence of the amount, a flat-rate amount is deducted for the various things the fuel is for: the amounts are given below. Whenever your local authority makes flat-rate deductions, it must write inviting you to provide evidence of the actual amount. If you can provide reasonable evidence (which need not be from your landlord), your authority must estimate the actual amount and deduct that instead of the flat-rate.

Warning! It is not a good idea to seek out evidence that your fuel costs more than the flat-rate. You'll be worse off if you do!

Exceptions – A fuel charge for a communal area (including communal rooms in sheltered accommodation) is included as part of your eligible rent so long as it is separately specified in your rent book or letting agreement. The same is true for a separately specified charge for providing a heating system.

The flat-rate deductions – If you rent more than one room (not counting any shared accommodation), the flat-rate deductions per week are:
- £9.25 for heating
- £1.15 for hot water
- £0.80 for lighting
- £1.15 for cooking.

If you rent only one room (not counting any shared accommodation), the flat-rate deduction for heating is lower: it is £5.60. And if you get a flat-rate deduction for heating, there is no further deduction for hot water or lighting. But the figure for cooking is as above.

Meal charges
If your rent includes meals (including the preparation of food, or the provision of food even if it is not prepared for you), a flat-rate amount is deducted for these. The flat-rate is always used, regardless of how much you are actually charged for meals. One flat-rate deduction is made for each person (even if not a member of your family) whose meals are included in your rent. The amount for each person depends on his or her age and on what meals he or she gets.

The weekly deductions	For each person: aged 16+	under 16
For at least three meals every day	£17.55	£8.85
For breakfast only	£2.10	£2.10
For any other arrangement	£11.65	£5.85

Note that for these purposes, a person does not count as 'aged 16 +' until the first Monday in the September following his or her 16th birthday.

Other services
Cleaning (including window cleaning) – A charge for cleaning is included in your eligible rent if it is for communal areas (including common rooms in sheltered accommodation). A charge for cleaning your own room(s) is included only if neither you nor anyone in your household is able to do it. In all other cases, the amount of the charge (estimated if necessary) is deducted.
Furniture and household equipment – A charge for these is included in your eligible rent so long as your landlord has not agreed that they will become part of your personal property.
Counselling and support – A charge for these is included in your eligible rent if they *relate to the provision of adequate accommodation* (what this means has been debated a great deal: it may well be worth seeking advice about the current interpretation): or if they are provided personally by your landlord (so long as he or she spends more time providing other eligible services); or if they are provided by someone employed by your landlord (so long as they spend more time providing other eligible services). In any other case, the amount of the charge (estimated if necessary) is deducted.
Medical, nursing and personal care – A charge for any of these (estimated if necessary) is deducted.
Wardens and caretakers – A charge for services provided by a warden or caretaker is included in your eligible rent so long as those services are eligible (eg under the next heading).
Communal or accommodation-related services – Most charges for these are included in your eligible rent. Examples are TV/radio aerial and relay (with exceptions for satellite or cable), refuse removal, portering, lifts, communal telephones, entry phones, children's play areas, garden maintenance necessary for the provision of adequate accommodation, communal laundry facilities, and emergency alarm systems in accommodation specifically designed or adapted or particularly suitable for elderly, sick or disabled people.
Day-to-day living expenses, etc – Charges for day-to-day living expenses (estimated if necessary) are deducted. Examples are TV/radio rental and licence, laundering (ie if washing is done for you), transport, sports facilities, leisure items, and any other service which is not related to the provision of adequate accommodation.

9. Rent restrictions
There are two sets of rules about how your local authority can reduce your 'eligible rent'. We have called these the 'old rules' and the 'new rules'. The new rules were introduced on 2.1.96 but do not apply to everyone from then.

Several changes to the rules may apply from October 1997 – see our *Disability Rights Bulletin*.

The old rules; and do they apply to you?
The old rules (which are often more generous than the new ones) are described in the 20th edition of the *Disability Rights Handbook*. All the circumstances in which the old rules apply to you are listed below.

The old rules apply to you if you meet all the following four conditions:
- you were entitled to HB on 1.1.96; and
- you have been receiving (and entitled to) HB continuously since then; however gaps of no longer than 4 weeks are ignored; and
- you have not moved since then, unless the move was because your former home was uninhabitable due to a fire, flood, explosion or natural catastrophe; and
- if you are in a couple, the same one of you has been the claimant since then.

The old rules also apply to you if, after 1.1.96, you took over claiming HB on your home from someone who fell within the old rules and who was:
- your partner if s/he left you – and either you are no longer a couple, or s/he has gone long-term into a hospital or a residential care or nursing home;
- your partner if s/he was convicted and detained in prison or similar;
- someone whose household you were in if s/he has died.

But in each of these cases, the old rules apply to you only if you make your claim for HB within 4 weeks of the event described above, and only for as long as you continue to receive (and be entitled to) HB continuously; however gaps of no longer than 4 weeks are ignored.

The old rules also apply to you if your home is:
- a resettlement hostel; or
- any accommodation provided by a non-metropolitan county council, housing association, charitable body or non-profit-making voluntary organisation who provide you with *'care, support or supervision'* or have arranged for you to be provided with this.

The new rules; and do they apply to you?
If the old rules do not apply to you (see above) the new rules do!

If the new rules apply to you and you rent from a private landlord
In this case, your local authority must pass details of your rent and other circumstances to the rent officer before determining your claim for HB. (There is an exception: see 'Lettings begun before January 1989' below.) Whether your 'eligible rent' must be restricted depends on the following figures. You will see that there are several different names for the figures. The examples towards the end may help.

The 'reckonable rent' for your home – To calculate this, start with the weekly amount of the rent you actually pay your landlord. Then subtract any charges included in your rent for ineligible counselling and support, and medical, nursing and personal care (see 8). Then subtract the rent officer's valuation of charges for any other service included within your rent except for fuel, meals and water charges.

The 'appropriate rent' for your home – This is the figure given to your local authority by the rent officer. It is his or her valuation of a reasonable market rent for your home. The rent officer makes a lower valuation if your home is larger than you need or is exceptionally expensive. If the rent officer accepts your 'reckonable rent' as reasonable, this is the 'appropriate rent' for your home.

The 'local reference rent' – This is a figure given to your local authority by the rent officer. It is the midpoint for all rents in your 'locality' (ignoring extreme cases) for homes in a category appropriate to your needs and which are in a reasonable state of repair. The categories depend on the total number of living-rooms and bedrooms you need, except that for one-room accommodation there are further sub-categories. However if the 'local reference rent' is higher than (or equals) the 'appropriate rent' for your home, the rent officer does not inform your local authority of it and it is not used in calculating your HB.

The 'single room rent' for 'young individuals' – This is a figure given to your local authority by the rent officer, but only if your local authority tells the rent officer that you count as a 'young individual'. The 'single room rent' is the midpoint for all rents in your 'locality' (ignoring extreme cases) for accommodation in a reasonable state of repair which is just one room (eg a bedsit) with the shared use of a toilet and either shared use of a kitchen or no kitchen. This is the case even if you live in larger accommodation than what has just been described.

You count as a 'young individual' if you are single (not a lone parent or in a couple) and are under the age of 25. However, there are three exceptions.
- You do not count as a 'young individual' if you are under the age of 22 and were previously in local authority care under a court order (so long as the court order applied, or continued to apply, to you after your 16th birthday).
- You do not count as a 'young individual' if you are under the age of 22 and used to be accommodated by your Social Services Department at any time before your 18th birthday.
- If you were entitled to HB on 6.10.96, and have not moved home since then, you do not count as a 'young individual' until the first time after that date when you make a renewal claim for HB – see 15 (look at 'Your benefit period').

Note that you do not count as a 'young individual' if you rent from a registered housing association.

Your 'maximum rent' if you are not a 'young individual' – Your 'maximum rent' is the crucial thing. There are two possibilities if you are not a 'young individual'.
- If the rent officer *did not* give your local authority a 'local reference rent': the 'appropriate rent' for your home is your 'maximum rent' – but it is reduced by amounts for any fuel, meals or water charges in your rent (see 8).
- If the rent officer *did* give your local authority a 'local reference rent': it will be lower than the 'appropriate rent' for your home. To find your 'maximum rent': add together the 'local reference rent' and the 'appropriate rent' then divide the result by two. This is your 'maximum rent' (unless it is more than twice the 'local reference rent', in which case twice the 'local reference rent' is your 'maximum rent') – but it is reduced by amounts for any fuel, meals or water charges included in your rent (see 8).

Your 'maximum rent' if you are a 'young individual' – Your 'maximum rent' is the crucial thing. If you are a 'young individual', it is whichever is the lower of:
- the 'single room rent'; and
- the 'maximum rent' which would apply to you if you were not a 'young individual' (see above).

More information – You can get full information about all the above figures, categories, etc (but only those which have been used in calculating your HB entitlement) from your local authority by asking for a written statement (see 20 'Getting more information'). If you appeal at the internal review stage (see 20) about any of the figures supplied by the rent officer used in the calculation of your claim, the appeal will be referred to the rent officer to deal with. If you ask for reasons (and this is recommended), the rent officer's reply should be included when your local authority responds to your appeal.

Example 1 – A claimant and her family rent a flat for £70 a week. This does not include any service charges, so her 'reckonable rent' is £70. The rent officer gives a valuation of £60 for the flat, so the 'appropriate rent' is £60. The rent officer also gives a 'local reference rent' of £50.

Calculation: Adding the 'local reference rent' and the 'appropriate rent' and dividing by two gives £55. Because there are no fuel, meals or water charges, the 'maximum rent' is £55 a week.

Example 2 – A claimant and his family rent a flat for £80 a week. This includes only a charge of £10 for fuel and £2 for water charges, so his 'reckonable rent' is £80. The rent officer gives a valuation of £75 for the flat, so the 'appropriate rent' is £75. The rent officer does not give a 'local reference rent'.

Calculation: Since there is no 'local reference rent', the 'appropriate rent' (£75) is used. After deducting the £10 for fuel and the £2 for water charges, the 'maximum rent' is £63 a week.

Example 3 – A 'young individual' rents a flat for £80 a week. This does not include any charges for services, so her 'reckonable rent' is £80. The rent officer does not give a valuation for the flat itself, so the 'appropriate rent' is also £80. The rent officer does not give a 'local reference rent', so the 'maximum rent' would be £80 if she was not a 'young individual'. But the rent officer does give a 'single room rent' of £75.

Calculation: If she was not a 'young individual' the 'maximum rent' would be £80. The 'single room rent' is £75. Of these two figures, the 'single room rent' is the lower. So her 'maximum rent' is £75 a week. (But once she reaches 25, she will stop counting as a 'young individual', so – if there are no other changes – her 'maximum rent' will go up to £80 a week.)

Will your rent be restricted? – Your local authority must restrict your eligible rent to the 'maximum rent' as calculated above (though see 'Protections for certain people' and 'Increases for exceptional hardship' below). It can restrict it further if it considers the 'maximum rent' is unreasonable in all the circumstances of your case. If this happens, seek advice.

Protections for certain people – Your local authority must not use the 'maximum rent' figure described above in the following two cases.
- If you and/or any member of your household could afford the financial commitments of your home when you first entered into them, and you have not received HB during the 52 weeks before your current claim, your authority must not use the 'maximum rent' figure for the first 13 weeks of your claim.
- If any member of your household has died, and you have not moved since then, your authority must not use the 'maximum rent' figure until a year after the date of that death (unless there was already a 'maximum rent' figure which applied before that death, in which case that continues).

Although your local authority cannot use the 'maximum rent' figure in the above circumstances, it can restrict your eligible rent if it considers it is unreasonable in all the circumstances of your case. If this happens, seek advice.

For the purposes of the above protections, all the following count as a member of your household:
- each member of your family: yourself, your partner if you are in a couple, children under 16, and children aged 16, 17 or 18 for whom child benefit is payable – see 25 (look at 'Your family');
- any other relative of yourself (or your partner) who lives with you but does not have an independent right to do so. A 'relative' means only a parent, parent-in-law, step-parent, son, daughter, son/daughter-in-law, step-son/daughter, sister, brother or the (married or unmarried) partner of any of those; or a grandparent, grandchild, uncle, aunt, niece or nephew.

Increases for exceptional hardship – If the effect of restricting your eligible rent to the 'maximum rent' is that you or a member of your family (as defined above) will suffer 'exceptional hardship', your local authority can agree to remove the restriction wholly or partly. It can do this only until it has reached its annual budget limit, known as a 'permitted total'. This is fixed each year by law. In considering whether to remove the restriction, your local authority may ask for detailed information about your circumstances and those of your household. You should explain these fully. For example, it could take into account disability needs; but it could also take into account the fact that you receive state benefits such as disability living allowance for these (even if the HB rules would normally ignore these). The availability of these increases (and how they are administered) varies widely from authority to authority. It is often worth getting advice about this.

Lettings begun before January 1989 – If your letting began before 15.1.89 in England and Wales or 2.1.89 in Scotland, your details are not referred to the rent officer and there is no 'maximum rent' in your case. However your local authority can restrict your eligible rent if it considers it is unreasonable in all the circumstances of your case. This is unlikely to happen if you have a rent registered by the rent officer as binding on your landlord. If it does happen, seek advice.

If the new rules apply to you and you rent from a housing association

If you rent from an unregistered housing association, all the rules for people who rent from a private landlord also apply to you.

If you rent from a registered housing association, the situation is different. If your local authority considers that your rent is unreasonably expensive or your accommodation is unreasonably large, they may decide to refer your details to the rent officer, in which case all the rules for people who rent from a private landlord also apply to you (except for the rules about 'single room rents' for 'young individuals'). If they do not do this, your local authority should not restrict your 'eligible rent' at all.

If the new rules apply to you and you rent from your local authority

In this case, it is very unlikely indeed that your rent will be restricted.

Getting information before you sign up for a letting

Are you thinking of taking up a letting at a new address? Or are you considering whether to sign a new letting agreement with your landlord (and at least 11 months have passed since you last signed an agreement with him or her)? And would you like to know whether your 'eligible rent' is likely to be restricted if you claim HB? If 'yes', you have the right to a 'Pre-tenancy determination'. Get a form from your local authority (in some areas the forms may be available from your landlord or a local advice agency, too). Fill it in, sign it, get the landlord of the accommodation to sign it, and give it or send it to your local authority.

Either the rent officer or your local authority will then write to you (and the landlord of the accommodation) to say whether there will be a 'maximum rent' in your case. You should hear within nine days in most cases (quicker in some areas).

The 'maximum rent' will apply for a year (as long as your circumstances, such as family size, do not change). Though this is not a guarantee of the amount of your HB, it can be a good guide. Your local authority will usually be able to give you further advice about this.

Note – The form you fill in asking for a 'Pre-tenancy determination' is *not* a claim for HB. You must make a claim for HB separately. As always: do not delay; make an HB claim as soon as you can to avoid losing any HB.

You cannot get a 'Pre-tenancy determination' for a council letting. In practice, it is unlikely that the landlord will agree to you getting one if the landlord is a registered housing association.

10. What is council tax benefit?

Council tax benefit (CTB) helps people pay their council tax. There are two types of council tax benefit, but you can only get one type at a time: see 26 (look at 'The better buy'). 'Main council tax benefit' (Main CTB) is the more common type: it is described below. 'Second adult rebate' is much less common – see 26.

In all cases, local authorities run the CTB scheme, though in some areas local authorities have contracted out part of the administration to private firms. Local authorities are paid central government subsidy for much of the CTB they award and for some of their administration costs. (There is no council tax, and so no CTB, in Northern Ireland.)

Rules and regulations – The framework for the scheme is in the Social Security Contributions and Benefits Act 1992 and the Social Security Administration Act 1992. The details are in the Council Tax Benefit (General) Regulations 1992 as amended. Local authorities have a duty to allow members of the public to inspect the Acts and regulations.

11. Who can get Main council tax benefit?

You can get Main CTB if you satisfy all the following conditions:
- you are not excluded from getting Main CTB – see below;
- you are liable to pay council tax on your normal home – see 12;
- your capital is no more than £16,000 – see 23;
- you are on IS or income-based JSA or have fairly low income – see 21;
- you claim and provide the information requested – see 14.

People who cannot get Main council tax benefit
If you are in either of the following groups, you are excluded altogether from getting Main CTB.

'Persons from abroad' – This does not include every non-UK national, but it does cover some UK nationals who do not habitually reside in the UK. The details are in Chapter 3(7). If you are in a couple, and only one of you is a 'person from abroad', the other one can get Main CTB (or second adult rebate) for you both.

Many full-time students – Full-time students cannot get Main CTB unless they fall within certain groups (though they can get second adult rebate). Many students with disabilities do, however, fall within one of those groups. The details are in Chapter 31(5). If you are in a couple and only one of you is a full-time student, the other can get Main CTB for you both.

12. Liability for council tax on your normal home

To get CTB, you must be personally liable to pay the council tax on your normal home. For most purposes, your 'normal home' means wherever you are treated as being *'resident'* under council tax rules – see Chapter 5(6). Most home owners and rent-payers are liable for council tax and so can get CTB. But there are some further points.

Exempt dwellings – If your dwelling is exempt from council tax (see Chapter 5(4)), you cannot get CTB on it.

If you rent non-self-contained accommodation – You are not liable for council tax (your landlord is). So you are not eligible for CTB.

Water charges – You cannot get CTB towards water charges or (in Scotland) towards the council water charge.

Couples – If you are in a couple, and you are jointly liable for council tax on your home, either one of you can get CTB towards this. If only one of you is liable, that one can get CTB on behalf of you both – see Chapter 5(5).

Joint occupiers – We use 'joint occupiers' to mean two or more people (other than a couple) who are jointly liable to pay the council tax on their home (see Chapter 5(5)). If you are a joint occupier, you can get Main CTB towards a share of the council tax on your home. This 'share' is always found by dividing the total council tax bill by the number of people who are liable (ignoring any who are students, in most cases).

Absences from home – The rules for whether you can get CTB during a temporary absence from home, or during a trial period in a residential care or nursing home, are the same as in HB – see 6.

Moving home and occupying two homes – You can only ever get CTB on one home at a time. This is wherever you are treated as being 'resident' under the council tax rules – see Chapter 5(6).

13. How much of your council tax is taken into account?

The whole of your liability for council tax is taken into account in calculating your entitlement to Main CTB. This means whatever you are liable to pay after you have been awarded any reduction for disabilities or discount – see Chapter 5.

Converting council tax to a weekly figure.
CTB is worked out on a weekly basis, so your council tax liability has to be converted. Divide the annual figure by 365 (giving a daily figure), then multiply by 7. If your bill is not for a full year, divide it by the number of days it covers, then multiply by 7.

14. How to claim HB and CTB

The following applies to HB for rent and CTB (both Main CTB and second adult rebate). For HB for rates in Northern Ireland, see 27.

Whether you get IS or not, you must make a written claim for HB and/or CTB. Even though you can phone your local authority to ask for a claim form, your benefit starts later – see below.

Getting someone to claim for you – If you are incapable of managing your own affairs, an 'appointee' can take over all the responsibilities of claiming for you and dealing with any further matters relating to your claim. That person (who must be aged 18 or more) should write to your local authority to request approval to act as your appointee. Permission should not be unreasonably withheld.

C.2 Why council tax benefit may not cover all your council tax

If you are eligible for CTB, your CTB may not cover all of your council tax. This could be because:
- you have one or more non-dependant(s) in your home and a deduction has to be made because of this – see 22;
- the level of your income means that you do not qualify for the whole of your council tax to be met – see 21;
- you have been awarded second adult rebate – see 26.

Keeping a record – If possible keep a copy, or at least a record including the date, when you send in any of the claim forms described below or any information you have been asked for. If you take forms in instead of posting them, get a receipt or an acknowledgement from whoever you give them to. Forms do sometimes go astray, and without a record it can be hard to convince your local authority that you submitted a form that has been lost. A form which your local authority accepts it has lost is treated as though it was received (though you may have to fill in a replacement for their records).

If you are claiming income support or income-based JSA
When you claim IS or income-based JSA, you should be given claim forms for HB and CTB, called 'NHB1 forms' (as well as your IS or JSA claim form). If possible, send the NHB1 forms with your IS or JSA claim form to your DSS office or Jobcentre. At the latest, make sure the NHB1 forms reach your DSS office or Jobcentre within 4 weeks of your 'date of claim' for IS or income-based JSA (this date is explained in Chapter 3(32)). You have to complete and send in both of the NHB1 forms if you want both HB and CTB. Your DSS office will send the NHB1 forms to your local authority once they have decided whether you qualify for IS or income-based JSA.

The NHB1 forms only ask for basic details about you and the people who live with you. Usually your local authority will send you another form to provide further details. Complete this and send it to the address shown on it. The form may ask you to provide various documents – such as your rent book in the case of a claim for HB. You should send the form back so that it reaches your local authority within 4 weeks of when it was sent to you. If you do not have all the information or documents requested, send the form in within this time limit, and write on it that you will send the further information or documents as soon as you can: it is a good idea to explain any reasons for the delay, too. Sometimes, your local authority may write with yet further questions. Always ensure your reply reaches them within 4 weeks of when they sent the letter out.

Your 'date of claim for HB/CTB', if you keep to the time limits – If you keep within the various time limits explained above, your 'date of claim for HB/CTB' will be the first day of your entitlement to IS or income-based JSA. Or, if you turn out not to be entitled to IS or income-based JSA, your 'date of claim for HB/CTB' will be the day the NHB1 form(s) reached your DSS office or Jobcentre (or your local authority if for any reason it got to them first).

Your 'date of claim for HB/CTB', if you don't keep to the time limits – The 4 weeks time limit for sending in the NHB1 form(s) is strict. If you do not keep within it, your 'date of claim' will be the day the NHB1 form(s) actually reach your DSS office or Jobcentre (or your local authority if for any reason it got to them first). If you do not keep within the 4 weeks time limit for sending the other forms and information back to your local authority, they can agree a delay of whatever period is *'reasonable'*. This will mean that you are treated as having claimed within the time limits (as above). However, in all cases, you may qualify for your claim for HB/CTB to be backdated under the 'good cause' rule – see 17.

Points to note
Sending in a claim form for IS or JSA does not entitle you to HB or CTB. To get these, you must fill in the NHB1 form(s) too.

Alternatively, to speed things, you can ask your authority for one of its own claim forms and use the method of claiming described below. Write on it that you are also claiming IS or income-based JSA. Your 'date of claim for HB/CTB' will still be worked out as above.

Your HB/CTB claim lasts for a fixed period only – see 15. If you do not then send in a further HB/CTB claim form to your local authority, you will no longer be entitled to HB/CTB.

If your circumstances change – especially if you come off IS or income-based JSA – you have a duty to notify your local authority. If you do not, you will probably have to repay any resulting overpayment – see 19. It is not enough just to notify your DSS office or Jobcentre.

If you are not claiming income support or income-based JSA
If you are not claiming IS or income-based JSA, you should ask your local authority for one of its own claim forms, complete it and send it to them as soon as possible. Your local authority may have one form for claiming both HB and CTB. Or it may have separate claim forms for the two benefits, which means if you want both you must complete both. You can phone and ask for the form(s), but this will not count as a claim. Your 'date of claim for HB/CTB' (see below) depends on your local authority receiving something in writing.

So if you cannot easily get the claim form(s), write a letter to your local authority: give your name and address, say you wish to claim HB and/or CTB, and date it. Your local authority should then send you the claim form(s): make sure you get them back to your local authority within 4 weeks of when they were sent out.

The claim form(s) may ask you to provide various documents – such as your rent book in the case of a claim for HB. If you do not have all the information or documents requested, send the form(s) in as soon as possible, and write on them that you will send the further information or documents as soon as you can: it is a good idea to explain any reasons for the delay, too. Sometimes, your local authority may write with further questions. Always ensure your reply reaches them within 4 weeks of when they sent the letter out.

Your 'date of claim for HB/CTB', if you keep to the time limits – If you keep within the various time limits explained above, your 'date of claim for HB/CTB' will be the day your form(s) (or your letter if you wrote as described above) reach your local authority.

Your 'date of claim for HB/CTB', if you don't keep to the time limits – If you do not keep within the 4 weeks time limit for sending information back to your local authority (or for sending in the form(s) if you originally sent a letter), they can agree a delay of whatever period is *'reasonable'*. This will mean that you are treated as having claimed within the time limits (as

---

C.3 For more information

Your local Citizens Advice Bureau has detailed information in their files on housing benefit, council tax benefit and the council tax rules. They should be able to advise you. If you want to look at the law, see CPAG's *Housing Benefit and Council Tax Benefit Legislation*, 9th edition. For further information see the *Guide to Housing Benefit and Council Tax Benefit 1997-98* and the other publications in our list of Useful Publications at the back of the Handbook.
See Section K if you enter a residential care or nursing home.
See Section L if you go into hospital.
See Chapter 54 if there are delays in dealing with your claim.

above). However, in all cases, you may qualify for your claim for HB/CTB to be backdated under the 'good cause' rule – see 17.

Points to note
Your HB/CTB claim lasts for a fixed period only – see 15. If you do not then send in a further HB/CTB claim form to your local authority, you will no longer be entitled to HB/CTB.

If your circumstances change, you have a duty to notify your local authority. If you do not, you will probably have to repay any resulting overpayment – see 19.

15. When your HB/CTB starts, changes and ends

Your first day of entitlement
The usual rule is that HB and/or CTB start on the Monday after your 'date of claim for HB/CTB' (this date was described above). Even if that date was itself a Monday, HB and/or CTB start the following Monday.

The exception is if your 'date of claim for HB/CTB' is in the same benefit week (Monday to Sunday) as you moved into your home (or first became liable for rent or council tax for any other reason). In that case, your CTB starts on the exact day you became liable for council tax; your HB starts on the Monday of that week (if your rent is due weekly, fortnightly or four-weekly) or on the exact day your rent liability began (if your rent is due daily or calendar-monthly).

Your benefit period
If you qualify for HB/CTB, it will be awarded for a fixed *'benefit period'* of up to 60 benefit weeks: your local authority will tell you how long it will last. You will then have to make a renewal claim – see below.

Changes of circumstances
At any point before your benefit period does run out, you have a duty to tell your local authority about any changes in your circumstances that might affect your HB/CTB: your local authority will tell you what sorts of changes you should inform them of. If you stop getting IS or income-based JSA or move out of your local authority's area, your local authority must end your benefit period early at that point, unless you are entitled to 'extended payments' – see below. You will then have to make a renewal claim – see below. Most other changes will only affect the *amount* of your housing benefit: in other words your benefit period will carry on for the period originally fixed but you will get a different amount of benefit.

Extended payments
If you stop getting IS or income-based JSA because you or (if you are in a couple) your partner get a job or an increase in hours or in pay, your HB/CTB will carry on for an extra four weeks – usually at the same rate as when you were getting IS. But you have to have been on IS or income-based JSA (or in some cases, signing on) for at least 26 weeks continuously for this to apply and there are further conditions for some people. You must make a special claim to get extended payments, on 'form NHB 1EP' (available from your DSS office) and your claim must reach the DSS office (or your local authority) within 8 days of the end of your IS or income-based JSA entitlement. A claim for extended payments cannot be backdated, so it is essential to claim as quickly as possible.

At the end of your benefit period
Your local authority should send you a renewal claim form towards the end of your benefit period (and also in cases where it is ended early because you come off IS). But if you wish, you can submit a renewal claim form (which you can get from your local authority) at any point in the 13 weeks before your benefit period is due to end. If you do not submit a renewal claim form by the last week of your benefit period, and you are either on IS or income-based JSA or qualify for the disability premium or higher pensioner premium (see 25: look at 'Your premiums'), your local authority can lengthen your benefit period by 4 weeks, the idea being that they can then send you a reminder to renew your claim.

Time limits for sending in your renewal claim
So long as your renewal claim is received by your local authority within 4 weeks after the end of your last benefit period (whether it is lengthened as described above or not), your new benefit period will run consecutively and there will be no gap in your entitlement to HB/CTB. This 4 weeks is a strict time limit. If you do not comply with it, there will be a gap in your entitlement to HB/CTB unless you have 'good cause' for your renewal claim to be backdated – see 17.

16. How your HB/CTB is paid

HB if you pay rent to the council
Your HB is awarded as a rebate towards your rent account – which is why it is also called a 'rent rebate'. In other words, the rent you have to pay will be reduced.

HB for everyone else
Your HB is paid in a cheque, giro, etc – which is why it is also called a 'rent allowance'. Your local authority must take into account your *'reasonable needs and convenience'* in choosing the method of payment: so it should not insist on paying you by crossed cheques if you do not have a bank account.

Your first payment of HB – The law says that your local authority should make your first payment with 14 days of when they receive your properly completed claim or, *'if that is not reasonably practicable, as soon as possible thereafter'*. This must either be of the correct amount of your entitlement or, if that is not yet known, of an estimated amount, known as a *'payment on account'* – which will be adjusted when the correct amount is known. The law is also clear that you should not have to ask for a prompt first payment; though of course if you do not get one, it is sensible to get in touch with them and remind them of their duties! They do not, however, have to make a prompt first payment if you have not supplied the information and documents they have requested, unless you can show that there is 'good cause' for your failure to do so (eg if the delay in providing these is outside your control).

Paying your HB to your landlord – Your HB is paid to your landlord, instead of you, in the following main circumstances:
- if you request or consent to this;
- if it is in your or your family's best interests;
- if your landlord requests it and can show your local authority that you have at least 8 weeks of rent arrears.

In the first two cases, your local authority does not have to agree. In the third case they have to agree (until the rent arrears reduce to below 8 weeks) unless there are overriding reasons for refusing. Your local authority can also choose to pay your first payment of HB to your landlord (regardless of whether you agree) if they consider this appropriate.

Council tax benefit
Your CTB is awarded as a rebate towards your council tax liability. In other words, your bill for council tax will be

reduced. If, however, by the end of the financial year (31st March) your authority owes you any outstanding CTB, you can ask for it to be paid to you in a cheque, giro, etc. If you do not do this, it is usually carried over and rebated against the new financial year's council tax bill.

17. Getting more benefit

Extra benefit in exceptional circumstances

Your local authority has a discretion to award you additional HB and/or CTB if it *'is satisfied'* that your circumstances are *'exceptional'*. You have to qualify for at least some HB/CTB under the ordinary rules before you can get this. There are limits on how much this can be. You cannot be awarded so much HB/CTB (including the addition for your exceptional circumstances) that your total HB exceeds your 'eligible rent' or your total CTB exceeds your council tax liability. For example, you cannot get additional HB to cover ineligible charges (see 8), but you can get additional HB and/or CTB to compensate for the effect of non-dependant deductions (see 22). (This increase is different from the increase for 'exceptional hardship' – see 9.)

Getting your benefit backdated

If you can show that you had continuous *'good cause'* for having delayed making your claim, your local authority must backdate your HB and/or CTB. You have to ask in writing for your claim to be backdated. And benefit can only be backdated for a maximum of one year before this written request is received by your local authority – see 14.

'Good cause' means some fact or facts, which *'having regard to all the circumstances (including the claimant's state of health and the information which he had received and that which he might have obtained) would probably have caused a reasonable person of his age and experience to act (or fail to act) as the claimant did'* CS/371/49(KL). For example, you may have good cause if you are ill and have nobody to help you make the claim, or if you are unable to manage your own affairs and you don't have an appointee. If you do have an appointee, they have to prove good cause for their delay, not you. Ignorance of the law on its own is not normally good cause unless there are exceptional circumstances (eg mental health or learning disabilities, educational limitations, youthfulness, language difficulties, or a combination of these and other factors). Generally you are expected to make reasonable enquiries about your right to benefit. You will normally be able to show good cause if you ask the DSS or local authority for advice and then act on the basis of their wrong or misleading advice; or if you reasonably misunderstood the advice you were given. This test of 'good cause' used to apply to almost all benefits, but from April 1997 only applies to HB and CTB.

If your claim was delayed for over a year due to your local authority's fault, you can ask for an ex-gratia compensation payment.

18. Underpayments

If for any reason your local authority has awarded you less HB or CTB than they should have, they must make up the difference. This is the case even if the reason is that you failed to declare something that was to your advantage. But they cannot make up the difference for underpayments which occurred more than 52 weeks ago – unless these were due to a purely *'accidental error'* by your local authority (such as copying information incorrectly from a claim form onto their computer).

19. Overpayments

Overpayments are amounts of HB/CTB which you were awarded but which you weren't entitled to – perhaps because you did not tell your local authority something you should have, or because your local authority (or DSS office or Jobcentre) made a mistake, or for some unavoidable reason. Different rules apply to different types of overpayment, as follows.

Overpayments of CTB due to a change in your council tax liability – If you get a backdated reduction for disabilities or discount (see Chapter 5), and you were getting CTB, you will have been overpaid CTB. When your local authority adjusts your council tax bill, they will adjust your entitlement to CTB at the same time to recover the overpayment.

Overpayments of HB payments on account – If you were granted a payment on account (see 16) and it turned out to be greater than your actual entitlement to HB, the overpayment will be recovered from your future HB entitlement. (But if you turn out not to be entitled to any HB, the following rules apply.)

Any other overpayments of HB or CTB which are due to official error – An *'official error'* means a mistake by your local authority or by your DSS office or Jobcentre. (The main example of a mistake DSS offices and Jobcentres make which counts as official error is telling your local authority that you qualify for IS or income-based JSA when in fact you do not. If they do not tell your local authority that you have come off IS or income-based JSA, this does not count as an official error – because the law says it is your duty to tell your local authority this.) Your local authority must not recover an overpayment due to official error unless you (or someone acting for you, or the person who received the payment – such as your landlord if your HB is paid to him or her) could *'reasonably have been expected to realise that it was an overpayment'* at the time the payment or any notification about it was received. Your local authority must take into account what you (or the other person) personally could have been expected to realise.

Overpayments due to a mistake about capital – An overpayment of more than 13 weeks of HB or CTB due to a mistake about capital is not recoverable in full. There are 'diminishing capital' rules which treat the capital as gradually reducing (described in Chapter 52(7)).

All other overpayments – Any overpayment of HB or CTB not mentioned above may be recovered by your local authority. This includes overpayments due to a failure or mistake by you, and even overpayments which were unavoidable (such as overpayments due to a backdated pay rise or a backdated social security benefit).

Discretion and hardship – Even if an overpayment is recoverable, your local authority can exercise their discretion not to recover it – for example if you can show that you would otherwise suffer hardship.

Notifications and appeals – In all cases, if your local authority decides to recover an overpayment, they must write notifying you of all the details and of your appeal rights. You can appeal (see below) about any aspect of their decision.

How are overpayments recovered?

If an overpayment is recoverable, it can be recovered from you, or your partner (so long as you were a couple both at the time of the overpayment and at the time of recovery), or the person who received the payment (eg your landlord), or the person who caused the overpayment. It can be recovered as follows.

❑ Overpaid HB may be recovered by reducing your future

HB entitlement (but not, if you are a council tenant, by simply turning the amount into arrears of rent).
- ❏ Overpaid CTB may be recovered by adding the amount back to your council tax account. So you will have more council tax to pay.
- ❏ If the above methods are not possible, overpaid HB or CTB may be recovered by asking the Secretary of State to make deductions from almost any other social security benefit.

In all cases, you can agree to repay the overpayment in cash or by cheques, giros, etc. As a last resort, your local authority can take action in the courts to recover an overpayment.

20. Decisions and appeals

Notice of decisions

Your local authority has a duty to send you a written notice about the decision it makes on your HB and/or CTB claim. It will cover all the main details – such as how much of your rent or council tax was taken into account, your normal weekly entitlement to benefit, enough information for you to make a rough check of the amount, and the start and end dates of your award. If you do not qualify, the notice will say why not. If your local authority makes further decisions during the course of your claim (eg about a change of circumstances or an overpayment), it must send you a written notice about that. In each case, it will also explain your right to get more information and to appeal.

Getting more information

If you want more information about how your entitlement to HB or CTB (or lack of it) was worked out, you can write to your local authority asking for a written statement. You can do this at any time (though if you are thinking about making an appeal as well, bear in mind the time limits mentioned below). You can ask about specific things or ask for full details of how your claim was assessed. Your local authority should reply in writing within 14 days or as soon as possible after that.

Internal reviews – the first stage of an appeal

You have the right to appeal about your HB and/or CTB claim. The first stage is to write to your local authority asking them to reconsider their assessment. This can be about any aspect of your claim. It is usually known as asking for an 'internal review'. If your letter arrives within the time limits, your local authority must reconsider their decision taking account of what you say. They should give you a written notice within 4 weeks, saying whether they are changing or sticking to their original decision, and giving their reasons. But if your appeal is about a 'maximum rent' fixed by the rent officer (see 9), it will take longer because it will be sent on to the rent officer to consider.

Time limits – Your letter should reach your local authority within 6 weeks of the day they sent out the notice about your claim; or if you are appealing about something your local authority decided during the course of your claim (for example, an overpayment), within 6 weeks of the day they sent out the notice about that. If you have asked for a written statement, the time they took to deal with that is ignored in adding up the 6 weeks. For example, if you asked for a written statement 2 weeks after your local authority's notice was sent out, you have 4 weeks left from the date they reply to ask for an internal review. Also, your local authority can agree to extend the 6 weeks for 'special reasons': if you make a late appeal, always give your reasons for the delay so that they can consider this.

Further reviews – the second stage of an appeal

After your local authority has made an internal review of its decision, you can, if you disagree, ask for a *'further review'*. You have to write asking for this, and give your reasons: these need not be detailed or legalistic. This time, your appeal will go before a Review Board. A Review Board is a panel of local councillors (or if your benefit is not administered by a local authority, by the equivalent). You will be invited to attend a hearing to put your case. Your local authority will also send someone to put their case. The hearing should normally take place within 6 weeks of your request. You should be given at least 10 days' notice of the hearing and can ask for the date to be changed if you cannot make it. The Review Board will consider the matter independently. It must be composed of at least 3 councillors, unless you agree to only 2.

You can ask a friend or relative to come with you for support. You can also ask someone to represent you if you wish: they need not be legally qualified to do so: often advice agencies such as Citizens Advice Bureaux or housing aid centres can to do this. It is wise to seek advice from them before the hearing even if they will not be able to represent you: they may well be able to help you with ideas and/or write a submission for you. You and/or your representative will have the right to speak to the Review Board, to call witnesses, and to question anyone else who gives evidence. You may get your reasonable travel expenses paid (and those of your representative or someone who goes with you). You should be told before the hearing starts how it will be run. Once the hearing is over you should be notified in writing of the Review Board's decision within 7 days. Your local authority is bound by the Review Board's decision (unless fresh factual evidence arises later which the Board was not informed of).

Time limits – Your written request for a further review before a Review Board must reach your local authority within 4 weeks of the day they sent out the result of your internal review. However, the Review Board can agree to extend the 4 weeks for 'special reasons': if you make a late appeal, always give your reasons for the delay so that they can consider this.

Exceptions – A Review Board cannot alter the amount of the 'maximum rent' if the rent officer fixed one for your home (see 9). Seek advice if you want to challenge this after the internal review stage.

Other appeal matters

Usually, after a Review Board has made a decision on your case, the only way you can appeal further is to apply to the courts for judicial review. You cannot get a judicial review merely about the facts of the case: there must have been some error of law or procedural unfairness for the courts to agree to a judicial review. It is essential to get advice at this stage. Normally you have up to 3 months to appeal to the courts. One alternative to going to the courts arises if the Review Board itself agrees to *'set aside'* its own decision and to hold a fresh hearing. This can be done if, for example, they held a hearing in your absence: get advice quickly if you think this might be a possibility.

The Ombudsman – You can make a complaint to the Ombudsman if you feel the council administered your claim unfairly or caused unreasonable delays. This is separate from the appeal procedures: for more information, see Chapter 54.

21. How much benefit?

We explain below how to work out your entitlement to housing benefit (HB) and 'Main council tax benefit' (Main CTB). We give the rules for people on IS or income-based JSA first; then the rules for other people. (For how to work out the other kind of CTB, second adult rebate, see 26. For how to calculate HB for rates in Northern Ireland see 27.)

People on income support or income-based JSA
If you (or your partner, if you are in a couple) are on IS or income-based JSA, there are a few simple steps to follow.

Step 1 – Your eligible rent and council tax
HB is worked out on your weekly 'eligible rent'. This can be less than your actual rent – see 8 and 9. Main CTB is worked out on your weekly council tax liability – see 13.

Step 2 – Deduct amounts for non-dependants
If you have one or more 'non-dependants' in your home, your HB and Main CTB are reduced by flat-rate amounts (though there are exceptions to this). For who counts as a non-dependant and the other details, see 22.

Step 3 – Amount of benefit if you are on IS or income-based JSA
The amount of your HB per week equals:
- your weekly eligible rent,
- minus any amounts for non-dependants.

The amount of your Main CTB per week equals:
- your weekly council tax liability,
- minus any amounts for non-dependants.

Examples if you are on IS or income-based JSA
HB – If your weekly eligible rent is £70, and you have no non-dependants, the weekly amount of your HB is £70. But if you had one non-dependant, and a flat-rate deduction of £39 applied, the weekly amount of your HB would be £31.
Main CTB – If your weekly council tax liability is £7, and you have no non-dependants, the weekly amount of your Main CTB is £7. But if you had one non-dependant, and a flat-rate deduction of £4 applied, the weekly amount of your HB would be £3.

People not on income support or income-based JSA
If you are not on IS or income-based JSA (and neither is your partner, if you are in a couple), there are several steps to follow.

Step 1 – Your capital
If your capital (including your partner's) is more than £16,000, you cannot get HB or Main CTB. Not all capital counts. For how to work out your capital, see 23. Even if your capital is over £16,000, you may be able to get second adult rebate – see 26.

Step 2 – Your eligible rent and council tax
HB is worked out on your weekly 'eligible rent'. This can be less than your actual rent – see 8 and 9. Main CTB is worked out on your weekly council tax liability – see 13.

Step 3 – Deduct amounts for non-dependants
If you have one or more 'non-dependants' in your home, your HB and Main CTB are reduced by flat-rate amounts (though there are exceptions to this). For who counts as a non-dependant and the other details, see 22.

Step 4 – Work out your weekly income
This includes your (and your partner's) income from some – but not all – sources. For how to work out your weekly income, see 24.

Step 5 – Work out your applicable amount
This figure represents your weekly living needs. For how to work out your applicable amount, see 25.

Step 6 – Have you got 'excess income'?
If your income is *less* than, or equal to, your applicable amount, you do not have 'excess income'. See Step 7.

If your income is *greater* than your applicable amount, you have 'excess income'. The amount of your excess income is the difference between your income and your applicable amount. See Step 8.

Step 7 – Amount of benefit if you do not have 'excess income'
The amount of your HB per week equals:
- your weekly eligible rent,
- minus any amounts for non-dependants.

The amount of your Main CTB per week equals:
- your weekly council tax liability,
- minus any amounts for non-dependants.

This is exactly the same as for people who are on IS or income-based JSA. The earlier 'Examples if you are on IS or income-based JSA' also apply to you.

Step 8 – Amount of benefit if you have 'excess income'
The amount of your HB per week equals:
- your weekly eligible rent,
- minus any amounts for non-dependants,
- minus 65% of your 'excess income'.

But if the answer is less than 50p you will not be awarded HB. For this and other points see after the examples.

The amount of your Main CTB per week equals:
- your weekly council tax liability,
- minus any amounts for non-dependants,
- minus 20% of your 'excess income'.

But you might get more using the second adult rebate calculation (see 26). For other points see after the examples.

Examples if you have 'excess income'
HB – If your weekly eligible rent is £70, and you have no non-dependants, and you have 'excess income' of £20, the weekly amount of your HB is:
£70 – £13 * = £57.
But if you had one non-dependant, and a flat-rate deduction of £7 applied, the weekly amount of your HB would be:
£70 – £7 – £13 * = £50.
(* £13 is 65% of the £20 'excess income' figure.)
Main CTB – If your weekly council tax liability is £7, and you have no non-dependants, and you have 'excess income' of £20, the weekly amount of your Main CTB is:
£7 – £4 * = £3.
But if you had one non-dependant, and a flat-rate deduction of £1.50 applied, the weekly amount of your Main CTB would be:
£7 – £1.50 – £4 * = £1.50.
(* £4 is 20% of the £20 'excess income' figure.)

Points to note
The percentages (65% in HB and 20% in Main CTB) are also called 'tapers' – because of how they work: as your 'excess income' goes up, your benefit goes down. You can have so much 'excess income' that you do not qualify for any benefit. You can also have so many non-dependant deductions that you do not qualify for any benefit.

The minimum award of HB is 50p per week. So if the calculation comes out at less than 50p, you will not get any HB. There is no minimum award of Main CTB: you can get as little as 1p per year!

22. Non-dependants
Whether or not you are on IS or income-based JSA, deductions are made from your HB and/or Main CTB if you have one or more 'non-dependants'. The law assumes they will contribute towards your rent and/or council tax, whether or not they actually do so. A deduction cannot be cancelled on the grounds your non-dependant pays you nothing. But there are cases when the law says that no deduction must be made.

Who is a non-dependant?
A non-dependant is someone who lives in your home on a non-commercial basis – usually an adult son, daughter, friend or relative. None of the following are your non-dependants (and so there is no deduction for any of them).
- Your *'family'* – see 25. For example, an 18-year-old who is still included in your 'family' is not your non-dependant.
- Foster children.
- Someone with whom you share just a bathroom, toilet, communal area (or in sheltered accommodation a communal room).
- Your joint occupier(s), tenant(s) or sub-tenant(s), resident landlord/landlady, and members of their households.
- Your or your partner's carer if he or she is provided by a charity or voluntary organisation who charge you for this (even if someone else pays the charge for you).

Almost anyone else who lives with you is your non-dependant.

No non-dependant deduction
Your (or your partner's) circumstances – There is no deduction for any non-dependants you have (no matter how many) if you or your partner:
- are registered as blind or ceased to be registered within the last 28 weeks; or
- get the care component of disability living allowance (any rate), or attendance allowance or constant attendance allowance.

Your non-dependant's circumstances – There is no deduction for any individual non-dependant you have if he or she:
- is under 18; or
- in calculating HB, is under 25 and is on IS or income-based JSA; or
- in calculating Main CTB, is any age and is on IS or income-based JSA; or
- gets a Youth Training allowance; or
- has been in an NHS hospital for over 6 weeks; or
- is detained in prison or a similar institution; or
- has his or her normal home elsewhere; or
- is a full-time student (see Chapter 31(5)) – but in calculating HB only, there is a deduction in the summer vacation if he or she takes up 'remunerative work' (see below); or
- in calculating Main CTB only, is in any of the groups who are 'disregarded' for the purposes of the council tax discount rules – see Box C.5.

The amounts of the deductions
Non-dependants aged 25 or over on IS or income-based JSA – The weekly amount of the deduction in calculating HB is £7, but there is no deduction in calculating Main CTB.

Other non-dependants who are not in remunerative work – Regardless of the level of your non-dependant's income, the weekly amount of the deduction is £7 in HB and £1.50 in Main CTB.

Non-dependants who are in remunerative work – The weekly amount of the deduction depends on the level of your non-dependant's weekly gross income:

Weekly gross income	HB	Main CTB
£250 or more	£39	£4.00
£200 to £249.99	£36	£3.50
£152 to £199.99	£33	£3.00
£116 to £151.99	£17	£3.00
£78 to £115.99	£13	£1.50
under £78	£7	£1.50

But if you cannot provide evidence of your non-dependant's gross income (and he or she is in remunerative work), your local authority will make the highest of the above deductions. If you later provide evidence which shows that the deduction should have been lower, your local authority should award you arrears of HB/Main CTB because you have been underpaid (see 18).

Which non-dependants are in remunerative work?
'Remunerative work' means work which averages 16 or more hours per week. If your non-dependant is on maternity leave or sick leave, he or she is not counted as being in remunerative work (even if paid full pay, statutory sick pay, or statutory maternity pay). If your non-dependant gets IS or income-based JSA for more than 3 days in any benefit week (Monday to Sunday), or is on a state training scheme, he or she is not counted as being in remunerative work.

Your non-dependant's gross income
Your non-dependant's income is relevant if he or she is in remunerative work. It is assessed 'gross'. In the case of earnings, this means before tax, National Insurance and any other deductions are made. Any other income is counted, except disability living allowance, attendance allowance, constant attendance allowance and payments from the Macfarlane Trusts, the Eileen Trust, the Independent Living Fund and the Fund. If he or she has capital, only the actual interest is counted as gross income. If he or she is in a couple, add in his or her partner's gross income – but see below.

Other points about non-dependants
You get a deduction for each non-dependant you have (apart from those for whom no deduction applies).

But if you have non-dependants who are a couple, you get only one deduction for the two of them. This is the higher figure of the two amounts which would have applied to them if each was single and each had the income of both.

If you are a joint occupier (see 5 and 12), and your non-dependant is also a non-dependant of the other joint occupier(s), the deduction is shared between you and the other joint occupier(s).

23. Capital
Your local authority needs to assess your capital if you are not on IS or income-based JSA. If you are in a couple, your partner's capital is counted in with yours. The rules about how capital is assessed for HB and Main CTB purposes are almost the same as in the IS scheme – see Chapter 3(30) and (31). Where they differ and this could make a difference to you, we say so.

If your capital works out at over £16,000, you cannot get HB or Main CTB (but you may still get second adult rebate – see 26). This is the main way in which HB/CTB differs from IS.

If a child in your family has capital of his or her own, this is not counted in with your capital. If his or her capital is more than £3,000, this instead affects your 'applicable amount' – see 25.

Tariff income from capital up to £16,000
If your capital works out at £3,000 or less, it is totally ignored in assessing your HB/CTB. If it works out at over £3,000 (but not over £16,000), you are treated as having income – known as *'tariff income'*. To calculate your tariff income: subtract £3,000 from your capital; then divide what is left by 250. The result is the amount of your weekly tariff income. If

the result is not a whole number, round it up to the next whole number. For example, if your capital works out at £6,083: subtracting £3,000 leaves £3,083; dividing by 250 gives £12.33; rounding this up means that you are treated as having £13.00 per week of tariff income.

Exceptions – A few people in residential care or nursing homes are entitled to HB – see Chapter 36. For them, the first £10,000 (instead of £3,000) of capital is ignored.

24. Income

Your local authority needs to assess your income if you are not on IS or income-based JSA. If you are in a couple, your partner's income is counted in with yours. The rules about how income is assessed for HB and Main CTB purposes are almost the same as in the IS scheme – see Chapter 3(24) to (28). Where they differ and this could make a difference to you, we say so.

If your income is greater than your applicable amount, this affects the amount of HB and Main CTB you get. It does not affect second adult rebate – see 26.

If a child in your family receives earned income of his or her own, this is only counted in with yours during the holiday after he or she leaves school for good. If a child receives unearned income, this is counted in with yours at any time. But in either case, if the amount is greater than the personal allowance and any disabled child premium for that child, only an amount equal to those two things is counted in with yours: the rest is ignored. If a child has capital of his or her own over £3,000, all his or her income is ignored.

Main differences from income support

Employees – Your earnings are taken into account whether you work full-time or part-time. Your average weekly earnings are estimated over the 5 weeks before your HB/CTB claim if you are paid weekly; or the 2 months before your HB/CTB claim if you are paid monthly. But in either case, your local authority should average them over another period if that would give a more accurate estimate.

Earnings disregards – Your earnings are assessed after deductions have been made for tax, National Insurance and half of contributions to occupational or personal pension schemes. Then an 'earnings disregard' is deducted of either £25, £15, £10 or £5. The details are the same as in income support (see Chapter 3(25)) except that in HB/Main CTB:
- lone parents (only) get a £25 disregard;
- there is no equivalent of the rule which allows some disabled school-leavers' earnings to be completely disregarded: the maximum disregard for a disabled child is always £15.

An extra earnings disregard for child care costs – In HB/Main CTB you can get an extra earnings disregard which applies in addition to the disregards we have just described. You can get this if:
- you are a lone parent who works at least 16 hours per week; or
- you are in a couple and you both work at least 16 hours per week; or
- you are in a couple and one of you works at least 16 hours per week and the other counts as 'disabled' in one of the ways which would satisfy the conditions for a disability premium – see 25 (look at 'Your premiums').

You must be paying a registered childminder (or a childminder provided on Crown premises or by schools, hospitals, etc where childminders do not have to be registered) for child care for at least one child under the age of 11, or paying an out-of-school-hours scheme (run on school premises or provided by a local authority) to look after at least one child aged 8 or more but under 11. If your child is age 11, you can get the disregard up until the day before the first Monday in September after his or her 11th birthday. The whole amount of these child care payments are deducted from your earnings – up to a maximum of £60 weekly per family (not per child).

Statutory sick pay (SSP) and statutory maternity pay (SMP) – In HB/Main CTB, SSP and SMP are counted as earnings. So when you go on sick leave or maternity leave, your SSP and SMP are added in with any actual earnings you continue to receive. All the above points about assessing earnings then apply. In particular, you get an earnings disregard even if you receive only SSP or SMP. If you do not get the equivalent of your full pay when you go on sick or maternity leave, and you are already getting HB/Main CTB, write informing your local authority, so that they can increase it. If you are not getting HB/Main CTB when you go on sick or maternity leave, your new lower income may entitle you to HB/Main CTB for the first time.

Leaving a job and strikers – There are no equivalents in HB/Main CTB to the rules which can prevent you from getting jobseeker's allowance if you leave a job or go on strike. So if you cannot get JSA, claim HB/CTB anyway.

Maintenance payments – In HB/Main CTB, any maintenance you receive is counted in full as your income – unless there is at least one child in your family, and the maintenance is paid by your former partner or the child's parent, in which case £15 is disregarded. There are no rules in HB/Main CTB like the income support rules about payments from 'liable relatives'.

War widow's and war disablement pensions – Local authorities can choose to run a 'local scheme' under which they disregard more than £10 of these in HB/Main CTB. Your local authority can tell you if it runs a 'local scheme' and how much more it disregards.

Family credit and disability working allowance – If you get an extra £10.55 in either of these because of working at least 30 hours a week (the figure is £10.30 for awards which began before 8.4.97), the extra £10.55 (or £10.30) is disregarded in HB/Main CTB. Apart from that, these benefits count as your income for HB/Main CTB.

Guardian's allowance – This is completely disregarded in HB/Main CTB.

If you support a student son/daughter – In HB/Main CTB if you make parental contributions to a student son or daughter, the same amount as you pay is deducted from your income – unless the student gets a discretionary grant or no grant, in which case the disregard from your income is limited to £38.90 per week.

25. Applicable amounts

Your local authority needs to assess your applicable amount if you are not on IS or income-based JSA. An *'applicable amount'* is a figure set by Parliament which is intended to reflect your weekly living needs and those of your family. Your applicable amount is made up of:
- *'personal allowances'* – you get one or more of these for the various members of your family; plus
- *'premiums'* – many, but not all, people get one or more premiums to take account of family responsibilities, age, disabilities and responsibilities as a carer.

You have to satisfy conditions for each part of the applicable amount. The premiums for disabilities are the most complex. It can be a good idea to ask for a written statement from your local authority about what premiums you have been awarded and why. You can check these and, if you think any have been missed, appeal – see 20.

Your family

Applicable amounts are based on the circumstances of your 'family'. *'Family'* is used in a technical sense in HB/CTB. It means:
- you (the claimant), and
- your partner of the opposite sex, if you are married and are members of the same household or if you are unmarried and living together as husband and wife, and
- any dependent child(ren) who are members of your household, and are either under the age of 16, or are aged 16, 17 or 18 if child benefit is still payable. The definition of a dependent child includes not only your natural children but also other children for whom you are responsible (eg a grandchild). Adopted children are included. But foster children usually are not. For more on this, see Chapter 3(9).

If a child who is normally in local authority care spends time with you at home, your local authority can either include that child or not as a member of your family for the benefit week(s) (Monday to Sunday) when he or she does so. Unlike IS, this is an 'all or nothing' rule: your local authority cannot give you just part of a personal allowance or family premium.

Your personal allowance(s)

You get one personal allowance for yourself – or, if you are in a couple, for both of you; plus a personal allowance for each child in your family (but not for any child who has capital over £3,000).

The weekly rates are the same as in income support with just one exception: in HB/Main CTB, if you are single and under 18 you do not get a lower personal allowance than a single person aged 18 or more.

Weekly rates

Couple:	both aged under 18	£58.70
	at least one aged 18+	£77.15
Lone parent:	aged under 18	£38.90
	aged 18+	£49.15
Single claimant:	aged under 25	£38.90
	aged 25+	£49.15
Each dependent child: *	aged 0–11	£16.90
	aged 11–16	£24.75
	aged 16–18	£29.60

* The allowance is increased from the first Monday in September following the 11th or 16th birthday. If a child reaches his or her 11th, 16th or 18th birthday before April 1997, the figure can be higher – see Chapter 3(10).

Your premiums

The detailed conditions for the premiums are the same as in income support – see Chapter 3(11) to (19). The following summarises the main points.

You get:
- a family premium if you have at least one child in your family – either at the ordinary rate (if you are in a couple) or at the lone parent rate (if you are a lone parent); plus
- a disabled child premium for each child in your family who is disabled (but not if he or she has capital over £3,000); plus
- a carer premium if you or your partner are a carer – or two carer premiums if both you and your partner are carers.

You may also get one of the following premiums. But you can only get one of them: if you satisfy the conditions for more than one of them, you only get the one which is worth most. And if you are a lone parent and get one of the following, your family premium (see above) will be at the ordinary rate, *not* the lone parent rate:
- a disability premium if you or your partner are disabled and both of you are under 60;
- a pensioner premium if you or your partner are aged 60 or more, but both are under 75;
- an enhanced pensioner premium if you or your partner are aged 75 or more, but both are under 80;
- a higher pensioner premium if you or your partner are disabled and at least one of you is aged 60 or more, OR if you or your partner are aged 80 or more.

Finally, if you get a disability premium or a higher pensioner premium, you may also get
- a severe disability premium at either the single rate or the double rate.

Points to note – Don't forget that there is a special definition of who counts as a member of your 'family', including rules about who counts as a 'child' – see above. There are also special rules about who counts as 'disabled' or a 'carer', and really technical rules about who can get severe disability premium. See Chapter 3(13).

The weekly rates are the same as in income support with just one exception: the lone parent rate of the family premium is higher in HB/Main CTB than in income support.

Weekly rates

Family premium	ordinary rate	£10.80
	lone parent rate	£22.05
Disabled child premium		£20.95
Carer premium		£13.35
Disability premium	single	£20.95
	couple	£29.90
Pensioner premium	single	£19.65
	couple	£29.65
Enhanced pensioner premium	single	£21.85
	couple	£32.75
Higher pensioner premium	single	£26.55
	couple	£38.00
Severe disability premium	'single rate'	£37.15
	'double rate'	£74.30

26. Second adult rebate

This type of council tax benefit is known in the law as *'alternative maximum council tax benefit'* – but we use the more common term 'second adult rebate'. It is completely different from 'Main council tax benefit' (Main CTB) described earlier. One of the unique features of second adult rebate is that you can get it regardless of how much income and capital you have. You cannot get second adult rebate and Main CTB at the same time; but if you satisfy the rules for both, your local authority will grant whichever is the higher amount.

A rule of thumb – If you qualify for Main CTB equal to at least 35% of your council tax liability, you need not consider second adult rebate, because you could never get second adult rebate of this much.

Claims – You should not have to make a separate claim for second adult rebate: your claim for CTB should be treated as a claim for both Main CTB and second adult rebate. However, some local authorities do have a special claim form you can use if you want to be considered only for second adult rebate (eg if your capital is way over £16,000).

Who can get second adult rebate?
You can get second adult rebate if you satisfy all these conditions:
- you are not excluded from getting council tax benefit by the rule about 'persons from abroad' – see 11;
- you are liable to pay council tax on your normal home – see Chapter 5(5);
- there are one or more 'second adult(s)' in your home – see below;
- the second adult(s) are on IS or income-based JSA or have fairly low income – see below;
- you meet conditions to do with certain types of households – see below;
- your entitlement to second adult rebate is greater than your entitlement (if any) to Main CTB – see below (look at 'The better buy');
- you claim and provide the information requested – see 14.

Note that if you are a student you can get second adult rebate, even if you are excluded from getting Main CTB – see Chapter 31(5).

Who is a 'second adult'?
You must have at least one 'second adult' in your home to get second adult rebate. A person is a 'second adult' if he or she:
- is aged 18 or more; and
- is your non-dependant – see 22; and
- is not in any of the groups who are 'disregarded' for the purposes of the council tax discount rules. Those groups are listed in Box C.5.

If your non-dependant is in one of the 'disregarded' groups, this should have been taken into account in considering whether you qualify for a council tax discount (see Chapter 5(9)): that is why you can only get second adult rebate if you have a non-dependant who is not 'disregarded'. (The note on carers under the 'Extra rules' below gives the one exception to the above definition of a 'second adult'.)

Extra rules for certain types of households
Single claimants and lone parents – If you alone are liable for the council tax on your home, there are no extra rules. But if you are jointly liable for the council tax, see below.
Couples – If you are in a couple, there is an extra rule. Either you or your partner (or both of you) must be 'disregarded' for the purposes of the council tax discount rules – see Box C.5. And if you are jointly liable for the council tax with someone other than just your partner, see below.
Jointly liable for council tax – If you and others are jointly liable for the council tax on your home, there is an extra rule. Either all, or all but one, of the jointly liable people must be 'disregarded' for the purposes of the council tax discount rules – see Box C.5. The amount of second adult rebate is worked out for the whole dwelling, and you will get a share – calculated by dividing the total amount by the number of jointly liable people.
All claimants who have tenants, sub-tenants or boarders in their home – In addition to the rules mentioned above, there is an overriding rule that you cannot get second adult rebate if you personally receive rent from a tenant, sub-tenant or boarder in your home.
Carers – Many carers are 'disregarded' for the purposes of the council tax discount rules – see Box C.5 – so they cannot be second adults. But if you or your partner have a carer who is not 'disregarded' and who is provided by a charity or voluntary organisation who charge you for this, the carer is a 'second adult'. This is the only case in which someone who is not a non-dependant can be a 'second adult'.

How much second adult rebate?
The amount of your second adult rebate depends only on the income of your second adult(s).
- If you have just one second adult, you get the highest amount of second adult rebate if he or she is on IS or income-based JSA. In all other cases the amount depends on his or her gross income.
- If you have two or more second adults, you get the highest amount of second adult rebate if they are all on IS or income-based JSA. In all other cases, the amount depends on the combined gross income of all of them apart from any who are on IS or income-based JSA.

Weekly amounts	%
If second adult(s) are on IS or income-based JSA	25 *
If weekly gross income of second adult(s) is:	
■ under £116	15 *
■ £116 to £151.99	7½ *
■ £152 or more	nil

* This means 25%, 15% or 7½% of your weekly liability for council tax. But if you also qualify for a council tax discount, it means 25%, 15% or 7½% of your weekly liability for council tax calculated as though you did not qualify for that discount. (You do not lose the discount: it is ignored only for the purposes of this calculation.) For how to convert council tax figures to a weekly amount, see 13.

Your second adult's gross income
Your second adult's income is relevant whether or not he or she is in remunerative work (though not if he or she is on IS or income-based JSA). It is assessed 'gross'. In the case of earnings, this means before tax, National Insurance and any other deductions are made. Any other income is counted, except disability living allowance, attendance allowance, constant attendance allowance and payments from the Macfarlane Trusts, the Eileen Trust, the Independent Living Fund and the Fund. If he or she has capital, only the actual interest is counted as gross income. If he or she is in a couple, add in his or her partner's gross income (even if the partner is not personally a second adult).

The 'better buy'
If you qualify under the above rules for some second adult rebate, and you also qualify under the earlier rules for some Main CTB, there is one final step – often known as a 'better buy' calculation. This is because you cannot get both Main CTB and second adult rebate at the same time: you will only get the one which is worth most. You should get a full notification explaining this if it applies to you, and can ask for a written statement if you want more information – see 20.

27. Rate rebates in Northern Ireland
Rates are payable on domestic properties in Northern Ireland: there is no council tax. You can get HB, also known as a 'rate rebate', towards the rates you are liable to pay on your normal home – whether you pay rent for your home (in which case you can get a rate rebate as well as HB for your rent) or whether you own your home (in which case you can get only a

rate rebate). The conditions for getting a rate rebate are similar to those for getting HB for rent, described at the start of this chapter. The method of claiming a rate rebate is also similar to that for HB for rent – see 14. Your rate rebate is awarded towards your rates liability, so your bill will be reduced. However, if you rent accommodation from a private or housing association landlord, and your landlord (not you) pays the rates, your rate rebate is usually paid to you – along with your HB for rent – in a cheque, giro, etc. Recoverable overpayments may be recovered by adding the amount back to your rates bill. Other rules (eg about appeals) are similar to the rules about HB for rent – see 20.

How much rate rebate for people on IS or income-based JSA? – If you (or your partner) are on IS or income-based JSA, your rate rebate equals:
- 80% of the weekly amount of your rates liability,
- minus any amount for non-dependants.

Note that only 80% of your rates liability is taken into account. You will have to pay the other 20% yourself. The amounts for non-dependants are the same as the figures used in England and Wales for council tax benefit – see 22.

How much rate rebate for people who are not on IS or income-based JSA? – If you are not on IS or income-based JSA (and nor is your partner), your rate rebate equals:
- 80% of the weekly amount of your rates liability,
- minus any amount for non-dependants,
- minus 20% of your excess income.

Note that only 80% of your rates liability is taken into account. You will have to pay the other 20% yourself. The amounts for non-dependants are the same as for council tax benefit – see 22. For whether you have 'excess income', see 21.

5 Council tax

In this chapter we look at:

What is council tax?	see 1
Your dwelling	see 2
How much council tax?	see 3
Exempt dwellings	see 4
Summary of council tax exemptions	see Box C.4
Who is liable to pay?	see 5
Who is a resident of a dwelling?	see 6
How to pay less council tax	see 7
The disability reduction scheme	see 8
The discount scheme	see 9
People who are disregarded for discount purposes	see Box C.5

1. What is council tax?
Council tax is a property-based tax paid to the local authority to help pay for services they provide. It exists in England, Wales and Scotland. Council tax does not exist in Northern Ireland, where domestic rates are still payable. This chapter summarises the rules about council tax. There are several ways in which council tax bills can be reduced if you or someone in your home is disabled.

Rules and regulations – The framework and some of the details of council tax are contained in the Local Government Finance Act 1992. Further details are contained in numerous Regulations and Orders made mainly in 1992 but which have in many cases been amended since then. You can get details of the rules which you are interested in from your local authority or an advice agency.

2. Your dwelling
Council tax is only for domestic properties, referred to in council tax law as dwellings. A *'dwelling'* is a self-contained unit of living accommodation. It could be a house, bungalow, flat, maisonette, houseboat, mobile home, residential care or nursing home or hostel (though not all types of hostel count as a dwelling: some are subject to non-domestic rates). One council tax bill is due on each dwelling, unless it is exempt – see 4.

Points to note – If a property is divided into self-contained units (eg flats), each self-contained unit is a separate dwelling and gets a separate bill (unless it is exempt). If a property contains non-self-contained units (eg a house with a number of rooms with different people in each, but they all share some accommodation), the property is one dwelling and gets only one bill (unless it is exempt). If a property contains both living and business accommodation, one amount of council tax is due for the domestic part (unless it is exempt) and the business part is subject to non-domestic rates.

3. How much council tax?
The amount of your council tax bill depends on the band which your dwelling has been placed in, which in turn depends on the value of your dwelling. Your bill will usually be payable by instalments.

Values – The value of a dwelling is always based on April 1991 property values, and on several other assumptions, such as that it is in a reasonable state of repair. Even if your dwelling has to be revalued, it is still valued by reference to April 1991 values. In England and Wales, dwellings are valued by the Valuation Office. In Scotland, they are valued by the local assessor. (The Valuation Office or local assessor also decide about what counts as a dwelling and how many dwellings there are in a property.)

Council tax bands – The Valuation Office or local assessor place all dwellings into one of eight 'bands' called band A (the lowest value band) to band H (the highest value band). The higher the band, the more council tax you are liable to pay.

Appeals – You have the right of appeal about the correct band for your dwelling in two circumstances: if you have become liable for council tax on your dwelling in the past 6 months (eg because of moving), or if your dwelling has had to be revalued (eg because of a partial demolition). In these cases, your appeal goes first to your Valuation Office or local assessor then to the Valuation Tribunal (England and Wales) or Valuation Appeal Committee (Scotland).

In other circumstances, you can ask your Valuation Office or local assessor to reconsider the band for your dwelling and, if it is clearly wrong, they may alter it. But if they do not agree, you do not have the right of appeal.

4. Exempt dwellings
If your home is an exempt dwelling, no council tax is due on it. Most of the exemptions are for unoccupied dwellings. The main conditions for the exemptions are given in Box C.4: in most cases there are further technicalities.

Getting an exemption, and backdating – Your local authority can award an exemption based on information it has. Or you can ask for one. If you should have been given an exemption in the past, but were not, it should be backdated. There is no time limit at present.

Appeals – Appeals about whether a dwelling is exempt go first to your local authority, then to the Valuation Tribunal (England and Wales) or Valuation Appeal Committee (Scotland).

5. Who is liable to pay?

Unless a dwelling is exempt, someone will be liable to pay council tax on it. This usually depends on who is *'resident'* there – see 6. The details for the dwelling in which you are resident are given below. If you own or rent a dwelling which has no residents, you are usually liable for council tax there (whether or not you are also liable on the dwelling where you are resident).

Backdating – If you were liable for council tax in the past, but were not billed, a bill can be backdated. There is no time limit at present.

Appeals – Appeals about who is liable for council tax on a dwelling go first to your local authority, then to the Valuation Tribunal (England and Wales) or Valuation Appeal Committee (Scotland).

General rules for the dwelling where you are resident

These rules apply to the dwelling where you are 'resident' – see 6.

If you own it – You are liable for council tax there. Your partner, if resident with you, is jointly liable with you (even if not a joint owner). Any other joint owners resident with you are also jointly liable.

If you rent it and do not have a resident landlord – You are liable for council tax there. Your partner, if resident with you, is jointly liable with you (even if not included on the letting agreement). Any other residents who rent it on the same letting agreement are also jointly liable.

If you rent from a resident landlord – Your landlord is liable, not you.

If you rent non-self-contained accommodation and/or any others who rent it have separate letting agreements – Your landlord is liable, not you – even if the landlord is not resident there.

If it is a residential care or nursing home, or (in most cases) a hostel – The landlord is liable, not you.

Special cases

If you are 'severely mentally impaired' (See Box C.5 for what this means.) – Since 1.4.95, the dwelling where you are resident is exempt (see Box C.4) if you and any other occupiers are all 'severely mentally impaired' and no-one else could be liable under the ordinary rules (described above) for council tax there. Note that if a carer lives with you, your dwelling is not exempt. In broad terms, if your dwelling is not exempt, you are liable for council tax even if you are 'severely mentally impaired', except if there is someone else who could be liable instead of you under the rules, described above, about joint

---

C.4 Summary of council tax exemptions

❑ **A dwelling which is unoccupied and (except for a boat or caravan) substantially unfurnished, is exempt if:**
- it needs or is undergoing structural or other major repair works to make it habitable, or the works were substantially completed within the last 6 months;
- it is undergoing structural alteration, or the alteration was substantially completed within the last 6 months; or
- it is unoccupied for any other reason (which could be that it has just been built), and has been for less than 6 months.

❑ **A dwelling which is unoccupied (though it does not need to be unfurnished), is exempt if the previously-resident owner or renter:**
- is in prison or a similar institution;
- is in a hospital, or a residential care or nursing home, or a hostel where personal care is provided;
- is resident anywhere else (which could be a friend's or relative's home) in order to receive or provide personal care for old age, disablement, illness, past or present alcohol or drug dependence, or past or present mental disorder; or
- has died and the bill would otherwise go to that person's estate – but only until the grant of probate or letters of administration and for 6 months after that.

❑ **A dwelling is also exempt if it is:**
- wholly occupied by people who are 'severely mentally impaired' (see Box C.5) and no-one else could be liable for council tax there;
- wholly occupied by people under the age of 18;
- unoccupied, and is part of a property containing a dwelling where someone resides, and letting it separately would be in breach of planning controls (for example an annex);
- in Scotland and is a housing association trial flat for pensioners or for people with disabilities;
- unoccupied and occupation is prohibited by law because it is uninhabitable or due to a compulsory purchase order or similar;
- unoccupied and satisfies conditions to do with charitable ownership, ministers of religion, repossession by a mortgage lender, bankruptcy, or empty caravan sites and boat moorings;
- used as forces accommodation;
- a student hall of residence; or
- currently wholly occupied by students (including students temporarily absent from their course), or is now unoccupied and was last occupied by students.

❑ **From 1.4.97, in England and Wales, there is a new exemption** – It is for cases when a person is 'resident' (see 6) in one part of a property and is a *'dependent relative'* of someone who is 'resident' in another part of the property. The exemption applies only to the part where the dependent relative is resident; and only if the two parts are self-contained units (in other words, they are counted as different dwellings for council tax purposes). For these purposes a 'relative' (see below) counts as a 'dependent relative' only if he or she is:
- aged 65 or more; or
- 'severely mentally impaired' (see Box C.5); or
- is *substantially and permanently disabled (whether by illness, injury, congenital deformity or otherwise)*. The exact meaning of this phrase is open to interpretation. Most people who are registered disabled with the Social Services Department will meet this condition.

A 'relative' means any of the following:
- a parent, child, brother, sister, grandparent, grandchild, uncle, aunt, nephew or niece;
- the parent or child of any of the above (eg great grandparent, cousin, etc);
- a husband or wife;
- relationships by marriage equivalent to any blood relationships mentioned above;
- relationships equivalent to the above but treating unmarried couples of the opposite sex as though they were married;
- relationships equivalent to the above but treating stepchildren as children.

This lengthy list is hard to fathom in some cases. We think 'relative' would include (for example) a person's unmarried partner's grandfather's step-daughter!

liability. The exact rules are complex and can produce strange results: it is often worth getting advice.

If you are under 18 – You are not liable for council tax on any dwelling in which you are resident. The other resident(s) aged 18 or more are liable instead. If there are none, the dwelling is exempt – see Box C.4.

6. Who is a resident of a dwelling?
You are a *'resident'* of a dwelling if it is your *'sole or main residence'*. You can only be a resident of one dwelling at a time. Deciding where you are resident is usually straightforward. In difficult cases, your local authority should take into account how much time you spend at different addresses, where you work, where your children go to school, how much security of tenure you have at different addresses, and your own reasonable views.

Appeals – Appeals about where you are resident go first to your local authority, then to the Valuation Tribunal (England and Wales) or Valuation Appeal Committee (Scotland).

7. How to pay less council tax
There are three different schemes for reducing council tax bills. You need to work through the details of each scheme separately. You can get help through all three schemes at the same

---

C.5 People who are disregarded for council tax discount purposes

People who are 'severely mentally impaired'
This means anyone who:
- *'has a severe impairment of intelligence or social functioning (however caused) which appears to be permanent'*; and
- has a certificate from a registered medical practitioner confirming this (which may cover a past or future period); and
- is entitled to one of the following:
  - DLA middle or higher rate care component;
  - attendance allowance, constant attendance allowance (or an equivalent benefit);
  - incapacity benefit (or formerly invalidity benefit);
  - severe disablement allowance;
  - IS including a disability premium, or whose partner has a disability premium for them included in their income-based JSA;
  - DWA (if your DWA 'qualifying benefit' is in the list above); or
  - is over pension age and would have been entitled to one of the above benefits if under pension age.

Carers
There are three different types of carer who are disregarded. The details for the three types are as follows.
First type of carer – All the following conditions must be met.
- The carer provides care for at least 35 hours per week on average. (The law refers to *'care'*; not *'support'*.)
- The carer is 'resident' (see 6) in the same dwelling as the person cared for.
- The carer is not the partner of the person cared for (ie neither married nor living together as husband and wife).
- The carer is not the parent of the person cared for, if the person cared for is aged under 18.
- The person cared for is entitled to one of the following: the highest rate of the care component of disability living allowance, the higher rate of attendance allowance, or constant attendance allowance.

Second type of carer – All the following conditions must be met.
- The carer provides *'care or support'* or both for at least 24 hours per week.
- The carer is employed by the person cared for.
- The carer is paid no more than £30 per week for the work.
- The carer is 'resident' (see 6), for the better performance of the work, in accommodation (not necessarily the same dwelling) provided by the person cared for.
- The carer was introduced to the person cared for by a local authority, government department or charity.

Third type of carer – All the following conditions must be met.
- The carer provides *'care or support'* or both for at least 24 hours per week.
- The carer is paid no more than £30 per week for the work.
- The carer provides the care or support on behalf of a local authority, government department or charity.
- The carer is 'resident' (see 6), for the better performance of the work, in accommodation (not necessarily the same dwelling) provided by or on behalf of the body just mentioned.

People in a hospital, a residential care or nursing home, or certain kinds of hostel
In the case of hospital, the person must be 'resident' there (see 6); so short stays are rarely sufficient. In the case of a residential care or nursing home, it is sufficient that the person is receiving care or treatment there. In the case of a hostel, the person must be receiving care or treatment, and it must be a hostel where the owner is liable for council tax (not the residents) or a bail or probation hostel.

Anyone who is 'resident' elsewhere
For where someone is 'resident', see 6.

Young people, students, student nurses, youth trainees, apprentices, and others
This means any of the following. The full details are not given except in the first two cases:
- everyone under the age of 18;
- 18-year-olds for whom child benefit is payable – see Chapter 27;
- education-leavers under 20 (but only if they left after 30th April, and then only until 31st October inclusive that year);
- school or college-level students, if their term-time study normally amounts to 12 or more hours per week;
- students at university or an equivalent level of study, if their study amounts to 21 hours or more per week for 24 or more weeks per year;
- student nurses studying under Project 2000, or whose academic course means they count as a 'student', or who are studying for their first nursing registration in hospital-based training;
- foreign language assistants;
- Youth Training trainees under the age of 25;
- apprentices doing a National Vocational Qualification, subject to limitations on pay;
- people in prison or similar institutions;
- members of a religious community;
- members of some international organisations or visiting forces.

time, if you satisfy the relevant conditions for all of them. The three schemes are:
- the disability reduction scheme – see 8;
- the discount scheme – see 9;
- the council tax benefit scheme – see Chapter 4.

Also some dwellings are exempt altogether from council tax – see 4. (If your local authority changed on 1.4.96 or 1.4.97 due to local government reorganisation, you may have a separate 'transitional reduction' shown on your council tax bill. Apart from that, there is no longer any transitional reduction scheme.)

8. The disability reduction scheme

Conditions – You can get a disability reduction if you or any other *'resident'* (see 6) in your dwelling is *'substantially and permanently disabled'*: this can be an adult or a child of any age, whether or not they are related to you. And at least one of the next three conditions must be met:
- you have a second bathroom or kitchen needed by that person; or
- you have a room (other than a bathroom, kitchen or toilet) needed by and predominantly used by that person; or
- you have enough space in your dwelling for that person to use a wheelchair which he or she needs indoors.

Disability reductions are available in all types of dwellings, including residential care and nursing homes and hostels.

Comments – There is no general test of who counts as 'substantially and permanently disabled', though it is clear that it includes people who have been disabled for life and also those who have become disabled later in life. There is also no general test of what it means for the disabled person to 'need' the room or the wheelchair, except that they must be *'essential or of major importance to [his or her] well-being by reason of the nature and extent of [his or her] disability'*. However, it is clear that disability reductions are not limited to dwellings which were specially constructed or adapted to provide a room or wheelchair space.

How much is it worth? – If you qualify for a disability reduction, your council tax bill is reduced to the amount payable for a dwelling in the valuation band below yours. So if your home is in band F, the bill will be reduced to the amount for band E. But if your dwelling is in band A, you cannot get a disability reduction (because band A is the lowest band).

Getting a reduction, and backdating – The person liable for council tax (not the disabled person if different), has to make an application: local authorities usually have standard forms for this. You usually have to make a separate application for each financial year. If you should have been given a disability reduction in the past, but were not, it should be backdated. There is no time limit at present.

Appeals – Appeals about disability reductions go first to your local authority, then to the Valuation Tribunal (England and Wales) or Valuation Appeal Committee (Scotland).

9. The discount scheme

Conditions – and how much is it worth? – The council tax discount scheme is for dwellings where less than 2 adults are 'resident' (see 6). But the way in which the residents are counted is unusual (see below). You can get a discount if:
- there is only one resident in your dwelling: in this case your discount will equal 25% of your council tax liability; or
- there are no residents in your dwelling: in this case your discount will equal 50% of your council tax liability (except in Wales, where local authorities can set the discount at 50%, 25% or nil).

Counting the residents – Several groups of people are disregarded when counting up the number of residents in your dwelling. They are sometimes called (in a rather vivid way) 'invisible people'. The groups are outlined in Box C.5. This is important because it can mean that you qualify for a discount even if there are several people in your dwelling – so long as enough of them are 'disregarded'.

Example – If you are in a couple and have two children aged 17 and 20 at home, you might not expect to get a discount. But if your partner was severely mentally impaired or a carer (as defined in Box C.5), and the 20-year-old was a student or a Youth Training trainee, they would both be 'disregarded'. So would the 17-year old (because of being under 18). That would leave you as the only resident who would be counted. Your discount would be 25% of your council tax.

Getting a discount, and backdating – Your local authority may grant a discount based on information available to it. So you may get a discount without doing anything. But you can also apply for one: local authorities usually have standard forms for this. If you should have been given a discount in the past, but were not, it should be backdated. There is no time limit at present.

Appeals – Appeals about discounts go first to your local authority, then to the Valuation Tribunal (England and Wales) or Valuation Appeal Committee (Scotland).

This section of the Handbook looks at the following:
Regulated social fund   Chapter **6**
Discretionary social fund   Chapter **7**

Social fund

6 Regulated social fund

1. What is the social fund?
The social fund encompasses two very different systems: the regulated social fund and the discretionary social fund.
Regulated social fund – Under the regulated social fund, your right to a maternity payment, funeral expenses or to a cold weather payment is clearly based on legal entitlement. If you pass the various tests in the law you must receive the particular payment. Decisions on payments are taken by the Adjudication Officer. If you disagree with any decision, you have the right to appeal to the Social Security Appeal Tribunal.
Discretionary social fund – Chapter 7 deals with the discretionary social fund. This part of the social fund can make interest-free loans or grants. Loans are usually repayable out of weekly benefit. Decisions are taken by social fund officers, and may be reviewed by social fund inspectors. These decisions are based on discretion.

2. Maternity payments
You will be entitled to a maternity payment of £100 for each expected child, including a stillborn child if:
- you or your partner are getting income support (IS), income-based jobseeker's allowance (JSA), DWA, or family credit at the time you claim. Thus someone under 16 cannot claim in her own right. Her right to a maternity payment depends on her parent's or carer's situation; and
- your capital is no more than £500, or £1,000 if you or your partner are aged 60 or over. Capital is worked out in the same way as for IS – see Chapter 3(31). If your husband died less than 12 months ago, any widow's payment is ignored as capital. A maternity payment is reduced by the amount of any capital above £500 (or £1,000); and
- you claim no earlier than 11 weeks before the week the baby is expected, and no later than 3 months after s/he is born (or after the date of an adoption order, or parental order to married couples who have a child by a surrogate mother). If you've adopted a child, s/he must be under 1 year old on the day you claim.

Claim on form SF100. You can get this from the DSS or your antenatal clinic. Make sure you claim within the time limit even if you're waiting for a decision on your qualifying benefit. If you make a further claim within 3 months of the decision on the qualifying benefit, it can be backdated to the date of the original claim for a maternity payment (or to the date from which the qualifying benefit is awarded if that is later).

3. Funeral expenses
The rules below apply for deaths which occur on or after 7.4.97. If the death occurred before 7.4.97 and the funeral takes place before 8.7.97, the old rules apply (see the 21st edition of the *Disability Rights Handbook*).
You will be entitled to a payment for funeral expenses if:

- you or your partner get a qualifying benefit at the time of your claim – IS, income-based JSA, family credit, DWA, housing benefit or council tax benefit; and
- the funeral takes place in the UK and the deceased was ordinarily resident in the UK when s/he died; and
- you claim any time from the date of death up to 3 months after the funeral. Make sure you claim within the time limit even if you are waiting to hear about a qualifying benefit. So long as you put in a *further* claim for funeral expenses within 3 months of the decision on the qualifying benefit, your claim will be backdated to the date of your first claim (or to the date from which the qualifying benefit is awarded if that is later); and
- you accept responsibility for the costs of the funeral (or you've already paid them) and either:
  - you were the partner of the deceased (of the opposite sex, married and part of the same household or unmarried and living together as husband and wife, or you were partners living in the same household before either or both of you entered a residential care or nursing home); or
  - you were a close relative or close friend of the deceased and there is no surviving partner nor any immediate family member not getting a qualifying benefit, and it is 'reasonable' for you to take responsibility for the funeral costs (see below); or
  - you are claiming for the funeral of a child who lived with you or a still born child, and there is no 'absent parent' who gets a qualifying benefit.

If there is no surviving partner – You may be eligible as a close relative or close friend of the deceased if it is 'reasonable' for you to take responsibility for the costs, given the nature and extent of your contact with the deceased. But first of all the DSS will look at the circumstances of any immediate family.

In most cases you will not be entitled to a funeral payment where there is a parent, son or daughter of the deceased who does not get any of the qualifying benefits. You will only be eligible if that person was estranged from the deceased, or a full-time student, or a wholly maintained member of a religious order; or if they are in hospital or in prison and had been getting a qualifying benefit immediately before they went in.

If there isn't an immediate family member whose circumstances exclude you from entitlement, where there are one or more 'close relatives', the DSS will go on to look at your level of contact with the deceased compared with that of any close relatives. If there is a close relative whose contact was greater, you will not be entitled. If the close relative's contact was equally close, you will only be entitled if they or their partner do not get any of the qualifying benefits, and their savings are no higher than yours (but only if they have savings over £500, or £1,000 if aged over 60; under the limit their savings don't affect your entitlement).

A 'close relative' means a parent, parent-in-law, stepparent, daughter, son, daughter/son-in-law, step-daughter/

son, step-daughter-in-law/son-in-law, sister, brother, sister/brother-in-law.

The amount of the funeral payment – The following costs can be met.
- For a burial:
  - the necessary costs of purchasing a burial plot with an exclusive right of burial;
  - the necessary costs of the burial.
- For a cremation:
  - the necessary costs of the cremation including medical references;
  - the cost of any necessary registered doctor's certificates;
  - the amount of a doctor's fee for the removal of a pacemaker or other active implanted medical device, or up to £20 if it is removed by a funeral director.
- In addition to the above costs, for either a burial or a cremation, the following costs can be met:
  - the cost of any documentation required to release assets which may be deducted from a funeral payment;
  - the reasonable costs of transport over and above 50 miles, if it is necessary to transport the deceased more than 50 miles within the UK to the funeral director's premises or place of rest;
  - the reasonable costs of transport for the coffin and bearers and one additional car over and above 50 miles, if it is necessary to travel more than 50 miles from the funeral director's premises or place of rest to the funeral;
  - the reasonable expenses of one return journey within the UK for you or your partner if they are responsible for the funeral costs, to either arrange or attend the funeral;
  - up to £600 for any other funeral expenses (up to £100 if items or services are provided for under a pre-paid funeral plan or similar arrangement).

Deductions – Certain deductions are made from the payment to you. Any funeral payment is recoverable from the estate of the deceased. The following are deducted from the funeral payment:
- any savings you have above £500, or £1,000 if aged over 60, (capital is worked out in the same way as for income support). However, if you claim funeral expenses within 12 months of the death of your husband, any of your widow's payment is also ignored as capital. It makes no difference whose funeral you are arranging;
- any of the deceased's assets which are available to you without probate, letters of administration or confirmation having been granted;
- any sum due to you because of the death: from an insurance policy, occupational pension scheme, burial club, or similar arrangements;
- any contribution towards funeral expenses from a charity or relative (yours or of the deceased);
- any war pension funeral grant;
- any amount paid for funeral expenses from a pre-paid funeral plan or similar arrangement.

Any payments from the MacFarlane Trusts, the Fund or the Eileen Trust are disregarded.

4. Cold weather payments

If the Met office declares a period of cold weather in your area and you get income support or income-based JSA for at least one day during that period, you may qualify for the cold weather payment. You will not be entitled if your income support or income-based JSA includes a residential allowance, payable to people who live in a residential care home or nursing home. Otherwise, you will qualify if you pass the following tests:
- there must be a period of cold weather which means that the average of the actual or forecasted mean daily temperature for seven days in a row must be at or below freezing; and
- you get a disabled child premium; or
- you are responsible for a child under 5 years; or
- you get a disability or severe disability premium; or
- you get a pensioner or higher pensioner or enhanced pensioner premium.

Payments are made automatically by the DSS – you do not have to claim. The payment is £8.50 for each week that counts as a period of cold weather.

5. Appeals

Decisions on payments from the regulated social fund are taken by Adjudication Officers. If you aren't satisfied with any decision, you have the right to appeal to the Social Security Appeal Tribunal. Chapter 52 gives full details.

7 Discretionary social fund

1. What is the discretionary social fund?

The discretionary social fund provides lump sum payments for needs that are difficult to meet from weekly benefit. Payments can be made in the form of non-repayable grants or interest-free loans.

Unlike other social security benefits, there is no legal entitlement to help. Within the rules laid down in the law and the Secretary of State's Directions, social fund officers have discretion to decide which applications get priority taking into account local and national guidance. The scheme is cash limited and district offices are not allowed to overspend their annual budget for grants and loans.

The procedure for challenging decisions is based on a review system, rather than appeal to an independent tribunal.

There are three types of discretionary payments available.
- **Community care grants** – These are not repayable. Grants are intended to assist people on income support or income-based jobseeker's allowance (JSA) facing difficulties arising from special circumstances. In particular, grants are meant to promote Community Care by helping vulnerable people to live as independent a life as possible in the community.
- **Budgeting loans** – These are interest-free, repayable loans. Budgeting loans are intended to help people on income support or income-based JSA to meet important intermittent expenses for which it may be difficult to budget. This allows you to spread the cost over a period of time.
- **Crisis loans** – These are interest-free, repayable loans. Crisis loans are for people unable to meet their immediate short-term needs either in an emergency or as a consequence of a disaster. A crisis loan will only be awarded where it is considered to be the only means available of preventing serious damage or serious risk to the health or safety of you or your family. You don't have to be on income support or income-based JSA to qualify.

2. Who can get a payment?

To get a grant or loan you must:
- meet the basic rules of eligibility – see 4 below;
- the payment must be for something that is not in the list of excluded items – see Box D.1;
- your circumstances or need must come within the qualifying conditions – see 5 and 6 below;

- your need for the item(s) must have sufficient priority – see 5 and 6 below.

When you fill in your application form, try to give as much detail as you can to show why you should qualify and why your needs are high priority. It is better to apply for a grant rather than a loan if you are eligible. If a grant is refused, you will be considered for a loan. Even if you do just apply for a loan, the social fund officer must consider whether a grant would be more appropriate.

3. The legal framework

Acts and regulations

The main legal framework of the discretionary social fund is detailed in the Social Security Contributions and Benefits Act 1992. The Act provides that in deciding to make an award, or its amount or value, the social fund officer must take into account all the circumstances of the case and in particular:
- the nature, extent and urgency of the need;
- the existence of resources from which the need may be met (DLA mobility component cannot be taken into account);
- the possibility that some other person or body may wholly or partly meet it;
- where the payment is repayable, the likelihood of repayment and the time within which repayment is likely;
- the local office's social fund budget for grants and loans;
- social fund Directions and guidance.

s.140(1), (2) SSCBA

The Social Security Administration Act 1992 gives the framework for reviews. The Social Fund (Application for Review) Regulations 1988 set out the basic rules and time limits for reviews of decisions. The Social Fund (Recovery by Deductions from Benefits) Regulations 1988 list the social security benefits from which a social fund loan can be recovered.

Directions

Directions are issued by the Secretary of State. They give the eligibility and qualifying conditions for grants and loans, list the items that are excluded from help, and give the rules on repeat applications, minimum and maximum awards, the review procedure and managing the budget. Directions are legally binding.

Guidance

The Secretary of State issues national guidance on the practical application of the law and Directions. The guidance covers the circumstances in which an award may be made, the items and services considered and the way in which priority need is assessed. The guidance is not binding but must be taken into account.

Local guidance is issued by social fund district managers. It gives information about the balance of the budget for the district, and whether high, medium or low priority needs can be met. For most districts, only high priority needs can be met consistently throughout the year.

Advice Notes are produced for social fund inspectors by the legal adviser to the social fund Independent Review Service. These interpret aspects of the law and Directions taking into account relevant judicial review cases.

Both the Directions and national guidance are contained in the *Social Fund Guide* (available from The Stationery Office). Advice centres should have a copy and you may also find copies in a good reference library. The Acts, regulations, case law and Advice Notes are included in *The Social Fund – Law and Practice* by Trevor Buck (Sweet & Maxwell). You can get a copy of the local guidance from your local DSS office.

You should use the guidance wherever this helps to support your application, in particular to help you argue for a grant rather than a loan. Social fund officers must take account of national and local guidance. But, unlike the Directions, guidance is not legally binding. Social fund officers should consider circumstances that are outside the scope of the guidance. The absence of Directions or guidance applying to a particular circumstance, item or service does not mean that help should be refused. In your application, ask for all the help you need unless it's clearly specifically excluded from help.

The budget

The amount available in the district budget allocation is a major factor in deciding whether an award can be made. The annual budgets for grants and loans for a district are managed through a monthly profile to ensure that help is available on a consistent basis throughout the financial year (April to March). As the state of the district office's budget is reviewed each month, local guidance may also change on what levels of priority can be met. Social fund officers must not exceed the annual budget allocation. The Secretary of State has the power to make additional allocations during the year.

4. The basic rules

To be considered for a social fund grant or loan you must satisfy the following basic rules laid out in the Directions. If you do meet these rules, the next step is to look at the qualifying conditions outlined in 5 and 6 below.

Repeat applications

You cannot get a grant or loan for an item or service within 26 weeks of a previous social fund payment or refusal for the same item or service unless:
- there has been a relevant change in your circumstances; or
- you are applying for a budgeting loan and at the time of your last application you did not satisfy the budgeting loan condition of being in receipt of income support or income-based JSA for 26 weeks.

You are not excluded from a payment if the previous application was made by your partner.

Community care grants

To be eligible for a grant you must satisfy all the following conditions.
- ❑ You are in receipt of IS or income-based JSA when you apply (or you are leaving institutional or residential care in the next 6 weeks and are likely to get IS or income-based JSA when you leave). You satisfy this condition if your IS or income-based JSA is backdated to include the date of your social fund application.
- ❑ The item you apply for is not excluded – see Box D.1.
- ❑ You don't have too much capital. Any grant is reduced by capital or savings that you or your partner have above £500 (or £1,000 if you or your partner are aged 60 or over). Capital is worked out in the same way as for IS except that Family Fund payments are disregarded for grants.

Budgeting loans

To be eligible for a budgeting loan you must satisfy all the following conditions.
- ❑ You are in receipt of IS or income-based JSA at the date the social fund officer makes a decision on your application.
- ❑ You or your partner have been in receipt of IS or income-based JSA throughout the 26 weeks before the decision is made on your application. You are treated as still in receipt

of IS or JSA during one break in your claim of 14 days or less. But you are not treated as in receipt of JSA during the 3 waiting days at the beginning of the claim.
- Neither you nor your partner are involved in a trade dispute and thus ineligible for JSA.
- The item you apply for is not excluded – see Box D.1.
- You don't have too much capital. The amount of the loan is reduced by any capital or savings that you or your partner have above £500 (or £1,000 if you or your partner are aged 60 or over). Capital is worked out in the same way as for IS except that Family Fund payments are disregarded for loans.
- The amount to be awarded must not be more than you can afford to repay – see 8 below.

Crisis loans
To be eligible for a crisis loan you must satisfy all the following conditions.
- You are aged 16 or over.
- The item you apply for is not excluded – see Box D.1.
- The amount to be awarded must not be more than you can afford to repay – see 8 below.
- You are without sufficient resources to meet the immediate short-term needs of yourself and/or your family.

All your available resources are taken into account including most types of savings, if it is reasonable to do so in the circumstances. Guidance gives examples of resources which should normally be ignored, including housing benefit, social fund payments, business assets, personal possessions, Independent Living Fund and MacFarlane Trust payments. DLA mobility component must be ignored. Help from any other source can be taken into account if there is a realistic expectation that help would be available in time. Possible sources of help might be charities and benevolent funds which are known to be likely to provide the required assistance. Social fund officers should not routinely refer applicants to employers, relatives or close friends unless there is reason to believe that an offer of help will be forthcoming. Credit facilities can only be taken into account if you are not getting IS and are likely to be able to afford the repayments.

Who cannot get a crisis loan? – You cannot get a crisis loan if you are:
- resident in a residential care home, nursing home or hospital, unless you are going to be discharged within the following two weeks;
- a prisoner or in custody or released on temporary licence;
- a member of, and fully maintained by, a religious order;
- in full-time relevant education (or would be treated as such) for the purpose of IS or JSA and as a result are not entitled to IS or income-based JSA.

5. Qualifying for a grant
Community care grants can be awarded for expenses which will promote community care by:
- helping you (or a member of your family or someone you will be caring for) to re-establish yourself in the community after leaving institutional or residential care – see below; or
- helping you (or a member of your family or someone you are caring for) to remain in the community rather than enter institutional or residential care – see below; or
- easing exceptional pressures on you and your family – see below; or
- allowing you or your partner to care for a prisoner or young offender on release on temporary licence; or
- helping you or your family with travel expenses, including any reasonable charges for overnight accommodation within the UK to visit someone who is ill; or attend a relative's funeral; or ease a domestic crisis; or move to suitable accommodation; or visit a child who is with the other parent pending a court decision.

These qualifying conditions are laid out in Direction 4. To qualify for a grant, your own situation and need for a grant must come within at least one of these five conditions. We look at these in more detail below.

Within each category, guidance gives examples of the kind of items or expenses that may be covered. But there is no fixed list and you can ask for whatever you need so long as this is not specifically excluded (see Box D.1).

If the social fund officer decides a grant would meet one of the conditions in Direction 4, they will then go on to assess whether your application has sufficient priority for an award to be made.

Priorities
The social fund officer takes account of the national guidance to decide on the level of priority of your need for the items applied for within broad categories of high, medium and low priority according to the extent to which a grant would improve or resolve your circumstances and fulfil the aims of Direction 4 (ie the qualifying conditions above). The local guidance is used to decide whether an award can actually be made for that level of priority given the current state of the district budget.

Guidance advises that high priority should normally be given if a grant will have a significant and substantial impact in resolving or improving your circumstances and be very important in fulfilling the aims of Direction 4. Medium priority should be given if a grant is less important in fulfilling these aims. Low priority should normally be given if the need is indirectly linked to your circumstances or a grant will be of minor importance in fulfilling the aims of Direction 4.

Vulnerable groups – Guidance advises social fund officers to identify circumstances which might give the application a higher priority than would otherwise be given for a particular need, eg:
- frailty;
- restricted mobility;
- mental or physical disability;
- mental illness;
- chronic physical illness;
- unstable family circumstances, eg if a parent behaves irrationally or relationships are at breaking point;
- behavioural problems (eg associated with drug or alcohol misuse);
- experience of physical or social abuse or neglect (eg young people from broken homes or who never had a home).

These examples are not exhaustive.

Your need for each item should be considered in the context of your individual circumstances. When you are completing the application, consider which one or more of the situations in Direction 4 could apply and show how important a grant would be in improving your situation, eg how much more likely it would be that you could remain living independently in the community if you got the grant. If you are in one of the vulnerable groups above, you should say so.

However the guidance is not binding. Social fund officers must use their discretion within the law and Directions in deciding the priority of an application.

Leaving institutional or residential care
A grant can be made to help you, a member of your family

or other person for whom you or a member of your family will be providing care to *'re-establish [yourself] in the community following a stay in institutional or residential care'* (Direction 4(a)(i)).

Guidance advises that 'institutional or residential care' means places like hospitals, residential care homes, nursing homes, hostels, supported lodgings, prisons, youth centres and foster care, where there is a significant amount of care or supervision provided to residents because they cannot live independently or might be a danger to others. Other kinds of accommodation can count if they provide a substantial element of care. If the accommodation would not usually be classed as institutional or residential care, you can still come within this provision if you personally received a high level of care. If not, you might instead qualify on the grounds that a grant will help you to stay in the community rather than go into care – see below.

Try and get a letter of support from the accommodation you are leaving to help explain the kind of services provided and the level of care you received while you were resident.

Your stay in care should normally have been 3 months or more, or else a pattern of frequent or regular admission. But this is not defined in law so you could argue that shorter stays could count. *'Undue importance should not be attached to the reference to a three month period in . . . the guidance'* (*R v Secretary of State, ex p. Stitt, Sherwin and Roberts*, 23.2.90 TLR).

To qualify you must be moving back into the community, so you cannot get a grant under this provision if you are transferring from one care home to another.

You should apply for whatever you need to help you set up and live independently, eg furniture, household equipment, connection charges, bedding, clothing, removal expenses, storage charges.

Staying out of institutional or residential care
A grant can be made to help you, a member of your family, or someone you or a member of your family are caring for *'to remain in the community rather than enter institutional or residential care'* (Direction 4(a)(ii)).

The risk of care does not have to be immediate but you should show how a grant would improve your independent life and therefore lessen the risk of admission into care.

Guidance suggests that a higher priority should be given to applications where the threat of care is immediate or imminent or there is a direct link between the threat of care and the need in question.

If you have a history of admission into care, it should be easier to argue that the risk is likely. If you are elderly or have a disability and your medical condition or home circumstances are deteriorating, a grant should be considered.

Guidance gives examples of situations where a grant may be appropriate:
- improving living conditions;
- moving to more suitable accommodation;
- moving nearer relatives or close friends who will provide support (including moving to another household);
- moving in with or nearer to a vulnerable person to provide greater support;
- moving within the community to set up home for the first time.

Remember this list is not exhaustive. You can ask for whatever you need to help you to remain independent. For example, to improve living conditions you may get a grant for redecoration, refurbishment, bedding (particularly for those who are housebound and need extra warmth, or are incontinent), reconnection charges, heaters, washing machine (particularly for those who are bedridden, incontinent or can't wash by hand because of a disability), minor repairs and improvements. If you are moving home you may get a grant for removal expenses, fares, furniture and household equipment, connection charges and installation charges, etc.

Families under exceptional pressure
A grant can be paid *'to ease exceptional pressures'* on you and your family (Direction 4(a)(iii)).

Having a low income or being a single parent is not regarded as a situation which by itself creates exceptional pressure. Guidance gives examples of circumstances in which a grant may be appropriate:
- breakdown of a relationship;
- reconciliation of a relationship;
- moving home;
- high washing costs because of a disabled child;
- repair or replacement of items damaged by behavioural problems within the family – priority is likely to be given to families with a disabled child;
- minor structural repair to keep the home habitable or for the safety of a child (priority should be given to families with a disabled child);
- clothing and footwear for disabled children, eg if there is excessive wear and tear or rapid weight gain or loss;
- reconnection charges, meter installation for families with a disabled child, or a child under age five.

These are only examples. In your application you should give details of the effect on your family of the pressure you are under, eg health problems, sleeping difficulties, difficulties at school, accommodation problems, financial difficulties, etc.

Guidance advises that the term 'family' generally means couples with or without children, people caring for children, or women over 24 weeks pregnant. However, it is not defined in law. Social fund officers are advised to be flexible in their interpretation, and to give higher priority to cases involving domestic violence. You could argue that you are a family if for example you live with a parent, or adult child, or a sister or brother, or if you live with a lesbian or gay partner.

6. Qualifying for a loan

Budgeting loans
A budgeting loan may be paid to help you spread the cost of *'important intermittent expenses . . . for which it may be difficult to budget'* (Direction 2). They are not limited to people facing special difficulties arising from special circumstances.

Priorities – The guidance gives examples of high, medium and low priority needs. But these are not exhaustive, and social fund officers should consider the need for the item in the context of your own situation before deciding the priority for the application as a whole.

High priority needs include essential items of furniture and household equipment, bedclothes, essential minor home repairs, fuel meter installation and reconnection and removal charges if a move to more suitable accommodation is essential.

Medium priority needs include non-essential items of furniture and household equipment, redecoration, hire purchase and other debts, and clothing where stocks are inadequate.

Crisis loans
A crisis loan may be paid to meet expenses *'in an emergency, or as a consequence of a disaster, provided that the provision of such assistance is the only means by which serious damage or*

serious risk to the health or safety of that person, or to a member of his family, may be prevented' (Direction 3). If you are awarded a community care grant to enable you to return to the community after a stay in institutional or residential care, you can also get a crisis loan to cover rent in advance (without having to show there would otherwise be a risk to your health or safety).

The need for help will generally be for a specific item or service or for immediate living expenses for a short period not normally exceeding 14 days.

The *Social Fund Guide* does not define the terms 'emergency', 'disaster' or 'serious risk to health or safety'. It is important that you argue that your individual circumstances should be considered fully as people may be affected differently by the same situation. Guidance gives a number of situations where a crisis loan may be considered:

- loss of money;
- hardship due to payment of regular income in arrears;
- disaster, eg fire or flood which has caused significant damage;
- emergency travel expenses, eg if you are stranded away from home;
- hardship due to compulsory unpaid holiday;
- fares to hospital for patients;
- reconnection charges;
- people without accommodation.

You don't have to be on IS or income-based JSA to apply for a crisis loan.

Where a crisis loan is considered to be appropriate it is unlikely that a payment would be refused on priority grounds.

Restrictions for certain groups – Some groups of people whose circumstances exclude them from entitlement to IS or income-based JSA are also excluded from claiming a crisis loan for emergency living expenses.

You can get a crisis loan but only to alleviate the consequences of a disaster, if you are a full-time student not on IS or income-based JSA, or a 'person from abroad' who has no entitlement to IS or income-based JSA.

If your JSA is sanctioned or disallowed – For the first two weeks you can only get a crisis loan for items needed for cooking or space heating or to meet expenses arising from a disaster. This restriction applies only to those who are not in receipt of JSA hardship payments for the first two weeks of the sanction or disallowance. If you are in a vulnerable group (see Chapter 14(10)), you can get JSA hardship payments during the first two weeks and can claim a crisis loan under the normal rules. Your partner is not subject to this restriction and can claim a crisis loan in the normal way although s/he cannot get living expenses for you.

If you or your partner are involved in a trade dispute – You can get a crisis loan only for items needed for cooking or space heating or to meet expenses arising from a disaster.

7. How to claim

You must claim in writing to the local DSS office. SF300 is the form for community care grants and budgeting loans. You don't have to fill in the SF300 at the DSS office, but can take it away and get advice, or think about the best way to write

---

D.1 Which items are excluded?

You cannot get help from the social fund for certain items or needs listed in Directions 12, 23 and 29.

Common exclusions – grants and loans

You cannot get a community care grant, budgeting loan or crisis loan for:
- any need which occurs outside the UK;
- an educational or training need including clothing and tools;
- distinctive school uniform or sports clothes of any description for use at school or equipment of any description to be used at school;
- travelling expenses to or from school;
- school meals and meals taken during school holidays by children who are entitled to free school meals;
- expenses in connection with court (legal) proceedings (including a community service order) such as legal fees, court fees, fines, costs, damages, subsistence or travelling expenses (other than a crisis loan for emergency travelling expenses where an applicant is stranded away from home);
- removal or storage charges where an applicant is rehoused following the imposition of a compulsory purchase order, or a redevelopment or closing order, or a compulsory exchange of tenancies, or pursuant to a housing authority's statutory duty to the homeless under the Housing Act 1996 or Part II of the Housing (Scotland) Act 1987;
- domestic assistance and respite care;
- any repair to property of any body mentioned in section 80(1) of the Housing Act 1985 or section 61(2)(a) of the Housing (Scotland) Act 1987 and, in the case of Scotland, any repair to property of any housing trust in existence on 13.11.53;
- work related expenses;
- debts to government departments;
- investments;
- council tax, council water charges, arrears of community charge, collective community charge contributions or community water charges;
- a medical, surgical, optical, aural or dental item or service – see below.

Medical items – You can't get a grant or loan for a 'medical' item. An item of ordinary everyday use can't be regarded as a medical item (*R v SFI ex p. Connick*, 8.6.93). So you can apply for things like cotton sheets, non-allergic bedding or curtains, built-up shoes, incontinence pads, beds with adaptations or lactose-free foods. If the item is not one of ordinary everyday use, it is excluded from help if it counts as 'medical'. This term is not defined but an Advice Note to inspectors suggests that 'medical' means *'an item that can be reasonably regarded as dedicated to the cure, alleviation, treatment, diagnosis or prevention of a medical condition'*, eg nebulisers or insulin guns. If it's not clear, the applicant must be given benefit of the doubt (Advice Note 7). Wheelchairs are not medical items (Advice Note 13) so you can apply for a grant or budgeting loan to help with the cost. However, you won't get help if someone else such as the NHS or Motability can meet the need.

Community care grants only

You cannot get a community care grant for:
- costs of purchasing, renting or installing a telephone and of any call charges;
- any expenses which the local authority has a statutory duty to meet;
- costs of fuel consumption and any associated standing charges;
- housing costs, including repairs and improvements to the dwelling occupied as the home, including any garage,

down your answers to the questions.

The form for crisis loans is usually filled in during an interview at the DSS office. However, if you or your adviser wish to complete it, ask for form SF401.

Filling in the form
Your application is to the social fund as a whole so the social fund officer must consider whether you can be awarded a grant even if you have only asked for a loan. However, if you are eligible for a grant it is best to concentrate on showing how your circumstances meet the qualifying conditions for a grant and why your grant application should be high priority (see 5).

❑ Ask for all the help you need. Check to see if your need is specifically excluded from help (see Box D.1) or if your situation excludes you from help. If you are not sure, go ahead and ask for help just in case.
❑ Check the qualifying conditions to see which one or more could apply to your situation (eg staying out of institutional care, etc) and use the relevant parts of the *Social Fund Guide* that are helpful for your case.
❑ Detail the size, quantity, cost, etc of the items you need. For example, if you need bedding say what it is you need, eg 2 single sheets, 1 single duvet cover, 2 pillows, etc. If you need carpets, which rooms are they for, what size are the rooms, what is the condition of any existing carpet? If you need curtains, what size do you need, for which rooms, are the rooms overlooked? For less common items, such as an orthopaedic bed, it is best to back up your application with an estimate from a specialist supplier.
❑ For each item applied for, show how getting a grant would significantly improve your circumstances and fulfil the purpose of the qualifying condition(s) that applies to you.
❑ Show how your need for each item is a high priority (use the guidance where this helps) and point out if you are in a vulnerable group.

8. How much do you get?

General rules
If you qualify for help with an item or service, guidance says that the amount you ask for should normally be allowed unless it is inappropriate. The social fund officer often uses a shopping catalogue or local price list of common items to check whether the cost is within the broad range of prices appropriate for an item of serviceable quality.

Community care grants
There is no maximum amount that can be awarded but the minimum amount is £30, apart from travelling expenses and daily living expenses where there is no minimum.

The amount of the award is reduced if you have savings over the limit – see 4 above.

Budgeting loans
The minimum award is £30. The maximum is £1,000 less any amount of social fund loan already outstanding.

The amount of the award is reduced if you have savings over the limit – see 4 above.

---

garden and outbuildings, and including deposits to secure accommodation, mortgage payments, water rates, sewerage rates, service charges, rent, and all other charges for accommodation, whether or not such charges include payment for meals and/or services, other than:
– minor repairs and improvements; or
– charges for accommodation applied for under direction 4(b) – [ie overnight accommodation included in a grant for travel expenses (see 5)];
■ any daily living expenses such as food and groceries, except:
– where such expenses are incurred in caring for a prisoner or young offender on release on temporary licence . . .; or
– where a crisis loan cannot be awarded for such expenses because the maximum loan limit has been reached.

Budgeting loans only
You cannot get a budgeting loan for:
■ the cost of mains fuel consumption and associated standing charges;
■ housing costs, including repairs and improvements to the dwelling occupied as the home, including any garage, garden and outbuildings, and including deposits to secure accommodation, mortgage payments, water rates, sewerage rates, service charges, rent, residential charges for hostels, and all other charges for accommodation, whether or not such charges include payment for meals and/or services other than:
– payments for intermittent housing costs not met by housing benefit, income support or income-based JSA or for which direct payments cannot be implemented such as the cost of emptying cess pits or septic tanks; or
– rent in advance which is payable to secure fresh accommodation where the landlord is not a local authority; or

– where such charges are payable in advance to secure board and lodging accommodation, or residential accommodation in hostels, but not any part of such charges not relating to accommodation, for example, meals, services, deposits; or
– minor repairs and improvements.

Crisis loans only
You cannot get a crisis loan for:
■ installation, rental and call charges for a telephone;
■ mobility needs;
■ holidays;
■ a television or radio, or license, aerial or rental charges for a television or radio;
■ garaging, parking, purchase, and running costs of any motor vehicle except where payment is being considered for emergency travelling expenses;
■ housing costs, including repairs and improvements to the dwelling occupied as the home, including any garage, garden and outbuildings, and including deposits to secure accommodation, mortgage payments, water rates, sewerage rates, service charges, rent and analogous charges for accommodation, other than:
– payments for intermittent housing costs not met by housing benefit, income support or income-based JSA or for which direct payments cannot be implemented such as the cost of emptying cess pits or septic tanks; or
– rent in advance which is payable to secure fresh accommodation where the landlord is not a local authority; or
– charges for board and lodging accommodation and residential charges for hostels, but not deposits, whether included in the total charge or not; or
– minor repairs and improvements.

The social fund officer can only award an amount that you are likely to be able to repay. They will take into account your other continuing commitments as well as any current social fund loans. The amount you can afford is usually taken to be the weekly repayment rate multiplied by the maximum repayment period (usually 78 weeks) – see 10 below.

Crisis loans
The amount of any crisis loan awarded is the smallest amount needed to tide you over or remove the crisis. There is no minimum amount. The maximum amount that can be paid is the lesser of the cost of repair or replacement of the item needed. But the amount cannot be more than £1,000 less any other social fund loan outstanding.

If you are applying for immediate living expenses, eg because of lost or stolen money, the maximum loan is:
- 75% of the IS personal allowance for you and your partner; plus
- the 'under 11' personal allowance for each child regardless of age.

If you are in a trade dispute, or disallowed or sanctioned for JSA, special rules apply.

9. Payment of awards

You should get a written decision within 28 days (or one day for crisis loans). This time limit is not specified in law, although it is in the guidance. If there are unreasonable delays you can complain to the social fund manager at the district office or ask your MP to intervene.

Grants and loans are normally paid by girocheque which you can cash or pay into a bank or building society. Payment can be made to a supplier if they have already provided the service for which the award is made.

If you are not successful or you don't get what you want, you can ask for a review – see 11 below.

10. Repayment of loans

When you are sent a decision awarding a loan, the letter will include an explanation of the repayment terms and procedures. There are three normal rates for weekly repayment: 15%, 10% or 5% of your IS or income-based JSA applicable amount excluding housing costs. The rates are:
- 15% if you have no other debts;
- 10% if you have medium debt repayments;
- 5% if you have high debt repayments.

The most that can be deducted is 25%.

The repayment period is worked out by dividing the amount of the award by the weekly repayment rate. The maximum repayment period is normally 78 weeks but this can be extended to 104 weeks in special circumstances.

The loan can be rescheduled where hardship could result if you had to keep on paying the current rate; where a change in your income allows you to repay the loan more quickly; and where it is necessary to keep a number of loans within overall limits for the rate and period of repaying loans.

If you want to change the rate at which you are repaying a loan, write to your local DSS office. Explain why you cannot afford the current rate of repayment and ask them to reconsider that decision. You cannot challenge the decision by review, since repayment decisions are made by the Secretary of State.

Loans are deducted from your or your partner's IS or income-based JSA. If you don't get enough IS or JSA, or your benefit stops, deductions can be made from most other social security benefits. Deductions cannot be made from DLA, attendance allowance or child benefit.

11. Reviews

If you are not happy with the decision of the social fund officer, you can ask for a review. You must do this in writing within 28 days of the date the decision was given or posted to you. The time limit can be extended if there are *'special reasons'*. There is no definition of, or guidance on, what counts as 'special reasons' so each case should be considered on its merits. The restrictive rules for late appeals (see Chapter 52(13)) do not apply to social fund reviews.

If you are unhappy with the amount of an award, or you were awarded a loan instead of a grant, you can accept payment of the award while still challenging the decision.

Your letter should give enough details to make it clear why you disagree with the decision. The review is carried out by a social fund officer in the local DSS office. If they can't decide in your favour, you will be asked to attend an interview at the local office. The interview can be held at your home if you are unable to attend the office. In most cases interviews take place in a private interview room. You can take a representative with you to help you present your case. During the interview the social fund officer will explain the law, Directions, budget and guidance used to make the decision, and then summarise the reasons for the decision. You'll have the chance to put forward your own case and any extra evidence. You'll be asked to agree the record of the interview. Don't sign unless you are happy that it is an accurate reflection of what was said.

Review by social fund inspectors
If you are not happy with the first review decision made by the local social fund officer, you can ask for a further review. This is carried out by the social fund inspectors. Inspectors are based at the Independent Review Service in Birmingham and are independent of the DSS.

You must write to the local DSS office within 28 days of the day the social fund officer's decision was posted to you. The local DSS send your review letter and all the papers to the Independent Review Service. The social fund inspector can agree to a late request if there are 'special reasons' (see above).

In your review letter give as much detail as you can to show why you are not happy with the decision. You can accept any grant or loan that has already been offered while you are asking for this further review.

The Independent Review Service will send you a copy of all the papers. If there are any mistakes or gaps in the record, write a further letter to correct the picture. The social fund inspector won't normally see you in person. The inspector is concerned with the reasonableness of the social fund officer's review decision and whether it was properly taken, and whether the decision was the right one in all the circumstances. S/he can ask for more information, from you and from the social fund review officer.

The social fund inspector may confirm the original decision; or revise it in your favour; or refer it back to the local office with a list of points which the social fund review officer should take into account. The social fund review officer must also remedy any defects which the inspector draws to their attention. If the inspector refers a decision back to the local office and you are still unsuccessful, it is worth asking for a second review by the inspector. If you are still unsuccessful, it may be possible to apply for judicial review of the inspector's decision. You must act quickly.

Unable to work?

This section of the Handbook looks at the following:

Incapacity for work	Chapter **8**
Contributions and credits	Chapter **9**
Statutory sick pay	Chapter **10**
Incapacity benefit	Chapter **11**
Transitional rules	Chapter **12**
Severe disablement allowance	Chapter **13**

8 Incapacity for work

In this chapter we look at:

Introduction	see 1
What help can you get?	see 2
What is 'incapacity'?	see 3
When are you 'treated' as incapable of work?	see 4
What work are you allowed to do while claiming?	see 5
Disqualification	see 6
How is your incapacity assessed?	see 7
The 'own occupation' test	see 8
The 'all work' test	see 9
Filling in the all work questionnaire	see 10
The all work test – physical disabilities	see Box E.1
The all work test – mental disabilities	see Box E.2
Medical examinations	see 11
Appeals	see 12
Appeal tactics	see Box E.3
What if you fall ill again?	see 13

1. Introduction

On 13 April 1995, incapacity benefit replaced sickness benefit and invalidity benefit. Along with incapacity benefit came a new system of assessing incapacity for work, including the 'all work' test. The all work test affects most people who make a claim for incapacity benefit. It will also be applied to most people who moved onto incapacity benefit from invalidity benefit. There are transitional rules which preserve levels of benefit for people entitled to invalidity benefit before the changes.

In this chapter we describe the current rules for assessing incapacity for work. If you were entitled to invalidity benefit before 13.4.95 or your incapacity for work started before then, Chapter 12 gives details of how the changes might affect you.

2. What help can you get?

If you are unable to work through ill health or disability, there are a number of benefits you might be able to claim depending on your situation.

❑ **Are you an employee?**

If you have an employer and earn at least £62 a week, you are likely to get statutory sick pay (SSP). SSP can last for up to 28 weeks off sick – Chapter 10 gives details. If you don't get SSP for any reason, you may get incapacity benefit instead.

❑ **Are you self-employed or unemployed?**

If yes, you cannot get SSP. Instead you may get incapacity benefit – see Chapter 11.

❑ **Do you have the right amount of contributions?**

These do not matter for SSP. But they do matter for incapacity benefit (unless you are claiming under special rules for widows and widowers). You must have paid or been credited with enough National Insurance contributions in the right tax years – see Chapter 9. Severe disablement allowance has no contribution conditions – see Chapter 13.

❑ **Are you off sick because of an industrial accident or disease?**

Claim SSP or incapacity benefit under the normal rules. You might also be able to get industrial disablement benefit – see Chapter 21. There are transitional rules which protect people who were claiming no-contribution sickness or invalidity benefit before 13.4.95 – see Chapter 12.

❑ **Are you a widow or widower?**

If you are a widow and were incapable of work before your husband's death or before the end of your widowed mother's allowance, and continue to be incapable of work, you may get incapacity benefit even if you do not have the right contributions. A widower may also qualify – see Chapter 46.

❑ **Is your household income low and savings no more than £8,000?**

You might qualify for income support to top up other benefits or provide a basic household income – see Chapter 3. If you have a partner, s/he must not be working for 24 or more hours a week. A disability premium may be included in your assessment if you receive a qualifying benefit, or you pass the 'incapacity condition' – see Chapter 3(12). Income support can provide help with mortgage interest. For help with the rent or council tax see Chapter 4. For help with NHS costs see Chapter 48.

❑ **Do you need help with personal care or mobility?**

Check to see if you might get disability living allowance (DLA) – see Chapter 17. This is paid on its own or on top of other benefits to disabled people who need help with personal care or supervision. DLA is also paid to people with mobility difficulties. You can get DLA in work or out of work; it does not depend on your income or savings, or on NI contributions.

3. What is 'incapacity'?

Not all sickness and disability benefits you might claim depend on being incapable of work. For example, DLA, disability working allowance and industrial disablement benefit each have quite different qualifying tests. The rules and assessment of incapacity for work described in this chapter apply to:

- incapacity benefit – see Chapter 11;
- severe disablement allowance – see Chapter 13;
- disability premium under the 'incapacity condition' with income support, housing benefit and council tax benefit – see Chapter 3(12) and Chapter 4;
- eligibility for income support on grounds of incapacity for work – see Box B.1 in Chapter 3;
- National Insurance credits for incapacity for work – see Chapter 9(2).

The individual chapters describe the specific rules and conditions for each benefit. Note that, although entitlement to statutory sick pay does depend on being unfit for work, the way this is assessed is different – see Chapter 10.

Your 'incapacity for work' must be *'by reason of some*

specific disease or bodily or mental disablement'. 'Specific' is not the same as 'specified', so it is not essential that the cause of the disease or disablement is identified (CS/7/82). For example, you may suffer pain, the cause of which has not yet been diagnosed. A normal pregnancy does not count as a disease or disablement, but conditions such as high blood pressure arising because of the pregnancy do count.

To show you are incapable of work you must satisfy either the 'own occupation' test or, unless you are exempt, the 'all work' test. We look at how incapacity is assessed under these tests in 7–11 below. But, before applying these tests, the DSS will check to see if your circumstances are such that you can be 'treated' as incapable of work.

4. When are you 'treated' as incapable of work?

You may be 'treated' as incapable of work even if you are able to work. While you come into one of the groups below, you do not have to pass any further tests of incapacity – but you do have to satisfy all the other conditions for benefit, including the requirement that you do not actually work on the days for which you are claiming benefit (note that some work is exempt – see 5 below).

You are treated as incapable of work on any day:
- you are an in-patient in hospital;
- you are under medical observation because you are a carrier, or have been in contact with an infectious disease, and a Medical Officer for Environmental Health has issued a certificate excluding you from work;
- you receive regular weekly peritoneal or haemodialysis for chronic renal failure; or weekly parenteral nutrition for gross impairment of enteric function; or treatment by plasmapheresis, parenteral chemotherapy with cytotoxic drugs, anti-tumour agents or immuno-suppressive drugs or radiotherapy; days of treatment can include any necessary recuperation specified in the treatment. If you are not able to work on the other days in the week, your incapacity on those days is assessed under either the 'own occupation' or 'all work' test. If you work on other days of the week, you are only treated as capable of work on the days you work, not for the whole week (see Chapter 11(2));
- you are pregnant and, to avoid serious risk of damage to your health or the baby's health, you must not work in your own occupation if the 'own occupation' test applies, or in any work if the 'all work' test applies;
- you are pregnant but not entitled to maternity allowance or statutory maternity pay from 6 weeks before the baby is due to two weeks after the birth – see Chapter 26(5).

Regs 11 to 14, Social Security (Incapacity for Work) (General) Regs 1995

5. What work are you allowed to do while claiming?

Generally if you do any work, whether or not you expect to be paid, you are treated as capable of work for the week in which you do any work (Sunday to Saturday) and thus are not entitled to benefit. But you are allowed to do some kinds of work and still receive incapacity benefit or severe disablement allowance, or still be counted as incapable of work for other purposes (eg the disability premium).

The decision on whether or not the work you do is allowed is made by an Adjudication Officer at the DSS. You should tell the DSS beforehand if you intend to work. For 'therapeutic work' you need your doctor's approval and the DSS will write to your doctor asking for more information. Although work that falls into the categories below is allowed, it may not be ignored completely in the assessment. The sort of activities or tasks you are able to do, whether they are connected with the work or not, could be taken into account when deciding whether you pass the all work test or the own occupation test. The following kinds of work are allowed:
- caring for a 'relative'. This means caring for a *'close relative'*, ie parent, parent-in-law, step-parent, son, daughter, son/daughter-in-law, step-son/daughter, brother, sister, or the partner of any of these; or caring for the following other relatives: a spouse or unmarried partner, grandparent, grandchild, uncle, aunt, nephew or niece;
- domestic tasks in your own home;
- any activity undertaken during an emergency, to protect another person or to prevent serious damage to property or livestock;
- duties undertaken as a member of a Disability Appeal Tribunal or the Disability Living Allowance Advisory Board – but only one day a week is allowed;
- voluntary work of less than 16 hours a week – see below;
- 'therapeutic work' done on the advice of a doctor, provided your earnings are no more than £46.50 a week – see below;
- work done as a councillor – see below.

Regs 16 and 17, Social Security (Incapacity for Work) (General) Regs 1995

Voluntary work
You are classed as a volunteer if you do voluntary work for someone other than a 'close relative' (see above). You must not be paid for your work, other than expenses *'reasonably incurred by [you] in connection with that work'*. Permitted expenses could include travel, childminding or the costs of caring for another dependant, equipment needed for work and use of a telephone. You may be treated as a volunteer if you're doing community service.

16 hour limit – You must work for less than 16 hours a week. If you work for 16 or more hours in a particular week, in calculating your hours for that week, your hours are averaged over the current week and the 4 preceding weeks, or over the period of a 'recognisable cycle' of work.

'Therapeutic work'
Work of less than 16 hours a week (see above) may be allowed if it helps to *'improve, or to prevent or delay deterioration in, the disease or bodily or mental disablement which causes [your] incapacity for work'*.

Or you may work, without limit on the weekly hours, as part of a treatment programme, done under medical supervision while you are an in-patient or out-patient at a hospital or similar institution. You may also work while attending an institution which provides sheltered work; this is intended to include placement schemes arranged and supervised by an organisation but not necessarily at their own premises.

In each case the work must be undertaken on the advice of a doctor and you must earn no more than £46.50 a week, after any allowable deductions (see Chapter 11(4)). If your earnings are below the limit, your incapacity benefit or SDA is not affected. But if you get income support, housing benefit or council tax benefit, earnings are taken into account as income and may reduce your benefit.

There is transitional protection for people who were getting invalidity benefit or SDA and doing therapeutic work before 13.4.95 – see Chapter 12(5).

Councillors
Any work you do as a councillor is disregarded when deciding whether or not you are capable of work. This applies to members of county, district, parish or community councils, to London borough and City of London councils, to regional or

islands councils and to the Council of the Isles of Scilly.

Your allowances as a councillor are taken into account, even if you do not claim them. You can deduct expenses incurred in connection with your membership. If your net allowance is £46.50 a week or less, your incapacity benefit or SDA is not affected. If your net allowance is over £46.50 a week, the excess is deducted from your benefit. Note that allowances of any amount (other than for travel and subsistence) are taken into account as earnings for income support, housing benefit and council tax benefit.

It is possible for your allowance to be high enough to completely cancel out your benefit. But you keep your underlying entitlement to benefit, so you would not break your period of incapacity for work even if your benefit was cancelled out for over 8 weeks.

S.171F Social Security Contributions and Benefits Act 1992

6. Disqualification

You can be disqualified from incapacity benefit or severe disablement allowance, or treated as capable of work for other purposes (eg disability premium), for up to six weeks in the situations outlined below. Six weeks is the maximum; the Adjudication Officer can decide on a shorter period. You have the right to appeal against the disqualification itself, or to argue that a shorter period is appropriate.

You may be disqualified if:
- you become incapable of work through your own misconduct (but not if incapacity is due to pregnancy or sexually transmitted disease). Misconduct is a wilful act, perhaps recklessly and knowingly breaking accepted safety rules;
- you do not accept medical or other treatment (not including vaccination, inoculation or major surgery) recommended by a doctor or hospital that is treating you – but only if the treatment would be likely to make you capable of work, and you do not have 'good cause' for your refusal;
- you behave in a way calculated to slow down your recovery, without having 'good cause';
- you are absent from home without leaving word where you can be found, without having 'good cause'.

Reg 18, Social Security (Incapacity for Work) (General) Regs 1995

7. How is your incapacity assessed?

There are two tests of incapacity:
- the **'own occupation'** test which looks at your ability to do your usual work; and
- the **'all work'** test which assesses your capacity to do any work. The test looks at your ability to carry out a range of activities such as walking, standing and sitting, and includes an assessment of mental health where appropriate.

The decision on whether or not you are incapable of work on any day depends on passing these tests, unless either you are 'treated' as incapable of work (see 4 above) or, if the all work test applies, you are in an exempt group (see 9 below). Some people already receiving benefit before 13.4.95 are covered by transitional protection which exempts them from the test – see Chapter 12(7).

When you make a claim for benefit, the DSS will decide which of the tests to apply by looking to see whether you have done enough recent work. If you have, then the own occupation test applies for the first 28 weeks of incapacity. It is based on medical certificates provided by your doctor. See 8 below for more details. After 28 weeks of incapacity, the all work test applies.

If you have not worked recently, the all work test will apply from the start of your claim. Firstly, the DSS will check to see if they have enough information in their records and from your medical certificates to decide whether you are exempt from the test – they may write to your doctor for more details of your condition. If you are not exempt, you are sent a questionnaire to fill in to assess your physical abilities and you may also be called in for a medical examination. If you have a 'severe' mental health problem, you are exempt from the test and will not be sent a questionnaire. If your mental health problem is not 'severe', you will first be sent a questionnaire to assess any physical disabilities you may have and then you may be asked in for a medical examination.

Until you have passed the all work test, or the DSS have decided you are exempt, you must continue to send in medical certificates.

See 9 below for details of the all work test.

8. The 'own occupation' test

When does the own occupation test apply?

If you have worked for more than 8 weeks out of the last 21 weeks in one occupation, before the first day for which a decision on incapacity needs to be made, then the own occupation test is applied. The work you do must be for at least 16 hours a week. The 8 weeks do not need to be consecutive. You can be employed or self-employed provided you are paid or the work is done in expectation of payment. But it still counts if you are on paid or unpaid leave (eg sick leave).

Reg 4 Social Security (Incapacity for Work) (General) Regs 1995

More than one job? – The 16 hours a week can be made up of work in more than one job if it is the same kind of work. Or they can be made up of different contracts with one employer even if in this case it is different types of work. These jobs count as one occupation so you cannot be found capable of doing one job and not the other.

But if you have more than one type of job (which qualifies as 16 or more hours a week for more than 8 weeks) during the 21 weeks and you're not working for the same employer, the own occupation test applies to the most recent, unless they both ended in the same week, in which case, the test must be satisfied in each. For example, if you worked for ten years full-time as a builder, followed by nine weeks full-time as a taxi driver, the own occupation test will be applied to the work you did as a taxi driver.

What is the own occupation test?

The own occupation test is whether you are incapable *'by reason of some specific disease or bodily or mental disablement of doing work which [you] could reasonably be expected to do in the course of the occupation in which [you were] engaged'*.

S.171B(2) Social Security Contributions and Benefits Act 1992

Normally the Adjudication Officer who is responsible for the decision on your claim, will accept your statement and your doctor's statement as proving you are incapable of work. However, sometimes they might want a second opinion and may ask you to attend a medical examination by a DSS doctor. Box E.5 in Chapter 10 gives some idea of the stage at which a second opinion may be required.

After your 23rd week of incapacity, the DSS will write to you about the all work test, and, if you are claiming incapacity benefit, advise you that you may claim additions for your dependants. If you get DLA higher rate care component, make sure the local DSS office know about this (it exempts you from the test and entitles you to be paid at the long-term rate of incapacity benefit after 28 weeks instead of 52).

The all work test will be applied after 28 weeks (196 days) of incapacity. If you are not exempt from the test you will receive a questionnaire some time after your 28th week of incapacity. You must continue to send in medical certificates.

If you make a fresh claim for benefit before the 196 days are up, and the break between claims is less than 8 weeks, the own occupation test will continue to apply for the remainder of the linked spell of 196 days.

9. The 'all work' test

When does the all work test apply?
If the own occupation test does not apply (ie you haven't worked for more than 8 weeks in the last 21 weeks – see above) the all work test applies from the first day of incapacity for which you claim.

If your incapacity is first tested under the own occupation test, the all work test applies after 28 weeks (196 days) of incapacity. The 196 days may start before you actually claim: days on statutory sick pay (SSP), days within the maternity allowance period and days when you are treated as incapable of work (see 4 above) are included.

The 196 days need not be continuous. Four or more consecutive days (or 2 days, which need not be consecutive, out of 7, if you receive certain specified treatment, such as dialysis – see 4) separated by 8 weeks or less are linked together.

So, if you transfer from SSP after less than your maximum 28 week entitlement, you could be tested on your own occupation initially, followed by the all work test once 28 weeks have passed from the start of your SSP. If you transfer to incapacity benefit (or SDA) after 28 weeks of statutory sick pay, the all work test applies from the first day of your incapacity benefit (or SDA) claim.

Until you are assessed under the all work test, you must carry on sending in medical certificates.

Are you exempt from the all work test?
When the all work test applies, the DSS will check to see if you are in a group exempt from the test.

❑ **You are exempt from the all work test if you satisfy any one of these conditions:**
- you get DLA higher rate care component, or constant attendance allowance (intermediate or exceptional rate);
- you are assessed (or passported) as 80% disabled for the purposes of your claim for SDA; or are entitled to industrial injuries disablement pension or war pension on the basis of 80% disablement (this exemption applies from 1.4.97);
- you are terminally ill and your death can *'reasonably be expected within 6 months'* (see Box G.4 in Chapter 17 for details of the legal definition);
- you are registered blind;
- you have any of these conditions: tetraplegia; persistent vegetative state; dementia; paraplegia or *'uncontrollable involuntary movements or ataxia which effectively renders [you] functionally paraplegic'*.

❑ **You are exempt if there is medical evidence that you are suffering from any of the following conditions:**
- severe learning disability – this is defined as a *'condition which results from the arrested or incomplete physical development of the brain, or severe damage to the brain, and which involves severe impairment of intelligence and social functioning'* (this is less restrictive than the 'severe mental impairment' test for DLA higher rate mobility component, in that it includes conditions which arise later in life, eg a later head injury – see Chapter 17(23));
- severe and progressive neurological or muscle wasting disease (eg advanced multiple sclerosis, Huntington's disease, Parkinson's disease, motor neurone disease);
- active and progressive form of inflammatory polyarthritis;
- progressive impairment of cardio-respiratory function which severely and persistently limits effort tolerance (eg from heart disease, emphysema);
- dense paralysis of the upper limb, trunk and lower limb on one side of the body (eg from a severe stroke);
- multiple effects of impairment of function of the brain or nervous system causing severe and irreversible motor, sensory and intellectual deficits (eg from a severe stroke, brain tumour);
- manifestations of severe and progressive immune deficiency states characterised by the occurrence of severe constitutional disease (eg loss of weight, CD4 count below 500, fever, night sweats) or opportunistic infections or tumour formation;
- severe mental illness involving the presence of mental disease which severely and adversely affects mood or behaviour, and severely restricts social functioning or awareness of immediate environment – see below.

Reg 10 Social Security (Incapacity for Work) (General) Regs 1995

If you were receiving benefit or incapable of work before 13.4.95, see also Chapter 12(7).

Severe mental illness – Where your medical certificates show that you have mental health problems, the DSS will write to your doctor for more information about the severity of your disability arising from your mental health condition.

The *Incapacity Benefit Handbook for Medical Services Doctors* advises that severe mental health problems are suggested by a need for ongoing psychiatric care which may include sheltered residential facilities where the person receives regular medical or nursing supervision, day care at least one day a week in a centre where qualified nursing care is available, care at home with intervention, at least one day a week, by a qualified mental health care worker and long-term medication with anti-psychotic drugs including depot neuroleptics or mood modifying drugs.

If your condition is not assessed as 'severe' enough to declare you exempt, you will be sent a questionnaire to assess any physical disabilities you may have and then, if necessary, be offered a medical examination to test your incapacity for work under the mental health assessment.

Decisions on exemption – If there is enough information to decide you are exempt, then a decision is issued that you are incapable of work. You do not have to fill in the questionnaire and, in most cases (see Chapter 12(7) for exceptions), you do not need to send in any further medical certificates. If there is not enough information on your medical certificates, they may write to your GP for more details. The Adjudication Officer may make the decision on whether you have an exempt condition based solely on medical evidence from a DSS doctor. But where there is also evidence from your own doctor, the Adjudication Officer must decide on the basis of the most 'reliable' medical evidence available.

If you do not fall into an exempt group, or there is still doubt whether you could be exempt, you will be sent a questionnaire to fill in.

If you are not exempt but think you should be, and you are found capable of work, you can appeal against this when you are sent the decision on your capacity for work.

Note that before 6.1.97, you could only be declared exempt on the grounds of having certain of the severe medical conditions above if a *DSS doctor* certified that you had the condition – see Chapter 8(9) of the 21st edition of the *Disability Rights Handbook*. There was no right of appeal against the refusal of the doctor to do this. However, the High Court has decided that a similar rule that applied to the 'exceptional circumstances' rule was unlawful – see 11 below. Arguably, it was also unlawful to make decisions on exemption dependent on the DSS doctor. If therefore you were found fit for work before 6.1.97, think that you should have been declared exempt, but did not appeal or lost your appeal, seek advice about whether you can now challenge that decision.

What is the all work test?
If you are not exempt, you will be sent a questionnaire which you must fill in. The questionnaire is mainly intended to ask you about the effects of any physical disabilities or health problems you may have, but does also ask about mental health problems. If you do have a mental health problem, you should fill in the questionnaire – unless you are found incapable of work on physical disability or ill-health grounds, you will be asked to attend a medical examination so that an additional mental health assessment can be carried out – see 11.

In the questionnaire, you are asked to tick the boxes which most closely match how difficult you find it to perform certain activities. These activities are walking, walking up and down stairs, sitting in a chair, getting up from a chair, standing, bending and kneeling, using your hands, lifting and carrying, reaching with your arms, speech, hearing, seeing, continence, and fits and blackouts. Under each of these activities is a list of related tasks of varying degrees of difficulty. These tasks are called 'descriptors'. The descriptors are ranked so that within each activity there is a threshold at which you are found to be incapable of work and thus pass the test, and a lower threshold at which it is judged that the effects of your condition begin to impair your ability to work. For a list of the activities and descriptors used in the questionnaire, see Box E.1.

For example, under the activity of walking are seven descriptors, ranging from 'cannot walk at all' to 'no walking problem'. If you cannot walk more than 50 metres, you are above the threshold and pass the test. If you cannot walk more than 800 metres, this is below the lower threshold and is judged to have no effect on your ability to work. If your walking ability lies somewhere in the middle, this will not be enough on its own to pass the test, but can be combined with your ability under other activities to bring you above the qualifying threshold.

How many points do you need? – The questionnaire does not tell you where the threshold lies. A points system is used by the DSS to determine whether you pass the test. Each descriptor is allocated a fixed number of points, ranging from 0 points to 15 points. These points are not shown on the questionnaire. To pass the test you need a score of at least 15 points. Points are added together from the descriptor with the highest score which applies to you under each activity. Only the higher score from the two activities 'walking' and 'walking up and down stairs' may be counted, together with one descriptor for each other activity.

You don't have to score points in every activity. You will pass the test if you score 15 points in just one activity; or if the points under two or more different activities add up to 15 or more.

There is a different way of adding the points and different thresholds where you are tested under the mental health assessment – see 11 below.

For a complete list of the activities and points allocated to each descriptor, see Box E.1.

10. Filling in the all work questionnaire
For each different activity (walking, sitting, etc), you are asked to tick whichever boxes apply to you. The boxes correspond to the descriptors for that activity. When deciding which descriptor most closely matches your situation, there are a number of factors which should be taken into account.

Mental or physical disability? – To score points in the mental health assessment, the problem must arise from *'some specific mental illness or disablement'*. To score points in the physical disability assessment, the problem must arise from *'a specific bodily disease or disablement'*. So if, for example, you have a mental health problem that means you are too frightened to go up a flight of stairs, you may not score points in the physical disability assessment for that. However sometimes the same condition will give rise to both physical and mental disablement. For example, a physical health problem like tinnitus can affect both your hearing and your ability to concentrate, in which case you could score points in both the physical and mental health assessments.

Artificial aids – The test takes into account your abilities when using any aid or appliance that you would normally use, or a prosthesis.

Work – The rules themselves say nothing about whether your abilities should be considered in the context of a work setting. However, if you cannot do an activity reliably, safely and at a reasonable speed, you should say so. If the difficulty is sufficiently serious or common, argue that because of this you cannot do the activity at all. The DSS has said that if you can only work in special circumstances such as sheltered or supported employment schemes or specially adapted workplaces, you would not count as being capable of work.

Pain and fatigue – When assessing your questionnaire, the DSS doctor should take into account pain, fatigue, stiffness, breathlessness and balance problems. If you cannot perform a task effectively because of pain, you should be regarded as just as incapacitated as someone who cannot perform the activity at all. Similarly, if you find it so tiring to do a particular task that you could not repeat it, or could only do it so slowly that you could not effectively complete the task, you should be regarded as if you cannot do it at all.
Incapacity Benefit Handbook for Medical Services Doctors, p61 and p92

Problems you might have in travelling to work are not taken into account. But you could argue that after travelling you would be too exhausted to do particular tasks. Or it may be that you would not be able to get to work on time consistently.

There is space on the questionnaire to give extra information, so give details of how it effects you if you attempt to do a task. Say how often you would need to rest and explain the cumulative effects of exhaustion on your ability to perform the tasks.

Variable conditions – You may find it difficult to show you are incapable of work if your condition varies in severity. You may have days when you can work and days when you cannot. The DSS has said that the test is not a snapshot of your abilities on a particular day, but an assessment of your abilities over time. If there are some occasions when you cannot perform tasks then you should give full details in the questionnaire. It is best to tick the boxes in the questionnaire based on what you can or can't do on your bad days. Then use the space below to explain more fully how your condition affects you.
The Medical Assessment for Incapacity Benefit (BA consultation document)

DSS doctors are under very clear guidance to take into account variations in symptoms. If factors like pain, fatigue, stiffness etc mean that you cannot perform an activity predictably, repeatedly and efficiently, say so. If the difficulty is sufficiently serious or frequent, argue that you cannot do the activity at all.
Incapacity Benefit Handbook for Medical Services Doctors, p61, p92–3

Your ability should be assessed with regard to *'reasonableness and some regularity'* so that, if, for example, you can only perform a task slowly, or need to take breaks, then it may be that you should not be regarded as capable of it (CSIB/17/96).

Mental health problems – The questionnaire mainly takes account of physical disabilities. The DSS may know from your medical certificates whether you have a mental health problem. If your condition is not severe enough to be exempt from the test, you are sent the questionnaire to determine the effects of any physical disability you may have. However, the questionnaire does ask if you have any mental health problems, so you should also mention those. If the questionnaire is not enough on its own for you to pass the test, you are offered a medical examination, so that a DSS doctor can go through the mental health assessment with you. You should make sure when filling in the questionnaire that you give information about the way your condition affects your ability to work. There is space at the back of the form for extra information.

Sending back the questionnaire

With your questionnaire you are required to send in a medical statement which you get from your doctor. This is a specific

E.1 The all work test – physical disabilities

To pass the test you need 15 points. Add together the highest score from each activity that applies to you. The first two activities (walking on level ground and walking up and down stairs) count as one activity so if you score on both, just count the highest. See 9 for more details.

The test shown here includes a number of changes made on 6.1.97. For the test that applied before this date, see the 21st edition of the *Disability Rights Handbook*.

Descriptors	Points
Walking on level ground with a walking stick or other aid if such aid is normally used.	
■ Cannot walk at all.	15
■ Cannot walk more than a few steps without stopping or severe discomfort.	15
■ Cannot walk more than 50 metres without stopping or severe discomfort.	15
■ Cannot walk more than 200 metres without stopping or severe discomfort.	7
■ Cannot walk more than 400 metres without stopping or severe discomfort.	3
■ Cannot walk more than 800 metres without stopping or severe discomfort.	0
■ No walking problem.	0
Walking up and down stairs.	
■ Cannot walk up and down one stair.	15
■ Cannot walk up and down a flight of 12 stairs.	15
■ Cannot walk up and down a flight of 12 stairs without holding on and taking a rest.	7
■ Cannot walk up and down a flight of 12 stairs without holding on.	3
■ Can only walk up and down a flight of 12 stairs if he goes sideways or one step at a time.	3
■ No problem in walking up and down stairs.	0
Sitting in an upright chair with a back, but no arms.	
■ Cannot sit comfortably.	15
■ Cannot sit comfortably for more than 10 minutes without having to move from the chair because the degree of discomfort makes it impossible to continue sitting.	15
■ Cannot sit comfortably for more than 30 minutes without having to move from the chair because the degree of discomfort makes it impossible to continue sitting.	7
■ Cannot sit comfortably for more than 1 hour without having to move from the chair because the degree of discomfort makes it impossible to continue sitting.	3
■ Cannot sit comfortably for more than 2 hours without having to move from the chair because the degree of discomfort makes it impossible to continue sitting.	0
■ No problem with sitting.	0
Standing without the support of another person or the use of an aid except a walking stick.	
■ Cannot stand unassisted.	15
■ Cannot stand for more than a minute before needing to sit down.	15
■ Cannot stand for more than 10 minutes before needing to sit down.	15
■ Cannot stand for more than 30 minutes before needing to sit down.	7
■ Cannot stand for more than 10 minutes before needing to move around.	7
■ Cannot stand for more than 30 minutes before needing to move around.	3
■ No problem standing.	0
Rising from sitting in an upright chair with a back but no arms without the help of another person.	
■ Cannot rise from sitting to standing.	15
■ Cannot rise from sitting to standing without holding on to something.	7
■ Sometimes cannot rise from sitting to standing without holding on to something.	3
■ No problem with rising from sitting to standing.	0
Bending and kneeling.	
■ Cannot bend to touch his knees and straighten up again.	15
■ Cannot either, bend or kneel, or bend and kneel as if to pick up a piece of paper from the floor and straighten up again.	15
■ Sometimes cannot either, bend or kneel, or bend and kneel as if to pick up a piece of paper from the floor and straighten up again.	3
■ No problem with bending or kneeling.	0
Manual dexterity.	
■ Cannot turn the pages of a book with either hand.	15
■ Cannot turn a sink tap or the control knobs on a cooker with either hand.	15
■ Cannot pick up a coin which is 2.5 cm or less in diameter with either hand.	15
■ Cannot use a pen or pencil.	15
■ Cannot tie a bow in laces or string.	10
■ Cannot turn a sink tap or the control knobs on a cooker with one hand, but can with the other.	6
■ Cannot pick up a coin which is 2.5 cm or less in diameter with one hand, but can with the other.	6
■ No problem with manual dexterity.	0

form, Med 4, in which your doctor is asked to give a diagnosis of your condition, its disabling effects and an opinion on your ability to carry out your usual occupation. The doctor is not asked to look at your questionnaire or make any comment on it.

Your completed questionnaire should reach the DSS within 6 weeks (starting from the day after it was sent out). After 4 weeks, you will be sent a reminder. If you have not returned it within the time limit, you will be treated as capable of work unless you can show you have *'good cause'* for failing to return it. The DSS must take into account your health, disability and whether you were outside Britain, when deciding whether you have good cause. But other reasons could be valid. This decision is taken by an Adjudication Officer and you have a right of appeal. If you return your form late and the DSS does not accept you have 'good cause', it may be treated as a new claim for benefit.

It is very important that you do return the form. If you're not sure how to complete the questionnaire and you have time, seek advice from a local Citizens Advice Bureau or other

Lifting and carrying by the use of upper body and arms (excluding all other activities specified in Part I of this Schedule [ie this box]).
- Cannot pick up a paperback book with either hand. 15
- Cannot pick up and carry a 0.5 litre carton of milk with either hand. 15
- Cannot pick up and pour from a full saucepan or kettle of 1.7 litre capacity with either hand. 15
- Cannot pick up and carry a 2.5 kg bag of potatoes with either hand. 8
- Cannot pick up and carry a 0.5 litre carton of milk with one hand, but can with the other. 6
- Cannot pick up and carry a 2.5 kg bag of potatoes with one hand, but can with the other. 0
- No problem with lifting and carrying. 0

Reaching.
- Cannot raise either arm as if to put something in the top pocket of a coat or jacket. 15
- Cannot raise either arm to his head as if to put on a hat. 15
- Cannot put either arm behind his back as if to put on a coat or jacket. 15
- Cannot raise either arm above his head as if to reach for something. 15
- Cannot raise one arm to his head as if to put on a hat, but can with the other. 6
- Cannot raise one arm above his head as if to reach for something, but can with the other. 0
- No problem with reaching. 0

Speech.
- Cannot speak. 15
- Speech cannot be understood by family or friends. 15
- Speech cannot be understood by strangers. 15
- Strangers have great difficulty understanding speech. 10
- Strangers have some difficulty understanding speech. 8
- No problems with speech. 0

Hearing with a hearing aid or other aid if normally worn.
- Cannot hear sounds at all. 15
- Cannot hear well enough to follow a television programme with the volume turned up. 15
- Cannot hear well enough to understand someone talking in a loud voice in a quiet room. 15
- Cannot hear well enough to understand someone talking in a normal voice in a quiet room. 10
- Cannot hear well enough to understand someone talking in a normal voice on a busy street. 8
- No problem with hearing. 0

Vision in normal daylight or bright electric light with glasses or other aid to vision if such aid is normally worn.
- Cannot tell light from dark. 15
- Cannot see the shape of furniture in the room. 15
- Cannot see well enough to read 16 point print at a distance greater than 20 cm. 15
- Cannot see well enough to recognise a friend across the room at a distance of at least 5 metres. 12
- Cannot see well enough to recognise a friend across the road at a distance of at least 15 metres. 8
- No problem with vision. 0

Continence (other than enuresis (bed wetting)).
- No voluntary control over bowels. 15
- No voluntary control over bladder. 15
- Loses control of bowels at least once a week. 15
- Loses control of bowels at least once a month. 15
- Loses control of bowels occasionally. 9
- Loses control of bladder at least once a month. 3
- Loses control of bladder occasionally. 0
- No problem with continence. 0

Remaining conscious without having epileptic or similar seizures during waking moments.
- Has an involuntary episode of lost or altered consciousness at least once a day. 15
- Has an involuntary episode of lost or altered consciousness at least once a week. 15
- Has an involuntary episode of lost or altered consciousness at least once a month. 15
- Has had an involuntary episode of lost or altered consciousness at least twice in the 6 months before the day in respect to which it falls to be determined whether he is incapable of work for the purposes of entitlement to any benefit, allowance or advantage. 12
- Has had an involuntary episode of lost or altered consciousness once in the 6 months before the day in respect to which it falls to be determined whether he is incapable of work for the purposes of entitlement to any benefit, allowance or advantage. 8
- Has had an involuntary episode of lost or altered consciousness once in the 3 years before the day in respect to which it falls to be determined whether he is incapable of work for the purposes of entitlement to any benefit, allowance or advantage. 0
- Has no problems with consciousness. 0

Part I, Schedule, Social Security (Incapacity for Work) (General) Regs 1995

E.2 The all work test – mental disabilities

Descriptors	Points
Completion of tasks	
■ Cannot answer the telephone and reliably take a message.	2
■ Often sits for hours doing nothing.	2
■ Cannot concentrate to read a magazine article or follow a radio or television programme.	1
■ Cannot use a telephone book or other directory to find a number.	1
■ Mental condition prevents him from undertaking leisure activities previously enjoyed.	1
■ Overlooks or forgets the risk posed by domestic appliances or other common hazards due to poor concentration.	1
■ Agitation, confusion or forgetfulness has resulted in potentially dangerous accidents in the 3 months before the day in respect to which it falls to be determined whether he is incapable of work for the purposes of entitlement to any benefit, allowance or advantage.	1
■ Concentration can only be sustained by prompting.	1
Daily living	
■ Needs encouragement to get up and dress.	2
■ Needs alcohol before midday.	2
■ Is frequently distressed at some time of the day due to fluctuation of mood.	1
■ Does not care about his appearance and living conditions.	1
■ Sleep problems interfere with his daytime activities.	1
Coping with pressure	
■ Mental stress was a factor in making him stop work.	2
■ Frequently feels scared or panicky for no obvious reason.	2
■ Avoids carrying out routine activities because he is convinced they will prove too tiring or stressful.	1
■ Is unable to cope with changes in daily routine.	1
■ Frequently finds there are so many things to do that he gives up because of fatigue, apathy or disinterest.	1
■ Is scared or anxious that work would bring back or worsen his illness.	1
Interaction with other people	
■ Cannot look after himself without help from others.	2
■ Gets upset by ordinary events and it results in disruptive behavioural problems.	2
■ Mental problems impair ability to communicate with other people.	2
■ Gets irritated by things that would not have bothered him before he became ill.	1
■ Prefers to be left alone for 6 hours or more each day.	1
■ Is too frightened to go out alone.	1

Part II, Schedule, Social Security (Incapacity for Work) (General) Regs 1995

See 11 for details of the mental health assessment.
The test shown here includes changes made on 6.1.97. For the test that applied before that date, see the 21st edition of the *Disability Rights Handbook*.

---

advice centre before sending it back. But don't worry if you can't do this. You will not be found capable of work just on the basis of your answers. Before any such decision is made, you will always be offered a medical examination where you get a chance to talk to the doctor in person about how your condition affects you.

Normally, your completed questionnaire is sent to a DSS doctor (from BAMS – the Benefits Agency Medical Services) to assess, but if it is clear that you are in an exempt group that does not require supporting medical evidence, the Adjudication Officer will make a decision without a further medical opinion. The DSS doctor considers all the evidence on your claim and may request further information from your own doctor.

If the Adjudication Officer cannot make a decision in your favour, you will be offered a medical examination.

11. Medical examinations

The DSS must give you at least 7 days notice of the time and place for the examination. If you do not attend, you will be treated as capable of work unless you can show you have 'good cause' for not attending – see above. If you cannot attend, you should inform the office which arranged the examination as soon as possible. You can claim travel expenses.

When the doctor is ready to see you, s/he will probably come to get you from the waiting area to take you into the examination room. Note that this gives them a chance to watch how you manage to rise from a chair and to walk. The doctor will ask you questions about your everyday activities and give you a clinical examination. The doctor's opinion should not be based on a snapshot of your condition on the day of the examination, nor should the assessment simply involve asking you to perform the activities in the questionnaire. They should consider the effects of your condition over time. Explain your abilities as fully as you can; do not assume the doctor will know that you can only perform the activity with discomfort, that your ability varies, etc. You should tell the doctor about any pain or tiredness you suffer, or would suffer, while carrying out these activities, both on the day of the examination and over time. How would you feel if you had to do the same activity repeatedly? Try not to overestimate your ability to do these tasks. Focus on the problems and difficulties you have, rather than the ways that you manage to deal with those difficulties. You might like to make a note of such things in advance to help you when speaking to the doctor. You can also be accompanied by a relative or friend if you need someone to jog your memory or simply want reassurance.

The examination should last about 20 to 30 minutes. The doctor will identify the 'descriptors' which apply and should provide a full explanation of their choice to the Adjudication Officer, particularly where their opinion differs from yours. The doctor must also consider the exceptional circumstances outlined below. The decision on entitlement is taken by the Adjudication Officer.

In some cases it will be appropriate for the doctor to carry out a 'mental health assessment' not only if you have a mental health problem, but also for example where your ability to complete tasks is affected by medication you take, you have a physical condition which affects your alertness or cognition, you have mild or moderate learning difficulties or you have an alcohol or drug dependency problem which impairs your mental abilities. See below for an outline of the mental health assessment.

Mental health assessment
At the medical examination, the doctor will ask you how your condition affects your ability in four main areas of activity:

- completion of tasks;
- daily living;
- coping with pressure;
- interaction with other people.

Like the questionnaire for physical abilities (see 9 above), there are a series of tasks ('descriptors') related to each activity, and a points system for determining whether you pass the test or not. For a list of the activities and points allocated to each descriptor, see Box E.2. For each of the descriptors that applies to you, you score either 1 or 2 points.

How many points do you need? – **All** the points are added together to see if you pass the threshold of 10 points for this assessment. If you have scored at least 6 points but you have not scored enough to pass the test, the mental health assessment and the physical/sensory assessment can be combined: 9 points are added (whatever your actual score was) to the score on your physical/sensory assessment to see if you can meet the combined threshold of 15 points.

The doctor will interview you to assess how your medical condition affects your day to day life. From the interview, the doctor will decide which descriptors are appropriate. The interview will not consist of the doctor simply asking you whether or not each of the descriptors applies to you. Instead the doctor will ask about everyday activities and experiences, as well as experience of work and training. Try and explain to the doctor if you can only manage things under certain conditions. For example, the doctor might ask if you read books. If you just say yes, the doctor might decide you have no problems concentrating to read. But it might be that it takes you a long time to read a book because you can't concentrate on it for any length of time. You can take someone with you to the examination for support.

The doctor should also consider whether any of the exceptional circumstances below apply. The doctor then provides a report for the Adjudication Officer who makes a decision on your entitlement.

E.3 Appeal tactics

If you are found capable of work under the own occupation test, carry on sending in medical certificates while you are appealing. Your doctor is not bound by the decision of the DSS, but is free to form his or her own opinion.

If you are found capable of work under the all work test, you will be sent a summary of the Adjudication Officer's assessment telling you the activities in which they decided you had some limitation, and the total number of points allocated. It is not necessary to send in medical certificates while you are waiting for your appeal to be heard.

For information on appeal procedures, see Chapter 52. For information on claiming benefit while appealing, see 12 and Chapter 14(8).

Your appeal will be heard by a Social Security Appeal Tribunal. Where it involves the all work test, the tribunal will sit with a medical assessor, who is a doctor there to give the tribunal factual advice about medical matters – s/he will not examine you. Although the tribunal should be conducted in an informal manner, there are several things you can do to increase your chances of success.

❑ Make sure you get a copy of the DSS doctor's medical report. This will allow you to see where you might need to dispute it, or point out misunderstandings.
❑ Seek advice from a Citizens Advice Bureau or other advice centre. They can help you prepare your case and may be able to represent you at the tribunal.
❑ Think about how your condition affects your capacity for work. If you have been assessed under the own occupation test, think about the tasks involved in the job – a job description may help, if you have one. If you have been assessed under the all work test, use Box E.1 and/or Box E.2 to see which descriptors apply to you, and add up the points score. Remember to think about your ability to perform the task reliably, safely and at reasonable speed, and the effects of pain, fatigue, etc – see 10. You can use this information to gather good medical evidence (see below) and to be clear to the tribunal about exactly where in the test you should score points.
❑ If you think one of the exempt categories or exceptional circumstances should apply, seek medical evidence (see below) to back up what you say about this. Argue that your doctor's evidence is the most reliable medical evidence. For example, your doctor probably knows you and how your condition affects you much better than the DSS doctor, or may be an expert or specialist in the field.
❑ If your medication affects your ability to complete tasks, or your physical condition affects your alertness, check whether this has been properly assessed under the mental health assessment. Perhaps you have a mental health problem that has not been taken into account. For example you may suffer from depression or anxiety but not seen your GP about it.
❑ If you have walking problems, remember that any distance you can walk after you begin to suffer 'severe discomfort' should be ignored. See if the descriptor you have been given reflects this. Case law relating to DLA mobility component has interpreted the phrase 'severe discomfort' – see Chapter 17(22) for details.
❑ Seek medical evidence in advance. An advice centre may be able to help you with this. Your doctor may want to charge a fee for providing evidence for you, so check on this first – you may be able to get Legal Aid to pay for it (see Chapter 52(15) and Chapter 53). Ask your doctor, consultant, physiotherapist, etc to comment on what is at issue in your appeal, eg the descriptors that you think should apply, whether or not you come under the exemption or exceptional circumstances rules. It is very important that your evidence focuses on these things, not simply on what condition you have and the treatment you receive.
❑ Regarding the effects of pain, fatigue, variable symptoms etc, you may want to refer the tribunal to the case law (CSIB/17/96) and DSS guidance (see 10). The guidance is not binding, but you can argue that it should be taken into account. There is likely to be more case law on this and other issues in the near future, so check with an advice centre about this.
❑ Remember however that you know your abilities better than anyone. The DSS doctor will only have seen you briefly so cannot know everything about you. What you say will count as evidence as long as it is not self-contradictory or implausible – R(I)2/51, R(SB)33/85. A doctor can offer an opinion on whether or not what you say is consistent with your condition.
❑ If you think a medical point needs clarifying at the tribunal, you can ask the Chair to consult the medical assessor; but if you think you need more evidence from your own doctor, ask for an adjournment.

Exceptional circumstances
Even if you do not score enough points to satisfy the all work test, you will be treated as incapable of work if any of the following circumstances apply to you:
- you are suffering from a severe life threatening disease and there is medical evidence that this disease is uncontrollable or uncontrolled by recognised treatment, and if uncontrolled there is reasonable cause for this; or
- you suffer from a previously undiagnosed potentially life threatening condition, discovered during your examination by the DSS doctor; or
- there is medical evidence that you require major surgery, or other major therapeutic procedure, and it is likely that this will be within 3 months of the DSS doctor's examination.

Reg 27, Social Security (Incapacity for Work) (General) Regs 1995

There is no definition of 'major surgery' or 'therapeutic procedures', but DSS guidance suggests as examples things like a hip replacement, hysterectomy, a major cartilage operation on the knee and an open cholecystectomy.

Incapacity Benefit Handbook for Medical Services Doctors, p187

Before this rule was changed on 6.1.97, you were also treated as incapable of work if there would be a substantial risk to your, or somebody else's mental or physical health if you were found capable of work. This still applies if your incapacity is being assessed for a period before 6.1.97.

Decisions on exceptional circumstances – The Adjudication Officer decides whether any of the exceptional circumstances apply based on the report from the DSS doctor who examined you. But if there is also medical evidence from your own doctor they must consider this too and decide on the basis of *'the most reliable evidence available'*. You can appeal against the Adjudication Officer's decision.

Before the rules were changed on 6.1.97, the Adjudication Officer had to follow the opinion of the DSS doctor, and there was no right of appeal against the doctor's opinion. However, in a judicial review case of 12.9.96 (*R v Secretary of State for Social Security, ex p Moule*), it was decided that it was unlawful for the DSS doctor's opinion to be binding on the Adjudication Officer. If therefore you ask for a review or appeal of a pre-6.1.97 decision, the AO or SSAT does have the discretion to decide whether any of the exceptional circumstances applied to you.

12. Appeals
You can appeal against a decision that you are capable of work within 3 months of the decision being sent to you. Chapter 52 gives more information on the procedure for appeals. If you don't agree that you are fit for work it is well worth appealing – at the time of writing, 47% of those appealing against a decision under the all work test were successful. See Box E.3 for some ideas of points to consider in your appeal.

While you are appealing, you can sign on as available for work for jobseeker's allowance – see Chapter 14. This does not prejudice your chance of winning an appeal on incapacity for work. By signing on, you will protect your right to National Insurance credits, whether or not your appeal is successful.

You can, however, choose to claim income support without signing on while you are waiting for your appeal (send in medical certificates only if it is an own occupation test appeal) but there are disadvantages. Your income support personal allowance is reduced by 20% while you are awaiting an appeal against an *all work test* decision. But this reduction won't be applied if you were continuously incapable of work for 28 weeks, or getting invalidity benefit or severe disablement allowance, immediately before 13.4.95, and this is the first time the all work test has been applied in your case. Nor will the reduction apply to own occupation test appeals. Note that your right to National Insurance credits is not protected unless your appeal is successful. See Box B.1 in Chapter 3.

Reg 22A Income Support (General) Regs 1987

13. What if you fall ill again?
If you reclaim benefit on the grounds of incapacity for work, within six months of a decision that you are capable of work, and your incapacity is due to be assessed under the all work test, medical certificates from your doctor will be sufficient evidence of your incapacity until the all work test can be applied, provided you are suffering from a different condition, or your condition has worsened since the decision. This allows benefit to be paid pending a new decision on the all work test.

If your condition is the same as before and you reclaim within 6 months, you won't be accepted as incapable of work while you are due to be assessed under the all work test until you have actually passed the test, or the AO has decided you are exempt, or you are treated as incapable of work (see 4).

9 Contributions and credits

1. National Insurance contributions
There are four different classes of National Insurance contributions. Only Classes 1, 2 and 3 count towards contributory benefits. Class 4 contributions are extra contributions paid by self-employed people on profits or gains above a certain level. The table below shows which class of contribution counts towards which benefit.

Benefit	Class 1	Class 2	Class 3
contribution-based JSA	Yes	No	No
incapacity benefit	Yes	Yes	No
maternity allowance	Yes	Yes	No
widows' benefits	Yes	Yes	Yes
retirement pension	Yes	Yes	Yes

Class 1 contributions
Class 1 contributions are paid by employees (not if you are self-employed) and employers.

You are only liable to pay Class 1 contributions once your gross earnings reach £62 a week (in the 1997–98 tax year). This is called the 'lower earnings limit'. If you are not contracted-out of the state retirement pension scheme (see Chapter 44(8)), your contribution will be 2% on the first £62 of your earnings and 10% on the rest of your earnings up to £465 a week. This last figure is called the 'upper earnings limit'. The limits usually change each April.

If you are a married woman or widow and have kept your right to pay reduced rate contributions and earn at least £62 a week (in 97/98), you will pay Class 1 contributions of 3.85% on all your earnings up to £465. If you earn £80 a week, or less, you'll be paying more in contributions than you would if you paid full rate contributions. But reduced rate contributions do not count towards contributory benefits. So, if you are not contracted-out of the state pension scheme, it is worth considering giving up your right to pay reduced-rate contributions – ask a Citizens Advice Bureau or the Contributions Agency section at the DSS for advice.

Class 2 contributions
Class 2 contributions are flat rate contributions paid by

self-employed people. In the tax year 1997–98 they are £6.15 a week.

If your net profits or gains are below (or you expect them to be below) £3,480 in the 1997–98 tax year, you can apply for a certificate of exception on form CF 10 which comes with DSS leaflet CA 02 (*For self-employed people with small earnings*). If (and only if) you get this certificate, you do not have to pay Class 2 contributions. However, even if your net profits are below £3,480 and you have the certificate, you still have the right to pay Class 2 contributions. If you have low earnings from self-employment and want to pay contributions voluntarily, it is sensible to pay Class 2, rather than Class 3, contributions. However, if you get disability working allowance or family credit, you may get credits if you have a certificate of exception.

A married woman or widow who has kept her reduced-rate election, does not have to pay Class 2 contributions. However, if her taxable profits from self-employment are £7,010 a year or more, she will nevertheless be liable to pay Class 4 contributions.

Class 3 contributions

Class 3 contributions are flat-rate contributions and are completely voluntary. In the 1997–98 tax year they are £6.05 a week. You may want to pay them if the other contributions you have paid (or been credited with) in a tax year are not enough to make that year count as a 'qualifying year' for retirement pension or widows' benefits – see Box M.1 in Chapter 44 and Chapter 46. If you are covered by home responsibilities protection for that complete tax year, you won't need to pay Class 3 contributions – see Chapter 45.

2. Contribution credits

Credits can count only towards the second contribution condition for any contributory benefit. They usually help towards the second contribution condition for retirement pension and widows' benefits. Most types of credits also count for incapacity benefit and jobseeker's allowance. If you are a married woman and have kept your right to pay the reduced-rate NI contributions, you cannot get Class 1 contribution credits. Class 1 credits are equal to the lower earnings limit.

In any tax year (April to April) you can only get credits up to the minimum required for the benefit contribution condition.

Credits for incapacity for work

You will be credited with a Class 1 contribution for each complete week of incapacity for work, ie on each day of the week you are entitled to:
- incapacity benefit; or
- severe disablement allowance; or
- income support on grounds of incapacity for work; or
- maternity allowance.

If you are not entitled to any of these benefits or you claim late, you can still get credits if you are accepted as incapable of work. The rules for assessing incapacity for work are described in Chapter 8. Note that if you are applying for a period before 13.4.95 when incapacity benefit replaced sickness and invalidity benefit, old rules on assessment of incapacity apply (see the 19th edition of this Handbook).

If you were getting statutory sick pay (SSP), you will usually have paid Class 1 contributions on your SSP – so you won't need credits. But if you did not pay enough contributions and your NI contribution record is deficient, the DSS will tell you. You can then apply for credits.

You can also get a credit for each week for any part of which you received an unemployability supplement.

A week for NI contribution purposes begins on a Sunday and ends on a Saturday.

Incapacity credits can help meet the second contribution condition for any benefit, but for incapacity benefit your credits only count in certain circumstances – see below.

Credits for unemployment

You will be credited with a Class 1 contribution for each complete week you are paid jobseeker's allowance (JSA).

If you are not entitled to JSA, you can protect your NI contribution record by signing on at the Jobcentre for credits only. You will get a credit for each week in which you meet all the basic JSA rules (other than the specific contribution-based or income-based conditions for receipt of benefit), eg you are available for and actively seeking work – see Chapter 14(2).

However, you will not a credit for any week in which your JSA is not paid because of a sanction, or you get JSA hardship payments, or you are on strike. If there is a gap in your contribution record, you can protect your pension entitlement by paying voluntary Class 3 contributions.

Unemployment credits help meet the second contribution condition for any benefit, but for incapacity benefit your credits only count in certain circumstances – see below.

Before 7.10.96 – For credit entitlement before 7.10.96 when JSA replaced unemployment benefit, the rules are slightly different. You get a credit for each week of 6 days of unemployment. If you worked for less than 8 hours a week, you get a credit so long as you were available for full-time work and the job was not in your main occupation unless it was for a charity. Or you get a credit for 5 days unemployment provided that you worked in employed earners' employment and earned less than the lower earnings limit (see 4) on the 6th day.

When do incapacity or unemployment credits count for incapacity benefit?

Incapacity and unemployment credits only help you pass the second contribution condition for incapacity benefit if you also pass one of the tests below. This is intended to make it more difficult for people receiving SDA, a non-contributory benefit, to use their past credits in order to get into the contributory system.

❑ Your credits count if you paid Class 1 or Class 2 contributions on earnings of 25 times the lower earnings limit in either of the two complete tax years before the start of your 'benefit year' (see 3). OR

❑ Your credits count if, in the tax year before your benefit year:
- you were entitled to higher rate short-term incapacity benefit, long-term incapacity benefit (invalidity benefit before 13.4.95), invalid care allowance or unemployability supplement for at least one day in that tax year; or
- you claimed short-term incapacity benefit (sickness benefit before 13.4.95), disability working allowance, jobseeker's allowance (unemployment benefit before 7.10.96) or maternity allowance for at least a day in that tax year – and you satisfied the contribution conditions for incapacity benefit, or would have satisfied them had the earlier claim been an incapacity benefit claim; or
- for people covered by SSP, you would have met the contribution conditions for incapacity benefit, had you claimed it, at any time in that tax year; or
- you were credited with a contribution in that tax year for approved training (see below).

Invalid care allowance credits
You get a Class 1 credit for each week in which you were paid invalid care allowance, or in which you would have been paid ICA if you had not received widow's benefit. ICA credits count for any benefit.

Credits for disability working allowance
You can get a Class 1 credit for each week in which you were paid disability working allowance and were employed, or self-employed and excepted from Class 2 contributions because of small earnings. DWA credits count for any benefit.

Credits for family credit
To help meet the second contribution condition for retirement pension, widowed mother's allowance or widow's pension only, you may get a Class 3 credit for each week in which you got family credit. You must be employed, or self-employed and excepted from Class 2 contributions because of low earnings. The earliest tax year in which you could get these credits is the 1995–96 tax year, and only if you are due to reach pension age after 5.4.99.

Maternity pay period credits
If you were getting statutory maternity pay and did not pay contributions on your SMP, you can apply for Class 1 credits. These credits count for any benefit.

Jury service credits
If you were at Court on jury service for all or part of any week, you can apply for Class 1 credits if you need them. Jury credits count for any benefit.

Starting credits
To help meet the second contribution condition for retirement pension, widowed mother's allowance or widow's pension only, you can get Class 3 credits for the tax year in which you reached 16 and for the two following years. The earliest tax year in which you can get these credits is 1974–75.

Termination of full-time education/training credits
To help meet the second contribution condition for contribution-based JSA or incapacity benefit only, you can get Class 1 contribution credits for one of the two tax years before your benefit year if in that tax year you were aged 18 or over and in full-time education, or on a training course, or in an apprenticeship and the course (or apprenticeship), which must have begun before you became 21, has now ended. In the other year, you must have passed the second contribution condition in a different way.

Approved training credits
To help you meet the second contribution condition for any benefit, you can get Class 1 credits for each week you are on an approved training course. You must meet the following conditions.
The course must be full-time; or 15 or more hours if you are disabled; or it is an introductory course to one of those courses. It must not be part of your job. It must be intended to run for no longer than one year (unless it is a course provided by, or on behalf of, the Employment Service and a longer period is reasonable because of your disability). ES training courses automatically count. For other courses, you must apply for credits – ask the DSS for form CF 55C. You can only get credits for courses that are vocational, technical or rehabilitative.
You yourself must have reached 18 before the start of the tax year in which you require the credits.

60 or older credits
Since 6 April 1983, men can get credits automatically for the tax year in which they reach 60 and the next 4 years. These cover any gaps in your NI record and count for all benefits. If you are unemployed, you don't have to sign on to get these credits. You must continue to pay Class 1 or 2 contributions for weeks where you are liable.

Credits for widows
To help meet the second contribution condition for JSA or incapacity benefit when your widowed mother's allowance ceases, you can get Class 1 credits for each year in which you received widowed mother's allowance or widow's allowance (abolished in 1988), except where your benefit stopped because of remarriage or cohabitation. You are also deemed to satisfy the first contribution condition.
The Social Security (Benefit) (Married Women and Widows Special Provisions) Regulations 1974 contain these provisions. The government forgot to amend them on the introduction of JSA, so contribution-based JSA payments must now be made on an extra-statutory basis to widows who satisfy the above conditions.

3. Benefit year and contribution years
Your entitlement to incapacity benefit or jobseeker's allowance depends on two things:
- which 'benefit year' you are in;
- which are the relevant tax years (or contribution years) for your 'benefit year'.

A 'benefit year' always starts on the first Sunday in January. It ends on the Saturday before the first Sunday in January in the following year. The 1997 benefit year started on Sunday, 5 January 1997. It will end on Saturday, 3 January 1998.

Once you know which is the correct benefit year for your claim, you will also know the right contribution years for your claim.

Contribution years for incapacity benefit
For incapacity benefit, the contribution years are the two complete tax years (6 April to 5 April) before the beginning of the benefit year which includes the start of the 'period of incapacity for work' that contains your claim.

Usually the period of incapacity for work begins on the first day you are incapable of work for which you claim incapacity benefit. In this case, you count three years back from the start of your claim to work out the right contribution years. For example, if your claim starts in June 1997, your contribution years are 6 April 1994 – 5 April 1995 and 6 April 1995 – 5 April 1996. These are the years in which you must have paid or been credited with enough contributions to pass the second contribution condition.

However, there are linking rules that mean in some circumstances your period of incapacity for work begins before you actually claim. These are important since it is the beginning of this period that determines which are the right contribution years for your claim.

Period of incapacity for work – A 'period of incapacity for work' is made up of at least 4 consecutive days of incapacity for work (or 2 days out of 7 if you receive certain regular treatments) and includes days of entitlement to maternity allowance – see Chapter 11(2). It lasts for as long as you remain incapable of work.

Any two periods of incapacity for work separated by no more than 8 weeks are joined together into one single period. It is the beginning of the first linked period that determines which years are the contribution years. This linking rule allows you, for example, to reclaim incapacity benefit within 8 weeks of the end of a previous claim and get the same rate as before without serving any waiting period or resatisfying any contribution conditions.

❏ Example – you've been off work for 6 months and your SSP runs out on 3 June 1997. You claim incapacity benefit on 4 June 1997. Your period of incapacity for work begins on 4 June 1997 so your contribution years are 1994–95 and 1995–96. You return to work on 1 December 1997 for 6 weeks, and reclaim incapacity benefit on 12 January 1998. The two periods of incapacity are linked so your contribution years are still 1994–95 and 1995–96.

An exception to the 8-week linking rule helps you if you've failed the second contribution condition for incapacity benefit but you would have passed had you waited and claimed the following benefit year. You can reclaim in the next benefit year without waiting 8 weeks to break the link. The first claim is simply ignored.

If you were incapable of work before going on a training course, or getting disability working allowance, a 2-year linking rule provides a bridge between your earlier period of incapacity and a new claim for incapacity benefit – see Chapter 15(12) and Chapter 16(6).

Linking rules before 13.4.95 – Periods of incapacity for work were introduced on 13.4.95. Before this, 'periods of interruption of employment' (PIE) were used for both unemployment and sickness benefit and linked together both days of incapacity and days of unemployment. There is a transitional rule to link a PIE with a period of incapacity for work. If a period of incapacity for work started no more than 8 weeks after the last day of incapacity which was part of a PIE (which ended before 13.4.95), the two periods are linked. So, the contribution conditions for incapacity benefit would need to be met in the two tax years before the benefit year that includes the start of the PIE. A PIE is made up of at least two 'days of unemployment' which don't need to be consecutive as long as they are within a period of 6 consecutive days (not including Sundays), or a period of incapacity for work. Any two PIEs separated by no more than 8 weeks are treated as one PIE.

Contribution years for jobseeker's allowance

For contribution-based JSA, the contribution years are the two complete tax years before the beginning of the benefit year which includes either the start of the 'jobseeking period' that contains your claim, or the start of a 'linked period' if that is earlier – see below. The start of the jobseeking period is usually just the day you claim JSA, and you count 3 years back from there to work out your contribution years. So if you claim in July 1997, your contribution years are 1994–95 and 1995–96. But there are linking rules that mean the jobseeking period may start earlier.

Jobseeking period and linking rules – The jobseeking period is any period for which you claim and satisfy the basic conditions of entitlement to JSA (see Chapter 14(2)), or you get a hardship payment, or you're not paid JSA but are signing on to protect your NI contribution record. A period where you lose entitlement due to failing to sign on or attend an appointment, or you are not entitled because you are involved in a trade dispute, is not included in the jobseeking period.

Any two jobseeking periods link together and are treated as one single jobseeking period if they are separated by:
■ 12 weeks or less; or
■ one or more 'linked periods'; or
■ a period on jury service.

Gaps of 12 weeks or less in between jobseeking periods and linked periods, or in between linked periods are ignored. '*Linked periods*' are periods when you are incapable of work,

or entitled to maternity allowance, or training and getting a training allowance.

It is the beginning of the jobseeking period or any linked period that is used to decide which years you must satisfy the contribution conditions for JSA.

For example, if your incapacity benefit ends and you sign on for JSA instead, so long as you claim JSA within 12 weeks of the end of your incapacity benefit claim, your contribution years for your JSA claim will be the same as they were for your earlier incapacity benefit claim.

Another linking rule helps people who gave up work to care for someone, to qualify for JSA on the basis of the contributions they paid when they were working. If you were getting invalid care allowance and this ended within 12 weeks of the beginning of your jobseeking period (or linked period), the period of ICA entitlement also links to the jobseeking period – if this would help you satisfy the contribution conditions for JSA. So your 'benefit year' would be the year in which your ICA entitlement began.

4. Contribution conditions for benefit

The first condition – paid contributions

❏ **For contribution-based jobseeker's allowance** you must actually have paid Class 1 contributions on earnings 25 times the lower earnings limit, in either one of the two complete tax years before the start of the benefit year in which you make your claim or in which your jobseeking period (or 'linked period') began – see 3 above.

So if you claim in the 1997 benefit year, you pass the first condition if you paid Class 1 contributions on earnings of £1,425 between April 1994 and April 1995, or on earnings of £1,450 between April 1995 and April 1996.

❏ **For incapacity benefit** you must actually have paid in *any* complete tax year:
■ Class 1 contributions on earnings of 25 times the lower earnings limit for that tax year; or
■ 25 Class 2 contributions; or
■ a mixture of Class 1 and Class 2 contributions, totalling 25 times the lower earnings limit for that year; or
■ before 6 April 1975, 26 flat rate Class 1 or Class 2 contributions.

A Class 2 contribution counts as a contribution on earnings of the amount of the lower earnings limit for that tax year (ie £62 for 1997–98).

Lower earnings limits

1988–89	£41	1993–94	£56
1989–90	£43	1994–95	£57
1990–91	£46	1995–96	£58
1991–92	£52	1996–97	£61
1992–93	£54	1997–98	£62

The second condition – paid or credited contributions

In each of the two tax years before the start of your benefit year you must have paid or been credited with contributions. For incapacity benefit and contribution-based JSA you must have paid, or been credited with, Class 1 contributions (Class 1 or Class 2 for incapacity benefit) on earnings of 50 times the lower earnings limit for that tax year in each of the two tax years.

If your benefit year is 1996, you meet this condition if you paid contributions on earnings of £2,800 in the 1993–94 tax year and of £2,850 in the 1994–95 tax year.

If your benefit year is 1997, you meet this condition if you paid contributions on earnings of £2,850 in the 1994–95 tax year, and of £2,900 in the 1995–96 tax year.

A credited contribution counts as a Class 1 contribution on earnings of the amount of the lower earnings limit for that tax year (see above). You can combine credits and paid contributions.

Maternity
Most employees will get statutory maternity pay (SMP). SMP does not depend on contributions. If you don't get SMP, for whatever reason, you may qualify for maternity allowance. This does have a contribution test, explained in Chapter 26.

10 Statutory sick pay

1. What is statutory sick pay?
Statutory sick pay (SSP) is paid to employees by their employers for up to 28 weeks in any period of sickness.

SSP does not depend on National Insurance contributions. You can work full or part-time, but you must earn at least the lower earnings limit for NI contributions (£62 from April 1997). SSP is taxable and is itself subject to NI contributions. There are no additions for dependants.

SSP is primarily the responsibility of employers. An outline of the scheme is in the *Employer's Quick Guide to Pay As You Earn and National Insurance Contributions*, CWG1. Much more detail is in CA30, *Employer's Manual on Statutory Sick Pay*.

Unemployed and self-employed people are not covered by SSP. If you cannot get SSP, you can claim incapacity benefit instead – see Chapter 11.

If your SSP and any other income is below your income support 'applicable amount', you can claim income support to top it up – see Chapter 3. If you don't get income support, you may nevertheless get housing benefit because SSP is treated more generously under that scheme – see Chapter 4.

2. Do you qualify?
There are three key terms that describe the qualifying conditions for SSP:
❑ SSP Period of Incapacity for Work (PIW);
❑ Period of Entitlement (PE);
❑ Qualifying Days (QD).

You can only be paid SSP if you are sick on a Qualifying Day and your days of sickness form part of a SSP Period of Incapacity for Work that comes within a Period of Entitlement. These three different qualifying conditions are explained in 3 to 5 below.

3. SSP 'Period of Incapacity for Work'
The first qualifying condition for SSP is that there must be a SSP 'Period of Incapacity for Work' (PIW). This means that you must be incapable of doing the job you're employed to do, because of sickness or disability for at least 4 days in a row. Sundays and Public Holidays count – therefore, every day of the week can count towards a SSP PIW, including days when you wouldn't have worked anyway even if you had been fit. SSP PIWs that are separated by 8 weeks or less are 'linked' and count as one PIW.

Your employer is entitled to ask for reasonable evidence of your incapacity for work. For the first 7 days of a spell of sickness, you may need to provide some type of self-certification, for example, DSS form SC2 or a special form provided by your employer. During the first 7 days of any spell of sickness you cannot be asked to produce a doctor's sicknote. But after the first 7 days you will usually be expected to get a doctor's sicknote.

Note that there are some situations when you'll still qualify even if you are not actually sick on a particular day. You can be treated as incapable of work for days when you are under medical care, or a doctor has advised you not to work for precautionary or convalescent reasons, provided you do not work on those days. You are also treated as incapable of work if you are under medical observation because you are a carrier, or have been in contact with an infectious disease, and a Medical Officer for Environmental Health has issued a certificate excluding you from work.

The term 'period of incapacity for work' is also used for other benefits, in particular, incapacity benefit. But the rules are different for SSP. If you are receiving certain types of treatment, eg radiotherapy, you may find that days of treatment do not form a SSP PIW, even though they do form a 'period of incapacity for work' for incapacity benefit purposes. So you might qualify for incapacity benefit instead. Days on SSP do count for some incapacity benefit purposes (eg deciding when you move onto the higher rate) but do not count towards 'periods of incapacity for work' for any other benefit other than SSP.

4. Period of entitlement
The second qualifying condition for SSP is that there has to be a 'Period of Entitlement' (PE). This just means the actual period of time when you are entitled to SSP. It begins with the start of the SSP Period of Incapacity for Work and ends when your employer's liability to pay you SSP ends.

Your employer's liability to pay SSP ends if:
- you are no longer sick; or
- you have had 28 weeks of SSP, either in one go or 'linked'; or
- your contract of employment comes to an end (unless your employer has dismissed you solely or mainly to avoid paying you SSP); or
- for pregnant women, you are at the start of the 'disqualifying period'. This is the 18 weeks during which you are entitled to SMP or maternity allowance. If you are entitled to neither then the start of the 18 week disqualifying period depends on whether or not SSP is being paid to you:
  – if you are getting SSP, it cannot be paid beyond the day your baby is born or, if earlier, beyond the first day you are off work sick with a pregnancy related illness on or after the start of the 6th week before the expected week of confinement;
  – if you are not getting SSP, it cannot be paid from the earlier of either the start of the week your baby is born or the start of the week you are first off sick with a pregnancy related illness if this is after the beginning of the 6th week before your expected week of confinement; or
- you are taken into legal custody; or
- your 'linked' SSP Period of Incapacity for Work has spanned 3 years.

SSP will also end if your employer no longer considers you to be incapable of work. In this case, you can appeal against the decision – see 10 below.

People who cannot get SSP
In some circumstances, you won't be entitled to SSP at all (so no Period of Entitlement can start). These circumstances are listed in Box E.4 but remember that they have to apply on the first day of a SSP Period of Incapacity for Work for you to be excluded from SSP altogether.

5. Qualifying days

SSP is only paid for days that are 'qualifying days'. These are normally the days you would have been required to work under the terms of your contract if you hadn't been sick – but they don't have to be.

If your working pattern varies from one week to another, for example, if you work on a rota system, you and your employer can come to some other arrangement as to which days will be the qualifying days. As long as you and your employer reach agreement, you have a free choice of qualifying days – so long as they are not fixed by reference to the actual days you are off sick, and that there is at least one qualifying day in each week.

If you can't reach agreement with your employer, the qualifying days are the days your contract would have required you to work if you hadn't fallen sick. If it isn't clear which days would be working days in a particular week, the law says that every day of that week, except days you and your employer agree are rest days, should be SSP qualifying days.

If you wouldn't normally have worked in a particular week and don't have an agreement on qualifying days with your employer, the law says that the Wednesday of that week will be a qualifying day regardless.

If there are any doubts about qualifying days, it is important to sort this out with your employer.

SSP is not paid for the first three qualifying days of a SSP Period of Incapacity for Work (PIW) – these are known as 'waiting days'. However, you do not need to wait another three days if you reclaim SSP and your second spell of sickness starts no more than 8 weeks after the end of the first PIW. The different PIWs are linked together and count as one continuous PIW. If different PIWs are linked in this way, your right to SSP in the later linked PIWs depends on your circumstances at the start of the first one.

6. How much do you get?

SSP is £55.70 a week. There are no additions for dependants.

To qualify, your average weekly earnings must be at least the level of the lower earnings limit for NI contributions (£62 from 6.4.97). To arrive at an average weekly figure, gross earnings are averaged over the 8 weeks ending with the last pay day before the start of the SSP Period of Incapacity for Work.

SSP is subject to deductions for income tax and NI contributions. However, no NI deductions are due if SSP is the only payment you receive when you are sick because SSP is below the lower earnings limit for NI contributions. Other normal deductions, such as union subs, can also be made from SSP. It is important to make sure that your payslip details any SSP payments you have received, together with any deductions made by your employer, so you can check that it's all correct.

Payment of SSP

You should normally be paid SSP at the same time and in the same way as you would have been paid wages for the same period. Note that SSP cannot be paid in kind, or as board and lodging, or through a service.

If there has been some disagreement with your employer about your entitlement to SSP and the Adjudication Officer (AO) based at the DSS states you are entitled to it (provided you pass all the other tests), your employer must pay SSP within a certain time limit. These time limits are laid down in the law – see also 11. In certain circumstances, if your employer defaults on payment of SSP or becomes insolvent, liability for any outstanding SSP transfers to the Secretary of State.

Occupational sick pay

If your employer runs an occupational sick pay scheme, any sick pay you get under that scheme usually counts towards your SSP entitlement for a particular day (and vice versa). But if the occupational scheme pays less than your full SSP, your

---

E.4 Who cannot get SSP?

You are not entitled to SSP if on the first day of your SSP Period of Incapacity for Work, any of the following apply.

- ❏ You are over 65. But if you become 65 during a Period of Entitlement and don't plan to retire immediately, SSP should continue to the end of that Period of Entitlement.
- ❏ Your contract of employment is for a set period of 3 months or less – unless your employer has extended your contract beyond 3 months before your Period of Incapacity for Work (PIW) begins, or you've been employed continuously for over 3 months on a series of short contracts. Special rules apply if you have more than one contract of employment with the same employer.
- ❏ Your average earnings are below £62 a week. But remember the PIW linking rule – the first day of the first linked PIW should be used when working out your average earnings. If a new tax year starts while you're receiving SSP, this makes no difference (but you will get any increase in payment).
- ❏ You've received incapacity benefit, severe disablement allowance or maternity allowance within the previous 57 days.
- ❏ There is a stoppage of work at your workplace due to a trade dispute and you have a direct interest in the outcome.
- ❏ You have already received SSP for 28 weeks in the same PIW from your employer. If you moved jobs, see 14.
- ❏ You are pregnant and already into the 'disqualifying period' – see 4.
- ❏ You are in a country which is outside the European Economic Area (but you are entitled if your employer is liable for Class 1 contributions for you or would be if your earnings were high enough) – see Chapter 41.
- ❏ You are in legal custody.
- ❏ You have not yet done any work for your employer.

Remember that PIWs with the same employer which are separated by 8 weeks or less count as one continuous PIW – they are 'linked' together.

What happens if you cannot get SSP?

You won't be entitled to SSP if you come into one of these groups. Once you have been off sick for 4 days in a row and your employer decides you cannot get SSP, s/he is required by law to complete form SSP1 (or their own version of this form), and send it to you within 7 days, or if payroll arrangements make this impracticable, by the first payday in the following tax month. There is a legal penalty for failing to do so.

Form SSP1 tells you and the DSS why your employer is not paying you SSP. When you're sent this form, you should also be sent back any sicknotes you sent to your employer. The rest of form SSP1 is a claim for incapacity benefit for you to complete and send to your local DSS office with any sicknotes you have – see Chapter 11. If your employer gives you their own version of the SSP1, they must also give you a blank DSS form SSP1. You should fill in the incapacity benefit claim section and send this together with your employer's version of the SSP1.

E.5 Lengthy absences

If you are off work for a long time, your employer may ask the DSS for an opinion on your continuing incapacity for work. S/he can do this if your absence seems unduly lengthy, given the cause of incapacity. Employers are expected to try and resolve any problem themselves. The DSS only help where the employer has been unable to make their own arrangements to get more medical advice. If a serious illness or injury has been diagnosed, the DSS would not expect to help the employer – they consider that 'control action would not be appropriate in such cases'.

Your employer can only refer your case to the DSS if you consent. The DSS will only assist if you give your consent and if they agree that the absence does seem unduly long. The table below gives the DSS's guide on the more common and less serious ailments. This suggests the time by which your employer should have started some form of control action – but there is nothing in law to stop them taking action sooner.

If the DSS agree to help, they will consult your doctor and may ask you to attend for a medical examination. The DSS report will not be sent to your employer – s/he will only be told whether or not you are considered to be capable of work. This is not a decision, it is only to help your employer decide whether payment of SSP should continue. If your employer stops SSP and you disagree see 10.

Illness or diagnosis	Control (by months)
Addiction (drugs or alcohol)	6
Anaemia (other than in pregnancy)	4
Arthritis (unspecified)	6
Back and spinal disorders (PID – slipped disc, sciatica, spondylitis)	6
Concussion	1
Fractures of upper limbs	2
Fractures of lower limbs	6
Gastroenteritis, gastritis, diarrhoea and vomiting	1
Haemorrhage	3
Headache, migraine	1
Hernia (strangulated)	6
Inflammation and swelling	1
Joint disorders, other than arthritis and rheumatism	3
Kidney and bladder disorders, cystitis, UTI	3
Menstrual disorders, menorrhagia, D&C	3
Miscellaneous symptoms & diagnoses, anorexia, debility, fainting, giddiness, insomnia, investigation, not yet diagnosed, obesity, observation, tachycardia	1
Mouth and throat disorders	1
No abnormality discovered	Immediate
Nervous illnesses	3
Post-natal conditions	6
Respiratory illness ■ cold, coryza, URTI, influenza	1
■ bronchitis	2
■ asthma	6
Skin conditions, dermatitis, eczema	2
Sprains, strains, bruises	1
Ulcers ■ peptic, gastric, duodenal, corneal	2
■ perforated	9
■ varicose	6
Wounds, cuts, lacerations, abrasions, burns, blisters, splinters, foreign bodies	1

employer must make up the balance so that you get all the SSP you are due. From April 1997, employers are no longer obliged to operate the rules of the SSP scheme provided that they pay remuneration or occupational sick pay at or above the SSP rate. Employees retain an underlying right to their SSP.

7. Does anything affect what you get?

Other benefits
You cannot get SSP while you are receiving incapacity benefit, severe disablement allowance or maternity allowance. Other benefits do not affect your entitlement to SSP. See Box E.4 for other circumstances when you cannot get SSP.

Earnings from another job
If your employer accepts you are incapable of doing the work s/he employs you to do, you can earn money from a different type of work while receiving SSP. For example, if a milkman injures his leg and can't deliver milk, he may still be fit enough to, say, call Bingo. If so, he can do that and get SSP from his first employer. There is no limit on what you can earn from a different type of job while receiving SSP. However doing other work may lead an employer to doubt you are genuinely incapable of doing your usual job.

Hospital
Going into hospital won't affect entitlement to SSP.

8. How do you get SSP?

To obtain SSP, you need to notify your employer that you're off sick and you may be asked to provide evidence that you're incapable of work.

It is up to your employer to decide what kind of evidence is needed – but s/he cannot ask for a doctor's sicknote for the first 7 days. DSS leaflet CA30 states that an employer is entitled *'to ask for reasonable evidence of incapacity, eg a self-certificate for spells of 4 to 7 days, or a doctor's statement, ie sick note, for periods after the first 7 days'*. You can get a self-certificate form SC2 from a doctor's surgery or DSS office if your employer doesn't have a special form.

Notification of sickness absence
This just means letting your employer know you are sick and incapable of work. To get SSP, you have to provide evidence that you are incapable of work if your employer requires you to do so – see 9.

These are the rules on notification of sickness laid down in the law. Your employer's procedures for SSP must conform to them. But, if you also get occupational sick pay, you'll have to keep to the rules of that scheme to safeguard those payments.

❑ Your employer has to make the rules clear to all the workforce in advance.
❑ Your employer cannot demand notification before the end of the first qualifying day of a Period of Incapacity for Work.
❑ Your employer cannot demand notification in the form of medical evidence. But if you use medical evidence to notify your employer, it should be accepted as OK.
❑ Your employer can't insist you use a special form.
❑ If you post your notification, your employer should treat it as having been given on the day it was posted.
❑ Your employer can't demand notification more than once a week during a spell of sickness.

❑ Your employer must accept notification from someone else on your behalf.
❑ If your employer doesn't make any rules about notification of sickness absence, or the rules don't conform with SSP law, your employer must nevertheless accept notification of sickness on a qualifying day, if it's given in writing no later than 7 days after that day.

Late notification – If your notification of sickness is late according to your employer's rules (and these rules comply with SSP law) you could be disqualified from SSP for any day of incapacity notified late. But SSP can be paid if your employer accepts you have 'good cause' for late notification provided this is given within a month of the normal time limit. This can be extended to 91 days from the day of incapacity if the employer accepts that it was not reasonably practicable for you to contact them within the month. After that time, your employer need not pay SSP for that day even if you have good cause for late notification.

If your employer withholds SSP as s/he does not accept there is good cause for late notification, you can ask the Adjudication Officer at the DSS for a decision.

9. Supporting evidence

DSS leaflet CA30 says that a doctor's sicknote is *'strong evidence of incapacity and should usually be accepted as conclusive unless there is evidence to the contrary'*. (It gives an example of someone said to be incapable of work through an ankle injury who is seen playing football!) A sicknote may be accepted from someone who is not a registered medical practitioner, eg an osteopath, acupuncturist, homeopath, etc.

It is up to your employer to decide whether to accept the evidence that you are incapable of work. If s/he does not accept it, SSP can be withheld. But you can write and ask the DSS for a formal decision.

Employers can decide to use their own self-certificates as evidence of incapacity. Some of these forms are very lengthy and require detailed information. Others will accept a written note from an employee as evidence for the first 7 days of sickness. So it is important to come to some arrangement as to what type of evidence will be acceptable.

For SSP purposes, your employer cannot require initial notice of your sickness in the form of medical evidence, private or otherwise. But after the first 7 days of any spell off-sick they have discretion to ask for supporting medical evidence – eg a doctor's sicknote. If your employer wants more medical evidence s/he must arrange and pay for it – unless the DSS agree to help (see below). S/he can only do this with your consent.

Frequent short spells of sickness
If you are frequently off sick for periods of 4 to 7 days, you may not have seen your doctor, and all your absences will probably be self-certificated.

If you've had at least 4 self-certificated sickness absences over 12 months, and your employer isn't satisfied you've really been incapable of work, s/he should discuss the matter with you, and try and resolve any problem internally. This could involve sending you (with your consent) to a company doctor. If your employer still has any doubts, s/he can refer your case to the DSS for help, but only with your consent.

The DSS should then contact you directly, and will ask you to visit your doctor next time you're sick. If you do fall sick again, your doctor will be asked to give a medical report to a DSS doctor. This can only be done with your consent.

The DSS doctor will be asked to give an independent

E.6 Transfers to incapacity benefit

After 28 weeks on SSP
After 28 weeks on SSP you can go on to higher rate short-term incapacity benefit if you meet the National Insurance contribution conditions – see Chapter 9. If you only pass the contribution conditions part way through your 28 weeks on SSP, you will go on to lower rate short-term incapacity benefit.

Once you have spent a total of 28 weeks on SSP (from the day you satisfied the contribution conditions) together with lower rate short-term incapacity benefit, then you can move on to the higher rate of short-term incapacity benefit. If you are terminally ill, you will be paid the long-term rate of incapacity benefit at this stage.

The higher rate lasts for a further 24 weeks. So if you are still unable to work after 52 weeks altogether, you can then go on to long-term incapacity benefit.

An age addition may be paid with long-term incapacity benefit – see Chapter 11. If you transfer from SSP, it is your age at the beginning of your SSP entitlement that counts.

For any rate of incapacity benefit, after 28 weeks on SSP, you must also pass the 'all work' test to show you are incapable of work, unless you are exempt – see Chapter 8 for details.

SSP ends before 28 weeks
If your SSP ends before your employer has paid the maximum 28 weeks of SSP, you will go on to lower rate short-term incapacity benefit, if you pass the contribution conditions.

When you send in your SSP1 form, the DSS will check to see whether the 'own occupation' or the 'all work' test of incapacity should be applied. It will be the own occupation test if you have worked at least 16 hours a week for more than 8 weeks in the 21 weeks before the first day for which you are claiming incapacity benefit. This means you qualify if you are unable to do your usual work, and you need only send in doctor's sicknotes. Otherwise the all work test will apply straight away, unless you are exempt.

You move on to higher rate short-term incapacity benefit once you have spent 28 weeks in total on SSP and lower rate short-term incapacity benefit. Only the days on SSP after you have passed the contribution conditions count when working out when to move on the higher rate. If you have not already had the all work test applied, it will apply after you have had a total of 28 weeks on SSP and the lower rate. In this case even SSP days before you passed the contribution conditions count.

Transfers to SDA
In order to qualify for SDA, you must have been incapable of work for a continuous period of 196 days. So it is only possible to transfer straight to SDA if you have received SSP for 28 weeks with no breaks at all. You may also need to pass the 80% disablement test and you will have to pass the 'all work' test of incapacity unless you are exempt. See Chapter 13.

Disability working allowance
If you were getting DWA at work, you might be covered by the two year linking rule that allows you to pick up your incapacity benefit at the same rate you left it. Transitional rules also protect levels of benefit for those who got invalidity benefit before 13.4.95. See Chapters 12 and 16.

medical opinion. This will be sent to the Adjudication Officer (AO) at the DSS. The AO takes the decision on whether you're incapable of work. The doctor's report will not be sent to your employer – s/he will only be told whether or not you're considered to be incapable of work. If you are held to be capable of work, and want to appeal – see Chapter 52.

See Box E.5 if you have been off-sick for a long time given the cause of your sickness.

10. Fit for work?

If your employer doesn't accept you are incapable of work, you have the right to ask for a written statement setting out the reasons for this, and details of the dates when you won't receive SSP. You also have the right to apply to the Adjudication Officer at the DSS for a decision – write to your local DSS office. The DSS will expect you to have discussed the matter with your employer where it is reasonable to do so, and to have gone through the agreed grievance procedure if one exists where you work.

Both you and your employer will be asked to send comments in writing to the DSS. You can provide other evidence eg further medical statements. A copy of the decision will be sent both to you and your employer. If the decision says you are incapable of work, your employer must pay you the correct amount of SSP within fixed time limits, providing that you pass the other tests for SSP.

Both you and your employer have the right to appeal against the decision to a Social Security Appeal Tribunal. If your employer appeals, s/he does not have to pay SSP until a final decision has been given.

11. Enforcing a decision

If an Adjudication Officer, SSAT or Social Security Commissioner has issued a formal written decision that you are entitled to SSP, and your employer doesn't pay it within the time laid down by law, tell your DSS office. In this situation, the responsibility for paying SSP transfers to the Secretary of State. The DSS will pay any SSP to which you are entitled.

12. What information will the DSS give?

In order to decide whether you are entitled to SSP, your employer can ask the local DSS office for limited information about you. Before disclosing it, the DSS should be satisfied that the enquiry actually comes from your employer and no one else. The DSS has told employers that detailed personal information about employees will continue to be treated as confidential, and not be disclosed.

13. What happens when SSP ends?

If you're still sick at the start of the 23rd week of your Period of Entitlement to SSP, your employer has to complete and send you DSS form SSP1 (the Changeover Form) to help you transfer to incapacity benefit. In some cases, your employer will have to issue the SSP1 earlier. For example, if your employer's liability to pay SSP is due to end before the 23rd week of sickness, or SSP ends unexpectedly, or if you are off sick for 4 or more days in a row but you are not entitled to SSP. The employer should issue the SSP1 within 7 days of notification of sickness, or if payroll arrangements make this impracticable, by the first payday in the tax month after the one in which the reason for issuing the SSP1 arose.

On the form, your employer has to tick off the reasons why s/he considers you're no longer entitled to SSP. The SSP1 also has a section for you to complete and send to the local DSS office so that you can claim incapacity benefit. The employer can choose to issue their own version of the SSP1. If they do, they must also send you a blank DSS form SSP1. You should fill in your part of the DSS form and send it to the DSS together with your employer's version.

Box E.6 explains the rules for transferring to incapacity benefit. When your employer gives you the SSP1, you should fill in the incapacity benefit claim form and send it to your local DSS office. If you are not sure of being off-sick after 28 weeks, complete the form anyway and send it in. If you wait right until the end of the SSP period before claiming incapacity benefit, you are likely to have a gap in payments. Sending the form to the DSS in advance gives them time to check your NI contribution record, process your claim, and make sure you can be paid incapacity benefit without a break.

If your employer is holding any of your doctor's statements (sicknotes) which cover days beyond the last day of your SSP entitlement, these should be returned to you, with form SSP1. Send them on to the DSS with your completed form.

After 28 weeks on SSP, you will go on to higher rate short-term incapacity benefit if you satisfy the NI contribution conditions at the beginning of your SSP period and the DSS accept you are incapable of work. The DSS will assess your incapacity under the 'all work' test – see Chapter 8(9). Higher rate short-term incapacity benefit is the same amount as SSP, £55.70 a week, but you may be able to claim additions for adult and/or child dependants.

14. What if your job ends?

If you have had a SSP Period of Incapacity for Work (PIW) which ended no more than 8 weeks before your current contract of service ends, and were paid SSP for at least a week, your employer must give you a leaver's statement, on DSS form SSP1(L) or their own version of this form. You must ask your employer to give you the SSP1(L); they don't need to give it to you automatically. They must then supply the form within 7 days of your request, or if payroll arrangements make this impracticable, by the first payday of the following tax month.

This statement will give the date of your first day of sickness in that PIW. If you have a linked PIW, it will state the very first day of incapacity in that linked PIW. The leaver's statement will also state the last day for which SSP was payable and the number of weeks of SSP payable during that PIW. Where you have some odd days of SSP, 3 days will round down and 4 will round up, both to the nearest whole week.

Starting a new job

If you go to a new employer and fall sick again no later than 8 weeks after the end of your previous PIW, your position is partly protected. This happens where you have given your new employer a leaver's statement from your last job within 7 days of your first qualifying day for SSP in the new job. Your employer may have set a longer time limit. If you hand over your leaver's statement late (but within 91 days of the first qualifying day of sickness in the new job) your employer can take it into account if you have 'good cause' for your delay.

Your new employer can take into account the number of weeks of SSP you have already received in the previous PIW. If you have had, say, 15 weeks of SSP from your old employer, and the new spell off sick starts within 8 weeks of the previous spell, your new employer will only be liable to pay you 13 weeks of SSP during the PIW with the new employer. However, this is the only way in which a PIW can straddle a change of jobs. For all other purposes your right to SSP and the rate of payment depend on your situation on the first day of incapacity in the PIW with your new employer: eg you will have to serve 3 'waiting days' again and will be paid SSP from the 4th qualifying day.

No job to go to
If you had less than 28 weeks worth of SSP from your last employer, and are still incapable of work, you can claim lower rate short-term incapacity benefit on form SSP1. But note that if your employer is found to have dismissed you solely or mainly to avoid paying SSP, s/he remains liable to pay SSP until liability ends for some other reason. Whatever the reason for your dismissal you should claim incapacity benefit on the SSP1. Seek advice if you have difficulties or would not qualify for incapacity benefit. Lower rate short-term incapacity benefit is £8.60 a week less than SSP, but you might be able to claim an addition for an adult dependant – see Chapter 11(3).

After a total of 28 linked weeks on SSP and lower rate short-term incapacity benefit, you can go on to higher rate short-term incapacity benefit. Box E.6 gives details.

11 Incapacity benefit

In this chapter we look at:	
What is incapacity benefit?	see 1
Do you qualify?	see 2
How much do you get?	see 3
Does anything affect what you get?	see 4
Income tax	see Box E.7
What happens on retirement?	see 5
How do you claim?	see 6
How are you paid?	see 7
Reviews and appeals	see 8

1. What is incapacity benefit?
Incapacity benefit is for people unable to work because of illness or disability. It replaced sickness benefit and invalidity benefit from 13.4.95. You must have paid enough National Insurance contributions to qualify. Incapacity benefit is not means-tested, so the amount you get does not depend on your income or savings. You should claim if you can't get statutory sick pay (eg you are not employed or you are self-employed) or if your statutory sick pay has run out – see Chapter 10. Your incapacity for work is assessed for the first 28 weeks of incapacity under the 'own occupation' test which looks at your ability to do your usual job if you've worked recently. Otherwise, you are assessed under the 'all work' test, unless your circumstances exempt you from the test.

People who were getting sickness or invalidity benefit before 13.4.95 were transferred automatically on to incapacity benefit – see Chapter 12. There are transitional rules which protect the level of benefit for people claiming before the new benefit came in, but most people have to pass the 'all work' test of incapacity to continue to receive benefit.

2. Do you qualify?
You qualify for short-term incapacity benefit if:
- you are 'incapable of work' – see below and Chapter 8(3); and
- you are in a 'period of incapacity for work' – see below; and
- you cannot get statutory sick pay – see Box E.4 in Chapter 10; and
- you are under pension age (60 for women, 65 for men); and
- you satisfy the National Insurance contribution conditions – see Chapter 9(4) – (or you claim under the special rules for widows and widowers – see Chapter 46); or

- you are no more than 5 years over pension age, your 'period of incapacity for work' began before pension age and you would be entitled to retirement pension if you claimed it – see 5 below.

You cannot be paid benefit for the first 3 days of your claim. These are called waiting days. However, if your claim is linked to an earlier period of incapacity for work or a period on statutory sick pay (ie you have claimed not more than 8 weeks since the end of the last spell of sickness), you can be paid from the first day of your claim in the new period of incapacity for work.

For the first 28 weeks of incapacity you get the short-term lower rate. If you are transferring from statutory sick pay, see Box E.6 in Chapter 10.

After 28 weeks on the lower rate, you move on to the short-term higher rate. This is paid from week 29 to week 52.

If you are entitled to disability living allowance higher rate care component or you are terminally ill, you are paid at the long-term rate after 28 weeks of incapacity.

After 52 weeks of incapacity the long-term rate becomes payable. You are entitled to 364 days short-term benefit (which can include entitlement to statutory sick pay) before moving to long-term benefit. The days of incapacity may be consecutive or in linked 'periods of incapacity for work'.

Period of incapacity for work
To qualify for incapacity benefit, each day of your claim must be a 'day of incapacity for work'. These days must be part of a 'period of incapacity for work'. This means that you must have at least 4 days in a row before you can begin to qualify. The first 3 days of your claim are waiting days and you're not paid for these days. Once you've qualified, if you have a gap in your incapacity of up to 8 weeks (eg if you go back to work) you can reclaim when you have another 4 or more days of incapacity and go straight back on to incapacity benefit at the same rate without serving the 3 waiting days again. You can't be paid for odd days of incapacity. But if you receive certain kinds of regular treatment such as dialysis, you can be paid if you are treated for 2 or more days a week, including days of recuperation if that is part of the treatment. In this case, you don't need to be incapable of work for 4 days in a row. But you'll only be paid for the actual days of treatment unless the other days of the week are also days of incapacity.

What is a 'day of incapacity'? – A day of incapacity is a day on which you are 'incapable of work'. This depends on passing either the 'own occupation' test which looks at whether you are fit for your usual work if you have worked recently, or the 'all work' test which assesses your ability to do any work. These tests are explained in Chapter 8.

A day of incapacity also includes a day on which you are 'treated' as incapable of work (eg you're in hospital, or dialysing – Chapter 8(4)), or you are exempt from the all work test (Chapter 8(9)) or you are entitled to maternity allowance.

What is a 'period of incapacity for work'? – Your days of incapacity must link together in a 'period of incapacity for work' which is made up of:
- 4 or more consecutive days of incapacity; and/or
- 2 or more days of incapacity whether consecutive or not out of 7 consecutive days (including Sunday), when your incapacity results from:
  - regular weekly peritoneal or haemodialysis for chronic renal failure: or
  - treatment by way of plasmapheresis, chemotherapy with cytotoxic drugs, anti-tumour agents or immunosuppressive drugs or radiotherapy; or
  - regular weekly treatment by way of total parenteral

nutrition for gross impairment of enteric function.
Any two or more of these periods which are no more than 8 weeks apart are linked together and count as just one continuous period of incapacity for work. Sundays count towards a period of incapacity for work.

The rules for SSP are different. SSP periods of incapacity for work are explained in Chapter 10. Days on SSP don't count towards an incapacity benefit period of incapacity for work – see Box E.6 in Chapter 10 for details of transferring from SSP to incapacity benefit.

Why are periods of incapacity for work important?
Periods of incapacity for work are important for a number of reasons. We outline some key points below. If your period of incapacity for work is linked with a period on SSP – see Box E.6.

- Incapacity benefit is not paid for the first three days of a period of incapacity for work (waiting days) but if you fall sick again within 8 weeks, the two spells are linked together and you don't have to wait another three days.
- The first day of your current period of incapacity for work determines which tax years are the ones in which you must have met the contribution conditions for incapacity benefit – see Chapter 9(3).
- If you are still in the same period of incapacity for work as when you last got incapacity benefit, you can go straight back on at the same rate if you fall sick again.
- If the first day of your period of incapacity for work is before you reach pension age, you can claim short-term incapacity benefit beyond pension age.
- Your age on the first day of your current period of incapacity for work determines entitlement to an age allowance with long-term incapacity benefit.

3. How much do you get?

Short-term

Week 1–28	lower rate	£47.10
	adult dependant	£29.15
Week 29–52	higher rate	£55.70
	adult dependant	£29.15
	child dependant	
	first child	£9.90
	each other child	£11.20

Long-term

After 52 weeks	basic rate	£62.45
(or 28 weeks*)	adult dependant	£37.35
	child dependant	
	first child	£9.90
	each other child	£11.20
	age addition	
	under 35	£13.15
	35–44	£6.60

* Long-term rate is payable after 28 weeks, if you are entitled to DLA higher rate care component or are terminally ill.

If you were getting invalidity benefit before 13.4.95, your level of benefit is protected – see Chapter 12.

Additions for dependants
You may be able to get extra benefit for any children living with you once you move on to the higher rate of short-term incapacity benefit or the long-term rate. If you are over pension age, you can claim for children when you're on the lower rate as well. If you have any children living with you, you may also be able to get extra benefit for your partner or someone who looks after your children. If you don't have children, you may be able to claim extra for your husband or wife if they are aged over 60. Your partner's (or other dependant's) earnings may affect the additions – see 4.

You must claim separately for the dependant's additions. You have 3 months to make a claim. If you claim after this time, you will lose benefit. The incapacity benefit claim pack has a section to fill in if you want to claim extra benefit for an adult or children.

Adult dependants – You qualify for an adult dependant's addition if:

- your wife or husband is 60 or over and they either live with you, or you contribute to their maintenance at least to the level of the adult dependant's addition; or
- you live with your wife or husband (of any age) and you are also entitled to an addition for a dependent child; or
- you live with an adult (who may be your unmarried, or lesbian or gay partner or a relative or friend) who looks after a child for whom you are entitled to an addition; or
- you contribute to the maintenance of, or employ, an adult who does not live with you, to look after a child for whom you are entitled to an addition, and you pay at least the amount of the adult dependant's addition to the person's maintenance or for caring for the child.

While you are on lower rate short-term incapacity benefit, where the qualifying conditions above depend on you being entitled to an addition for a dependant child, you satisfy this if you fulfil the conditions for receipt of an addition for a child even though child dependant additions are not payable with the lower rate.

Child dependants – You qualify for an addition for any dependent child if:

- you are entitled to child benefit for that child and either the child lives with you or you contribute at least the amount of the addition to their maintenance (and more than the amount of child benefit); or
- you live with the child and the child's parent who gets child benefit, and;
  – you are also the child's parent; or
  – you maintain the child at least to the level of the addition and before you were incapable of work you contributed more than half the actual cost of maintenance for the child if s/he was a dependant (eg you are a step-father).

See Chapter 27 for details of child benefit entitlement.

Age addition
Age additions are payable only with the long-term rate. It is your age on the first day of your 'period of incapacity for work' that counts for determining whether an age addition is payable – see 2 above. If you are under 35 on the first day of your period of incapacity for work, you get the higher amount of £13.15. If you are at least 35 but have not reached your 45th birthday on the first day of your period of incapacity for work, you get the lower amount of £6.60. The addition is paid at the same rate while you are in the same period of incapacity. So if you are 45 or over and have a break in your claim of over 8 weeks, you cannot regain the age addition. If you are transferring from statutory sick pay, see Box E.6 in Chapter 10.

Over pension age
You may be able to claim short-term incapacity benefit – the rates are higher – see 5 below. You cannot receive long-term incapacity benefit beyond pension age, but see 5.

Terminal illness
If you are terminally ill, you are paid at the long-term rate after 28 weeks, instead of 52. You count as terminally ill if you *'suffer from a progressive disease and [your] death can reasonably be expected within 6 months'*. (Box G.4 in Chapter 17 looks at the legal definition of terminal illness.)

Disability living allowance
If you are entitled to DLA higher rate care component you are paid at the long-term rate after 28 weeks instead of 52.

DWA or training schemes
There are special linking rules for people reclaiming incapacity benefit after a spell on disability working allowance (see Chapter 16(6)) or on a training scheme (see Chapter 15(12)).

4. Does anything affect what you get?

Other benefits
You cannot get incapacity benefit as well as retirement pension or jobseeker's allowance. Other benefits such as maternity allowance, severe disablement allowance, invalid care allowance and unemployability supplement are known as overlapping benefits. You can receive an amount equal to the highest of these benefits. Widows' benefits also overlap – see Chapter 46.

Other benefits can be paid on top, including disability living allowance, attendance allowance and disablement benefit. Disability working allowance can be paid on top, but incapacity benefit is taken into account in the DWA assessment.

If your income is low, you might get income support to top it up. If you get long-term incapacity benefit, you could get the disability premium or higher pensioner premium with income support, or with housing or council tax benefit – see Chapters 3 and 4.

Other income
Incapacity benefit is not means-tested so it is not affected if you receive wages or an occupational pension or sick pay while you are off sick. You might have more income tax deducted from your pay or pension if you get the taxable short-term higher rate or long-term incapacity benefit – see Box E.7.

Work
Generally if you do any work you are treated as capable of work and thus cannot get incapacity benefit. However, some work is exempt from this rule – see Chapter 8(5).

Disqualification
You can be disqualified from benefit for up to six weeks in certain situations – see Chapter 8(6).

Income tax
Incapacity benefit is taxable after 28 weeks of incapacity – see Box E.7.

Hospital
You can carry on getting incapacity benefit while in hospital, but after 6 weeks the amount you get will be reduced – see Chapter 39(8).

Partner's earnings
Your partner's earnings do not affect your basic benefit, but can affect the additions for children and dependent adults. Occupational and personal pensions count as earnings.

Earnings are taken into account after deductions for tax

E.7 Income tax
Higher rate short-term and long-term incapacity benefit are taxable (but see below for exceptions), as are any additions paid with these rates other than the child dependant's addition.

Who does not have to pay tax?
- The lower rate of short-term incapacity benefit is tax-free.
- Any child dependant's addition is also tax free.
- If you transferred in April 1995 from invalidity benefit to long-term incapacity benefit, your incapacity benefit remains tax-free. But if you reclaim after a break of over 8 weeks, you lose this protection and benefit will be taxed as normal.
- If you get a transitional award of long-term incapacity benefit under the linking rules for DWA or training schemes, your benefit remains tax-free – see Chapter 12(4).
- You do not have to pay tax if your total taxable income, including incapacity benefit, is below a certain level. This level depends on your tax allowances – see Chapter 51.

How do you pay tax?
If you have other income – If you get an occupational pension or are still being paid by an employer, your tax code is adjusted to take into account the amount of your taxable benefit. Your incapacity benefit is paid in full, but the tax is taken off your pay or pension.

If incapacity benefit is your main income – Where incapacity benefit is your main or only taxable income, any tax due is taken off your benefit by the DSS before it is paid to you.

The DSS will calculate any tax due using a tax code, similar to the way employers do. This code gives your tax allowances. You will be sent a form P2, *Notice of your income tax code*, by the Inland Revenue. It is important to ensure that this includes all the allowances you are entitled to, otherwise you could pay too much tax. Chapter 51 outlines the different types of tax allowances and explains what the tax codes mean.

The incapacity benefit claim form can be used to claim the Married Couple's Allowance and the Blind Person's Allowance. If you have a form P45 given to you by your last employer, you should give this to the DSS, unless they have told you that your incapacity benefit is not taxable, or you need to claim a tax refund. If you think there are other allowances you should be getting, or you think the DSS are deducting the wrong amount of tax, you should contact the Tax Office at the address below.

For more information
Leaflet IR 144, *Income Tax and Incapacity Benefit* and leaflet P3(IB), *Incapacity Benefit: Understanding Your Tax Code*, give more information.

If you already pay tax under PAYE on a pension or by your employer, you should contact your local Tax Office for advice or assistance. If incapacity benefit is your only or main income, there is a special tax office which you should contact: *HM Inspector of Taxes, Leicester 4 District, Attenborough House, 109-119 Charles Street, Leicester, LE1 1FZ; telephone 0116 242 5963, Minicom 0116 251 3764.*

and NI contributions, and certain other disregards (see 'Calculating earnings' below).

Child dependant's addition – If you are living with your husband or wife, or co-habiting, your partner's earnings may affect the amount you get for dependent children.

If your partner earns £135 or more a week, you lose one addition for a dependent child. For each extra £17 that your partner earns above £135, you lose an addition for one other child.

Adult dependant's addition – For short-term incapacity benefit, you lose the addition if your partner earns more than £29.15 a week (or £35.90 if you are over pension age). For long-term incapacity benefit (including those paid the long-term rate due to terminal illness or receipt of DLA higher rate care component), you lose the addition once your partner earns over £49.15 a week, if your partner lives with you. If you maintain someone who does not live with you, you lose the addition paid with the long-term rate if they earn over £37.35.

You can get an addition for an adult who you employ to care for your child. If the person lives with you, any wages you pay them for caring for the child are disregarded. If the person does not live with you, all their earnings from any source are disregarded.

If your partner's earnings are over the limit, you lose the addition in the following week. If earnings are not over the limit, the addition is not affected at all, you will get it in full.

If your adult dependant gets a benefit in their own right, your addition for them may be reduced or not paid at all. This is because of the overlapping benefit rules. For example, if your partner gets invalid care allowance this cancels out the addition paid with long-term incapacity benefit.

Calculating earnings
In working out how much of a partner's earnings are taken into account, certain deductions and disregards can be taken from gross earnings. The same rules apply when working out earnings from 'therapeutic' work if you get incapacity benefit or SDA – see Chapter 8(5). Count any payment from your employer as earnings, eg bonus, commission, payments for childminding, retainer, pay in lieu of notice. Occupational and personal pensions count as earnings for dependant's additions. If you're self-employed, the rules on working out net profit follow the income support rules – see Chapter 3(25). From your gross weekly earnings (or net profit) deduct:

- income tax and NI contributions (Class 1, 2 or 4);
- half of any contribution to an occupational or personal pension;
- expenses *'wholly, exclusively and necessarily incurred in the performance of the duties of the employment'*, eg equipment, special clothing, travel between workplaces;
- advance of earnings or a loan from your employer;
- childcare charges of up to £60 a week for children under 11 – the rule is the same as for disability working allowance (see Chapter 16(3));
- fostering allowance;
- payments from a local authority, health authority or voluntary organisation for someone temporarily in your care;
- £4 from rent paid to you by a subtenant plus £9.25 if heating is included;
- £20 a week plus half the rest of the income from a boarder;
- the whole of any contribution towards living and accommodation costs from someone living in your home (other than boarders and subtenants);
- earnings from employment payable abroad where transfer to the UK is prohibited;
- charges for currency conversion;
- annual bounty paid to part-time members of the fire brigade or lifeboat service, or to auxiliary coastguards or members of a territorial or reserve force.

The Social Security (Computation of Earnings) Regs 1996 (SI 1996/2745)
If earnings paid in one week are over the limit, the dependant's addition is lost the following week. Monthly earnings are worked out on a weekly basis and affect benefit for the month ahead. If earnings fluctuate, they are averaged over a recognisable cycle of work or over 5 weeks. One-off payments that are not for any specific period are divided by the relevant earnings limit to work out how many weeks benefit will be affected for.

5. What happens on retirement?

Long-term incapacity benefit
If you are over pension age (60 for women, 65 for men), you cannot normally receive long-term incapacity benefit. Your benefit stops the day you reach pension age. You can only receive long-term incapacity benefit after pension age if you are entitled to a transitional award because you were previously entitled to invalidity benefit and you reached pension age before 13.4.95 – see Chapter 12(2).

If you were getting an age addition with your incapacity benefit within 8 weeks of reaching pension age, this will be paid with your retirement pension (but the SERPS additional pension and the age addition overlap) – see Chapter 44(4) 'Extra pension'.

See Chapter 43(3) and (10) for further information.

Short-term incapacity benefit
You can make a claim for short-term incapacity benefit up to five years beyond pension age if you are in a 'period of incapacity for work' (see 3) which began before you reached pension age. Or you can stay on short-term benefit beyond pension age rather than draw your pension if you choose. You cannot get incapacity benefit and retirement pension at the same time, so you will not get short-term benefit if you draw your pension. You don't have to satisfy the NI contribution conditions for incapacity benefit once you reach pension age. But you will only qualify for, or continue to receive, short-term benefit if you would be entitled to a Category A or B (for widows and widowers) pension if you claimed. Short-term benefit is paid for a maximum of one year.

The basic short-term benefit is £59.90 (both lower and higher rate) a week and you can claim an addition of £35.90 for an adult dependant and £9.90 for the first child, £11.20 for each other child. However, if you would not be entitled to the full rate of retirement pension, your incapacity benefit is cut proportionately. Short-term benefit is tax free for the first 28 weeks, then it is taxable. The amount of short-term benefit is less than the basic retirement pension so you are likely to be worse off if you choose to stay on incapacity benefit. However, you may wish to claim short-term benefit in any case, if you will be going back to work and have deferred claiming retirement pension in order to earn extra increments.

If you get DLA higher rate care component, or you are terminally ill, your short-term benefit is paid at the full long-term rate of £62.45 (see 3 above) after 28 weeks of incapacity but benefit still ends after a year. In this case, if you would not be entitled to a full rate retirement pension, you are better off staying on short-term incapacity benefit.

6. How do you claim?

You claim using the incapacity benefit claim pack, SC1, available from a doctor's surgery, hospital, or the DSS. You should send this to your local DSS office. For the first seven days you do not need a medical certificate. If you are incapable of work for more than seven days, you must also send a medical certificate (form Med 3) from your doctor.

If you work for an employer and do not get statutory sick pay, you will need to send in form SSP1 which you get from your employer.

It is important to keep your medical certificates up to date. Ask your doctor for a new certificate in plenty of time before the old one runs out. If you are not covered by medical evidence for each day of your claim, benefit could be withheld. Until you have passed the all work test or the DSS has decided you are exempt from the test, you must carry on sending in certificates. The DSS will let you know if this is no longer required.

The procedure for assessing your incapacity is explained in Chapter 8(7).

Backdating claims – You can send in your claim form up to three months after the first day for which you wish to claim. Ask your doctor for a backdated medical certificate, form Med 5. Your claim cannot be backdated for longer than this.

However if you were found capable of work and your incapacity benefit entitlement ended, and before it ended you had claimed DLA or constant attendance allowance (CAA), then your next incapacity benefit claim, if made within 3 months of a decision to award you DLA higher rate care component or CAA at the intermediate or exceptional rate, will be backdated to the end of your earlier entitlement (or to the day from which DLA or CAA is first payable if that is later).

If you claimed incapacity benefit before 7.4.97, you had one month to send in your claim form. But if you were later than this, your benefit could be backdated for up to 12 months if you could show you had 'good cause' for not claiming earlier. For claims made from 7.4.97, there is no provision to backdate benefit even if you have good cause. See Chapter 52(4).

7. How are you paid?
Incapacity benefit is usually paid fortnightly in arrears. The DSS can consider weekly payments if fortnightly payments are causing hardship. If you get a transitional award (see Chapter 12) benefit is still paid weekly in arrears as before. You may be paid by an order book, by direct credit transfer into a bank or building society, or by girocheques. Over the next three years there are plans to replace giros and order books with a new plastic payment card.

8. Reviews and appeals
The decision on your claim is made by an Adjudication Officer at the DSS. If you disagree with the decision, you have the right of appeal to an independent tribunal – Social Security Appeal Tribunal – within 3 months of the decision being sent to you. If you are appealing against a decision on your capacity for work, see Chapter 8(12) and Box E.3. For more details on reviews and appeals, see Chapter 52.

Reviews by the DSS – When an Adjudication Officer makes a decision on your claim, a date for a review of your incapacity for work may be fixed, depending on your illness or disability. You are not informed of this date. On review, you may be asked to complete a further all work questionnaire and/or attend a medical examination.

12 Transitional rules

Incapacity benefit was introduced on 13.4.95 to replace sickness benefit and invalidity benefit. In this chapter we look at the rules for people who were on sickness benefit or invalidity benefit before 13.4.95.

The tests of incapacity introduced in April 1995 affect not just claims for incapacity benefit, but also any benefit (but not statutory sick pay) where your incapacity for work needs to be assessed. Some people are exempt from the all work test – see 7 below. For those who are not exempt, their continued entitlement depends on passing the test. We look at the tests of incapacity in detail in Chapter 8. You have the right to appeal if you are found capable of work. See Chapter 8(12) and Box E.3 for how to go about your appeal.

1. Transferring from sickness benefit
If you were entitled to sickness benefit on 12.4.95, you automatically moved on to incapacity benefit. Your benefit became a 'transitional award of short-term incapacity benefit'. The amount of benefit payable is the same as for short-term incapacity benefit – see Chapter 11(3). A transitional award ends when you move on to long-term benefit. If your short-term benefit stops, you can regain a transitional award if you claim again within 8 weeks.

Dependant's addition – You can no longer claim an addition for a wife or husband under the age of 60 unless you have children. But if an addition for an adult dependant was payable with your sickness benefit at any time in the 8 weeks immediately before 13.4.95, you could keep the addition with your transitional award. This protection is lost if the addition is not payable for more than 8 weeks. Once you move on to long-term incapacity benefit, you lose this protection.

Industrial injuries – If you were getting sickness benefit because of an industrial accident or disease, you can move on to long-term incapacity benefit after 52 weeks of incapacity even if you don't satisfy the contribution conditions – see 2.

Over pension age – If you reached pension age while you were getting short-term incapacity benefit and you would be entitled to a retirement pension, you could choose to stay on the short-term rate for up to the maximum 52 weeks. You cannot move on to the long-term rate.

2. Transferring from invalidity benefit
You automatically moved on to long-term incapacity benefit if you were entitled to invalidity benefit on 12.4.95. Your benefit became a 'transitional award of long-term incapacity benefit'. If your invalidity benefit stopped at any time between 15.2.95 and 12.4.95 and you became incapable of work again no more than 8 weeks after your last day of incapacity in that period, your new award is also a transitional award of long-term incapacity benefit.

A transitional award means the amount of benefit you were entitled to is protected. But you must pass the 'all work' test of incapacity unless you are exempt – see 7 below. Until the test is applied you must continue to send in medical certificates.

The rules for transitional awards continue to apply until you have a break in your claim of over 8 weeks. If you are claiming after a spell on DWA or on a training scheme see 4.

How much do you get?
Your transitional award is paid at the same rate as your invalidity benefit. The basic pension and any invalidity allowance and additions for dependants you get are uprated each year as normal. If you get an additional SERPS pension, the amount is frozen at your 1994/95 level if you are under pension age. Your benefit is not taxable.

The rates for 1997/98 are:

- **long-term incapacity benefit** £62.45
- **invalidity allowance**
  - higher rate £13.15
  - middle rate £8.30
  - lower rate £4.15
- **adult dependant** £37.35
- **child dependent**
  - first child £9.90
  - for each other child £11.20
- **additional pension (SERPS)** *

* amount based on your contribution record.

Dependant's addition
You can no longer claim an addition for a wife or husband under the age of 60 unless you have children. But if an addition for an adult dependant was payable with your invalidity benefit at any time in the 8 weeks immediately before 13.4.95, you could keep the addition with your transitional award. This protection is lost if the addition is not payable for more than 8 weeks (eg if it is overlapped by your dependant's own personal benefit, or if payment of the addition is extinguished by earnings).

If you were not getting an addition with your invalidity benefit, or you lose the transitional protection, you can claim an addition with your transitional long-term award if you qualify under the ordinary rules – see Chapter 11(3). There is no change to the rules for child dependants' additions.

Partner's earnings – The adult dependant's addition is not paid if your partner, who lives with you, earns more than £49.15 in a week – see Chapter 11(4) for the earnings rules.

Before 16.9.85 there was a *tapered earnings rule*. Under this rule, if your dependant earns £45.09 a week or less, you get the full £37.35 addition. The addition is cut by 5p for each 10p she earns between £45 and £49, and then cut by 5p for each 5p earned above £49. If earnings reach £84.35 in any week, the addition stops the next week. If you've been getting an addition for a wife, or a woman looking after a child, continuously since before 16.9.85, the old tapered earnings rule still applies. It stops applying if there is a continuous period of more than 8 weeks in which your incapacity benefit is not paid, or the dependant's addition is paid in full or not at all.

Over pension age?
If you reached pension age (60 for women, 65 for men) before 13.4.95 and you are entitled to a transitional award of long-term incapacity benefit, you can stay on the long-term rate for up to five years beyond pension age. See Chapter 43(3).

The amount of benefit is based on the amount of retirement pension you would be entitled to. So if there are gaps in your contribution record, your incapacity benefit is reduced. The unequal treatment of women and men because of the difference in pension ages at which this reduction is applied has been ruled to be lawful by the European Court (*Graham v Secretary of State*). See Chapter 43(10).

If you reach pension age on or after 13.4.95, your transitional award will end the day you reach 60 (women) or 65 (men). You can claim retirement pension instead.

Any invalidity allowance is carried over and paid on top of the retirement pension, although it is offset against the additional pension – see Chapter 44(4) 'Extra pension'.

Industrial injuries
If you received invalidity benefit on the grounds of industrial injury or disease (ie without having to pass any contribution conditions), your transitional award ends if your incapacity for work is no longer a result of that injury or disease. But you can pick up the transitional rate again if you become incapable of work within 8 weeks through the same injury or disease. The provision to receive sickness benefit without passing the contribution conditions has not been carried forward to incapacity benefit. So if your benefit is cut off, you can only requalify if you are able to pass the contribution conditions. You get National Insurance credits while on invalidity benefit or incapacity benefit and these could help you to pass the second contribution condition for incapacity benefit.

If you are already over pension age by 13.4.95, you keep the full rate of benefit (up to five years beyond pension age) even if you would not qualify for a full retirement pension.

3. Severe disablement allowance

If you were getting severe disablement allowance (SDA) before 13.4.95, your benefit is not generally affected by the changes. You do not have to pass the new 'all work' test of incapacity, but you must carry on sending in medical certificates. If you stop claiming SDA but reclaim within 8 weeks, exemption from the test still applies.

If you make a new claim on or after 13.4.95, or you put in a claim before then but your SDA did not start till afterwards, you must pass the 'all work' test as a condition of benefit, unless you are in one of the exempt groups – see Chapter 8(9). From 1.4.97, you are exempt if you've passed the 80% disablement test for SDA or you are passported to the 80% test.

The transitional rules that apply to adult dependant's additions also apply to SDA – see 2 above.

4. DWA and training schemes – the linking rules

If you were on a transitional award of short-term higher rate incapacity benefit or long-term benefit before going to work and receiving DWA, or starting a training scheme, you regain your transitional award if you reclaim within 2 years.

Your level of sickness or invalidity benefit is also protected if you claim incapacity benefit under the special DWA 2-year linking rule. Benefit is paid on the same basis as a transitional award of short-term or long-term benefit. See Chapter 16(6).

If you were on a training scheme during the period from 8 weeks before to 8 weeks after 13.4.95, you can regain your previous level of sickness or invalidity benefit if you claim within 8 weeks of the end of the course. Benefit is paid on the same basis as a transitional award. See Chapter 15(12).

5. Therapeutic work

You may have been doing some therapeutic work while on invalidity benefit, sickness benefit or severe disablement allowance. Under the rules from 13.4.95, therapeutic work must be under 16 hours a week. If you were deemed incapable of work under the therapeutic earnings provisions on 12.4.95, the 16 hours a week restriction does not apply until you stop work for at least 8 weeks and 1 day, or your period of incapacity for work ends. The earnings limit of £46.50 a week applies.

6. Income support, housing benefit and council tax benefit

The disability premium paid with these means-tested benefits is affected by the April 1995 changes. You may get the premium because you receive one of the qualifying benefits, such as DLA or DWA. Invalidity benefit has been replaced by long-term incapacity benefit as a disability premium qualifying benefit. This means that if you receive no other qualifying benefit other than incapacity benefit, the premium will only be paid after 52 weeks of incapacity.

If you do not receive a qualifying benefit, you may get the disability premium if you pass the incapacity condition. Before April 1995, you needed to be incapable of work for the qualifying period of 28 weeks, after which the premium would be paid. From 13.4.95 you must be incapable of work for 52 weeks before the disability premium is payable. This includes people already on income support, housing or council tax benefit but who had not reached the 28th week of incapacity by 13.4.95. See Chapter 3(12).

Your incapacity is assessed under the 'all work' test unless you are in one of the exempt groups – see 7 below.

7. Do the new incapacity tests apply?
From 13.4.95, there are two tests of incapacity for work: the 'all work' test and the 'own occupation' test. The own occupation test assesses your ability to do your normal work, if you have worked recently. It is based on medical certificates provided by your doctor. The all work test assesses your ability to carry out a range of activities such as walking, sitting and standing, and includes an assessment of mental health where appropriate. For the all work test you are sent a questionnaire to fill in and you may be asked to attend a medical examination by a DSS doctor. These tests are described in more detail in Chapter 8(7) to (11).

Unless you are in one of the exempt groups, you must pass the 'all work' test to continue to qualify for your transitional award of incapacity benefit or the disability premium paid with income support, housing benefit and council tax benefit. Until the all work test is applied, you should carry on sending in your medical certificates.

If your incapacity for work is assessed for a period before 13.4.95, the new tests do not apply to that period. Incapacity must be assessed under the rules that applied at the time. See Chapter 11 in the 19th edition of the *Disability Rights Handbook* if you are challenging a decision on a pre-13.4.95 period of incapacity.

Once you are found incapable of work under the all work test you no longer need to send in medical certificates. But your benefit could be reviewed at a later date and you may be asked to fill in a further questionnaire.

If you are found capable of work, your entitlement to benefit will stop. You have the right to appeal against the decision. You may be able to sign on for jobseeker's allowance. If your disability premium stops, you may still be able to get income support, housing benefit or council tax benefit nevertheless, but the amount you get will go down.

Who is exempt from the all work test?
You may be exempt from the all work test. The DSS may be able to make a decision on whether you are exempt from their records and the information on your medical certificates. If not, they may write to your doctor for more information on your condition. You may be asked to fill in a questionnaire if there is still doubt about your exemption and could be called in for a medical examination.

The groups listed below apply to transitional awards of incapacity benefit as well as to other benefits where you were incapable of work before 13.4.95. The exempt groups which apply to claims made on or after 13.4.95 are identical to those below (apart from the first 4 transitional groups). These are described in more detail in Chapter 8(9).

❑ You are exempt from the all work test if you are in one or more of these groups:
■ you were aged 58 or over on 13.4.95 and were entitled to **invalidity benefit** between 1.12.93 and 12.4.95 (breaks off benefit of 8 weeks or less are allowed);
■ you were aged 58 or over on 13.4.95 *and*
  – you were in receipt of a **disability premium** on incapacity grounds on 12.4.95; *and*
  – you were getting income support, housing benefit or council tax benefit on 1.12.93; *and*
  – you were incapable of work for at least the 28 weeks before 1.12.93; *and*
  – between 1.12.93 and 13.4.95, you were incapable of work (not counting breaks of 8 weeks or less);
■ you were in receipt of **severe disablement allowance** on 12.4.95 (the exemption ends if your spell of incapacity stops);
■ you've been getting **DLA higher rate care component** (or an equivalent constant attendance allowance) since before 13.4.95;
■ you are terminally ill;
■ you are registered blind;
■ you have any of these conditions: tetraplegia; persistent vegetative state; dementia; paraplegia or *'uncontrollable involuntary movements or ataxia which effectively renders [you] functionally paraplegic'*;

❑ You are also exempt if you have any of these conditions:
■ severe learning disability;
■ severe and progressive neurological or muscle wasting disease;
■ active and progressive form of inflammatory polyarthritis;
■ impairment of cardio-respiratory function;
■ dense paralysis of the upper limb, trunk and lower limb on one side of the body;
■ multiple effects of impairment of function of the brain or nervous system;
■ severe and progressive immune deficiency state;
■ severe mental illness.

If you come under one of the first three groups (ie the invalidity benefit, disability premium or SDA conditions) you must continue to send in medical certificates unless you also fall into any of the other exempt groups.

13 Severe disablement allowance

In this chapter we look at:	
What is severe disablement allowance?	see 1
The four routes to SDA	see 2
Do you qualify for SDA?	see 3
Route 1 – People who were entitled to NCIP	see 4
Route 2 – Incapable of work on 20th birthday	see 5
Route 2 – The work trial concession	see 6
The work trial concession – an example	see Box E.8
Route 3 – Passported to the 80% test	see 7
Route 4 – The 80% disablement test	see 8
How is disablement assessed?	see Box E.9
The listed conditions	see Box E.10
How much do you get?	see 9
How do you claim?	see 10
Does anything affect what you get?	see 11
For more information	see Box E.11

1. What is severe disablement allowance?
Severe disablement allowance (SDA) is a weekly cash benefit for people who have been incapable of work for at least 28

weeks but who do not have enough National Insurance contributions to qualify for incapacity benefit. It cannot normally be paid for the first time after you reach 65. SDA is not means-tested. Nor is it taxable.

SDA has an extra test. Some people (those who have to take Routes 3 or 4 to SDA) also have to prove they are at least 75/80% disabled and have been so for at least 28 weeks.

2. The four routes to SDA
There are four possible routes along which different groups of people can qualify for SDA:

Route 1 – people who were entitled to non-contributory invalidity pension (see 4);
Route 2 – people who first became incapable of work on or before their 20th birthday (see 5 and 6);
Route 3 – people who can be passported to the test of 80% disablement (see 7);
Route 4 – people who have to be assessed as at least 75% disabled (see 8).

3. Do you qualify for SDA?
In this section we look at the general qualifying conditions for SDA which all claimants must meet. If you meet these qualifying conditions, go on to the section for the route to SDA you have to take.

You qualify if:
- you are at least 16 (or 19 if you are in full-time education) and under 65 when you claim;
- you have been continuously incapable of work for 196 days and are still incapable of work;
- you satisfy the residence and presence conditions;
- you qualify under one of the Routes 1 to 4.

Age
You must be aged at least 16, and under 65 when you claim in order to qualify for SDA. If you are over 65, see Chapter 43(5).

The upper age limit was equalised at 65 for men and women on 28.10.94, following a ruling of the European Court of Justice. Women who were refused SDA or did not claim because they were over 60, may now qualify.

Incapacity for work
The key qualifying condition for SDA, which all claimants must meet, is that you are incapable of work.

You must also have been incapable of work for a continuous period of 196 days before the first day you are paid SDA. These 196 days can be the days before the day you could first claim SDA, including days before your 16th birthday. Once you have met this initial qualifying condition, you won't have to meet it again while your claim to SDA is still in the same 'period of incapacity for work' – see Chapter 11(2). If you have a break in your claim of no more than 8 weeks, you are still in the same period of incapacity for work and thus do not need to pass the 196 day test, but you do have to pass each of the other qualifying conditions.

Chapter 8 describes how incapacity for work is defined and the way it is assessed (the rules are the same as those for incapacity benefit). The tests of incapacity introduced on 13.4.95, also apply to SDA.

When you claim SDA, send in a current medical certificate and a backdated medical certificate covering the 28 weeks before the date you are claiming from. If you pass the 80% SDA disablement test under Route 4, or you are passported to the 80% test under Route 3, there are no extra tests of incapacity for work (you are exempt from the all work test of incapacity).

However, if you get SDA under Route 1 or Route 2, you must also pass the all work test of incapacity to qualify for SDA unless you are in one of the exempt groups – see Chapter 8(7) to (11). Before the rules changed on 1.4.97 those getting SDA under Route 3 and Route 4 also had their incapacity for work assessed under the all work test.

If you are already in receipt of SDA by 12.4.95, you are exempt from the all work test (whatever route to SDA you qualified under) and you should simply carry on sending in medical certificates to the DSS. This exemption continues provided there is not a break in the claim of more than 8 weeks.

Full-time education
If you are 19 or older, you cannot be excluded from SDA solely because you are in full-time education. However, the sort of tasks and activities you are able to do in attending the course may be taken into account when deciding whether you pass the all work test of incapacity, if you are not exempt from the test.

If you are 16, 17 or 18 you will be usually be excluded from SDA if you are in full-time education. Chapter 30(3) explains what this means.

Residence in Great Britain
You must be ordinarily resident and present in Great Britain to be paid SDA. You must have been present in Britain for at least 26 weeks in the year before your claim.

You are not entitled if you have any restriction on your right to reside in the UK unless you or a member of your family is an EEA national (see Chapter 41) or lawfully working and a national of Algeria, Morocco, Slovenia or Tunisia, or you have refugee status or exceptional leave to remain. This test applies to claims made on or after 5.2.96 where entitlement begins on or after 5.2.96. If your entitlement began before 5.2.96, the test does not apply unless your SDA is reviewed.

Some people may be able to get SDA even though they are abroad. Presence in an EEA country may count as presence in Britain. The residence and presence conditions don't apply if you are serving in HM forces; or you are an airman or mariner; or are living with someone who is in the forces. If you are going abroad temporarily, you may be able to keep your SDA – see Chapter 41 for details.

4. Route 1 – People who were entitled to non-contributory invalidity pension
SDA replaced non-contributory invalidity pension (NCIP) which was abolished on 29.11.84.

If you were paid NCIP on 28.11.84, you were automatically transferred to SDA under Route 1. Under Route 1, you do not have to prove you are 80% disabled. You simply have to continue to prove that you are incapable of work.

The protection of Route 1 lasts as long as your claim to SDA is linked to your earlier award of NCIP because it is still in the same period of incapacity for work.

Route 1 also covers former NCIP claimants who are still in the same 'period of incapacity for work' (see Chapter 9(3)) as when they were last paid NCIP – no matter how long ago this was.

Married women – Married women and women who lived with their male partner had to pass an extra household duties test to qualify for Housewives NCIP. If you were refused NCIP because of this test, or you did not claim, you may be entitled to SDA now, without having to pass the 80% disablement test, if:

- you would have been entitled to NCIP immediately before 29.11.84, apart from the household duties test; and
- you have been continuously incapable of work since then.

You need a backdated medical certificate from your doctor going back to 1984 to qualify under this provision, but if this is not possible, the DSS may accept your own statement unless there is some reason to doubt it. You may be able to claim SDA on these grounds now even if you are over 65. If you did claim NCIP and were refused, you could try asking for a late appeal. If an appeal is successful, you can get benefit paid from the date of your original claim.

5. Route 2 – Incapable of work on 20th birthday

Route 2 covers everyone who is incapable of work while aged under 20; or who has been incapable of work from and including their 20th birthday. Under Route 2, you simply have to prove you are incapable of work and that you have been incapable of work for a continuous period of 196 days before the first day you are paid SDA. These 196 days can be the days before your 16th birthday.

Route 2 also covers you if:
- your first day of incapacity for work occurred on or before your 20th birthday; and
- you were incapable of work for a continuous period of 196 days (so you served the whole of the qualifying period for SDA – even if you did not claim it); and
- you are now older than 20, and although you must have been incapable of work for 196 days before being paid SDA, you are protected by the 'work trial' concession see 6 below; or
- you were getting SDA before by Route 2 and are still in the same period of incapacity for work. So, you do not have to wait another 196 days before getting SDA again.

You do not have to be paid SDA by your 20th birthday to be able to take Route 2. It is enough if the very first day of the 196 day qualifying period is the day of your 20th birthday. If you can provide evidence that you have been continuously incapable of work since on or before your 20th birthday, you can get SDA under Route 2 even if you claim it when you are, say, 34 or 54.

6. Route 2 – The work trial concession

If you have been getting SDA under Route 2 and then manage to work in an 'ordinary' job for a period of 8 weeks and 1 day or longer, you will always have to requalify for SDA when making a fresh claim. This is because you will have broken the 8 week period of incapacity for work linking rule. However, if you claimed disability working allowance (DWA) to top up low earnings, there is a special 2 year linking rule. If you are covered by the DWA 2 year linking rule, days on DWA do not count as days on which you were capable of work for the work trial concession – see Chapter 16(6). There is a similar 2 year linking rule for people on specified training schemes – see Chapter 15(12).

If you reached your 20th birthday before the start of the 196 day qualifying period on your fresh claim (or a very first claim) to SDA, you might have to prove that you are also 80% disabled. However, the 'work trial' concession may allow you to keep the right to SDA under Route 2 (and avoid the test of 80% disablement) even though you are now over 20.

Former NCIP claimants who receive SDA under Route 1 may also benefit from the work trial concession. It will apply to them if (and only if) their first day of incapacity for work occurred on or before their 20th birthday – see below.

The work trial concession allows a total of no more than 182 days (including Sundays) on which you were capable of work to be ignored for the purpose of deciding whether or not you can get SDA for your fresh claim under Route 2, even though you are now older than 20.

When can you use the work trial concession?
To make effective use of the work trial concession you must meet the following conditions.
- You must have to serve (or re-serve) the 196 day qualifying period for a fresh claim to SDA.

E.8 The work trial concession

The following example illustrates the key points about the work trial concession.

Under 20

Sharon first qualified for SDA when she was 16. When she was 18 she got an ordinary job and worked for 10 weeks (70 days). She had to give up work because she found she could not manage it.

She reclaimed SDA. As she had broken the 8 week link she had to serve the 196 day qualifying period again. As she was younger than 20 she can reclaim SDA under Route 2. The days she has spent working make no difference to her new claim for SDA. And as she has had to requalify for SDA while aged under 20, these 10 weeks of capacity for work cannot affect her in the future.

If she had claimed disability working allowance (DWA) when she started work, and re-claimed SDA as soon as she gave up work, she would be covered by the DWA 2 year linking rule. She would not have to requalify for SDA because the days on DWA are treated as days of incapacity for work when she makes a fresh SDA claim. She would also keep the rest of the 26 weeks DWA award – on top of her SDA!

At the age of 19, Sharon goes on youth training (YT) for 26 weeks. She loses SDA for those 26 weeks. But at the end of the course she reclaims SDA. She is covered by the 2 year linking rule and does not have to requalify for SDA.

Over 20

When she is 25, Sharon decides to sign on for work. She signs on for 4 weeks. She then gets an ordinary job and manages to work for 4 weeks and 2 days. She finds she cannot cope and reclaims SDA.

Sharon has now broken the 8 week link. If she did not claim DWA, she cannot be protected by DWA's 2 year linking rule. This means she has to serve the 196 day qualifying period before she can be paid SDA once again.

Can she still claim SDA under Route 2? The answer is yes. For she has had only 8 weeks and 2 days on which she has been capable of work (58 days in all). The only days of capacity for work that count towards the work trial concession are the days between the beginning of the current 196 day qualifying period for SDA, and the end of a continuous stretch of 196 days of incapacity for work which started on or before the 20th birthday.

However, if Sharon had signed on for work for 18 extra weeks before getting a job, she would not have been able to make use of the work trial concession (nor could she be covered by the DWA linking rule – for that to apply, she must have received SDA at some time in the 8 weeks before claiming DWA). The extra 18 weeks of capacity for work makes the total days of capacity for work add up to 26 weeks and 2 days (184 days in all). She would have to requalify for SDA under Route 3 or Route 4.

If you've been getting SDA previously, you only ever have to re-serve the 196 day qualifying period if you break the 8 week period of incapacity for work linking rule and are not covered by the DWA or training scheme 2 year linking rules.

and

❏ You were already over 20 on the first day of incapacity for your fresh claim to SDA.

and

❏ You were previously incapable of work. That previous spell of incapacity must have started on or before your 20th birthday. And it must have lasted for at least 196 days.

and

❏ Between the end of the continuous 196 days of incapacity for work which included, or came before, the day of your 20th birthday and the beginning of the new 196 day period, you have been capable of work for no more than a total of 182 days (26 weeks) in all.

What days count towards the work trial concession?
Only days on which you were capable of work can count towards the 182 day work trial concession. They include days when you are actually working – unless you were getting DWA on those days and are covered by the DWA linking rule for your current SDA claim – see Chapter 16. Days when you are signing on as available for work count as days on which you are capable of work. So too do days on which you receive a state training allowance unless you are covered by the 2 year linking rule.

7. Route 3 – Passported to the 80% test

If you cannot get SDA under Route 1 or under Route 2, you can only get SDA if you are assessed as being at least 75% disabled. An assessment of 75% is always rounded up to 80%.

You must be both 75% disabled and incapable of work on the day you claim SDA, and have been 75% disabled and incapable of work during the previous 196 days.

When you are serving the 196 qualifying days before you can be paid SDA, remember that just a one day break (perhaps a day trying to see if you can manage a job) is enough to put you back to the beginning and start the 196 days all over again.

To make the disablement test easier to administer, some groups of people are automatically accepted as 80% disabled. If you fall into one (or more) of these groups, you can be passported to SDA, and you will be exempt from the all work test of incapacity.

You can be passported to the 80% test if:
- you get disability living allowance (DLA) care component at the higher rate (or don't get it just because, say, you are in hospital); or
- you have an invalid tricycle or invalid car or private car allowance from the DSS; or
- you are covered by an assessment of 75/80% disablement for the purposes of the industrial injuries scheme, or war disablement pension, or for SDA on a previous claim; or
- you have had a Vaccine Damage Payment; or
- you are registered as blind.

Before April 1997, there were five more ways to be passported to the 80% disablement test. These have now been removed but there is protection for existing claimants. If you were entitled to SDA before 1.4.97 under one of these conditions, and you are still in the same period of incapacity for work, you continue to be passported to the 80% test if:
- you get DLA care component at the middle rate; or
- you get DLA mobility component at the higher rate; or
- you get war pensioners' mobility supplement; or
- you get attendance allowance; or
- you are registered as partially sighted.

If your period of incapacity for work ends, for example, if you come off SDA for more than 8 weeks, you cannot requalify for SDA on a new claim under any of these five conditions. For most people this will mean having to pass the 80% disablement test under Route 4.

Do note that some people may have to claim SDA under a combination of Routes 3 and 4. For example, if you were first paid DLA higher rate care component say 50 days ago, you can only be passported to SDA from the start of your DLA award – you must also show that you were 75% disabled (under Route 4) during the 146 days before you were first paid DLA.

8. Route 4 – The 80% disablement test

If you cannot get SDA under Routes 1, 2 or 3, you must claim under Route 4. Here you must satisfy an extra test.

You must also show that you suffer from *'loss of physical or mental faculty such that the extent of the resulting disablement amounts to not less than 80%'*. An assessment of 75% is always rounded up to 80%. You must also show that you have been at least 75/80% disabled during the 196 day qualifying period before you can be paid SDA.

You must also show that you are incapable of work and have been so for the past 196 days. Medical certificates from your doctor are enough until you've been assessed. Once you've been assessed as 80% disabled, you are exempt from the all work test of incapacity.

Who decides the 80% test?
The 80% test under Route 4 to SDA is decided by the adjudicating medical authorities – not by an Adjudication Officer. At the first stage, a single Adjudicating Medical Practitioner (AMP for short), or two AMPs sitting as a medical board, will make the decision. If you are unsuccessful, you have the right to appeal to a Medical Appeal Tribunal.

How is the 80% test decided?
When you claim SDA, your claim will go to an Adjudication Officer at your local DSS office. S/he will check to see if you can be covered by Route 3.

If you must take Route 4, the Adjudication Officer will pass on your claim to your local Disability Benefits Centre. They will arrange for an AMP to examine you. You'll be given the chance to make a statement during the examination. It helps if you have read Box E.9 and thought about your disabilities beforehand. Like the other disability benefits, success may depend on your ability to look at the negative aspects of your disability. Check that the AMP has written down what you want to say – before you sign your statement. The AMP can also get a detailed medical report from your GP, hospital or consultant.

If the medical issues in your case seem complex (or there are just lots of medical reports to look at), you may be referred to a medical board. This will often happen if you suffer from three or more different, or uncommon, conditions; or if you have a history of psychiatric illness.

If either a single AMP, or a medical board, decide you are 74% or less disabled, you have the right to appeal to a Medical Appeal Tribunal. You must appeal within 3 months of the date the decision was sent to you.

What does 80% disablement mean?
No one is completely sure what 80% disablement means in

E.9 How is disablement assessed?

The legislation uses three different terms for the disablement test. These are:
- loss of faculty;
- disability;
- disablement.

They are each used as different concepts and must not be confused. They are not defined in the law but have been considered by the Social Security Commissioners: particularly in R(I)1/81. The disablement test is different from the 'all work' test which assesses incapacity for work – see Chapter 8.

Loss of faculty

A 'loss of faculty' is any pathological condition or any loss (including a reduction) of the normal physical or mental function of an organ or part of the body.

This does include disfigurement, even though there may not actually be any loss of faculty.

A loss of faculty is not itself a disability. It is the starting point for the assessment of disablement. It is a condition that is either an actual cause of one or more disabilities, or a potential cause of disability.

For example, the loss of one kidney is a 'loss of faculty'. If the other kidney works normally, you may not notice any problems. But you will have lost your back-up kidney – so this is a potential cause of disability in the future. Medical Appeal Tribunals have assessed the loss of one kidney (the other functioning properly) at between 5% to 10%.

Disability

A 'disability' means an inability to perform a bodily or mental process. This can either be a complete inability to do something (eg walking); or it can be a partial inability to do something (eg you can lift light weights but not heavy ones).

For any disability to be assessable (and count towards the 80% test for SDA) it must result from something which the Adjudicating Medical Practitioner (AMP) accepts is a 'loss of faculty'. (For industrial disablement benefit only, the loss of faculty must be caused by an industrial accident or prescribed industrial disease.)

Disablement

'Disablement' is the sum total of all the separate disabilities you may experience. It represents your overall inability to perform the 'normal' activities of life – the loss of your health, strength and power to enjoy a 'normal' life. If the assessments of your various disabilities add up to a total of 75% or more, you will meet the 80% test of disablement for SDA. Every case is decided individually, so it is difficult (and risky) to give hard and fast examples – we can only give general guidelines.

What is taken into account?

The assessment is done by comparing your condition (all your disabilities) with that of a person of the same age and sex whose physical and mental condition is 'normal'.

So the AMP also has to make judgements about what is 'normal' for someone of your age and sex. For example, how much hearing loss is 'normal' for a 50 year old man? At what age does it become 'normal' to lose teeth and wear false teeth? Note that the availability of artificial aids may reduce the actual disability resulting from the loss of faculty. The only reported Commissioners' decisions on this, R(I)7/67 and R(I)7/63, concerned spectacles.

The assessment is made without looking at your own personal circumstances – except for your own age, sex, and physical and mental condition. Obviously they have to consider how your condition affects you, rather than just considering what is generally true of people with your condition, or taking the same drugs. Inconvenience, genuine embarrassment, anxiety, or depression can all increase the assessment.

However, the fact of your loss of earning power, or incapacity for work, cannot be taken into account in this assessment. Nor can the fact that your disabilities may lead to extra expenses. But the disabilities that lead to incapacity for work (or extra expenses) are taken into account, along with disabilities that do not affect your working capacity at all.

The assessment doesn't just depend on your condition on the day (or time of day) you are examined. If your condition varies, the AMP will work out an average assessment taking into account your 'good' and 'bad' spells. It is arguable that the AMP can take into account any loss of life expectancy, as well as the effect of your knowledge of the nature of your disability on your life.

Scheduled and non-scheduled assessments

Some types of disability have a fixed percentage. These 'scheduled assessments' are listed in Box E.10. They are fixed on the assumption that your condition has stabilised and there are no added complications. Other disabilities are assessed accordingly.

If your disability is not in the schedule (and most people claiming SDA will have non-scheduled disabilities), the AMP *'may have such regard as may be appropriate to the prescribed degrees of disablement'*. So the AMP should try to assess your disabilities so that your percentage assessment looks right in relation to the scheduled assessments.

When you look at the schedule of prescribed degrees of disablement, remember that 100% is not total and absolute disablement. It is just the legal maximum assessment. If the scale could go higher, some people would be assessed as 200% disabled – or more.

The Schedule says that if you are totally deaf, or severely facially disfigured, the fixed assessment is 100%.

If you have had either arm amputated just below the shoulder, you will be assessed at 80% – even if you cope perfectly well. If the amputation has not yet stabilised, or there are other complications with it, the AMP can make a higher assessment.

If a stroke or bad arthritis means that you cannot use one arm at all, you may well be assessed at 80% – as if you had actually lost your arm.

Several conditions

Four different disabilities may each be assessed as causing 10% disablement. But if one person has all four disabilities, the assessment will not always be the total of 40%. This is because the interaction of different conditions in one person may be far more disabling – so the final assessment could well be higher. But if you have several of the minor scheduled conditions, the total percentage assessment could be less than the actual total of the percentages for each of the scheduled conditions. It is up to the AMP to decide what is the appropriate assessment for you – given your age, sex and physical and mental condition as a whole. So even for the scheduled assessments, the AMP may increase (or decrease) the percentage(s) if that is reasonable in a particular case.

practice – apart from the fact that the assessment of 80% disablement must follow the same general principles of assessment which apply for industrial injuries disablement benefit. So the best advice is to claim SDA and find out. We give brief guidelines in Box E.9 and sources of more information in Box E.11.

The assessment of disablement for SDA purposes has two key differences from the assessments under the industrial injuries and war disablement schemes.

Firstly, with SDA, what caused your disability does not affect the assessment. The AMP will take into account all the disabilities which you may be expected to have to cope with during the period of the assessment.

Secondly, with SDA, you never have to worry about going

E.10 Listed conditions

Prescribed degrees of disablement

Description of injury	Degree
Loss of both hands or amputation at higher sites	100%
Loss of a hand and a foot	100%
Double amputation through leg or thigh, or amputation through leg or thigh on one side and loss of other foot	100%
Loss of sight to such an extent as to render the claimant unable to perform any work for which eyesight is essential	100%
Very severe facial disfiguration	100%
Absolute deafness	100%
Forequarter or hindquarter amputation	100%

Amputation cases – upper limbs (either arm)

Amputation through shoulder joint	90%
Amputation below shoulder with stump less than 20.5 centimetres from tip of acromion	80%
Amputation from 20.5 centimetres from tip of acromion to less than 11.5 centimetres below tip of olecranon	70%
Loss of a hand or of the thumb and four fingers of one hand or amputation from 11.5 centimetres below tip of olecranon	60%
Loss of thumb	30%
Loss of thumb and its metacarpal bone	40%
Loss of four fingers of one hand	50%
Loss of three fingers of one hand	30%
Loss of two fingers of one hand	20%
Loss of terminal phalanx of thumb	20%

Amputation cases – lower limbs

Amputation of both feet resulting in end-bearing stumps	90%
Amputation through both feet proximal to the metatarso-phalangeal joint	80%
Loss of all toes of both feet through the metatarso-phalangeal joint	40%
Loss of all toes of both feet proximal to the proximal inter-phalangeal joint	30%
Loss of all toes of both feet distal to the proximal inter-phalangeal joint	20%
Amputation at hip	90%
Amputation below hip with stump not exceeding 13 centimetres in length measured from tip of great trochanter	80%
Amputation below hip and above knee with stump exceeding 13 centimetres in length measured from tip of great trochanter, or at knee not resulting in end-bearing stump	70%
Amputation at knee resulting in end-bearing stump or below knee with stump not exceeding 9 centimetres	60%
Amputation below knee with stump exceeding 9 centimetres but not exceeding 13 centimetres	50%
Amputation below knee with stump exceeding 13 centimetres	40%
Amputation of one foot resulting in end-bearing stump	30%
Amputation through one foot proximal to the metatarso-phalangeal joint	30%
Loss of all toes of one foot through the metatarso-phalangeal joint	20%

Other injuries

Loss of one eye, without complications, the other being normal	40%
Loss of vision of one eye, without complications or disfigurement of the eyeball, the other being normal	30%

Loss of fingers of right or left hand

❏ **Index finger:**
Whole	14%
Two phalanges	11%
One phalanx	9%
Guillotine amputation of tip without loss of bone	5%

❏ **Middle finger:**
Whole	12%
Two phalanges	9%
One phalanx	7%
Guillotine amputation of tip without loss of bone	4%

❏ **Ring or little finger:**
Whole	7%
Two phalanges	6%
One phalanx	5%
Guillotine amputation of tip without loss of bone	2%

Loss of toes of right or left foot

❏ **Great toe:**
Through metatarso-phalangeal joint	14%
Part, with some loss of bone	3%

❏ **Any other toe:**
Through metatarso-phalangeal joint	3%
Part, with some loss of bone	1%

❏ **Two toes of one foot, excluding great toe:**
Through metatarso-phalangeal joint	5%
Part, with some loss of bone	2%

❏ **Three toes of one foot, excluding great toe:**
Through metatarso-phalangeal joint	6%
Part, with some loss of bone	3%

❏ **Four toes of one foot, excluding great toe:**
Through metatarso-phalangeal joint	9%
Part, with some loss of bone	3%

for a review of an assessment because of 'unforeseen aggravation'. If you have been refused SDA and then get worse, you simply put in a fresh claim. In some cases, though, you may be able to get a review of an AMP's decision because fresh evidence shows that it was mistaken – this is explained in Chapter 52.

9. How much do you get?

You get each week:
- for yourself — £37.75
- an age addition
  - under 40 — £13.15
  - 40–49 — £8.30
  - 50–59 — £4.15
  (age additions depend on the age at which your current period of incapacity for work began)
- for the first child — £9.90
- for each other child — £11.20
- for an adult dependant — £22.40

See Chapter 11(3) for when you can claim for an adult dependant (the rules are the same as those for incapacity benefit).

10. How do you claim?

Get claim pack SDA1 from the DSS, a Citizens Advice Bureau, or post office. Fill in the claim form and return it to your local DSS office. If you have not been sending doctor's certificates to your local DSS office, ask your doctor for one. Send it to the DSS along with your claim form. Leaflet NI 252 gives information about SDA. Your claim can be backdated automatically for up to three months if you satisfied the qualifying conditions from that earlier date.

11. Does anything affect what you get?

Other benefits
The rules are the same as for incapacity benefit. See Chapter 11(4) for details.

If you get SDA, you may qualify for a disability premium or higher pensioner premium under income support, council tax benefit, or housing benefit – see Chapters 3 and 4.

If you go on an employment rehabilitation course, you can stay on SDA – see Chapter 15(4).

Occupational sick pay
SDA is not means tested. So you could receive salary, wages or an occupational pension or sick pay while you are off sick and not working. If your partner has an occupational or personal pension, this counts as earnings when you claim an addition for him or her, or for your children.

Additions for children
Your partner's earnings may affect your right to get additions for children. If s/he earns £135 or more, you will lose the addition for one child. An occupational or personal pension counts as earnings. See Chapter 11(4) for more details.

Partner's earnings
Your partner's earnings do not affect your basic benefit but can affect entitlement to dependants' additions. The rules are the same as for incapacity benefit (see Chapter 11(4)) but note that the long-term rate earnings limit (£49.15) applies from the beginning of an SDA claim. Because the earnings limit for short-term incapacity benefit is lower, if your partner earns between £29.15 and £49.15 a week, you may qualify for SDA topping up short-term higher rate incapacity benefit.

Disqualification
You can be disqualified from SDA in certain circumstances – see Chapter 8(6).

Working while getting SDA
It is possible to do some limited work and still be counted as incapable of work. The rules are explained in Chapter 8(5). If you get income support topping up your SDA, note that any earnings above £15 will just be deducted from your IS.

E.11 For more information

The 80% test
You can read more about the 80% test in the *Severe Disablement Allowance Handbook for Adjudicating Medical Authorities* (£13, available from the Stationery Office).

The SDA Handbook has a useful section on the factors to be taken into account when assessing the following conditions:
- Haemophilia
- Dementia
- Cardiorespiratory disease
- Musculoskeletal disorders
- Neuromuscular disorders (including multiple sclerosis)
- Diabetes
- Mental illness
- Learning difficulties
- Cerebral palsy
- Epilepsy
- Cardiovascular diseases and disorders

If you have any of these conditions, try and read this section of the SDA Handbook before your medical examination. You may still find this section useful even if you have another condition. There is also a table of about 50 different conditions giving the range and most common percentage assessments for each; details are taken from a survey of cases considered by Medical Appeal Tribunals.

Much of the SDA Handbook is taken from the *Industrial Injuries Handbook for Adjudicating Medical Authorities* – see Box O.4 in Chapter 52.

The DSS's HB5, a guide to *Non-contributory Benefits for Disabled People*, includes a slightly different approach to the nature of the 80% test.

Non-contributory invalidity benefit
See our Disability Rights Handbook for 1984. If you do not have a copy, send us a stamped addressed envelope and we will send you a photocopy of the chapters on NCIP.

Young people with disabilities
Chapter 30 explains the 'full-time education' test for SDA. It also explains the relationship between SDA and income support.

F Unemployment to employment

This section of the Handbook looks at the following:
Jobseeker's allowance	Chapter **14**
Employment and training	Chapter **15**
Disability working allowance	Chapter **16**

14 Jobseeker's allowance

In this chapter we look at:

A. General conditions
What is jobseeker's allowance?	see 1
Transferring from UB or income support	see Box F.1
The basic rules	see 2
How do you claim?	see 3
Available for work	see 4
Actively seeking work	see 5
Jobseeker's agreement	see 6
Working 16 or more hours?	see 7
Back to Work Bonus	see Box F.2
Capable of work	see 8
Sanctions	see 9
Hardship payments	see 10

B. Contribution-based JSA
Do you qualify?	see 11
How much do you get?	see 12
Does anything affect what you get?	see 13
How long does contribution-based JSA last?	see 14

C. Income-based JSA
Do you qualify?	see 15
If you have any income	see 16
If you have savings or other capital	see 17
If your partner is working	see 18
If you are aged 16 or 17	see 19
How much do you get?	see 20

A. GENERAL CONDITIONS

1. What is jobseeker's allowance?

Jobseeker's allowance (JSA) is for people who are unemployed or working less than 16 hours a week, and are available for, and actively looking for work. JSA was introduced on 7.10.96 to replace unemployment benefit and income support for those required to sign on as available for work. Income support remains for people who don't have to sign for work, eg for those who are incapable of work or aged 60 or over – see Box B.1 in Chapter 3.

There are two routes into JSA:
- **contribution-based JSA** – this is a personal flat rate allowance with entitlement based on your National Insurance contribution record; it is payable for up to 6 months and is taxable;
- **income-based JSA** – this is means-tested and taxable, payable if you have no income or a low income, any savings are no more than £8,000 and your partner (if you have one) is not working or is working less than 24 hours a week. It can top up contribution-based JSA if that is not enough for your needs or the needs of your family.

One set of general 'labour market' conditions of entitlement applies to JSA as a whole, eg you must sign on as available for work, take active steps to look for work and complete a jobseeker's agreement.

If you transferred to JSA from unemployment benefit there are transitional rules that protected your rate of benefit, but only up to April 1997– see Box F.1.

2. The basic rules
You are entitled to jobseeker's allowance if:
- you are available for work – see 4; and
- you are actively seeking work – see 5; and
- you have entered into a jobseeker's agreement which remains in force – see 6; and
- you are not working 16 hours or more a week – see 7; and
- you are capable of work – see 8; and
- you are under pension age (60 for women, 65 for men); and
- you are not in full-time, non-advanced education if you are under age 19; (students of any age on full-time courses are usually excluded from JSA, but you may be able to study part time – see Chapter 31); and
- you are in Great Britain – see Chapter 41 for exceptions;

AND
- for contribution-based JSA you pass the contribution-based conditions – see 11;

OR
- for income-based JSA, you pass the income-based conditions – see 15.

If you satisfy the conditions for both, you may be entitled to contribution-based JSA topped up with income-based JSA – see 20.

3. How do you claim?
On the first day you become unemployed, call in to your nearest Jobcentre and ask to claim jobseeker's allowance. Don't delay otherwise you will lose benefit unless you can show you have 'special reasons' for the delay (see Chapter 52(4)). You'll find the address of your nearest Jobcentre in the phone book under 'Employment Service'.

The new jobseeker receptionist will register your claim and make you an appointment to come back for a New Jobseeker Interview. You'll be given a JSA claim pack to take away and complete at home. The first part of the pack, form JSA1, asks for details to check whether you pass the contribution-based conditions or income-based conditions. The second part, form ES2 *Helping You Back To Work*, contains detailed questions about the type of work you are looking for, the hours you are available for work, the pay you will accept, the distance you are prepared to travel to work and the types of steps you will take to find work or improve your prospects. You should take care when filling in this form. The form is not meant to trick you, but on the other hand, if you put 'unreasonable' restrictions on what you are prepared to accept, your answers could lead to a doubt about whether you are 'available for work'. We look at the basic requirements you must fulfil to be 'available for work' and the kind of restrictions that are permitted in 4 below. For the sort of jobseeking steps you are expected to take, see 5.

At the New Jobseeker Interview, the adviser will be checking to see if you meet the 'labour market' conditions for benefit, ie whether you are available for work, what you intend to do to look for work, and that you are capable of work. You will also be asked to complete and sign the *'jobseeker's agreement'* – see 6. This is compulsory and details the type of work you are looking for and what you are expected to do to find work or improve your prospects, as well as any restrictions on your availability for work that are agreed. It will be based on the answers you've given in the ES2 *Helping You Back To Work* form. Once it has been established that you meet the basic labour market conditions for benefit, your claim will be assessed for the specific contribution-based or income-based conditions of entitlement to benefit. If your health or disability means that you need specialist advice and help, you can be referred to a Disability Employment Adviser.

Problems? – If there is a delay in your claim being decided, or benefit is suspended or disallowed, or a sanction is applied, or you are told you can't sign on, seek advice. You should continue to sign on if possible while you are challenging any decision. You might be able to get hardship payments in the meantime – see 10. Decisions on entitlement to benefit are made by Adjudication Officers. If you are not happy with the decision you can appeal to a Social Security Appeal Tribunal. But see 6 below for details of the review procedure if you don't accept the proposed jobseeker's agreement. Chapter 52 looks at the rules on time limits for claiming JSA, when your JSA can be backdated, and the procedures for appealing.

During your claim – Normally JSA is paid every two weeks in arrears by a girocheque sent to your home, or it can be paid directly into a bank account. The government intends to gradually phase in the replacement of giros with a social

---

F.1 Transferring from UB or income support

If you are getting unemployment benefit (UB) immediately before JSA is introduced on 7.10.96, your award of UB is automatically treated as an award of contribution-based JSA. Similarly, if you are getting income support and signing on, your income support award is replaced by an award of income-based JSA.

Some of the new JSA rules applied immediately, in particular the requirement to satisfy the availability for work and actively seeking work rules. The requirement to sign a jobseeker's agreement was phased in over a 6 month period for existing claimants. But for some other rules there was a period during which the old rules continued to apply so there was some limited protection for the amount of benefit you are entitled to.

Unemployment benefit

Transitional protection applied if UB was payable to you for 5.10.96 or 6.10.96. The transitional protection ended on 6.4.97 or the end of your jobseeking period if that was earlier. If you reclaimed JSA within 8 weeks of a previous claim, you regained your transitional protection. After the cut-off date of 6.4.97 there is no more transitional protection, even if you have not exhausted your full 6 (or 12) months contribution-based JSA.

If you are entitled to transitional protection, the following rules apply.

❑ **Duration of contribution-based JSA** – Contribution-based JSA is only payable for 6 months. But, if transitional protection applies and UB was also payable for 6.4.96 or 7.4.96, and you had no breaks in your benefit of more than 8 weeks between April and October 1996, you are entitled to the balance of 312 days (ie one year) contribution-based benefit. If UB was **not** payable for 6.4.96 or 7.4.96, regardless of when you made your claim, you are only entitled to the balance of 156 days (ie 6 months) contribution-based benefit.

❑ **Dependants' additions** – There are no increases for dependants paid with contribution-based JSA. But if your UB included an addition for an adult dependant, this continued to be paid with your contribution-based JSA. If you are also entitled to income-based JSA, and you were getting an addition for an adult who does not live with you, the increase was added to your applicable amount.

❑ **Occupational and personal pensions** – If you were under 55 on 5.10.96, the old rules relating to occupational and personal pensions continued to apply while you were covered by transitional protection and still under 55. So the whole of any occupational or personal pension you received was disregarded. However if you are 55 or over, the new disregard of £50 a week applies.

❑ **Over pension age** – Contribution-based JSA is not payable beyond pension age. But if you were over pension age (60 for women, 65 for men) on 5.10.96 and getting the over pension age rate of UB, you continued to receive contribution-based JSA at the same rate while you were covered by transitional protection.

❑ **Earnings rules** – While you were covered by transitional protection, the old UB earnings rules continued to apply, ie if you earn more than £2 in a day, no benefit is paid for that day; if you earn £61 or more in a week, no benefit is paid for that week.

❑ **Under 25** – Contribution-based JSA is paid at a lower rate to young people. If you were entitled to transitional protection, you continued to get the same amount as you were getting on UB.

JSA (Transitional Provisions) Regs 1996/2567

Income support

The rates of benefit paid with income support and income-based JSA are the same. Some income support transitional protection rules are brought into JSA. Unlike the contribution-based JSA transitional protection, the income-based protection is not time-limited but continues so long as you satisfy the relevant transitional rule.

Old transitional additions – If you were getting a transitional addition with your IS (eg payable from the changeover from the old supplementary benefit) this continues to be paid under the old rules with your JSA (see Box B.2 in Chapter 3).

Housing costs – There are various protections for the amount of income support payable for mortgages and loans, mostly arising from the changes to these rules on 2.10.95 (eg the introduction of a ceiling on loans and a standard rate of interest). If your income support included such transitional protection, this continues to be paid with your JSA as though you were still on income support. See Chapter 3(20) for the rules on housing costs.

security card which you would take to the post office to get your fortnightly payment.

You are normally expected to sign on at the Jobcentre every fortnight. If you miss your signing-on day, your benefit entitlement will stop, unless you show within 5 working days that you have 'good cause' for failing to sign on, for example you had a doctor's appointment or job interview. If you are in one of the circumstances in which you are 'treated' as though you are available for work, you will have 'good cause' for not signing on (see 5, look under 'Absences, emergencies and other circumstances'). Each time you sign on you will be asked to explain what you have done to look for work or improve your prospects of finding work. You should keep a record of your 'jobseeking' steps so you can demonstrate that you meet the 'actively seeking working' conditions – see 5. Ask at the Jobcentre for a job search activity log (form ES4) to help you keep a record.

Periodically there will be more in depth interviews where, in particular, the jobseeker's agreement will be reviewed and updated if necessary. This is likely to happen every 6 months but you can be called in for an in depth interview at any time, for example, on referral from your fortnightly signing on interview. You must attend any interview notified to you in writing. If you do not, your benefit entitlement will stop, unless you can show within 5 working days that you had 'good cause' for not attending.

Jobseeker's direction – At these in depth interviews, the employment officer could decide to issue a 'jobseeker's direction' requiring you to undertake a specific activity related to improving your job prospects. For example you could be directed to attend a course to improve your skills or motivation, or to take steps to improve the way you present yourself to employers. If you don't comply with a jobseeker's direction, unless you have 'good cause', a sanction is applied stopping your benefit for 2 weeks, or 4 weeks if this is the second time a sanction has been applied – see 9.

4. Available for work

Generally, you must be willing and able to take up immediately any paid employment of at least 40 hours a week. However, in some circumstances you can place restrictions on the employment you are prepared to accept or the hours you are available to work. Your availability for work is first checked when you sign on and complete the ES2 form, *Helping You Back To Work*, and jobseeker's agreement.

You are not regarded as available for work and therefore are not entitled to jobseeker's allowance if:
- you get maternity allowance or statutory maternity pay; or
- you are a full-time student, unless your partner is also a full-time student and either of you are responsible for a child, in which case you won't be excluded from jobseeker's allowance during the summer vacation (if you are studying part-time, see Chapter 31); or
- you are a prisoner on temporary release.

At the start of your claim – For a period of up to 13 weeks from the beginning of your claim, you may be allowed to restrict your availability and jobseeking to your usual occupation and/or to your usual pay. After this 'permitted period' you must be prepared to widen your availability for work and jobsearching activity. You are still allowed to restrict your availability under the rules described below, as long as (in most cases) you have reasonable prospects of securing employment.

Can you restrict the hours you are available for work?
The 40 hours rule – Generally you must be prepared to take up employment of at least 40 hours a week. In most cases, you don't have to accept a job of less than 24 hours a week – see 9 below, under 'What is good cause'.

JSA is a 7-day benefit, so you must fulfil the conditions of entitlement on each day of the week. This does not mean you must be prepared to work 7 days a week. The 40 hours could be spread over 5 or 6 days for example. If you wish to specify the times in the week you are available to take up work (eg Monday to Saturday, 9am to 6pm) you must show that these times would give you 'reasonable prospects of employment' (see below) and that your job prospects are not considerably less than they would be if you were available at all times. The times you are available are recorded in the jobseeker's agreement. The hours you specify must be at least 40 a week, unless fewer hours are agreed as reasonable given your disability (see below) or because of caring responsibilities.

Carers – If you care for a child or an elderly person or someone *'whose physical or mental condition requires him to be cared for'* who is a 'close relative' or a member of your household, you may restrict the hours you are available for work to less than 40 hours, but not less than 16 hours a week. You must be available for as many hours, and at the times that your caring responsibilities allow, taking into account the times you spend caring, whether the caring is shared, and age and physical and mental condition of the person you care for. You must also show you have 'reasonable prospects of securing employment' – see below. A *'close relative'* means a partner, parent, parent-in-law, step-parent, son, daughter, son/daughter-in-law, step-son/daughter, grandparent, grandchild, brother, sister or the partner of any of those.

If you care for a disabled person, or you are a single parent you may be eligible for income support instead of JSA – see Box B.1 in Chapter 3. For income support, there is no requirement to look for or take up work. However it is means-tested, so if you have other income, you may be better off claiming contribution-based JSA. For carers who don't get invalid care allowance, you may need to sign on in order to protect your NI contribution record.

Laid off or short-time working – For the first 13 weeks, you are treated as available for work provided you are available to take on casual employment to top up any hours you actually work to at least 40 hours a week, or you are prepared to resume immediately the work you were laid off from and to take up any casual employment. After 13 weeks, this 'concession' no longer applies, so if you want to continue to restrict the hours you are available for work, you will have to show you have reasonable prospects of employment.

Can you put any other restrictions on the type of work you'll accept?
Provided you can show you have 'reasonable prospects of securing employment' (see below), you can restrict:
- the nature of the employment;
- the terms and conditions of employment;
- the rate of pay – but only for the first 6 months of your claim (but see below if you have a disability);
- the localities you will work in – generally you are expected to be prepared to travel for up to an hour both to and from work.

Disability-related restrictions – You can restrict your availability in any way (eg pay, hours, travel time, type of work), providing the restrictions are reasonable given your physical or mental condition. In this case, it is not relevant whether the restrictions affect your employment prospects, providing you do not put other non-disability-related restrictions on your availability as well. If you do, you will have to show you have reasonable employment prospects given all the restrictions. If you restrict the rate of pay you are prepared to accept, this is not subject to the general 6 months limit, but applies for so long as the restriction is reasonable. If you refuse a job offer where the hours of work or other conditions of the job are beyond your agreed restrictions, you won't generally be sanctioned for doing so – see 9.

Religious or conscientious objections – You can restrict the nature of the employment you are prepared to do, if you have a sincerely held conscientious or religious objection, providing you can show you have reasonable prospects of getting employment despite the restrictions.

Reasonable prospects of employment.
If you put any restrictions on your availability, unless these are solely disability-related, you must show that you have reasonable prospects of securing employment. This takes into account:
- your skills, qualifications and experience;
- the type and number of vacancies within daily travelling distance;
- how long you have been unemployed;
- your job applications and their outcome; and
- if the restrictions are on the nature of the work, whether you are prepared to move home to take up work.

No account is taken of the level of unemployment in the area, so in areas of high unemployment in particular, showing you have reasonable prospects of getting work is a tough test. It is important to consider carefully before you put any restrictions on your availability. If you can't show you have reasonable employment prospects, your benefit is disallowed.

Can you delay taking up an offer of employment?
Generally you must be able to take up employment immediately. But if you are a volunteer or a carer (see above) then you must be able to take up employment given 48 hours notice.

If you are providing a service (paid or unpaid) you must be able to take up work given 24 hours notice. If you are employed less than 16 hours a week, you must be able to take up work immediately after the statutory minimum notice period (rather than any contractual notice) that your employer is entitled to – usually one week.

Absences, emergencies and other circumstances
If you're on holiday in Great Britain, you must still be available for work during your time away (although you might not be expected to take active steps to look for work – see 5). You must show that you can be contacted regularly while you are away, and how, and be willing to return at once to start work. Before you go away send in the 'Going Away' form to the Jobcentre. If you go abroad on holiday, you are not usually entitled to JSA – see Chapter 41.

If you are in any of the situations below for a full week, you are treated as available for work, ie you're not expected to be willing and able to take up work during that week. If it is part of a week, then you are treated as available for 8 hours each day that the situation applies. Or if you have restricted your hours and have an agreed pattern of availability (set out in your jobseeker's agreement), you are treated as available for as many hours as you agreed to be available on each day that the circumstances apply. In each case, you are also treated as actively seeking work, ie you're not expected to take any jobseeking steps that week, provided that the situation applies to you for at least 3 days in the week.

❏ **Absences from home**
- you are at a work camp – for up to 2 weeks, once in 12 months;
- you are on a Venture Trust programme – for up to 4 weeks, once in 12 months;
- you are on an Open University residential course – for up to 1 week per course;
- you are absent from Great Britain to attend a job interview (up to 1 week); or for a child's medical treatment (up to 8 weeks); or your partner is over 60 or disabled and you are both abroad (up to 4 weeks) – see Chapter 41 for details.

❏ **Emergencies**
- you need time to deal with a death or serious illness or funeral of a close relative or close friend; or a domestic emergency affecting you, a close relative or close friend; or the person you have been caring for has died – for up to one week no more than 4 times in 12 months;
- you are working as a part-time fire fighter, or helping to run or launch a lifeboat;
- you are part of a group of people organised to respond to an emergency, eg part of an organised search for a missing person, or after a railway or other accident.

❏ **Other circumstances**
- you are sick for a short while, and treated as capable of work – see 8 below;
- you are on a full-time, employment-related course and have prior approval from the employment officer – for up to 2 weeks, once in 12 months;
- you are looking after your child while your partner is temporarily absent from the UK – for up to 8 weeks;
- you are temporarily looking after a child because the usual carer is ill, temporarily away from home, or is looking after a member of your family who is ill – for up to 8 weeks;
- you've been discharged from prison – for one week.

5. Actively seeking work
As well as being available for work, you are also expected to take such steps as you can *'reasonably be expected to have to take'* in order to have the best prospects of getting employment. You must take at least two steps a week, unless one step is all it is reasonable for you to do in that week. A 'week' is the 7 days that ends on the day of the week on which you sign on.

What jobseeking steps are you expected to take?
The employment officer can reasonably expect you to take steps each week from the following list:
- making written or verbal job applications;
- looking for vacancies in job adverts, from employers or employment agencies;
- registering with an employment agency;
- appointing a third party (eg an agency) to help you find work;
- on referral from an employment officer, seeking specialist advice on improving your prospects with regard to your particular needs or disability;
- drawing up a curriculum vitae, or getting a reference;
- drawing up a list of relevant employers, and seeking information from them;
- seeking information on an occupation.

This is not an exhaustive list. Other steps that improve your job prospects may also count. In deciding whether the steps you've taken are enough to satisfy the actively seeking work condition, all the circumstances of your case should be taken into account including, for example, disabilities.

When your jobseeking steps are disregarded – Even where you've taken reasonable steps to look for work, they can be disregarded where by your *'behaviour or appearance [you] otherwise undermined [your] prospects of securing the employment in question'*, or you acted in a violent or abusive way or you spoiled a job application. But it can't be held against you if these were due to circumstances beyond your control.

Absences, emergencies and other circumstances
In some circumstances for a limited time, you are not expected to have to look for work.
If you are also treated as available for work – In each of the situations in which you are treated as available for work (see 4, under 'Absences, emergencies and other circumstances'), you are also treated as actively seeking work (ie you don't have to take any jobseeking steps during that week), so long as the situation applies for at least 3 days in the week. For example, if you need 4 days to deal with a domestic emergency, you are not expected to look for work in that week. But if you need just 1 or 2 days to deal with the emergency, you are still expected to take jobseeking steps in that week, but it might be reasonable for you to take just one step rather than two.
If you are absent from home – There are other times when you are not expected to take any steps to look for work, although you must still be available to take up work. In any 12 month period, you are treated as actively seeking work for a maximum of:
- 2 weeks for any reason (eg a holiday) so long as you are away from home for at least a day each week; or
- 6 weeks if you are blind: the 6 weeks consists of a maximum of 4 weeks during which you are attending a training course in using a guide dog for at least 3 days a week, and a further 2 weeks for any reason so long as you are away from home for at least a day each week; or
- 3 weeks if you are attending an Outward Bound course for at least 3 days a week.

The weeks don't have to be consecutive. You can't use more than one provision in any one 12 month period. For example, if you have had one week away on holiday and then within 12 months you go on an Outward Bound course, you can only have one more week in which you are treated as actively seeking work (ie your second week for any reason).

You must give written notice in advance that you don't intend to actively seek work for a particular week (or weeks) and that you intend to stay away from home for at least a day in each week. For the 2 week 'any reason' provision, once you've notified your intention, you'll be treated as actively seeking work. If you change your mind and don't go anywhere you must give written notice withdrawing your intention before the start of the week you were due to be away to make sure you don't use up a week unnecessarily.
Training courses – You are treated as actively seeking work for any week in which you spend at least 3 days on a state-sponsored employment or training programme for which no training allowance is payable.
Becoming self-employed – You are treated as actively seeking work for up to 8 weeks during which you're taking active steps to establish yourself in self-employment, starting with the week you are accepted on a specified government scheme for assisting people into self-employment.

6. Jobseeker's agreement
A jobseeker's agreement contains a description of the type of work you're looking for, the action you're expected to take to look for work and to improve your job prospects, and details of any restrictions on your availability for work (see 3). It is a condition of entitlement to JSA that you and the employment officer sign the jobseeker's agreement.

What if you don't accept the proposed agreement?
Once you've attended an interview with the employment officer in order to draw up a jobseeker's agreement, until you both sign it, you're not entitled to JSA. But if you don't accept the proposed agreement, you have the right to ask the employment officer to refer it to an Adjudication Officer (AO). The employment officer cannot sign the agreement unless they believe you would satisfy the availability for work and actively seeking work conditions based on the terms of the agreement. So even where you are prepared to sign, the employment officer may decide to refer the proposed agreement to an AO. You will have an opportunity to set out the terms that you would be prepared to accept.
Referral to the Adjudication Officer – The AO will decide whether the availability for work and actively seeking work conditions would be satisfied were you to comply with the agreement, and whether it is reasonable to expect you to comply. The AO can alter the terms of the proposed agreement as they consider appropriate.

The decision should be made, 'so far as practicable' within 14 days. In the meantime, you are not entitled to benefit. Hardship payments of reduced rate income-based JSA may be made but only if you are in a vulnerable group and would otherwise suffer hardship – see 10. With the decision, the AO may decide to backdate the jobseeker's agreement but not necessarily back to your date of claim.
Further review – You have a right to a further review by a different AO if you don't accept the decision. You should request the review in writing within 3 months of the date the decision was notified to you, setting out your reasons. If you're not happy with the outcome of the further review, you have a right to appeal to a Social Security Appeal Tribunal within 3 months. Note that you can't go straight to an appeal from the first AO's decision.

Varying an existing jobseeker's agreement
Either you or the employment officer can propose to vary the agreement. This may be because your circumstances have changed, for example you have reached the end of your 'permitted period'. If there is a disagreement, or if the employment officer does not believe the terms satisfy the availability or actively seeking work conditions, the proposed agreement may be referred to an Adjudication Officer as above.

The AO will decide whether the agreement should be varied and what the terms should be. In the event that both your and the employment officer's proposals meet the availability and actively seeking work conditions, your preference must be taken into account. While the AO is considering a variation, your benefit will continue to be paid as the original agreement is considered to still have effect until the AO makes a decision. If the agreement is varied, you must sign within 21 days, otherwise the jobseeker's agreement may be terminated and your entitlement to benefit will stop. You have the right to a further review by a different AO as outlined above.

7. Working 16 or more hours?
To be eligible for JSA you must be unemployed or working for less than 16 hours a week on average. Work counts if you are paid, or you work *'in expectation of payment'*. So you are not regarded as working if you are doing, for example, voluntary work where you are only paid expenses, nor if you are off work sick or on maternity leave. In some situations you can work for more than 16 hours a week without this affecting your entitlement. These exceptions can assist disabled people whose earning power or hours of work are less than that of a non-disabled person doing similar work. The rules closely

follow the income support rules described in Chapter 3(6). Note though that if you stop work because of a trade dispute at your workplace, you are not eligible to claim JSA. Your partner can claim income-based JSA for the family but it is paid at a reduced rate.

Partners – For contribution-based JSA it makes no difference to your entitlement whether or not your partner works or how much s/he earns. For income-based JSA, if your partner works it must be for less than 24 hours a week (see 18), and earnings are taken into account in the assessment of your benefit.

Back to Work Bonus – If you get JSA or income support, and you or your partner have earnings from part-time work, you may be able to build up entitlement to a Back to Work Bonus – see Box F.2.

8. Capable of work

Generally you only need to state that you are capable of work and that is accepted as sufficient to satisfy the condition of entitlement.

If you are disabled or ill – If you are incapable of work through ill health (unless it is a short illness – see below) or disability, you are not eligible for JSA, but you may be able to claim incapacity benefit, severe disablement allowance or income support instead.

Under the rules for assessing incapacity (see Chapter 8) you may find you are regarded as incapable of work even though you wish to sign on and are willing and able to work. This may apply if you get disability living allowance higher rate care component, are registered blind, are terminally ill, or you are tetraplegic or paraplegic, or if you were assessed as incapable of work under the 'all work test' and your condition has not improved. In this case, to be regarded as capable of work and thus eligible for JSA, you must pass an extra condition. You must have worked, or been in education or training to prepare for work, while you had the same illness or disability, and show you have a reasonable prospect of getting employment. Once you have shown that you are eligible for JSA, any restrictions you wish to place on your availability for work because of your health or disability are treated as a separate issue.

Reg 17A, SS(Incapacity for Work)(General) Regs 1995

What if you are ill for a short while?

If you fall ill, you may choose to stay on JSA for up to 2 weeks instead of claiming incapacity benefit. You need to fill in a form to declare that you are unfit for work and for how long. You may only do this twice in each 'jobseeking period' (ie period of entitlement to JSA – see Chapter 9(3)). Or if you are entitled to JSA for over a year (ignoring breaks in entitlement of 12 weeks or less) you can only choose this option twice in each year. If you fall ill a third time or you are ill for longer than 2 weeks, you should claim incapacity benefit or income support instead.

If you fall ill within 8 weeks of the end of an entitlement to incapacity benefit, SSP, severe disablement allowance, or income support with a disability premium on incapacity grounds, you cannot stay on JSA. You should reclaim your previous benefit and, in most cases, you'll be entitled to your previous rate of benefit without re-serving any qualifying period.

Incapacity cut-offs

If your incapacity benefit or income support has been cut off because you have been found capable of work, you may claim JSA instead. You may disagree with the decision and have appealed, but unless your appeal is successful, for the purposes of JSA, you are regarded as capable of work. This does not prevent you making a new claim for incapacity benefit or income support if your condition gets worse, or if you begin to suffer from a different illness or disability.

Reg 19, SS (Incapacity for Work)(General) Regs 1995

When you claim JSA, while there will be no question about your capacity for work, you will be asked about your availability for work and the sort of work you are looking for. The rules allow you to impose any restrictions that are reasonable given your disability, eg the type of work you can do, the distance you can travel, or the hours of work. And you are not expected to take work that would cause significant harm to your health, or would be excessively stressful. It might be useful to discuss things with an adviser in the Placement, Assessment and Counselling Team. Unusually, you may find you fall between incapacity benefit and JSA if what you say about the restrictions imposed by your health and disabilities is not regarded as reasonable. Seek advice if this happens to you.

You do not prejudice your chance of winning an appeal on incapacity for work if you sign on as available for work. The advantage of claiming JSA is that you protect your right to NI contribution credits, whether or not your appeal is successful. But you may claim income support instead (without signing on) while you are appealing. The disadvantage of doing so is that it may be paid at a reduced rate (see Box B.1 in Chapter 3) and, if you lose your appeal, you won't be covered by contribution credits for this period.

9. Sanctions

If you don't fulfil the basic 'labour market' conditions to be available for work and actively seeking work, benefit is disallowed altogether – only if you are within a vulnerable group and would suffer hardship, will you be eligible for hardship payments. Even if you do satisfy the basic conditions, in some circumstances your benefit may be 'sanctioned' and payment stopped for a limited period. The period of the sanction normally runs from the beginning of the benefit week following the AO's decision to apply the sanction. If a sanction is applied, you may be eligible for hardship payments of reduced rate income-based JSA – see 10.

2 or 4 weeks sanction
JSA is not payable for 2 weeks, or 4 weeks if this is the second sanction within 12 months, in the following circumstances.
- You refuse or fail to carry out a reasonable 'jobseeker's direction'.
- You refuse or fail to apply for, or take up a place on a training scheme or employment programme notified to you by an employment officer.
- You give up a place on, or fail to attend, a training scheme or employment programme.
- You lose your place on a training scheme or employment programme through misconduct.

Jobseeker's direction – The sanction will not be applied if you have 'good cause' for your action. What counts as good cause is outlined below, under the '26 weeks sanction'. For the circumstances in which a jobseeker's direction may be issued, see 3.

Training schemes and employment programmes – These sanctions only apply to certain schemes: Jobplan workshop; 1-2-1; Workwise (Worklink in Scotland); Restart; YT, Jobfinder, Contract for Work, Project Work. (However, you could also be sanctioned for not attending other schemes if you've been referred under a jobseeker's direction and you don't comply with the direction.)

Unless you have lost your place through misconduct, no

sanction is applied if you have 'good cause' for your action. Regulations give circumstances in which you automatically have good cause, although other reasons could also be considered:
- you could not attend because of your disability or ill health, or attendance would put your health at risk;
- you have caring responsibilities, you could not make alternative arrangements and the person has no 'close relative' (see 4) or member of their household available to care for them;
- travel time would be more than an hour either way, or if there is no scheme within an hour's travel, the travel time would be longer than to the nearest appropriate scheme;
- you had to deal with a domestic emergency;
- you were arranging a funeral of a close friend or relative;
- you did not participate due to a sincerely held religious or conscientious objection;
- you were attending court as a party to the proceedings, a witness or juror;
- you were running or launching a lifeboat, or on duty as a part-time fire fighter, or part of a group organised to provide assistance in an emergency.

26 weeks sanction
JSA is not payable for up to 26 weeks in the following circumstances.
- You lose your job through misconduct.
- You voluntarily leave your job without 'just cause'.
- You refuse or fail to apply for a vacancy or accept a job offer, notified to you by an employment officer, without 'good cause' – see below.
- You did not take up a job opportunity with an employer for whom you worked within the last 12 months, where the terms and conditions of employment were at least as good as before (eg you do not exercise your right to return to work after maternity leave), without 'good cause' – see below.

Entitlement to contribution-based JSA lasts for a maximum of 26 weeks. This time continues to run while the sanction is applied, so you could be left with no entitlement at all if the maximum 26 week sanction is applied. The 26 week maximum period is discretionary and the AO must consider all your circumstances, including:
- any physical or mental stress connected with a job you left voluntarily, or with a job for a previous employer;
- the rate of pay and hours of work in a job you left voluntarily, if you worked 16 hours or less a week;
- the length of time a job was likely to have lasted, if this would be less than 26 weeks.

You have the right to appeal against the decision – see Chapter 52. The SSAT could very well reduce the period of the sanction. The minimum sanction is one week.

If you lose your job through misconduct – Being dismissed does not necessarily lead to a benefit sanction. When you claim benefit, your ex-employer will be sent a standard form asking whether you were sacked and why. If it looks as though a sanction may be applied, you will be sent a copy of your employer's reply. It is important to comment on this reply in detail. Your ex-employer will also see what you have said and can add further comments. A Citizens Advice Bureau can help you sort out the important facts so you can reply in the best way. You may also be making a claim of unfair dismissal to an industrial tribunal. If someone is helping with this, eg your union representative, you should ask them for advice. If a sanction is applied, you have the right of appeal to the SSAT – see Chapter 52.

If you leave your job voluntarily – 'Just cause' for leaving work is not the same as having a good reason for leaving. Your state of health (or the health of a close relative) may help you show just cause. Generally there must be something in the nature of your job, or in your own domestic circumstances, that meant it was no longer reasonable for you to continue working.

You should try and resolve any work-related problems (using the firm's grievance procedures if they have them) before handing in your notice. You should also try and look for other suitable work before leaving. Or explore whether it is possible to transfer you to lighter work. If possible, discuss your personal or domestic difficulties with your employer to see if there is any way you can resolve the difficulty without handing in your notice. It helps if you can show that handing in your notice was the only thing you could do, given all the circumstances, including your attempts to resolve the problems. If you can do all this, you are likely to escape the sanction altogether.

There is no sanction for agreeing to take voluntary redundancy; you are not regarded as having left your job voluntarily – but see Chapter 42(1) if you are considering taking early retirement.

Trial period – There is a trial period of 8 weeks to allow you to try out a new job without risking benefit sanctions if it does not work out. This is available if you have not worked as an employee, or been self-employed, or in full-time education during the 13 weeks before starting the job. You will not have a benefit sanction applied if you leave work voluntarily at any time from the start of the 5th week to the end of the 12th week in that job. Any week in which you work for less than 16 hours is disregarded when deciding the beginning and end of the trial period. For example, if you work for 3 weeks and then are off sick for a week, you would have to return to the job for a week before you could be covered by the trial period exemption.

What is 'good cause'?
If you fail to carry out a jobseeker's direction, or refuse employment, your benefit payment is stopped for the period of the sanction unless you have 'good cause' for your actions.

You are not expected to accept a job of less than 24 hours a week unless it has been agreed that you may restrict the hours you are available for work to less than 24 hours a week (eg because of a disability or caring responsibilities – see 4). In this case, you won't be sanctioned for refusing a job of less than 16 hours a week.

The level of pay cannot usually be taken into account in deciding whether you have good cause for refusing a job, even if the pay would not cover your financial commitments or would be less than your benefits. The only exception is where, under the availability for work rules, it has been agreed that you may restrict the level of pay you are prepared to accept (eg if this is reasonable given your disability, or during the 'permitted period' at the start of your claim – see 4). See below if there are high work-related expenses.

You will have 'good cause' if your reason for refusing a job, or carrying out a jobseeker's direction is that you are only looking for work in your usual occupation during your 'permitted period', or that you are not required to be able to take up a job at once, eg you are a carer or a volunteer – see 4.

The Adjudication Officer must take certain other factors into account when deciding whether you have 'good cause':
- any personal circumstances which suggest that a particular job or jobseeker's direction might cause significant harm to your health, or subject you to excessive physical or mental stress;

- any responsibility for caring for a 'close relative' (see 4) or someone in your household which might make it unreasonable for you to do a particular job, or carry out a jobseeker's direction;
- travel time to and from work, or to a place mentioned in the jobseeker's direction; but it won't count as 'good cause' if the travel time is normally less than an hour each way unless the time is unreasonable because of your health or caring responsibilities;
- any agreed restrictions in your availability for work (see 4), and differences between the work you are available for given those restrictions and the requirements of the job;
- any sincerely held religious or conscientious objections to taking the job or carrying out the jobseeker's direction;
- travel expenses and other necessary, exclusively work-related expenses if these are a high proportion of the income from the job, or your income while carrying out a jobseeker's direction. However, nothing else to do with your income and outgoings, or your family's, can be taken into account, unless you have been allowed to restrict the level of pay you are prepared to accept because of your disability, or you are still in the 'permitted period' at the start of your claim (see 4), or if the job is paid only by commission.

10. Hardship payments

If your benefit is 'sanctioned', suspended, disallowed, or there is a delay in making a decision on your claim, you may be entitled to reduced-rate hardship payments of income-based JSA. However payment is not automatic. In most cases you must show that you or your family will suffer hardship unless benefit is paid. Unless you fall into a particular vulnerable group, no benefit will be paid for the first 2 weeks.

The applicable amount is reduced by 40% of the single person's personal allowance applicable for your age. But if you, your partner or child is seriously ill or pregnant, the reduction is 20%. If your partner is entitled to income support (IS), s/he may be able to claim IS for both of you. It is not subject to any reduction.

You may be entitled to hardship payments if you have no JSA in payment for one of the following reasons.
- There is a delay in the decision on your claim for JSA, because of a question whether you satisfy the availability, actively seeking work and jobseeker's agreement conditions for benefit.
- Your benefit has been 'sanctioned', eg you have left work voluntarily without just cause.
- Your benefit has been suspended because of a doubt whether you satisfy the availability, actively seeking work or jobseeker's agreement conditions.
- If you're not available for work or actively seeking work or you don't have a current jobseeker's agreement, you may still get hardship payments, but you must also be in one of the vulnerable groups below even after the first 2 weeks. However, qualifying for a disability premium does not count here, you must fall into one of the other groups.

F.2 Back to Work Bonus

This is a new scheme which allows people claiming income support (IS) or JSA and their partners, who work part time while on benefit to build up entitlement to a lump sum of up to £1,000, payable when they move into work which removes their entitlement to IS or JSA.

While you are on IS or JSA, you keep the first £5 of any part-time earnings and anything you earn above this is deducted from your benefit. In some cases the amount you can keep (the 'earnings disregard') is higher than £5 – see 13 and 16. Under the bonus scheme, you build up a bonus amount equal to 50% of earnings not disregarded. Your partner's earnings also count if you get IS or income-based JSA.

The bonus amount begins to accumulate once you've been on IS or JSA for over 13 weeks (91 days). The earliest this 13 week *'waiting period'* can start is 1.7.96. Entitlement to unemployment benefit also counts towards the waiting period, however, any earnings received before 7.10.96 do not count towards the bonus amount.

For example, say you earn £30 a week. Your JSA is reduced by £25 a week. But £12.50 a week accrues under the Back to Work Bonus. If you return to work 33 weeks later (13 weeks waiting period then 20 more weeks), you get a lump sum of £250.

Once you've been on JSA or IS for longer than the waiting period, you'll get a statement every 13 weeks estimating the amount of bonus accumulated to date, for as long as you continue to accumulate a bonus. If you stop accumulating a bonus, you'll then get annual statements. The maximum amount you can accumulate is £1,000; the minimum bonus payment is £5.

The bonus is treated as capital for means-tested benefits, but is disregarded for 52 weeks for housing benefit, council tax benefit, family credit and DWA.

To qualify for a bonus payment, your JSA or IS entitlement must end because you have started work, or increased your hours or earnings. Or if you start work, etc within 14 days of your benefit ending, that counts so long as it would have taken you off benefit. You must be aged under 60 (if you were on IS) or below pension age (if you were on JSA). You must claim the bonus within 12 weeks of the end of your benefit entitlement. The time limit can be extended to up to a year if you can show you have good cause for not claiming earlier.

Trainees – If your benefit stopped because you started getting a training allowance, you can claim a bonus if, within 14 days of completing your training, you start work of either 16 hours or more a week, or that pays the same or more as the training allowance. You must claim within 12 weeks of completing the training.

Couples who separate – If you are the claimant, on separation any part of a bonus amount based on your partner's earnings becomes their's alone. The exception to this rule is where you've already become entitled to a bonus payment even though you may not yet have claimed it. In this case you keep your entitlement.

If you have a break in benefit entitlement – You won't have to start the 13 weeks waiting period again if you did not claim the bonus but can pick up where you left off providing you reclaim IS or JSA within 12 weeks of the end of your previous entitlement; or if there is a longer gap but in between your claims, you were:
- getting incapacity benefit, severe disablement allowance or invalid care allowance, for up to 2 years; or
- getting maternity allowance; or
- on training, in receipt of a training allowance and not under a contract of service with the training provider; or
- on jury service;

and you reclaim IS or JSA within 12 weeks of the end of this period.

SS (Back to Work Bonus) (No. 2) Regs 1996

For the first 2 weeks – Hardship payments are not payable for the first 2 weeks unless you or your partner are:
- responsible for a child; or
- pregnant; or
- a carer looking after someone who gets attendance allowance or DLA middle or higher rate care component (or has claimed but is waiting for a decision), and you cannot continue to care for them unless you receive hardship payments – in this case you need not show hardship would result; or
- qualify for a disability premium; or
- suffer from a *'chronic medical condition which results in functional capacity being limited or restricted by physical impairment'* which has lasted, or is likely to last, for at least 26 weeks, and the disabled person's health would probably decline during the first 2 weeks more than that of a healthy person; or
- under 18 and fall within one of the groups eligible for JSA while age 16 or 17 (see 19).

In each case, other than the exception for carers, you must satisfy the Adjudication Officer that the vulnerable person will suffer hardship unless payments are made.

After 2 weeks – If you don't fit into one of the groups above, you are eligible for hardship payments only after the first 2 weeks after the sanction has been applied, or suspension made, etc. You must show that you or your partner will suffer hardship unless payment is made.

What is 'hardship'? – You must fill in an application form and set out your grounds for applying for a hardship payment. In deciding whether or not you will suffer hardship if no payment is made, the Adjudication Officer must take into account any resources likely to be available to you and the shortfall between these and the reduced rate of hardship payments. They must also look at whether there is a substantial risk that you will have much less, or lose altogether, essential items such as food, clothing, heating and accommodation. It is also relevant whether a disability premium or disabled child premium is payable. But they may also take other factors into account.

B. CONTRIBUTION-BASED JSA

11. Do you qualify?
In order to qualify for contribution-based JSA you must have paid enough National Insurance contributions in the right tax years. This contribution condition is explained in Chapter 9. You must also satisfy the basic rules for JSA set out in 2 above. Contribution-based JSA is a flat rate personal benefit and is payable for a maximum of 6 months. If you don't have enough contributions you may be entitled to income-based JSA instead. You may also be entitled to income-based JSA to top up your benefit, eg if you have a dependent partner or child, or certain housing costs such as a mortgage – see 15.

12. How much do you get?
The weekly amounts of contribution-based JSA are:
- aged under 18   £29.60
- aged 18–24   £38.90
- aged 25 or over   £49.15

13. Does anything affect what you get?
The amount you get may be affected by earnings, payments at the end of a job, or by an occupational or personal pension. Only your own earnings are taken into account. Payment is not affected by any income your partner may have, nor by any savings you may have.

Earnings
Earnings are taken into account less any income tax, National Insurance contributions and half of any contribution towards an occupational or personal pension scheme. Your weekly earnings from employment or self-employment are deducted in full from the amount of benefit due, apart from £5 which is disregarded.

Some payments do not count as earnings, eg sick pay, maternity pay, redundancy payment, payments in kind, wholly work-related expenses. Payments that do count as earnings include holiday pay (unless this is paid to you more than 4 weeks after you left employment), bonuses, commission, travel expenses to and from work and expenses for childcare.

The assessment of earnings is essentially the same as for income support, other than the earnings disregards. For contribution-based JSA the disregard is £5 (unless you are working as a part-time firefighter, auxiliary coastguard, helping operate a lifeboat, or a member of any territorial or reserve force when the disregard is £15). For more details see Chapter 3(25).

Occupational or personal pension
Income from an occupational or personal pension of over £50 a week is deducted from the amount of benefit due. For example, if your pension is £55 a week, £5 is deducted from your benefit. A one-off lump sum payment does not affect your benefit.

Other benefits
You cannot get more than one contributory benefit at the same time. Nor can you get income support while claiming contribution-based JSA. If your benefit is not enough to live on, you should claim income-based JSA to top it up. However your partner can claim income support provided you only get contribution-based JSA and are not entitled to (ie you don't claim) income-based JSA.

14. How long does contribution-based JSA last?
You cannot usually be paid JSA for the first 3 days of unemployment – these are called 'waiting days'. But if you claim JSA within 12 weeks of the end of an earlier entitlement to JSA (contribution or income-based) or to income support, incapacity benefit or invalid care allowance, you can be paid from the first day of your new JSA claim.

Entitlement to benefit lasts for a total of 6 months (182 days). This can be in one spell of unemployment lasting for 6 months, or it could be in more than one spell of unemployment where you make shorter claims for JSA but your entitlement in each of those claims is based on the same two tax years. Once your 6 months are exhausted, you can only requalify when entitlement to benefit in your new JSA claim is based on different tax years (at least one of which is a later year). See Chapter 9 for details of the tax years on which your claim is based.

If you transferred to JSA from unemployment benefit, see Box F.1.

C. INCOME-BASED JSA

15. Do you qualify?
To qualify for income-based JSA, you must satisfy the basic rules for JSA set out in 2 above. In addition you must satisfy these income-based rules:
- you must have no income, or any income is below your 'applicable amount' (a set amount that depends on your circumstances) – see 16;

- your capital must be no more than £8,000 – see 17;
- if you have a partner s/he must not be working for 24 hours or more a week – see 18;
- you must be aged 18 or over; or aged 16 or 17 and pass other tests – see 19.

Income-based JSA is means-tested and taxable. You claim for yourself and for your partner and any dependent children in your household. If you are one of a couple, you can choose who should make the claim. But if your partner claims, s/he is the one who must sign on and satisfy all the basic rules.

Entitlement to income-based JSA gives you access to other benefits and entitlements without going through another means-test. So you may also be entitled to housing benefit, council tax benefit, free prescriptions, free dental treatment, and any other benefit to which income support would provide access.

People from abroad – If you are classed as a person from abroad, you are not entitled to ordinary income-based JSA but in limited circumstances you might be entitled to an 'urgent cases' payment. The rules are the same as those for income support – see Chapter 3(7).

16. If you have any income

If you are one of a couple (married or living together as husband and wife), your partner's income is added to your own. Otherwise only your own income is taken into account. Children's income may be partly taken into account.

The rules for income-based JSA are very much the same as for income support. Turn to Chapter 3(24) for details of the way your resources are assessed. The rules on 'earnings disregards' (the amount you can earn before your benefit is reduced) are also the same as in income support. Broadly, £5 is disregarded if you are single, £10 for couples, £15 for lone parents, or £15 if you satisfy certain conditions. See Chapter 3(25) for details.

There are some differences from the income support rules in the way earnings are taken into account following the termination of employment (we don't cover these rules in detail in the Handbook).

17. If you have savings or other capital

If you or your partner have capital of over £8,000, you won't be entitled to income-based JSA. (The only exception is for people who live in residential care homes for whom the capital limit is £16,000 – see Chapter 36(5).)

If your capital is from £3,000.01 to £8,000 it is treated as producing a 'tariff income' – £1 for every £250 you have in capital above £3,000 is deducted from benefit.

Your capital is worked out in the same way as for income support – see Chapter 3(24) and (29). Some types of capital are ignored partly or completely, and other kinds count towards the capital limit – see Chapter 3(31).

18. If your partner is working

You are not entitled to income-based JSA if your partner is working for 24 hours or more a week. However there are exceptions which allow the work that your partner does to be discounted, and conversely which may treat him or her as working even when they're not. For example, you are not excluded from income-based JSA if your partner's disability means that their earnings or hours are 75% or less of what someone without their disability would expect to earn or work in a similar job. The rules are almost the same as those for income support – see Chapter 3(6).

19. If you are aged 16 or 17

If you are aged 16 or 17, you are only entitled to income-based JSA if you pass extra tests. To be eligible you must usually register for work and training with the Careers Service. You'll find the nearest office in the phone book – look under 'Careers Service' or under the name of the local education authority. You must also satisfy all the basic rules of entitlement (set out in 2 above) including being available to take up work and taking active steps to look for work and training. Provided you haven't been subject to a JSA penalty in the past, you can restrict your availability to work where the employer is providing suitable training (ie you can turn down a job if no such training is offered).

If you don't fit into any of the circumstances outlined below in which JSA can be paid to you while age 16 or 17, you can still be paid JSA on a discretionary basis if you would otherwise suffer severe hardship. The direction to pay JSA will be for a temporary period (usually 8 weeks) and you must satisfy all the basic rules of entitlement. Things such as your health, vulnerability, threat of homelessness, training or job prospects should be taken into account. In some situations the amount you get is reduced by 40% of the personal allowance (or 20% if you are seriously ill, or pregnant) for the first 2 weeks, eg if you fail to complete a course of training without good cause. The jobseeker's agreement will outline these benefit penalties.

Until age 18 (without time limit)

You are eligible for income-based JSA while aged 16 or 17 if you fall into one of the groups of people who are eligible for income support (but you choose to claim JSA instead) – see Box B.1 in Chapter 3. You are also eligible if you are one of a couple and are treated as responsible for a child who lives with you, or if you are laid off or on short-time working (up to a maximum of 13 weeks).

If you are not covered by these rules, you may be eligible for a limited period which either ends with the date that child benefit finishes for school leavers, called the 'child benefit extension period', or begins with that date.

During the 'child benefit extension period'

The child benefit extension period starts with the first Monday after the end of the holiday after you left non-advanced education. It lasts for 16 weeks for summer school-leavers and 12 weeks for Christmas and Easter school-leavers – see Chapter 27 for more details.

To receive JSA during this period, you must fall into one of the following categories.
- ❏ You are married, without children, and your spouse is either aged 18 or older; or is entitled to JSA and registered for employment and training; or is eligible for income support until age 18 (see above).
- ❏ You have no parent nor anyone acting in place of your parents.
- ❏ You are not living with your parents, or anyone acting in their place, and:
  - before you reached 16 you were in local authority care (and not living with your parents or any 'close relative' while in care); or in custody; or
  - you moved into your accommodation under the supervision of the probation service or a local authority as part of a rehabilitation or resettlement programme; or in order to avoid physical or sexual abuse; or because of a mental or physical handicap or illness and need that accommodation because of your disability.
- ❏ You are living away from your parents (and anyone acting

in their place), they are unable financially to support you – and they are chronically sick or mentally or physically disabled, or detained in custody, or prohibited from coming into Great Britain.
- You *'of necessity'* have to live away from your parents (and anyone acting in their place), because you are estranged from them; or you are in physical or moral danger; or there is a serious risk to your physical or mental health.

After the 'child benefit extension period'
You are eligible for JSA once the child benefit extension period is over in the following circumstances.
- You have left local authority care and you have to live away from your parents or anyone acting as a parent – JSA is paid for up to 8 weeks from the date the care order is discharged.
- You have been discharged from custody, and your circumstances are the same as any in the list of people who can get JSA only during the child benefit extension period (see above) – JSA is paid for up to 8 weeks from the date of discharge.

20. How much do you get?
The amount you get is based on your 'applicable amount'. This is made up of:
- **a personal allowance**: for yourself, or for a couple, and for each dependent child – see Chapter 3(10); plus
- **premiums**: to take account of family responsibilities, disability, age and caring responsibilities (not everyone qualifies for a premium) – see Chapter 3(11); plus
- **certain housing costs** (eg mortgage interest) – see Chapter 3(20).

Your entitlement to all of these is taken into account when your JSA claim is assessed. If you have no income and your capital is below the limit, the amount of JSA you get is equal to your 'applicable amount'. If you have other income, this is assessed to see how much may be disregarded and how much to take into account. If the income to be taken into account is less than the applicable amount, the amount you get in JSA is equal to the applicable amount less your total income. If your income is above the applicable amount, you are not entitled to benefit.

The amounts for the personal allowance and premiums, and the rules for housing costs are the same as for income support. These are explained in detail in Chapter 3.

The first 3 days of your claim are 'waiting days' and you are not paid for these days, unless you are reclaiming JSA within 12 weeks of the end of an earlier entitlement to JSA or to IS, incapacity benefit or invalid care allowance.
If you also satisfy the contribution-based conditions – Your entitlement is first worked out separately for income-based and contribution-based JSA. You'll get the income-based amount if this is higher than the contribution-based amount.

For example, say you have no income but your partner works 10 hours a week earning £30. You have no children. The contribution-based amount is £49.15. This is the full amount since your partner's earnings are not taken into account.

The income-based amount is:

couple's personal allowance	£77.15
less earnings (minus the £10 disregard)	£20.00
giving a total of	**£57.15**

This is higher than the £49.15 contribution-based amount, so your JSA is £57.15 a week.

15 Employment and training

In this chapter we look at:
A. Employment services
B. Training

A. EMPLOYMENT SERVICES

1. Jobcentre services
Employment Service Jobcentre staff provide job finding and advisory services for all disabled people. If you have more complex employment problems because of your disability, you may be referred to a Disability Employment Adviser (DEA) in the Placement, Assessment and Counselling Team (PACT). As well as giving you specialist advice and assessment, DEAs can help you get into suitable employment by using a number of special schemes, as outlined below.
Registering disabled? – Since the introduction of the Disability Discrimination Act on 2.12.96, you can no longer register as disabled with the Employment Service. Instead, the Act introduces a new definition of disability (see 6). If you were registered with the Employment Service both on 12.1.95 and 2.12.96, you automatically count as disabled under the Act for a further three years without having to show that you meet the new definition.

Registering as disabled (including registering as blind or partially sighted) with the Social Services Department is different. This is not affected by the new Act and you can still register in the usual way – see Chapter 32.

2. Job Introduction Scheme
The Job Introduction Scheme is available to all disabled people who, in the opinion of the DEA, require a period of adjustment in a job to help them demonstrate their capabilities to a new employer. The Employment Service will pay £45 a week to a firm if it agrees to give a 6-week trial period to a disabled person. In some cases, the trial period can be extended to 13 weeks.

3. Access to Work
Access to Work is an Employment Service programme to assist with the extra costs involved in providing support in employment because of disability, such as:
- a communicator for people who are deaf or have a hearing impairment;
- a part time reader for someone with impaired vision;
- support workers if you need practical help either at work or getting to work;
- special equipment or adaptations to equipment to suit individual needs;
- alterations to premises or working environment so that an employee with disabilities can work there;
- help with travel to work costs, such as adaptations to a car, or taxi fares if you can't use public transport to get to work.

The programme is designed to be flexible to suit each person's needs within their job, and there are other kinds of support available. Your local PACT will supply further information.
Who can get help – You may be eligible if you are unemployed, employed or self-employed, and you are disabled (as defined under the Disability Discrimination Act – see 6 below). The amount of support available depends on what is required because of disability need, and is granted for a maximum 3 year period, after which you can reapply for support. For people

who have been in a job for less than 6 weeks or are about to start work, the Employment Service will pay all costs for a 3 year period. For employed people, the Employment Service will contribute up to 80% of costs up to £10,000 over a 3 year period, except for the first £300 per annum, and all costs over £10,000. All extra costs for Travel to Work and communicator support are funded by the Employment Service.

4. Rehabilitation

The Employment Service can provide employment rehabilitation to help disabled people to get work by addressing specific employment-related needs that result from their disability and prevent them from being able to enter employment or take up vocational training of a type which would otherwise be suitable for them.

Employment rehabilitation is contracted out by PACTs to a national network of agents who provide flexible programmes of rehabilitation to meet the needs of the person after assessment by the PACT. PACTs may also contract to provide work placements as part of the rehabilitation programme to allow experience of unfamiliar occupations or to test suitability or restore confidence.

You may be entitled to a Rehabilitation Allowance and other expenses. Or you may have the option of staying on your remaining benefits instead of claiming the allowance. The PACT can advise you on your best option. If you choose to claim the allowance, at the end of your course you can reclaim your incapacity benefit or SDA and regain your former rate of benefit without having to serve any qualifying periods, provided you are still 'incapable of work' (see 12 below).

5. Supported employment

Supported employment is for people with severe disabilities who are unable to get or keep jobs in the open market. There are different types of supported employment:
- Supported Placements;
- Workshops run by local authorities or voluntary organisations;
- Remploy Interwork – Remploy placements with outside firms;
- Remploy factories.

Supported Placements are available in all kinds of jobs. Jobs are expected to be permanent and should last at least six months. You work at your own pace and will get the training you need to do the job. You are paid the same wages as non-disabled colleagues doing similar work. A local authority or voluntary organisation contracts with the Employment Service to sponsor you in Supported Placements with a firm; the sponsor keeps in touch with you to ensure there are no problems. You are usually employed by the sponsor but you may be employed directly by the firm where you work if that is best for you.

The Disability Employment Adviser will advise you about suitable opportunities in Supported Placements and other supported employment.

6. Employment rights

All people with disabilities have the same rights as able-bodied employees to protection against unfair dismissal and redundancy, maternity leave and pay, time off for trade union and public duties, etc. For more information, see RADAR's information pack, *Employment Rights: A Guide for Disabled People* – see our Address List for RADAR's address. Your trade union can help with employment advice. If you are not in a union, try contacting a local law centre if you have an employment problem.

Disability Discrimination Act – The Disability Discrimination Act 1995 introduced new employment rights for disabled people on 2.12.96. The Act makes it unlawful to treat a disabled person less favourably than someone else because of their disability, unless the employer can show the discrimination is 'justified'. This applies to all employment matters, including recruitment, training, promotion and dismissal. Employers must also take reasonable steps to prevent their employment practices or premises from causing a substantial disadvantage to a disabled person.

Disability is defined as *'a physical or mental impairment which has a substantial and long-term adverse effect on [your] ability to carry out normal day-to-day activities'*. The government has issued guidance to help clarify who is intended to be covered by the definition, and a Code of Practice to give practical guidance on the employment provisions in the Act. These are available from The Stationery Office (HMSO) bookshops. None of the provisions apply to employers with fewer than 20 employees but these small employers are encouraged to follow guidance in the Code of Practice. Complaints of discrimination are heard by an industrial tribunal, and you can ask ACAS (the Advisory Conciliation and Arbitration Service) to help. For any employment problem, you should first contact your trade union. See Chapter 2 for more information on the Disability Discrimination Act.

B. TRAINING

7. Government sponsored training

Training is the responsibility of the Department for Education and Employment (DfEE) who contract with Training and Enterprise Councils (TECs), and in Scotland, Local Enterprise Companies (LECs) to ensure training within Departmental guidelines is delivered.

Complaints – TECs are required to record and investigate all allegations that the TEC has not discharged its obligations under YT Guarantees and under its Training for Work requirement, which are made by or on behalf of eligible persons resident or normally resident in the TEC's area. The TEC has to do its best to effect a remedy as soon as possible and notify the DfEE about all established failures to do so.

8. Youth Training

Recruitment to Youth Training (YT) is usually through the Careers Service. The Careers Service plays a crucial role in identifying and assessing people with special training needs (STN), and where appropriate endorse STN for funding that individual's training. They will advise about the extra help for people with disabilities.

Most 16 and 17 year olds are excluded from jobseeker's allowance in the expectation that they will take up a 'guaranteed' place on YT. Unemployed 16 and 17 year olds who are seeking youth training are entitled to be offered a suitable full-time YT place up to their 18th birthday, with a re-offer as many times as necessary.

You are also guaranteed an offer of a suitable place on YT if you are aged 18 to 24 (inclusive) and disability or ill health, language difficulties, pregnancy, custodial sentence, remands, or a care order meant that you could not take part in YT or were unable to complete a YT course.

YT combines work experience with training. When you start YT, you should be given an Individual Plan by the training provider with details of your training programme and the qualifications you are working towards. If appropriate, you may have a spell of initial training before joining a mainstream

YT programme.

TECs have discretion in setting terms and conditions, apart from minimum training allowances. However, if your entry and subsequent training is covered by the YT Guarantee and Extended Guarantee, and if you can only join, or continue in, suitable training if certain expenditure (eg lodging costs, travel, childcare, disability support, safety equipment, tools, clothing, etc) are incurred, those expenditures should be met or reimbursed up to a level which is reasonable and necessary to secure entry to the scheme, and/or to maintain training after entry.

The range of special help to enable people with disabilities to take part in YT encompasses all the help also available to adults entering work or TFW which can include an interpreter service for deaf people, a readership service for blind people, essential taxi fares, adaptations to premises and equipment, and loans of specialised equipment. If you need to keep a special aid in order to start a job, the TEC should allow you to do so.

Most people on YT will be 'trainees', but some will have employed status. Before starting a YT programme you should be told whether your status is that of a trainee or an employee as the difference affects your rights. This section deals only with the position of YT trainees. If you are an 'employee' on a YT scheme, this could give you far more legal rights than a 'trainee', and usually means that you will receive a higher 'wage' rather than the basic YT allowance. If there is a trade union in the workplace, they can advise you of your rights.

A 16 year old gets £30 a week. From your 17th birthday, the YT allowance is £35 a week. You can get more details about YT from Careers Offices.

Income support – A YT trainee can claim income support (IS) to top up their YT allowance. The whole £30 or £35 is taken into account as income. In practice a 16 or 17 year old is only likely to qualify for an IS top up if s/he is entitled to a premium or if s/he is entitled to the higher rate of IS personal allowance – see Chapter 3(10).

If getting severe disablement allowance (SDA) is the only way you can qualify for the disability premium, note that you lose SDA on starting YT. This is because days on which you receive a state training allowance cannot count as days of incapacity for work. However, if you have been getting IS with a SDA-based disability premium, that premium won't be withdrawn if you lose SDA because of getting a training allowance. A disability premium based on disability living allowance won't be affected as you can continue to get DLA while on YT. However, starting YT may suggest a lessening in your care needs, so your DLA care component can be reviewed – see Chapter 17.

If you leave a YT course, you will no longer be eligible for income support, unless you are covered by one of the other situations in which you are not required to sign on (eg you are incapable of work) – see Box B.1 in Chapter 3. You should claim jobseeker's allowance instead. If you don't complete the course and you don't have 'good cause' for leaving, your jobseeker's allowance may be paid at a reduced rate.

Bridging allowance – If you cannot get IS or jobseeker's allowance and are registered with the Careers Service for a YT place and/or looking for work, and you are disabled, you can get a bridging allowance of £15 a week from the end of the child benefit extension period up to your 18th birthday – see Chapter 14(19). Claim on form BA1, available from the Careers Office (or Jobcentre) where you register for YT. In all other cases, the bridging allowance is for a maximum of 8 weeks within a 52 week period and can apply only if you are between jobs/YT places.

9. Youth credits

These are aimed mainly at 16 and 17 year old school and college leavers to enable them to go on work-based training leading to National Vocational Qualifications (NVQ). Each youth credit has a financial value which varies according to the training and individual needs. If the value of the credit does not cover the training costs, the TEC or employer should meet the shortfall.

Youth credits are known by different names in different areas (eg Skillseekers in Scotland, Network in London). The TEC or Careers Service will explain how they work locally.

10. Modern Apprenticeships

These are available across a wide range of industry and service sectors and are designed to enable more young people to gain higher level vocational qualifications and skills at NVQ Level 3. Apprenticeships are available to 16 and 17 year old school or college leavers, and other young people aged 18 to 24 at the discretion of the TEC. Your youth credit gives you access to the scheme, and most Modern Apprentices are employed and receive a wage. If you have special training needs, you must be given suitable extra help. Advice about Modern Apprentices and details of local vacancies are available from the Careers Office.

11. Training For Work

The Training For Work (TFW) programme is delivered by local TECs in England and Wales, and LECs in Scotland. TECs may use their own local brand name when referring to training they deliver under TFW. To qualify for TFW you need to be
- unemployed and disabled; or
- unemployed continuously for 26 weeks (this includes time in receipt of incapacity benefit, severe disablement allowance, severe hardship allowance, Youth Training bridging allowance or income support; or
- someone requiring Foundation level literacy and/or numeracy training including English for Speakers of Other Languages; or
- discharged from the armed forces (your time in the services counts towards the 26 week qualifying period); or
- released from prison (your time in prison counts towards the 26 week qualifying period); or
- a returner to the labour market (for domestic reasons you have not been in the labour market for a continuous period of two years or more); or
- someone who has recently been made redundant in a large scale redundancy (determined by TEC) and has remained continuously unemployed for up to 26 weeks.

Eligibility for TFW is determined by the Employment Service.

When you join TFW, you agree an Individual Training Plan with the training provider. This sets out details such as your training needs, approved qualifications being aimed for, hours of attendance and any agreed support arrangements. If there is anything you are not sure about, query it and get a full explanation before you sign. Your Training Plan should be regularly reviewed in terms of your progress and any changes agreed with you.

If, while in training, you aren't satisfied with the training you are receiving, complain first to the training provider. A review of your Training Plan might be enough to resolve the issue, or you may have reasonable grounds to ask for a transfer to suitable alternative training. There may be help available if you have special training needs because of a disability. If there are personal reasons why you cannot train full time, it may be possible to do part time training of more than 15 hours a week. Other support includes residential training in specialist colleges.

A training allowance will be paid based on your weekly benefit entitlement increased by £10. Additional financial support may be available if it is reasonable and necessary for your participation, eg travel, childcare, clothing, disability support. Contribution credits will normally be awarded. For more details contact your Jobcentre or Disability Employment Adviser.

Note that TFW does not count as an 'approved' training scheme. This means that your jobseeker's allowance (JSA) is not affected automatically if you refuse the offer of a TFW place, or leave TFW without good cause. However, an ES Adviser will ask you about this when you claim JSA. For your actions may call into question your general availability for work. However, if you are required to take up a TFW place under a 'jobseeker's direction', your benefit can be sanctioned if you do not comply – see Chapter 14(9).

TFW can affect your entitlement to benefits. In most cases you will keep your existing benefits, and the £10 allowance will be 'disregarded' by the DSS when it calculates entitlement to benefits, such as family credit. Local authorities, too, will disregard the TFW allowance for the purpose of housing benefit or council tax benefit. You should also be allowed to keep your ES40 to help gain access to concessionary reductions. TFW can affect your entitlement or eligibility for disability benefits. You should check with an advice centre or the local TEC/LEC before participating in the scheme.

European Social Fund – If you are about to go on a European Social Fund training scheme, be aware that it is different from a 'state training scheme' or TFW. The rules can be quite complicated, so seek advice on how your benefit rights might be affected.

12. Benefits and training allowances

DLA mobility component is not affected if you get a training allowance. DLA care component is not affected if you are living at home and attending the course daily. However you will not be able to get the care component for the days you stay in residential accommodation in order to attend the course; nor if your training allowance includes a 'living away from home' allowance. The care component stops after 28 days in such accommodation – see Chapter 17(10). You can get it for any days spent at home. Although the care component can be paid at the same time as a training allowance, your ability to start a training programme may suggest a lessening in your care needs: so your care component can be reviewed – see Chapter 17.

If you are receiving incapacity benefit or SDA you have to give this up on starting your course (but see 4 above if you are going on an employment rehabilitation course). This is because a day in receipt of a state training allowance cannot, in law, count as a day of incapacity for work. At the end of your course you may be able to pick up your SDA or incapacity benefit at the rate you were getting before your course started – see below.

If you do not find a job at the end of your course, and are capable of work, you can sign on and claim jobseeker's allowance – see Chapter 14.

The 2 year linking rule
If you are unable to work because of illness or disability at the end of your course, there is a 2 year linking rule to help you pick up your incapacity benefit or SDA again. (See below if you were on invalidity benefit at the start of your course.)

During the 8 weeks before your course started, you must have been entitled to higher rate short-term or long-term incapacity benefit, or SDA for at least a day. The day after your course finishes must be within 2 years of the end of your benefit entitlement. You can pick up the same level of benefit (with annual increases) if you are incapable of work from the day your course ends. You have one month to make your claim. To show you are incapable of work, you must pass the 'all work' test of incapacity, unless you are exempt. The way of assessing incapacity for work is described in Chapter 8.

The same 2 year rule applies to protect your 'transitional award of incapacity benefit' paid to people who transferred from sickness benefit or invalidity benefit onto incapacity benefit in April 1995 – see Chapter 12.

The 2 year rule applies to certain Employment Service courses including Training for Work, Youth Training, Employment Rehabilitation and Community Action. But it also applies to non-government courses where the primary purpose is the teaching of occupational or vocational skills and you attend for 16 or more hours a week.

Sickness and invalidity benefit – A different 8 week linking rule applies if you were on sickness or invalidity benefit, rather than the new incapacity benefit when you started your course. This 8 week rule only applies to Employment Service courses and not to non-government courses – see above. You must have been on your course for at least a day during the period 15.2.95 to 9.6.95 (this is the 8 weeks before, and 8 weeks after, incapacity benefit came into force). During the 8 weeks before your course began, you must have been entitled to sickness or invalidity benefit for at least a day. If you make a claim for incapacity benefit within 8 weeks of the end of your course then your claims are linked and your previous rate of sickness or invalidity benefit is protected. You must be incapable of work at the end of your course and the 'all work' test of incapacity will apply to you unless you are exempt. See Chapter 12 for more about the transition from sickness and invalidity benefit to incapacity benefit.

16 Disability working allowance

In this chapter we look at:	
What is disability working allowance?	see 1
Are you 'better off' on DWA?	see 2
Do you qualify?	see 3
The 'disability' test	see Box F.3
How is DWA worked out?	see 4
Claims, payments and appeals	see 5
DWA and other benefits	see 6

1. What is disability working allowance?

Disability working allowance (DWA) is tax free and is paid on top of low wages or self-employed earnings for people whose disabilities put them at a *'disadvantage in getting a job'*. You must be working for 16 or more hours a week to qualify.

DWA is means tested and similar to family credit, although you can qualify for DWA whether or not you have children. If you do have children, you may get up to £29.90 a week more from DWA than from family credit (or more if you have a disabled child). Each DWA award, like a family credit award, normally lasts for 26 weeks – see 5 below for the exceptions to this rule.

The amount of DWA you might get depends on your capital, income, working hours, and on your family situation –

whether you are single, or have a partner, and whether you are responsible for any children and, if so, the ages of your children and whether any child is disabled. If your income is below or the same as your 'applicable amount', you may be entitled to the maximum disability working allowance for your family. If your income is above the threshold level of your 'applicable amount', 70% of that extra income is deducted from your maximum disability working allowance. The DSS technical guide to DWA, leaflet HB4, gives full details.

Disability working allowance is intended to encourage people with disabilities 'to return to or take up work by topping up low earnings'. The key incentive is aimed at people on incapacity benefit or severe disablement allowance (SDA). A special 2 year linking rule may enable you to return to incapacity benefit or SDA on the same terms as before – see 6 below.

2. Are you 'better off' on DWA?

Disability working allowance is taken fully into account as income for other means-tested benefits. However, it also entitles you to the disability premium or higher pensioner premium with income support, income-based jobseeker's allowance, housing benefit and council tax benefit.

DWA is also a gateway to social fund maternity and funeral payments (Chapter 6), home repair assistance (Chapter 49), free legal advice and assistance (Chapter 53), assisted prison visits, weekly payments of child benefit (Chapter 27), and health benefits (Chapter 48). DWA also gives you Class 1 or Class 2 contribution credits if you need them.

Each DSS office and Jobcentre has someone who has been nominated to deal with all DWA 'better off' calculations. For a given level of earnings and other income, they can work out how much DWA, housing benefit (HB) and council tax benefit (CTB) you might get. You will be able to compare your total income in work and out of work. If you are currently getting incapacity benefit, SDA, income support or jobseeker's allowance, and are considering working, it's worth making use of this service – or asking an advice agency to work through the options with you.

If you are working out whether you might be 'better off' on DWA, the following points may be important.
- ❑ You can earn up to £46.50 a week 'therapeutic earnings' on top of incapacity benefit (or SDA) (although only £15 of 'therapeutic' or other earnings are ignored for IS, HB and CTB) – see Chapter 8(5). You may well be 'better off' continuing on your incapacity benefit (or SDA) plus earnings from a job of under 16 hours a week which has been agreed as 'therapeutic' by the DSS.
- ❑ If you are a home-owner on income support (IS) or income-based jobseeker's allowance (JSA), your benefit may include mortgage interest payments (see Chapter 3(20)), whereas DWA has no allowance for mortgage costs. If you work for 16 or more hours a week, or your partner works for 24 or more hours a week, you are excluded from IS and income-based JSA, so you may have no choice. However, if your hours or earnings are reduced because of disability, you can continue to be eligible for IS or JSA while working more than 16 hours a week – see Chapter 3(6) for details.
- ❑ Your partner is excluded from income-based JSA if you work 24 hours or more a week. If you work under 24 hours and claim DWA, your DWA would be taken into account in full for income-based JSA, but would entitle your partner to the disability premium.

3. Do you qualify?

There are 7 key qualifying conditions for DWA. At the time you claim:

- ■ you must be aged 16 or older;
- ■ you must be in Great Britain without restrictions on your right to remain – see below;
- ■ you must normally be working for 16 or more hours a week – see below;
- ■ you must have a *'physical or mental disability which puts [you] at a disadvantage in getting a job'* see Box F.3;
- ■ you must either
  - – have been getting one of a range of qualifying benefits at any time in the 8 weeks before your claim to DWA, or
  - – be getting one of a different range of qualifying benefits at the time you claim DWA, or
  - – be on a training course in the 8 weeks before your DWA claim and getting a qualifying benefit in the 8 weeks before the start of your training – see below;
- ■ you (and your partner) must not have savings or capital of over £16,000 – see below;
- ■ your income must be within a set limit, which varies according to your family circumstances – see below.

All of the rules outlined below depend on your circumstances at the time you make any claim for disability working allowance.

In Great Britain

You must be both present and ordinarily resident in GB (England, Wales and Scotland). If you have a partner, s/he doesn't have to be present in GB, but s/he must be ordinarily resident in the UK (GB and Northern Ireland). Your (and your partner's) earnings must at least in part come from work in the UK.

DWA in Northern Ireland comes under separate legislation. The rules are the same but in NI, you must be ordinarily resident in NI. Any partner must be ordinarily resident in the UK; and earnings must come from work in the UK or the Republic of Ireland.

If you have any restriction on your right to reside in GB, you are not entitled unless you or a member of your family is an EEA national (see Chapter 41), or lawfully working and a national of Algeria, Morocco, Slovenia or Tunisia, or you have refugee status or exceptional leave to remain.

Working 16 or more hours a week

You must normally work as an employee or self-employed person for an average of 16 or more hours a week. A *'week'* is from Sunday to Saturday.

Note that if you work for 30 hours or more a week (or if your partner does) an extra allowance is added to the amount of the maximum DWA – see 4 below.

Paid breaks for meals or refreshments, and paid time off for *'visits'* to a hospital, clinic or *'other establishment'* in connection with your disability, both count towards the 16 hours.

However, time off sick, even if you are paid for that time, does not count towards the 16 hours. Work as a volunteer, or for a charity or for a voluntary body, does not count if you are only paid expenses (except where you are treated as having 'notional' earnings); nor does work on a training scheme when you get a training allowance. Work providing respite care in your own home for someone who does not usually live with you does not count as work for DWA if you are paid by a local authority, health authority or voluntary organisation.

On the date you claim you must be employed or self-employed and either have worked 16 or more hours in the week you claim; or in one of the two previous weeks; or be expected to work for 16 or more hours in the week after your week of claim. If your average hours were under 16 because you were (are, or will be) on a *'recognised, customary or other holiday'* in each of these 4 weeks, you'll pass this test if your employer expects you to work for 16 or more hours in the week after your return to work. In all cases, your job must be likely to last for at least 5 weeks, starting with your week of claim. If you have more than one job, the hours from each job count towards the 16 hours.

If during the 5 weeks before you claim DWA, you started a new job, changed your hours, or returned to work after a break of 13 or more weeks, your average weekly hours will be based on the number of hours (or average number) you are expected to work each week. In any other case, how your average hours are worked out depends on whether or not you have a *'recognised cycle of working'* at the date you claim DWA.

If you have a recognised cycle of working, the Adjudication Officer (AO) will look at one complete cycle and work out the average weekly hours you worked in that cycle. If your cycle involves periods when you don't normally work, your hours are averaged over the whole cycle; eg if you work 40 hours every other week, your average hours are 20 a week. But if you work in a *'school, educational establishment or other place of employment'*, the school holidays when you're not working, and other times that you're not required to work, are not counted when working out your average hours.

If you don't have an obvious pattern of work, the AO can look at the hours you worked over the 5 weeks before you claimed DWA, or s/he can take a shorter or longer period if that would give a better picture of your average weekly hours of work.

The 'disability' test
To get DWA, you must have *'a physical or mental disability which puts [you] at a disadvantage in getting a job'*.
Initial claims – If you are claiming DWA for the very first time, or haven't been paid DWA in the past two years, the 'disability' test is straightforward. On page 14 of the DWA1 claim form, it asks *'does your illness or disability put you at a disadvantage in getting a job?'* If you tick the 'yes' box, after reading Section 2 of the Advice Notes in the DWA claim pack, you'll pass the disability test. You could only fail it if, unusually, something else in your claim suggests you misrepresented or exaggerated things, or where the AO has other evidence which contradicts your 'disability' claim. The AO doesn't have power to ask for extra evidence or information in order to cast doubt on your 'disability' claim. Thus, in almost all cases, the 'disability' test only matters when you come to make renewal claims to DWA.
Renewal claims – Each DWA award lasts for 26 weeks, so you'll need to make a renewal claim every 6 months – see 5 below. On a renewal claim, you may be 'passported' through the 'disability' test if you get one of the benefits listed in Part 2 of Box F.3. If not, you'll be asked to complete a self-assessment form, DWA2, and name a person professionally involved in your care who can confirm your self-assessment (they don't have to sign your DWA2). You'll pass the 'disability' test if any one of the paragraphs in Part 1 of Box F.3 apply to you. The DWA2 doesn't repeat these legal tests word for word, so do seek expert help with a review if you fail the 'disability' test.

The 'qualifying benefit' test
To get DWA, you must either have been getting one of the range of benefits listed in Group A at any time in the 8 weeks before your initial claim to DWA; or be getting one of the range of benefits listed in Group B on the date you claim DWA. Or you can get DWA if you've recently been on a training course and getting a qualifying benefit before the start of the training – see below.

Group A – previous 8 weeks
- higher rate short-term incapacity benefit
- long-term incapacity benefit
- severe disablement allowance
- disability, or higher pensioner premium in either income support, income-based JSA, housing benefit or council tax benefit.

Group B – current benefit
- disability living allowance (either component, any rate)
- attendance allowance
- the industrial injuries or war pensions constant attendance allowance
- war pensions mobility supplement
- an invalid trike from the DSS.

If you receive a Group B benefit, such as disability living allowance, this 'qualifying benefit' test is easy. If you delay claiming DWA, you'll just miss out on some weeks of benefit (unless you have 'special reasons' for your delayed claim).

However, if the only way you can pass the 'qualifying benefit' test is through one of the benefits listed in Group A, **you must act fast or you could lose entitlement to DWA altogether**. You must have been receiving a Group A benefit at any time in the 56 days (8 weeks) before your initial claim to DWA. On a renewal claim to DWA you will still count as getting a Group A benefit if you make your renewal claim within 8 weeks of the end of your previous award to DWA. If you claim DWA outside either of these 8 week periods, it is only possible to get DWA on the basis of entitlement to a Group A benefit if you have special reasons for a delayed claim to DWA so that the claim can be treated as having been made within the 8 week period. Chapter 52(4) explains what counts as 'special reasons'.

Training
You may get DWA if, in the 8 weeks before your DWA claim, you were on a government training course, such as Training for Work, Youth Training or Employment Rehabilitation, or on a non-government course for 16 or more hours a week where you were taught occupational or vocational skills. You must have been getting higher rate short-term incapacity benefit, long-term incapacity benefit or SDA at any time in the 8 weeks before the start of your training.

The capital limit
If you (or your partner) have capital of over £16,000, you won't be entitled to DWA. A child's capital does not count, but if s/he has over £3,000 capital, s/he won't be included in the assessment; nor will any of his or her own income be taken into account. However, you would still be entitled to the £15 maintenance disregard.

If your capital is from £3,000.01 to £16,000, it is treated as producing a notional 'tariff' income – see Chapter 3(29). Your capital is worked out in the same way as for income support: some types of capital don't count, eg the home you live in or business assets. We give the main rules in Chapter 3(24) and (31). The main differences from income support are:
- the value of a property will be ignored if a relative is living there but only if s/he has been incapacitated throughout the 13 weeks immediately before you claim DWA or if s/he is aged 60 or over;
- if you have sold any business asset and intend to reinvest the proceeds in your business within 13 weeks of the sale

(or a longer period if that is reasonable) those proceeds will also be ignored as capital;
- a Back to Work Bonus and a Child Maintenance Bonus is ignored for 52 weeks from the date it is paid.

Income
Your income is taken into account net of tax and National Insurance contributions and half of any contribution to a personal or occupational pension scheme. Your earnings include statutory sick pay. As with any other means-test, some types of income count in full, while other types are ignored, wholly or partly.

The rules for DWA follow those for family credit (see Chapter 28), and for both benefits income is worked out broadly in the same way as for income support (see Chapter 3). But there are a number of differences from income support in the way in which your earnings and other income are treated for DWA purposes. We list the main ones below.

❑ **Normal weekly earnings** – The DWA calculation is slightly different from the family credit one. The AO will usually

---

F.3 The 'disability' test

Disability which puts a person at a disadvantage in getting a job

In this box we quote all the ways you can pass the 'disability' test for DWA. It is taken from Schedule 1 to the DWA (General) Regulations.

On an initial claim, you will pass the disability test if any one (or more) of the paragraphs in parts 1, 2 or 3 apply to you.

On a renewal claim, you will pass the test if any one of the paragraphs in parts 1 or 2 apply to you.

Part 1
1. When standing he cannot keep his balance unless he continually holds onto something.
2. Using any crutches, walking frame, walking stick, prosthesis or similar walking aid which he habitually uses, he cannot walk a continuous distance of 100 metres along level ground without stopping or without suffering severe pain.
3. He can use neither of his hands behind his back as in the process of putting on a jacket or of tucking a shirt into trousers.
4. He can extend neither of his arms in front of him so as to shake hands with another person without difficulty.
5. He can put neither of his hands up to his head without difficulty so as to put on a hat.
6. Due to lack of manual dexterity he cannot with one hand, pick up a coin which is not more than 2.5 cm in diameter.
7. He is not able to use his hands or arms to pick up a full jug of 1 litre capacity and pour from it into a cup, without difficulty.
8. He can turn neither of his hands sideways through 180 degrees.
9. He is registered as blind or partially sighted.
10. He cannot see to read 16 point print at a distance greater than 20 centimetres, if appropriate, wearing the glasses he normally uses.
11. He cannot hear a telephone ring when he is in the same room as the telephone, if appropriate, using a hearing aid he normally uses.
12. In a quiet room he has difficulty hearing what someone talking in a loud voice at a distance of 2 metres says, if appropriate, using a hearing aid he normally uses.
13. People who know him well have difficulty in understanding what he says.
14. When a person he knows well speaks to him, he has difficulty in understanding what that person says.
15. At least once a year during waking hours he has a coma or fit in which he loses consciousness.
16. He has a mental illness for which he receives regular treatment under the supervision of a medically qualified person.
17. Due to mental disability he is often confused or forgetful.
18. He cannot do the simplest addition and subtraction.
19. Due to mental disability he strikes people or damages property or is unable to form normal social relationships.
20. He cannot normally sustain an 8 hour working day or a 5 day working week due to a medical condition or intermittent or continuous severe pain.

Part 2
21. Subject to paragraph 24, there is payable to him –
    (a) the highest or middle rate of the care component of disability living allowance,
    (b) the higher rate of the mobility component of disability living allowance,
    (c) an attendance allowance under section 64 of the Social Security Contributions and Benefits Act,
    (d) disablement benefit where the extent of the disablement is assessed at not less than 80 per cent, in accordance with section 103 of and Schedule 6 to the Social Security Contributions and Benefits Act,
    (e) a war pension in respect of which the degree of disablement is certified at not less than 80 per cent; for the purposes of this sub-paragraph 'war pension' means a war pension in accordance with section 25(4) of the Social Security Act 1989,
    (f) mobility supplement, or
    (g) a benefit corresponding to a benefit mentioned in sub-paragraphs (a)-(f), under any enactment having effect in Northern Ireland.
22. Subject to paragraph 24, for one or more of the 56 days immediately preceding the date when the initial claim for disability working allowance was made or treated as made, there was payable to him severe disablement allowance (or corresponding benefit in N. Ireland).
23. Subject to paragraph 24, he has an invalid carriage or other vehicle provided by the Secretary of State under section 5(2)(a) of the National Health Service Act 1977 and Schedule 2 to that Act or under section 46 of the National Health Service (Scotland) Act 1978 or provided under Article 30(1) of the Health and Personal Social Services (Northern Ireland) Order 1972.
24. Paragraphs 21–23 are subject to the condition that no evidence is before the Adjudication Officer which gives them reasonable grounds for believing that in respect of an initial claim, none of the paragraphs in Part I or Part III of this Schedule apply to the claimant and in respect of a repeat claim, none of the paragraphs in Part I apply to the claimant.

Part 3
25. As a result of an illness or accident he is undergoing a period of habilitation or rehabilitation.

estimate your average earnings by looking at the 5 weeks (weekly paid) or 2 months (monthly paid) before the week in which your claim reaches the DSS. If you haven't been in your job for long enough, an estimate from your employer is used.

If you are self-employed, the AO will usually look at the last 26 weeks, or at your last set of accounts (if they cover a 6-15 month period which ended during the year before your claim). If you have been self-employed for under 26 weeks, the AO will ask you to estimate your likely earnings over the next 26 weeks.

If this doesn't give an accurate picture of your likely earnings the AO has discretion to choose a more appropriate period.

A child's earnings are ignored. But if the child has other income, that may affect the DWA assessment – see 4.

❑ **Earnings disregards** – Once you've worked out your net earnings, these are taken into account in full – there are no 'disregards' in DWA like the £5, £10 or £15 disregards in income support. But see below for the childcare disregard from earnings.

❑ **Childcare costs** – If you have children under 11 years, you may be able to have your childcare costs taken into account when your DWA is worked out. Up to £60 a week can be disregarded from your earnings if:
- the child (or children) are under 11 when you claim; and
- the childcare is provided by a registered childminder, or other registered provider, such as a nursery or playscheme (including for children aged 8 to 10, an after school club or holiday playscheme); and
- you are a lone parent, or your partner is also working 16 or more hours a week, or your partner gets one of the Group A or Group B qualifying benefits above.

You claim for childcare costs on form DWA3 which comes with the claim pack. This includes a section for the childminder to complete.

From 7.10.97, help with childcare costs is extended. If you claim DWA before the first Tuesday in September after your child's 11th birthday, the disregard will apply.

❑ **Benefits** – Child benefit, guardians allowance, statutory maternity pay, maternity allowance, income support, income-based JSA, family credit are all ignored as income – as well as the benefits also ignored for income support, eg disability living allowance, housing and council tax benefit (see Chapter 3(26)). Other benefits such as incapacity benefit and SDA are taken into account.

❑ **Maintenance** – If you are treated as responsible for a child, £15 of any maintenance payments will be ignored if they are from a former partner or the parent of the child. If maintenance isn't paid regularly it is averaged out over the previous 13 weeks. If maintenance has been assessed by the Child Support Agency and you receive more than the amount due, only the actual amount due is taken into account. If you pay maintenance, there is no disregard from your payments.

4. How is DWA worked out?

To work out how much DWA you could get, go through the following steps.

Step 1 – Work out your and any partner's total capital – see below for who counts as a 'partner'. If you have over £16,000, DWA is not payable.

Step 2 – Work out the maximum DWA for your household – see below for who is included in the means-test; see below (under 'maximum DWA') for the amounts.

Step 3 – Work out your normal weekly income. Remember to include any 'tariff' income if you have over £3,000 capital. Deduct eligible childcare costs (up to a maximum of £60) from your earnings.

Step 4 – If your normal weekly income is below, or the same as your 'applicable amount', you'll get the maximum DWA for your family. The applicable amounts are £57.85 for a single person and £77.15 for a couple or lone parent.

Step 5 – If your normal weekly income is above your applicable amount, deduct your applicable amount from your income.

Step 6 – Work out 70% of the result at step 5.

Step 7 – Deduct the result at step 6 from your maximum DWA (step 2). The amount you are left with is your DWA entitlement. If this is less than 50p a week, DWA is not payable.

Whose needs are included in the means-test?

Single claimants – If you have no dependent children, only your own income, capital and needs are taken into account.

Couples – If you have a partner of the opposite sex, married or unmarried, and normally live together as members of the same household, it is your joint income, capital and needs which will be taken into account. If you are living apart, you will still be treated as members of the same household unless you do not intend to live together again. However, whatever your intentions, you will not be treated as living with your partner if s/he has been in hospital for 52 weeks or more; or s/he is serving a custodial sentence of 52 weeks or more; or s/he has been detained in a special hospital.

Lone parent – If you have any dependent children who normally live with you, the means-test will include the maximum DWA for a lone parent even if you cannot get a DWA allowance for any children because of their own income or capital.

Children – Any child under 16, or a child under 19 who is still receiving full-time, non-advanced education, who normally lives with you will usually be included in the DWA means-test. If s/he has been in hospital or residential accommodation during the 12 weeks before your claim, you must still be in regular contact. However, if s/he has been there throughout the 52 weeks before your claim, you won't get a DWA allowance for that child. If you are a lone parent and s/he is your only child, you will get the single person's applicable amount and not the lone parent's one.

The maximum DWA for your family is increased by an allowance for each child, depending on his or her age. However, although a child's own capital is not added to your capital, you won't get any allowance for a child who has over £3,000 in capital. Maintenance payable to a child is treated as your income. Other types of income are taken into account in the means-test – but only where the child's own weekly income is no more than the DWA allowance for that child. If a child's income is higher than the DWA allowance for his or her age, the assessment won't include the allowance for him or her, but the child's own income will be completely ignored in the means-test.

Disabled child's allowance – The maximum DWA is increased by an extra £20.95 for each child who counts as disabled. Your child counts as disabled if s/he is registered blind (or has been in the last 28 weeks), or gets disability living allowance (either component, any rate). The rules are the same as those for the income support disabled child premium – see Chapter 3(15).

DWA applicable amount

- single person — £57.85
- couple or lone parent — £77.15

If your income is above your applicable amount, you deduct 70% of your extra income from the maximum DWA for your family.

Maximum DWA
- single person £49.55
- couple or lone parent £77.55
- child *
  - aged 18 £34.70
  - 16 or 17 £24.80
  - 11 to 15 £19.95
  - under 11 £12.05
- disabled child's allowance £20.95
- 30 hours allowance £10.55

* Changes from 7.10.97 – Currently the amount of the allowance for a child depends on whether they have reached their 11th, 16th or 18th birthday by the beginning of your DWA award. From 7.10.97 the amount depends on whether you claim before or after the first Tuesday in September following their 11th or 16th birthday:
- from birth £12.05
- from first Tuesday in September following 11th birthday £19.95
- from first Tuesday in September following 16th birthday until day before 19th birthday £24.80

The change does not apply to renewal claims until 1 September 1998 if your DWA includes an allowance for a child already aged 11, 16 or 18 on 6.10.97.

Working out maximum DWA – Just add up the appropriate amounts to reach the maximum DWA for your family. Add one disabled child's allowance for each child who counts as disabled – see above. Add one '30 hours allowance' if you work 30 hours or more each week, or if you are one of a couple, your partner works 30 hours or more. You can add together the hours worked in part-time jobs to make up the 30 hours, although you can't add your own hours to those of your partner.

Example – Maximum DWA for a couple or lone parent working 35 hours a week, with a disabled child aged 11 is £129. Their applicable amount is £77.15. If their weekly income is £177.15, that is £100 above their applicable amount. You work out 70% of their £100 extra income – which comes to £70. Deduct £70 from their maximum DWA of £129, which leaves £59 a week DWA payable.

5. Claims, payments and appeals

Who can claim?
If you are one of a couple, it is the person with the illness or disability who must make the claim and satisfy all the DWA tests. If both of you are disabled and satisfy all the DWA tests, either of you can claim.

When can you claim?
You must pass all the DWA tests on the day you make your claim – usually the day your completed claim form, the DWA1, reaches a DSS office. So you cannot claim DWA unless you have a job in which you are, or will be, working for 16 or more hours a week. But if you will satisfy the tests within the next 3 days, your claim can start from then. You can get advice beforehand about the likely amount of DWA, housing benefit and council tax benefit for a given level of income – see 2.

If you have started a new job on a Monday or Tuesday and claim DWA by the Saturday of that week, DWA is payable from the Tuesday. In this case, the DSS will do their best to process your claim within 5 working days of getting all the information they requested.

If you are already in a job, claim as soon as you can. DWA can only start from the Tuesday payday on or after the day your claim reaches the DSS.

If you first claim income support or JSA and are turned down because you or your partner are working too many hours, so long as you claim DWA within 14 days of the decision, it can be backdated to the date of the first claim.

Family credit – Although claims for family credit and DWA are interchangeable (see Box O.1 in Chapter 52), once you have an award of family credit, you cannot normally get DWA until the end of that award – even though you can get more from DWA than from family credit. If your family credit claim form suggests you would get DWA, (eg you have put down that you get disability living allowance), the Family Credit Unit will pass your claim to the DWA Unit. The DWA Unit will write to you.

If you (rather than a partner) claimed family credit and you yourself are disabled and satisfy all the DWA tests, the DWA Unit will invite you to tell them whether or not your disability puts you at a disadvantage in getting a job. If you write back answering 'yes' to this question, the DSS will treat your family credit claim as if it had been a claim for DWA. You should do this before the AO makes a decision on your family credit claim.

If, however, it is your partner who qualifies for DWA, the DWA Unit will write to invite him or her to make a formal claim to DWA and ask you to withdraw your own family credit claim. If you do this, your partner's DWA claim will be treated as having been made on the date of your own family credit claim.

If the DWA Unit haven't written to you and you realise you should have claimed DWA, phone or write to the Family Credit Unit (see our Address List) asking for your claim to be treated as one for DWA. If you pick the DWA option, you could get more each week from DWA than from family credit.

Renewal claims – The DWA Unit will automatically send you a fresh DWA1 claim form 8 weeks before your current award runs out. You can submit your renewal claim at any time from 6 weeks before your current award runs out. So long as it reaches the DSS up to 14 days after the last day of your previous award, payment can resume without a break. Remember that you must pass all the DWA tests on your date of claim. You have some flexibility, eg if you are off sick.

If your renewal claim is due shortly before the April 1998 uprating, you may miss out on the higher rates. If you claim earlier than uprating day, your DWA is based on the rates for the previous year. If you delay claiming, you will miss out on a week or more of DWA and may even fall foul of the linking rules.

Linking your claims – If you had a Group A benefit before your first DWA claim and reclaim DWA no later then 8 Sundays after the last day (a Monday) of your previous DWA award, you will be treated as receiving a Group A qualifying benefit – see 3 above. For the purpose of protecting your right to return to incapacity benefit or SDA if you stop work, you must either have been receiving DWA continuously, or the breaks between the end and start of each DWA award must be no more than 8 weeks. For this purpose, you must reclaim DWA successfully no later than the Tuesday, 8 weeks after the last day of your previous DWA award – see 6 below for more details.

Backdating claims – If you take longer then any of these time limits, you will have to show you have special reasons for your delayed claim if you want to have DWA backdated – see 6 below and Chapter 52(4). Box O.2 in Chapter 52 gives the general rules about time limits for claims, including DWA claims.

How can you claim?
Telephone claims – You can telephone the Benefit Enquiry Line on 0800 882200, free. The adviser will answer any questions and send you a claim pack. If you have problems filling in the claim pack, you can ring the Forms Completion Service on 0800 441144, free. The adviser can answer any questions about the form, or, if you prefer, they can go through the questions with you over the phone and fill in the form on your behalf. This form will be posted to you so you can check and sign it before posting it to the DWA Unit. The form is date stamped by the Forms Completion Service and this date is treated as your date of claim, so you will not lose any benefit by using this service. You can ask for the form to be sent in large print or braille.
Written claims – You can get a DWA claim pack from a DSS office, Jobcentre or by phoning the DWA leaflet line on 0800 444000. Your date of claim is the date you asked for the claim pack so long as you return the completed claim form within one month. If you have any queries at all, call the Benefit Enquiry Line on 0800 882200 – your call is free.
Employer's form – The DWA claim pack includes a form EEF 200. This is for an employer to complete. You only have to give your employer the EEF 200 if, during the 5 weeks before you claim DWA (or 2 months if you're paid monthly), you started a new job. If you changed your contracted hours of work, or went back to work after a continuous break of over 13 weeks, or just don't have your payslips, you can also use the EEF 200. Do not delay sending your own DWA1 claim form to the DWA Unit – if you delay, you could miss out on benefit. So, send the DWA Unit the EEF 200 form when your employer gives it back to you. The DWA Unit will link it to your DWA1 claim form and process your claim.

Who decides your claim?
An Adjudication Officer (AO) based at the DWA Unit in Preston makes the decision on your claim. The Unit will send you a written notice of the AO's decision. If you disagree with the decision for any reason at all, you can ask for a review within 3 months of the date the first decision was posted to you. This is called an 'any grounds' review. A different AO will review your claim. You'll be sent a written notice of the review decision. If you disagree with this decision, you have the right to appeal to an independent tribunal. If your appeal includes a question about whether or not you pass the 'disability' test – see 3 above – it will be sent to the Disability Appeal Tribunal. If it doesn't involve the 'disability' test, your appeal will be sent to a Social Security Appeal Tribunal – see Chapter 52 for more details.

If you did not ask for an 'any grounds' review of the initial decision within 3 months of the date the DWA Unit posted the notice of that decision to you, you can only have an 'any time' review if the original decision was taken in ignorance of a material fact, or was based on a mistake as to a material fact. However, if the award was based on an estimate of your earnings, and the AO had all the relevant information about your earnings, the fact that the estimate was wrong does not enable a review. If, though, you had claimed DWA when your SDA was suspended or disallowed while you were doing a therapeutic job, winning an appeal and getting SDA reinstated from the date of your DWA claim, does enable a review.

How long is a DWA award?
Each DWA award lasts for 26 weeks, regardless of any changes in your situation, or changes in benefit rates. You can make as many renewal claims as you need to, for as long as you continue to pass the DWA tests. However, if you want to protect your right to return to your pre-DWA incapacity benefit or SDA, see 6 below. A DWA award can end before the 26 weeks are up in 4 situations:
- the death of a single claimant or lone parent. But if one of a couple dies, the surviving partner continues to get DWA until the end of that award, so long as his or her needs etc were included in the DWA assessment;
- where a child who is included in your current DWA award leaves your household and someone else makes a successful claim for income support, income-based JSA, family credit or DWA which includes an allowance for that child;
- a reduced benefit direction from the Child Support Agency is given, ends or is suspended – see Chapter 50;
- your current DWA award is overlapped by a new award on review or appeal; or you make a successful backdated claim for family credit or DWA for a period earlier than your current award of DWA.

How is DWA paid?
DWA is paid on a Tuesday, in arrears. You can choose to have weekly payments in an order book. Or you can choose to have DWA paid direct into a bank or building society account every 4 weeks in arrears. If you are entitled to £4 a week or less, your DWA for the 26 week award will be paid in a lump sum of up to £104. Note that your actual weekly entitlement to DWA will still be taken into account as income for other means-tested benefits.

6. DWA and other benefits

Sickness and DWA
If you're off work sick, you can get DWA and statutory sick pay, or incapacity benefit, or SDA at the same time. The normal 'period of incapacity for work' linking rule applies – see Chapter 11(2).
Linked spells of sickness – If you're off work sick within 8 weeks of the end of your last SDA or incapacity benefit award, you'll go back on to your SDA or incapacity benefit.
Unlinked spells of sickness – If it has been 8 weeks and 1 day, or longer, since the end of your last incapacity benefit or SDA award, and you fall sick again while you are still employed, you would either get statutory sick pay from your employer, or lower rate short-term incapacity benefit if you are self-employed or do not qualify for statutory sick pay.

A spell of sickness which does not link back to your pre-DWA incapacity benefit starts a fresh 'period of incapacity for work' for state benefit purposes (see Chapter 11(2) for details of the 'period of incapacity for work' linking rules).

If you fall sick again and give up your job, the DWA linking rule described below may apply.

The DWA linking rule
The special DWA 2 year linking rule is intended to help you to return to your former incapacity benefit on the same basis as before. It does not help you return to the disability premium with IS, HB or CTB – you have to requalify for premiums.

If it applies, you go back on to the same level of long-term incapacity benefit, or higher rate short-term incapacity benefit (or SDA) as you got before you went on to DWA and you do not have to satisfy the National Insurance contribution conditions again. Your time on DWA counts as days of incapacity

for work and continues your pre-DWA 'period of incapacity for work'. For the special DWA linking rule to apply, you must:
- give up or lose your job – for any reason at all;
- be entitled to DWA for the week which includes your last working day (if you were not at work, this is the day on which your employment terminated);
- be incapable of work on the first day after your last working day; and
- there must be a gap of no more than 2 years between your last day of entitlement to your pre-DWA incapacity benefit and the first day after giving up your job or self-employment.

Once you give up your job, the normal rules about claiming incapacity benefits come into play. You have 3 months in which to claim – either on the claim pack SC1 or, if you were off-sick when your employment terminated, on the SSP 1 form your employer gave you.

Your incapacity for work is first assessed under the 'own occupation' test based on medical certificates from your doctor. After 28 weeks of incapacity, you are assessed under the 'all work' test, unless you are in an exempt group. See Chapter 8 for more details.

If you were on a 'transitional award of incapacity benefit' (see Chapter 12) because you transferred from sickness or invalidity benefit in April 1995, the DWA linking rule allows you to keep this transitional protection.

If you were on invalidity benefit before April 1995 and claimed DWA within 8 weeks of the end of your invalidity benefit, the 2 year linking rule allows you to go on to a 'transitional award of long-term incapacity benefit', so your benefit remains tax-free and paid at the same level as before (uprated as normal each year). Chapter 12 gives more information about transitional awards.

DWA and income support (IS)
If you work less than 16 hours in any week, for example, because of sickness, but not if the reduced hours are part of your normal working cycle, you may be eligible for IS in the normal way – see 2 above and Chapter 3. In some circumstances you may get DWA and work for 16 hours or more in any week and still be able to get income support – see Chapter 3(6).

Disability living allowance • 119

This section of the Handbook looks at the following:
Disability living allowance	Chapter **17**
Attendance allowance	Chapter **18**
Invalid care allowance	Chapter **19**
Help with mobility needs	Chapter **20**

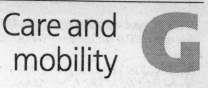

Care and mobility G

17 Disability living allowance

In this chapter we look at:
A. Introducing disability living allowance (DLA)
What is disability living allowance?	*see* 1
DLA and other help	*see Box G.1*
What happened to attendance and mobility allowance?	*see* 2
B. General points	
Do you qualify for DLA?	*see* 3
The non-disability tests	*Box G.2*
Age limits	*see* 4
Qualifying periods	*see* 5
Residence and presence	*see* 6
How much do you get?	*see* 7
Does anything affect what you get?	*see* 8
If you go into hospital	*see* 9
Special accommodation other than hospitals	*see* 10
Respite care	*see Box G.3*
C. The care component	
The disability tests	*see* 11
Terminal illness	*see Box G.4*
What is the 'cooking test'?	*see* 12
What is 'attention'?	*see* 13
What is 'continual supervision'?	*see* 14
What is 'watching over'?	*see* 15
Simpler methods?	*see* 16
Keeping a diary?	*see* 17
Attention or supervision?	*see* 18
Renal dialysis	*see* 19
D. The mobility component	
The disability tests	*see* 20
Other factors	*see* 21
Virtually unable to walk?	*see* 22
Severe mental impairment	*see* 23
The lower rate	*see* 24
Learning disabilities	*see Box G.5*
E. Claims, payments and reviews	
How do you claim?	*see* 25
Who decides your claim?	*see* 26
What happens after you claim?	*see* 27
How are you paid?	*see* 28
What if your condition changes?	*see* 29
For more information	*see Box G.6*

A. INTRODUCING DLA

1. What is disability living allowance?
Disability living allowance (DLA) is a benefit for people with disabilities, both children and adults. It is aimed at people who need help looking after themselves and at people who find it difficult to walk or get around. You don't need to have someone looking after you to qualify.

DLA is tax free, not means-tested and you don't have to have paid any National Insurance contributions. It is paid on top of any earnings or other income you may have. It is almost always paid in full on top of social security benefits.

DLA is divided into two parts:
- **a care component** – for help with personal care needs, paid at three different levels;
- **a mobility component** – for help with walking difficulties, paid at two levels.

You can be paid either the care component or the mobility component on its own. Or you can be paid both components at the same time. DLA is for you, not for a carer or parent. You can qualify for DLA whether or not you actually have someone helping you. What counts are the effects of your disability and the help you need, not whether you already get that help. If you get DLA you can spend it on anything you like.

Although DLA can be paid for life, there is an upper age limit for making your first claim. You can only get DLA if you first start to be disabled enough to pass the disability tests no later than the day before your 65th birthday – although if you are claiming before 6.10.97, you can put in a claim right up to the day before your 66th birthday. If you are claiming on or after 6.10.97, you must make your first DLA claim before your 65th birthday.

You can start off your claim by a free phone call to the Benefit Enquiry Line (BEL) on 0800 882200. They'll send you a claim pack and your claim can be backdated to the date of your call. Or you can phone the Forms Completion Service on 0800 441144. They can fill in the form for you over the phone and send the completed form for you to check and sign.

2. What happened to attendance allowance and mobility allowance?
Attendance allowance remains for people who are aged 65 or over when their need for care begins – see Chapter 18. When DLA was introduced in April 1992, it combined the old mobility allowance and attendance allowance for people under 65, into one benefit. The disability tests for the middle and higher rate care components of DLA are exactly the same as for attendance allowance. Mobility allowance became the higher rate mobility component of DLA. In addition, a lower rate was introduced for each DLA component.

Outstanding claims and appeals – Even though attendance allowance for people under 65 and mobility allowance disappeared from 6 April 1992, there are still claims and appeals being dealt with. No matter how long it takes to reach a final decision, your entitlement to attendance or mobility allowance is considered under the old law.

B. GENERAL POINTS

3. Do you qualify for DLA?

To qualify for DLA you have to pass a series of non-disability tests as well as satisfying at least one of the disability tests. Most of these non-disability tests have exceptions to the standard rules, so off-the-cuff advice may not always be correct.

To qualify for DLA, you must:
- pass at least one of the disability tests – see 11 and 20; and
- claim DLA – see 25; and
- pass the age test – see 4; and
- pass both the backwards and forwards qualifying period tests – see 5; and
- pass the residence and presence tests – see 6.

The Adjudication Officer (AO) must also be satisfied that there is nothing to prevent payment – see 8. If you pass all these tests you will be entitled to DLA. You will keep your underlying entitlement to DLA even if other rules mean that no payment is possible.

Box G.2 gives a summary of the non-disability tests. In Box G.6 we suggest sources of further information on DLA and explain the abbreviations used in our references to legislation.

4. Age limits

Lower age limit
There is no lower age limit for DLA care component. But there is an extra disability test for children under 16 and you cannot use the 'cooking test' until you reach age 16 – see 11.

To get mobility component, you have to be aged 5 or older. There is no extra disability test for higher rate mobility component for children, but there is an extra test for the lower rate – see 20.

Upper age limit
Although DLA may be payable for life, there is an upper age limit for first establishing entitlement and for first successful claims. The rules are changing in October 1997. Before 6.10.97, you can claim if you are not yet 66 and became disabled before your 65th birthday. But from 6.10.97, only those who make their first claim for DLA before their 65th birthday can be awarded DLA. So if you are already over 65 but haven't reached your 66th birthday, make sure you make your claim before 6.10.97.

If you claim before 6.10.97 – Your claim must be lodged with the DSS no later than the day before your 66th birthday. You must have passed the residence and presence tests and satisfied one of the disability tests for the DLA component(s) no later than the day before your 65th birthday. If you are now over 66 you cannot get DLA for the first time unless you count as having made a claim both before reaching 66 and before 6.10.97, or you are switching from the invalid vehicle scheme – see Box G.8 in Chapter 20.

If you claim on or after 6.10.97 – You must make your claim no later than the day before your 65th birthday. You don't need to pass the qualifying period before your 65th birthday, but you must satisfy all the other conditions of entitlement. If you reach age 65 on or after 6.10.97, you cannot get DLA for the first time unless you count as having made a claim before reaching 65, or you are switching from the invalid vehicle scheme.

Regs 3, 13, Sch 1 DLA Regs; regs 6, 12(3), Intro; reg 4(1) C&P

Renewal claims and reviews from age 65
If any DLA award ends after you reach 65, you can make a renewal claim within a year of the end of your previous award. However, for mobility component you can only regain your pre-65 rate of benefit, you cannot switch rates. If you leave it longer than a year, you will have to claim attendance allowance.

Care component – You can only maintain or renew the lower rate if you first began to qualify for it before reaching 65. If your care needs lessen, you cannot drop to the lower rate – you will lose the care component. However, you can regain the

---

G.1 Disability living allowance and other help

Disability living allowance acts as a gateway to certain other types of help. This table gives a list of the rates and components of disability living allowance which will entitle you to other types of help (if you pass any other tests for that help).

If you receive the middle or higher rate care component, you will also be eligible for the help available to people just receiving the lower rate. Similarly, if you receive the higher rate mobility component, you will also be eligible for the help available to people just receiving the lower rate.

The premiums are those included in the assessments of income support, income-based jobseeker's allowance, housing benefit, council tax benefit and health benefits.

Care component
❏ **Lower rate**
- Disability premium
- Higher pensioner premium
- Disabled child premium
- Christmas bonus
- DWA qualifying benefit
- No non-dependant deductions
- Home energy efficiency scheme grant
- Childcare disregard
- Disabled child's allowance (DWA)

❏ **Middle or higher rate**
- Disability test for DWA
- ICA carer test
- Home responsibilities protection
- IS – carer's exemption from signing on
- Carer premium test
- Severe disability premium
- Tax advantages for certain trusts

❏ **Higher rate**
- 80% disablement for SDA
- Independent Living Funds
- Exemption from all work test

Mobility component
❏ **Lower rate**
- Disability premium
- Higher pensioner premium
- Disabled child premium
- Christmas bonus
- DWA qualifying benefit
- Home energy efficiency scheme grant
- Childcare disregard
- Disabled child's allowance (DWA)

❏ **Higher rate**
- Exemption from road tax
- Orange Badge
- Motability
- Disability test for DWA

G.2 Non-disability tests

Age limits	Care component	Mobility component
■ to make your first claim	From birth to the day before your 66th birthday (from 6.10.97, to the day before your 65th birthday).	From 4 years 9 months to the day before your 66th birthday (from 6.10.97, to the day before your 65th birthday).
■ to pass the qualifying conditions	From birth to the day before your 65th birthday.	From 4 years 9 months to the day before your 65th birthday.
■ to be paid	From 3 months old (birth if terminally ill). No upper limit.	From 5 years. No upper limit.
■ extra tests for children	From birth to the day before your 16th birthday.	From 4 years 9 months to the day before your 16th birthday.
■ shorter presence in the country test for babies	Must claim and serve the 3 month qualifying period no later than the day before 6 months old.	Not payable to children under 5.
■ cooking test	From 16 years to the day before your 65th birthday.	Doesn't apply.
■ lower rate	The day before your 65th birthday. From 65 you can keep or renew your lower rate component or make a repeat claim within one year.	Same as care component.

Qualifying periods		
■ backwards test	If you're under 65 on the first day of entitlement, you must satisfy the disability tests throughout the 3 months before the award (payment) would start. If you're 65 or over – 6 months. No qualifying period if you're terminally ill.	If you're under 65 on the first day of entitlement, you must satisfy the disability tests throughout the 3 months before an award (payment) would start. If you're 65 or over and renewing a claim – 3 months. No qualifying period if you're terminally ill.
■ forwards test	6 months following first payday. No forwards test for attendance allowance.	6 months following first payday.

Residence and presence		
■ standard	Present for 26 out of the last 52 weeks. Present and ordinarily resident with unlimited right to reside in GB.	Same as care component.
■ babies	Present for 13 out of the last 52 weeks before award if less than 6 months old when claim made and qualifying period served. Present and ordinarily resident with unlimited right to reside in GB.	Not payable to children under 5.
■ terminal illness	Present and ordinarily resident with unlimited right to reside in GB.	Same as care component.

Other rules		
■ hospital and special accommodation	Payment may be stopped while in hospital or other special accommodation.	Payment may be stopped while in hospital but is not affected in special accommodation.
■ prison	Payment suspended while on remand, but arrears paid if you don't get a custodial or suspended sentence.	Same as care component.

lower rate if you reclaim within 12 months of the end of your previous award. If your care needs change after reaching 65, you can switch between the middle or higher rates, or move up from the lower rate – but after a 6 month qualifying period. So long as you have DLA mobility component, a change in your care needs after you reach 65 does enable a review of your DLA award. This means you can claim DLA care component (at the middle or higher rate), rather than attendance allowance, even if you are aged, say, 70. Because this type of top up claim is a review of your DLA award, it can be backdated for up to one month – see 27.

para 3(2), (3) and para 7 of Sch 1 DLA Regs

Mobility component – Once you reach 65 you stay with the rate you qualified for before reaching 65. You cannot move up or down a rate. If you have a current award of the care component which was made before you reached the age of 65, you can claim the mobility component after age 65 but only if your mobility difficulties began before age 65. If your mobility difficulties begin after you reach age 65, you cannot get the mobility component.

para 5, 6 and para 1 of Sch 1 DLA Regs

5. Qualifying periods

Backwards test

Under 65 – If you first start to qualify for DLA before reaching 65 you must have passed the disability test(s) throughout the 3 months before your claim. You can claim (or ask for a review) before the 3 months are up. If your condition starts to get worse when you are under 65, you can move up a rate from 3 months afterwards (even if you are over 65 at the end of this qualifying period).

Ss.72(2)(a), 73(9)(a) SSCBA; reg 3 Sch 1 DLA Regs

Over 65 – If your care needs change on or after your 65th birthday, the qualifying period is 6 months – the same as for attendance allowance.

If your mobility difficulties change on or after your 65th birthday, you cannot use that change to get mobility component for the first time, or to switch rates. On a post-65 renewal claim, the qualifying period for your former rate of mobility component remains at 3 months.

Terminal illness – Whatever your age, there is no qualifying period for DLA if you make a successful claim on the basis of terminal illness – see Box G.4. You will automatically get higher rate care component. Note that to get mobility component, you have to pass one of the disability tests from your date of claim.

Renal dialysis – If you've passed the dialysis test outlined in 19, during the 3 months before your claim, you have served the qualifying period. Spells dialysing at least twice a week in hospital, or as an out-patient getting help from hospital staff, always count for the purposes of this qualifying period.

Linked claims – If you've already served the 3 or 6 months backwards qualifying period on an earlier linked award, you do not have to re-serve it on a linked claim. If you re-claim DLA within 2 years of the end of your previous award, the claims are linked. This means if you have a relapse, you can get DLA just as soon as you claim. You can only regain your former rate and component of DLA under this rule.

If you are over 65, the 6 months qualifying period may apply but this shouldn't be a problem – the catch is you can only have up to one year off DLA – see 4.

Reg 6 DLA Regs

Forwards test

You also have to show that, all things being equal, you are likely to continue to satisfy the disability test(s) throughout the 6 months after your claim.

6. Residence and presence

You must be present and ordinarily resident in Great Britain, Northern Ireland, Jersey, Guernsey or Isle of Man, and have been present for not less than 26 weeks in the 52 weeks before your claim. Residence or presence in another EEA country may satisfy the test for EEA nationals and members of their families. Special rules apply for members of the forces and their families, certain airmen and mariners and continental shelf workers. If you go, abroad, see Chapter 41.

People from abroad – You are not entitled to DLA if your right to reside in Britain is subject to any limitation or condition, unless:
- you have refugee status; or
- you have exceptional leave to remain; or
- you or a member of your family is a national of a European Economic Area country (see Chapter 41); or
- you are covered by a reciprocal agreement with Jersey, Guernsey or the Isle of Man; or
- you are legally working in GB and you or a member of your family is a national of Algeria, Morocco, Slovenia or Tunisia.

If you were already receiving DLA before 5.2.96 when these restrictions were introduced, you continue to be entitled until your DLA is reviewed (under s.30 SSAA). So if you would not satisfy the new residency conditions, you should not ask for a review of your DLA.

Babies – If you claim for a baby and are entitled to the care component before s/he reaches 6 months, there is a shorter 13 week presence test. Once s/he reaches her 1st birthday, the standard 26 week test applies. If s/he becomes entitled to DLA after reaching 6 months, the 26 week test applies.

Terminal illness – The 26 or 13 weeks presence tests do not apply if you are terminally ill.

Foreign earnings – If you (or your spouse, or your parent if you are under 16) receive earnings exempt from UK income tax, you must have been present in the UK for not less than 3 years in the 4 years before your claim. This extra test also applies to people who are terminally ill.

7. How much do you get?

You can get one of the three possible rates of care component and one of the two possible rates of mobility component. You'll always get the highest rate to which you are entitled. Each person in your family who qualifies for DLA may claim it. Payment of DLA is affected in some situations – see 8.

DLA also acts as a 'passport' for some other types of help. Box G.1 lists the ways in which getting DLA can benefit you.

Care component	p/wk	Mobility component	p/wk
■ Higher rate	£49.50	■ Higher rate	£34.60
■ Middle rate	£33.10	■ Lower rate	£13.15
■ Lower rate	£13.15		

The disability tests for the care component are explained in 11 to 19 below. The disability tests for the mobility component are explained in 20 to 24.

8. Does anything affect what you get?

Earnings

DLA is not affected by earnings. It is payable whether you are in or out of work, and no matter how much you earn.

However, starting work may suggest your care needs have

lessened, or that you have found a simple way of cutting back on the help you need from another person so your care component can be reviewed on the basis of that change in your circumstances. If your care needs are unchanged, you should have little to worry about.

Tax
DLA is not taxable.

Other benefits or help
DLA is usually payable in full on top of any other social security benefit. The only exceptions are outlined below.

If you are awarded constant attendance allowance with industrial disablement or war pension, that overlaps with the care component. You'll be paid the higher of the two. War pensioners' mobility supplement overlaps with mobility component – so you'll get the supplement instead.

DLA is ignored as income for means-tested benefits. However, if you have a 'preserved right' to income support (IS) in a residential care or nursing home, your care component is taken into account by IS – see Chapter 38. If you are claiming IS on an 'urgent needs' basis, DLA is taken into account. In all other cases, DLA may trigger extra means-tested benefit. If you get awarded DLA, check to see if you now qualify for income support, housing benefit or council tax benefit, or higher amounts of any of these benefits – it can mean a lot more money. Box G.1 lists the ways in which getting DLA helps you qualify for other types of help – in cash or kind.

The care component may be taken into account in non-social security means tests, such as in charging for local authority services (discretionary rules) and residential care (national rules) – see Chapter 32(6) and Box K.2 in Chapter 37. However, the mobility component has specific protection against means testing – it can only ever be taken into account if the law (not the policy or practice) governing such a test of means specifically states that the mobility component should count. Always ask for a reference to the exact legal provision under which mobility component is said to count as income.
S.73(14) SSCBA.

If you go abroad
See Chapter 41 for details.

Refusing medicals
If the DSS or AO ask you to attend a medical examination but you refuse or don't attend, the claim, question, or review, will be decided against you – unless you have 'good cause' for your actions.
S.54(8) SSAA

If you go into prison
Payment of DLA is suspended if you go to into prison on remand to await trial. If you don't end up with a custodial sentence, including a suspended sentence, you'll be paid any arrears of DLA for the time you've spent on remand in prison.

If you go into hospital or special accommodation
Payment of the care component is affected by a period in hospital or in special accommodation. Payment of the mobility component is affected only by a period in hospital. See 9 and 10 below.

9. If you go into hospital
The general rule is that payment of both the care component and the mobility component stops after you've been in hospital or a similar institution for 28 days for adults, and 84 days for children under 16. But benefit may stop sooner if you are readmitted soon after an earlier stay in hospital or, for the care component only, if you go into hospital after staying in residential care or other special accommodation (see below).

Payment of benefit starts again from the first benefit pay day (usually a Wednesday) after you leave hospital. If you leave hospital temporarily and expect to return within 28 days you can be paid your DLA on a daily basis for each day out of hospital – see Chapter 39(10) for more details.

The mobility component can continue to be paid in hospital while you have a Motability agreement in force – see below.

The restriction on the mobility component in hospital was introduced in 1996. There is some protection for long-stay patients in hospital since before 31.7.96 – see below.

Hospital or similar institution? – Payment of DLA is affected if you are maintained free of charge and receive medical or other treatment as an in-patient in hospital or a similar institution. This includes special hospitals and secure units, and army, navy or airforce hospitals.

If you are a private patient paying the whole cost of accommodation and non-medical services, your DLA is not affected. Nor is it affected if you are residing in a hospice and are terminally ill. A hospice is defined as *'a hospital or other institution whose primary function is to provide palliative care for persons ... suffering from a progressive disease in its final stages'* (but not a NHS hospital).

The care component may also be affected by a stay in a residential care or nursing home and some other kinds of special accommodation – see 10 below. But the mobility component is **only** affected by a stay in hospital or a 'similar institution'. The term 'similar institution' is not defined in the regulations. However if your stay in a nursing home is arranged by the health authority and is therefore free of charge, this is normally regarded as a 'similar institution' to a hospital and so your mobility component is affected. This should only apply where you receive medical treatment or professional nursing care in the home.
See White v CAO, TLR 2.8.93, and Botchett v CAO, TLR 8.5.96 (discussed in the footnotes to reg 21 IS General Regs in Mesher – see Box O.4).

Readmission – Payment will stop before you've been in hospital for the full 28 days (or 84 days for children), if you are readmitted after spending 28 days or less out of hospital. Different spells in hospital are linked together and count as one continuous spell if the gaps between them are 28 days or less. For example if you've been in hospital for 10 days then go home for 3 weeks, when you are readmitted your payment will stop after another 18 days in hospital (or 74 days if you are under 16).

Claiming while in hospital – Because it is only the *payment* of benefit that is affected not actual entitlement, you can claim and establish entitlement to DLA while you are in hospital. You can then be paid as soon as you go home or for any days you spend out of hospital – see Chapter 39(10). Even if you return to hospital at any time within 28 days of leaving, you'll still be paid for the first 28 days (or 84 days) in hospital even though the two spells are linked.

If you go into hospital after a stay in residential care or other special accommodation
Mobility component – There are no special rules for the mobility component because payment is not affected by a stay in any accommodation other than a hospital or similar institution (but see above if the health authority arranged your place). So if you go into hospital after a stay in residential care, the mobility component stops after the first 28 days (or 84 days

for children) of your hospital stay and becomes payable again when you leave hospital, whether you go back into residential care or go home.

Care component – Payment of the care component is affected by a stay in certain types of special accommodation including residential care or nursing homes where the local authority helps with the fees, and local authority hostels and homes. We look at this in detail in 10 below. The care component stops being paid after 28 days in total of either a stay in hospital or a stay in special accommodation, or both if you've moved from one to the other with a gap of 28 days or less in between. Box G.3 explains how you can plan a pattern of relief or respite care that can allow you to keep the care component.

Care component for children – The position for children under 16 is more complicated if they have linked spells in both special accommodation and hospital. Payment of the care component for children continues for the first 84 days (12 weeks) in hospital but in special accommodation it stops after 28 days.

Three examples show how the linking rule works for children.

❑ If you have been in special accommodation for, say, 6 weeks, return home for a week, and then go into hospital, the care component is payable for your week at home and the first six weeks in hospital. This is because you have not yet had a linked spell in hospital or special accommodation of longer than 84 days – so you can be paid for the remainder of the 84 days which you spend in hospital.

❑ If you had been in special accommodation for 12 or more weeks and then go into hospital, the two spells are linked. Even though you were only paid the care component for the first 4 weeks in special accommodation, you cannot be paid the remainder of the hospital 12 week concession –

G.3 Respite care

As well as this box and Chapter 17(9) and (10), you should read Chapter 36, which looks at the effect on state benefits of a stay in a residential care or nursing home.

If a child under 16 also has spells in hospital, the position is more complicated – see 9. While s/he is in hospital (not in 'special accommodation'), s/he can be paid care component during the first 84 days (linked or consecutive) in hospital or in 'special accommodation'.

Careful Counting
If you keep a careful count of the days you (or your disabled child) are in hospital, a hostel, and/or other types of 'special accommodation', you can establish a pattern of respite care that will allow you to keep the care component. This depends on the 28 day linking rule – separate periods in hospital or special accommodation which are no more than 28 days apart are added together towards the 28 day limit on payment of the care component.

Example – If you have two full days of respite care every weekend (not counting the days of entry and discharge) you can continue like this for 14 weeks (2 × 14 = 28 days). For 14 weekends, you can go into respite care on a Friday and return home on a Monday. Only Saturday and Sunday count as days in hospital or special accommodation – the day you enter and the day you leave respite care count as days at home. If you keep on like this, the care component cannot be paid for the following days of respite care until you break the link between respite care stays.

Days of entry and leaving – Currently the day you enter and the day you leave residential care or hospital both count as days at home. There may be a change in the law in the near future which would alter this – see our *Disability Rights Bulletin*.

Break the link
If you spend 29 days in your own home (counting any days on which you return to your home and leave it), you will break the link between respite care stays. The next time you go into respite care, your care component can be paid for another 28 days (in one stay or in linked stays).

A pattern of respite care that is interrupted by a period of 29 days that count as days in your own home will allow you to keep the care component. You will not have to send your order book back to the Disability Benefits Unit. If you are paid by credit transfer (see 28), that arrangement will continue. But you must let the Unit have details of all dates you enter or leave respite care.

In our example above, you can break the link and at the same time continue to have some respite care. For the next 4 weekends, instead of going into respite care on a Friday and leaving on a Monday, you go in on the Saturday morning and return home on the Sunday evening. Because the day you enter and the day you leave respite care count as days at home, you'll have spent more than 28 days in a row at home and so you'll have broken the link. For the next 14 weekends, you can return to your main Friday to Monday pattern of respite care.

Let the Disability Benefits Unit know
When you first go into respite care (or any other 'special accommodation') always write to the Disability Benefits Unit. Let the Unit know the name and address of the place you are going to. Tell them what date you will be entering the home and what date you will be leaving to return to your own home. If you have planned a specific pattern of respite care in advance, let the Unit have details. Keep a copy of your letter.

If there are any changes from your planned pattern of respite care, write and let the Unit know. Remember that complete days in hospital link with days in special accommodation for the care component.

If you cannot break the link
Arranging or keeping to a pattern of respite care that allows you to keep the care component (by breaking the link every 28 days) will not always be possible. If it is not possible, you will eventually have to send your order book back. In this situation, credit transfer payments are the best bet. The Unit simply adjusts each credit transfer payment as necessary. You are unlikely to have to wait longer than your next pay day for what you are owed.

If you know that you cannot break the link, send your order book back to the Unit once you have had 28 'linked' full days of respite care. Until that link is broken you will not be entitled to the care component for any further full days spent in respite care from the 29th day onwards. However, you will be entitled to the care component for the days spent in your own home (including the day you enter respite care and the day you leave).

The Unit will let you know how you will be paid. Normally you will have to let the Unit have details of the dates you enter and leave respite care. If you have a planned pattern of respite care, you will just have to let the Unit know the dates of any changes from that pattern. The Unit will arrange for you to be paid the care component.

you have already been in either type of accommodation for over 84 days.
- If you have spent 29 days in your own home you have broken the link with any earlier spells in hospital or special accommodation. If you go into hospital, you can be paid for the first 84 days.

If you have a Motability agreement
Motability provides leased or hire purchase cars or wheelchairs paid for directly by the higher rate mobility component. If you have a Motability agreement in force at the time you go into hospital (or you were in hospital on 31.7.96 and the Motability agreement was in force at that time), payment of the mobility component continues to be made to Motability for the full term of the agreement. However, any balance that would otherwise be paid to you, stops after 28 days – unless you are entitled to be paid at the lower rate as a long-stay patient (see below).

Your mobility component will not be paid if you renew the Motability agreement while you are hospital. An exception allows the renewal of agreements under the Motability wheelchair scheme provided the new agreement is entered into the day after the old one ends. Note that the mobility component will be paid if you renew a Motability agreement during a temporary absence from hospital.

Transitional protection for long-stay patients
The restrictions to payment of the mobility component in hospital were introduced on 31.7.96. There is protection for people who had already been in hospital for 365 days or more when the rules were changed, either continuously or in linked spells no more than 28 days apart, and getting mobility component throughout (higher or lower rate). In this case, the mobility component is not withdrawn, but is only paid at a rate equal to the lower rate of £13.15 a week.

Once you've qualified for transitional protection, it continues to apply until either you've spent more than 28 consecutive days out of hospital or you lose entitlement to the mobility component. During a temporary absence from hospital of no more than 28 days, your full entitlement to the higher rate can be paid on a daily basis.

People committed to hospital under Part II or III of the Mental Health Act 1983, or Part V or VI of the Mental Health (Scotland) Act 1984 are excluded from this transitional protection. This means that payment of mobility component stopped altogether for long-stay patients detained in special hospitals or secure units, including committals without criminal proceedings.

10. Special accommodation other than hospitals
Payment of the care component may be affected if you stay in some kinds of 'special' accommodation (see below). The mobility component is not affected in any type of accommodation other than a hospital or similar institution (but see 9 above if the health authority arrange your place in a nursing home). **The rules below apply only to the care component.**

If you go into certain types of special accommodation such as a local authority hostel or home, or any independent residential care home or nursing home where the local authority is helping you meet the fees, your care component will stop after you have been in that accommodation for a total of 28 days. But it may stop sooner if you have been in special accommodation or in hospital within the past 28 days. In this case the different spells are lumped together and treated as one spell. So your care component will stop after a total of 28 days.

The Care in the Community changes in April 1993, affect the way the 'special accommodation' rule may apply to you. If you go into private or voluntary residential care now, it is very likely that the local authority will be helping towards the cost in a residential care or nursing home (rather than just DSS payments of income support). While the local authority is helping towards any funding of your accommodation, you will not be able to receive DLA care component after 4 weeks (see Chapter 36). If you were already in residential care before 31.3.93 you will be able to receive DLA care component, unless at any time the local authority takes over the funding (see Chapter 38).

Claiming while in special accommodation – Even though you can't be paid the care component while in special accommodation, you should apply for it to establish that you pass the disability tests. Then you can be paid it for any day you are not in 'special accommodation' ie in your own home or staying with relatives. Box G.3 explains how you can plan a pattern of relief or respite care that can allow you to keep the care component.

If you first claim the care component when you are already in special accommodation, it is not payable until the first day you leave. Even if you return to special accommodation at any time within 28 days of leaving, you'll still get the 4 week concession even though the two spells are linked.

What is 'special' accommodation?
Payment of DLA care component is affected in the following types of accommodation:
- a local authority owned or managed residential home (a Part III home, Part IV in Scotland);
- any home where *'the cost of [your] accommodation is borne wholly or partly out of public or local funds in pursuance of'* any legislation *'relating to persons under disability or to young persons or to education or training'*;
Reg 9(1)(b) DLA
- any home where *'the cost of [your] accommodation may be borne wholly or partly out of public or local funds in pursuance of'* any legislation *'relating to persons under disability or to young persons or to education or training'*. (But see below for the limitations to this rule – look under 'Paying your own fees'.)
Reg 9(1)(c) DLA

The rules for 'special accommodation' are very complex – this chapter only gives the main points. Chapters 36 and 38 also give some details about DLA care component in these situations. If you are entitled to DLA care component but are told you will not be paid, or if your DLA stops because of the 'special accommodation' rules, it is worth seeking expert advice. If you receive a form asking about your accommodation and how it is funded, seek advice as it is often not easy to know how your accommodation should be described.

People who are entitled to DLA care component in 'special accommodation'
In some situations, people are exempted from the rules that they are not paid DLA care component while in 'special accommodation'. In brief you will still be able to receive DLA care component even if you are in 'special accommodation' if:
- you are terminally ill and residing in a hospice (see 9); or
- you are a child (up to the age of 18 years) who has been accommodated in a private dwelling by the local authority (ie fostered); or
- you are a child living outside the UK and being, or may be, funded by the Education Act (such as at the Peto Institute Hungary); or
- you are a child who is privately fostered; or

- you are getting a student grant or loan; or
- you are housed as a homeless person; or
- you are living in a private dwelling and it is not a residential care home to which you were moved by the body which funded your previous accommodation (but see the note below); or
- you are living in a residential care home or nursing home and have 'preserved rights' (ie you were living in the home at 31.3.93) as long as the local authority is not funding your care – see Chapter 38 for more details; or
- you have moved into a residential care home or nursing home since 31.3.93 and are meeting the full fees out of your own resources or with the help of another person or charity (a person can mean an organisation but, in this context, if the organisation is a local authority, it will stop you getting DLA care component) – but see below.

Paying your own fees – If you moved into your residential care or nursing home after 31.3.93 and are paying the full fees out of your own resources (see above), you can receive the care component if you are not in receipt of IS or housing benefit. Even if you are getting IS, you can still receive the care component if you made your own arrangements with the care home so that the local authority has no contract for your place with the home. This is because of a flaw in the law. It was the policy intention that if you were in receipt of either IS or HB (or your partner got IS for you), you would not be able to get paid DLA care component after 4 weeks even if the local authority was not helping with the funding. This was because it was thought that the cost 'may be borne' by the local authority. However, it has been accepted that since the Care in the Community changes in April 1993 the local authority in England and Wales has no powers to fund in situations where you have made your own arrangements which meet your needs (see *Steane v CAO* [1996] 4 All ER 83). It is a power of last resort only. See Chapter 36(2) and Box K.3 for more details of how this may help you.

People who are not entitled to DLA care component in 'special accommodation'

You will not get paid DLA care component after the first 28 days if you:
- are living in a local authority owned or managed home even if in this case you are paying the full fee for the home;
- have been placed in a residential care or nursing home since 1993 by a local authority which is helping with the funding (but note you can get paid again if the funding stops);
- you are living in a residential care or nursing home since before April 1993 and the local authority is 'topping up' your fees (but seek advice if the local authority stops funding, eg because you come into capital, if your DLA is not made payable again);
- you are living in a non-registered home and the local authority is not funding your accommodation.

C. THE CARE COMPONENT

11. The disability tests

To qualify for DLA care component your care needs must ultimately stem from disability – but both physical and mental disabilities may help you qualify. You must need care, supervision or watching over from another person because of your disabilities.
You must be:
'so severely disabled physically or mentally that . . . you require [from another person]'

DURING THE DAY
No. 1 *'frequent attention throughout the day in connection with [your] bodily functions'*
or
No. 2 *'continual supervision throughout the day in order to avoid substantial danger to [yourself] or others'*
or
AT NIGHT
No. 3 *'prolonged or repeated attention in connection with [your] bodily functions'*
or
No. 4 *'in order to avoid substantial danger to [yourself] or others [you require] another person to be awake for a prolonged period or at frequent intervals for the purpose of watching over [you]'*
or
PART-TIME DAY CARE
No. 5 *'[you require] in connection with [your] bodily functions attention from another person for a significant portion of the day (whether during a single period or a number of periods)'*
or
No. 6 *'[you] cannot prepare a cooked main meal for [yourself] if [you have] the ingredients'.*
S.72(1) SSCBA

Higher rate care component – You'll pass the disability test for the £49.50 higher rate if you satisfy either (or both) of the No. 1 and No. 2 day time tests AND either (or both) of the No. 3 and No. 4 night time tests. Basically, your care or supervision needs are spread throughout both the day and the night.

If you are terminally ill, you qualify automatically for the higher rate even if you need no care at all when you claim – see Box G.4 for details.

Middle rate care component – You'll pass the disability test for the £33.10 middle rate if you satisfy either (or both) of the No. 1 and No. 2 day time tests OR either (or both) of the No. 3 and No. 4 night time tests. Basically, your care or supervision needs are spread throughout just the day or just the night.
or
If you are undergoing dialysis two or more times a week and normally require some help with the dialysis, you may qualify automatically for the middle rate – see 19 for details.

Lower rate care component – You'll pass the disability test for the £13.15 lower rate if you satisfy either (or both) of the No. 5 and No. 6 part-time day care tests. There is an upper age limit for the lower rate: you must be under 65 when you first start to satisfy either of the No. 5 or No. 6 lower rate disability tests. There is also a lower age limit: if you are under 16, you cannot use the No. 6 'cooked main meal' test at all – but you can use the No. 5 'significant portion' test. See 4 above.

Children
There is an extra disability test for children under 16. As well as satisfying any of the No. 1 to No. 5 disability tests, a child must show that either:
- her needs are *'substantially in excess of the normal requirements of persons [her] age'*;
or
- s/he has *'substantial'* care, supervision or watching over needs *'which younger persons in normal physical or mental health may also have but which persons of [her] age and in normal physical and mental health would not have'.*

Chapter 29 explains how the disability tests apply to children. To get payment from birth, a baby must be terminally ill – the qualifying period and the 26 week presence tests do not apply. In all other cases, a baby must need substantially more help than a healthy baby. For example, if your baby has severe feeding problems from birth, the qualifying period means that payment can only start from the first payday on or after the day s/he reaches 3 months old – see 9 if s/he is still in hospital. A shorter, 13 week, presence test applies if you are claiming for a baby who is under 6 months.

The starting point
The starting point for your attention, care, supervision and/or watching over needs must be that you are: *'so severely disabled physically or mentally that [you require] . . .'*. In most cases this poses no problem. However, if there is any suggestion that a 'personality problem', rather than a 'mental or physical disability', is the cause of your symptoms or care needs, get expert advice. In Commissioner's decision R(A)2/92, a claimant's anti- social behaviour was held to be a 'personality disorder' rather than a 'mental disability'. However this should not be taken to mean that a 'personality problem' can never be a 'mental disability'. Check R(I)13/75 and CS/7/82: they are relevant to this question, despite being given in different contexts.

12. What is the 'cooking test'?
This is the No. 6 disability test for the lower rate care component. You must be aged 16 or over to qualify for the lower rate on this basis. The upper age limit for starting to qualify for the first time is the day before your 65th birthday. But if you claim before your 66th birthday (65th birthday if you claim on or after 6.10.97), the lower rate can be maintained and renewed.

You have to show that you are *'so severely disabled physically or mentally that . . . [you] cannot prepare a cooked main meal for [yourself] if [you have] the ingredients'*.
S.72(1)(a)(ii) SSCBA

The cooking test is intended to be a hypothetical or abstract test. Passing or failing does not depend on the type of facilities or equipment you have or don't have, nor on what you do or don't do. It simply looks at whether or not your disabilities mean that you *'cannot prepare a cooked main meal'*.

The cooking test clearly covers people whose disabilities mean they cannot cook at all – even if they had help. But it also applies to people who don't normally cook, as well as to those who do cook but cannot prepare the type of cooked main meal at issue, or who need some help in order to carry out the tasks they are capable of.

What does the cooking test involve?
There are a number of different issues involved in the cooking test. The nature of the 'cooked main meal' which you have to show you 'cannot prepare' for yourself is clearly crucial. The questions in the DLA1 self-assessment form show that the DSS intend it to be a traditional, labour intensive, and, by implication, edible, main meal, freshly cooked on a traditional cooker. This approach was confirmed by the Commissioner in CDLA/85/94.

The use of the word 'prepare' in the law puts the emphasis on your ability to make all the ingredients ready for cooking. It shows that the meal at stake is not intended to be a main meal made up of convenience foods, such as pies and frozen vegetables involving no real preparation.

The use of the phrase 'for himself [or herself]' shows that the meal is intended to be for just one person – not for the rest of the household. In the context of the disability test and the qualifying periods, the 'main meal' at issue is a labour-intensive, main daily meal for one person, not a celebration meal or a snack. Because this is a hypothetical test, it is irrelevant that you would never wish to cook such a meal or that you cannot afford to do so. Nor is it relevant that you prepare, cook and freeze a number of main meals on the days that you actually have the help you need (and then defrost and heat them up in the microwave on the other days). We cannot emphasise enough that what you do or don't do is irrelevant. All depends on what you cannot do, without help, if you tried to do it on each day.

Intermittent disability – You don't have to show that you were unable to cook on every day of the 3 months before your claim and are likely to be unable to cook on every day of the next 6 months. The test is rather about what can be seen as the norm for you over a period of time. Taking the ordinary English language meaning of the words, and applying the test to the effects of your disabilities, is it true to say of you (over the 9 month period) that you *'cannot prepare a cooked main meal . . .'*?

The ability to cook a main meal on 4 out of 7 days each week does not mean, in law, that you must fail the test. All depends on the pattern of what you cannot do over the whole of the qualifying period. In practice, if you tick the box in the DLA1 self-assessment form to show that you need help on 1–3 days only, your chances of success are slim!

The approach taken in R(A)2/74, in looking at what help is normally required over a period of time, must be followed in preference to the unreported decision CA/593/89 which asserts, without considering earlier precedents, that the qualifying period requires a continuous run of bad days.

Help – Although s.72(l)(a)(ii) says nothing about the role of help or supervision from another person, it is clear that you 'cannot prepare a cooked main meal for [yourself]' if you could only do so with some help. The need for any type of help counts – it doesn't have to involve any effort or be at all substantial. But it must be crucial in enabling you to start or carry on with the tasks you are capable of doing all by yourself.

Reasonableness – The test is one of whether you cannot *reasonably* be expected to prepare a cooked main meal for yourself. Things like safety, tiredness, pain, and the time it would take you to do everything, may mean that although you can in fact prepare a cooked main meal, it is not reasonable to expect you to do so. See CDLA/902/94.

Practice and process
To produce an edible cooked main meal requires the ability to carry out, all by yourself, all of the physical and mental actions, tasks and stages involved in the process. If there is any part of the whole process which you are (or would be) unable to carry out by yourself, then you'll pass this test – even if you cope (or would cope) well with the rest.
See R(S)11/81 for support.

If you have a severe mental disability so that you cannot plan ahead or complete complex tasks then you would pass the cooking test. Or if lack of motivation is caused by, or is a symptom of, a mental disability, so that you cannot begin to prepare a meal or complete the preparations, then you could pass the test (CSDLA/80/96).

The process of preparing a cooked main meal includes:
- planning what to prepare for the cooked main meal, eg each type of food, seasoning, and the quantities required;
- the law says you already have the ingredients for the main meal, so it's debateable whether or not 'preparation' also includes getting them from their usual storage places;
- carrying out all the stages in the correct order and to the standard timings;
- lifting, carrying, washing, peeling and chopping fresh vegetables, meat etc;

- using taps, eg to fill a saucepan;
- using a cooker, eg lighting the gas, adjusting the heat, opening and closing an oven door;
- putting the vegetables etc into pans, stirring, tasting, checking whether properly cooked etc;
- lifting and moving full or hot pans on or off a cooker, or bending to lift pans into or out of the oven;
- draining cooked vegetables from hot pans; and
- dishing up your meal.

13. What is 'attention'?

This means active help from another person to do the personal things which you cannot do for yourself. It does not matter whether you actually get the help, what counts is the help you need.

To count for the 'attention' conditions, the help you need because of your disability must be in connection with your 'bodily functions'.

'Bodily functions' means personal things such as breathing, hearing, seeing, eating, drinking, walking, sitting, sleeping, getting in or out of bed, dressing and undressing, going to the toilet, getting in or out the bath, washing, shaving, communicating, speech practice, help with medication or treatment, etc.

Anything to do with your body and how it works can count. So too can things like help to avoid you making a mess in the toilet, to soothe you back to sleep, or change bedding after an 'accident': things closely linked to your bodily functions. Indirect or ancillary attention counts but is often forgotten.* Think about the beginnings and ends of particular activities. If there is some part of an activity you need help with (and you could not carry on if you didn't have that help) that help counts. For example, you may be able to dress yourself, but if you cannot get your clothes yourself, or maybe you need to be reminded to dress, you reasonably need help with 'getting dressed'. It is irrelevant that you can manage most of the activity by yourself. If it takes you a long time to do something, such as getting dressed for example, it may be that you reasonably require help even though you are able to manage by yourself.

* The general principle comes from R(A)2/74, p.13, which concerned help with dialysing.

If you need someone to wash clothes and bedding for you, this does not count as attention with a bodily function, but removing and handling of soiled articles does count.

Cockburn v CAO [1996] – but note that, at the time of writing, a decision on appeal to the House of Lords was pending.

You might need help with things that can't easily be seen as 'bodily functions', such as reading, guiding, shopping, cooking, housework, etc. In this case, the House of Lords decision in *Mallinson v Secretary of State for Social Security* (appendix to R(A)3/94)) might help.

Generally each separate activity you need help with has to count as a separate bodily function. But in *Mallinson*, the judge said *'where ... the function which is primarily impaired as a result of the disability can be readily identified ... it is preferable to focus on that function'*. So if you are blind, or deaf, or paralysed, the impaired bodily function could be seeing, or hearing, or movement. Thus each separate activity you need help with due to your disability, is 'attention in connection with' just one bodily function. For example, dealing with correspondence is not a bodily function, but in the case of a blind person then the 'primarily impaired' function is seeing. Therefore having your mail read to you counts as help with seeing. You must then go on to show that each activity has a sufficiently close connection; the help must be carried out in your presence and involve some personal contact with you – this need not be physical contact but can be talking or signing. Finally, the attention must also be *'reasonably required'* – see below.

The judgement specifically included guiding and reading to a blind person as attention in connection with the bodily function of seeing, but if you can demonstrate a close connection and show that the help needed is reasonable, then many everyday activities could be counted. Think about all the help you need from other people to do things you could do for yourself if you did not have a disability. Remember, you don't actually have to be getting help, it is enough that you need it.

Domestic tasks – The *Mallinson* judgement did not specifically say that help with housework can count as attention, and previous case law has clearly excluded domestic tasks. DSS guidance says that 'attention' does not include cooking, shopping or other domestic tasks – *'many domestic activities would not have the requisite close connection because they could be carried out without the disabled person being present'*. However, recent case law shows how help with domestic tasks can sometimes count as 'attention'. In CDLA/267/94 the Commissioner said *'if a claimant reasonably requires to be able himself to cook and can do so if he has assistance with, for example, seeing or lifting, that seems to me to show a requirement for attention in connection with his bodily functions'*. So although it would not count if someone does the cooking for you, if someone helps you to do the cooking for yourself – reading labels and recipes, checking cooker settings – this could count if it is reasonably required. You might argue it is reasonable for you to develop or maintain a level of independence. Similarly if someone does your shopping for you, this would not count, but if someone helps you with the shopping – reading labels, counting out money, using a cheque book – you can argue this help is reasonably required.

See also CDLA/450/95.

There is currently an extra section to the DLA1 claim form, to take account of *Mallinson* (and *Fairey* – see below). It tells you not to give details of domestic duties, but there is plenty of space at the back of the form for you to add anything you think relevant. So if you might need to include the help required with domestic duties in order to meet the 'frequent attention' condition, then give details of all the help you need, including domestic duties, but be prepared to appeal!

'Reasonably required' – The attention you need must be 'reasonably required' rather than medically required.

The Court of Appeal on 15.6.95 (*Secretary of State v Fairey*) held that *'it is right to include in the aggregate of attention that is reasonably required such attention as may enable the claimant to carry out a reasonable level of social activity'*. So help you need related to recreational, leisure, cultural or social activities may be taken into account. This may help you pass the 'frequent attention' condition – see below. However this may change – at the time of writing a decision on appeal to the House of Lords was pending (see our *Disability Rights Bulletin*). The DSS has already paid back benefit that was suspended pending the outcome of the House of Lords appeal.

In R v Secretary of State ex p Sutherland, TLR 2.1.97, it was held that reg 37A C&P was ultra vires, therefore such suspensions were unlawful.

During the day

Frequent attention – To pass the No. 1 disability test (see 11 above) for the middle rate, you have to show that during the daytime you need this help frequently and *'throughout'* the day – during the middle of the day, as well as in the morning and evening. But the fact you can manage the majority of your bodily functions without help does not mean you fail this test.

All depends on the pattern of your accepted care needs. For example, in CA/35/89 a child with cystic fibrosis required help at least 9 times a day (2 × physio and 7 × medication). The Commissioner said the Attendance Allowance Board's decision was perverse: in that no person acting judicially and properly instructed in the relevant law could have gone on to find that these facts did not pass the 'frequent attention' test.

'Frequent' means *'several times – not once or twice'*, and the pattern of help must be such that, looking at all the facts about your accepted care needs as a whole, it is true to say of you that you need *'frequent attention throughout the day'*. This means it is difficult to give a clear dividing line between success and failure. The best advice is to give as full a picture of your care needs as you can. The decision maker must then focus on what you need, and on the pattern of what you need, looking at the day and your needs as a whole, and at the pattern of days if your needs vary, rather than on the gaps between your needs and how long it takes to give that help.

See appendix to R(A)2/80, R(A)4/78, CA/140/85 and 12 above (under 'Intermittent disability').

Significant portion – To pass the No. 5 disability test for the lower rate (see 11 above), you must show that you need help from another person for a *'significant portion of the day'*. That help can be needed all at once, or on a number of times. You should pass this test if it would take 1 hour or more in total to give you the help you need. See CDLA/58/93.

This test for the lower rate is intended to cover people who, for example, just need help with getting up and going to bed and can manage on their own for the rest of the day. But it can also cover anyone whose care needs aren't sufficiently spread out over the whole day to fit the pattern required by the 'frequent attention' test.

If you need less than 1 hour's care, that may still be a 'significant portion' of the day. In deciding this, the position of the carer may be taken into account. If the carer's own life is disrupted by the need to give attention on a considerable number of small occasions in the day, then those periods of providing attention taken together may be 'significant', even though individually they may be relatively insignificant (CSDLA/29/94).

Depending on the frequency and pattern of your accepted care needs, it is also possible to pass the 'frequent attention' test for the middle rate even though it would take less than an hour in all to give you the help you need. If you need an hour's worth (or less) of help on and off several times over the whole course of the day, the pattern of your care needs should pass the 'frequent attention' test. If the pattern of your care needs isn't clear from the answers in your DLA1 self-assessment form, it is worth keeping a diary for a short time to make sure you are not wrongly awarded the lower rate.

During the night

During the night the help must either be *'prolonged'* (at least 20 minutes) or *'repeated'* (needed two times or more).

There is no fixed time for the start of the 'night'. It depends on your household's habits. 'Night' will normally start from the time your carer goes to bed (or midnight if your carer is up until the early hours and would go to bed earlier if s/he did not have to help you).

14. What is 'continual supervision'?

Supervision is more or less what it says: if you need someone to be around to prevent any accidents either to yourself, or other people. The words used are 'continual supervision' – this means frequent or regular, but not non-stop – so you can apply even if you don't need supervision every single minute. The supervision doesn't have to prevent the danger completely, but it must be needed *'in order to effect a real reduction in the risk of harm to the claimant'*, R(A) 3/92. Remember the golden rule – if in doubt claim.

The supervision must be *'reasonably'* required, rather than 'medically' required. For example, you may be mentally alert and know what you should not do without someone at hand to help. 'Medically' speaking, you could supervise yourself. But the question is whether or not you reasonably require supervision from someone else. In practice supervising yourself might mean that to avoid the risk of danger you would have to do nothing but stay in bed, or stay in an armchair. If you would have to restrict your lifestyle in order to supervise yourself without help from someone else, the question is whether or not those restrictions are reasonable. Do they allow you to carry on anything approaching a normal life? If the restrictions on your lifestyle are not reasonable, then you reasonably require help from another person to live a normal life.

The next question is whether you satisfy the other parts of the 'continual supervision' test. There are four parts to the 'continual supervision' test.

❑ You must show that your medical condition is such that it may (not will) give rise to substantial danger to yourself or to others. The danger to you could come from your own actions, or from the actions of other people. The danger to others could be wholly unintended – say, if you aren't able to care for a young child safely.

❑ The substantial danger must not be too remote a possibility. But the fact an incident may be isolated or infrequent does not rule this out. As well as looking at the chances of the incident happening, the AO must look at the likely result if it happens. If the results could be dire, then how often the incident is likely to happen becomes less and less relevant.

❑ You must need supervision from someone else in order to avoid the substantial danger.

❑ The supervision must be 'continual': but it doesn't always have to be alert, awake and active. Stand-by supervision, being ready to intervene and help, can also count.

If you suffer from epilepsy and the onset of an attack is unpredictable, with not enough warning to allow you to arrange for help to arrive, or to put yourself in a place of safety, then you may qualify for DLA care component; certainly at the middle rate for your day-time supervision needs. This is because of the case of *Moran v Secretary of State for Social Services* [appendix to R(A)1/88]. The principles in *Moran* also help other people whose needs for supervision and attention are unpredictable, and where the consequences of an unsupervised 'attack' would be grave. It particularly helps those who are mentally alert and can supervise themselves between 'attacks' but not during 'attacks'. *Moran* still applies to the day-time supervision test.

Supervision and falls

The risk of falls ranks alongside the care needs created by incontinence as being one of the main general indicators for entitlement to the care component. In the past, if you were mentally alert and sensible, it was often said that you could supervise yourself and so avoid the risk of falling without help from another person. This simplistic approach has been ruled out by R(A)3/89 and R(A)5/90(T) in particular.

AOs must consider the evidence, must properly evaluate the risk of falling in any case, and give sufficient reasons for their conclusions. In particular, it is not enough to say you are 'sensible'. AOs must identify any precautions you could take and/or any activities you should not do if you are to avoid the risk of falls by yourself without help from someone else. It is only if it is *'possible to isolate one or two activities which alone* might give rise to a fall, and which could be avoided except for one or two occasions during the course of the day, and [you would] still be left to enjoy a more or less normal life, [that] it would be justifiable to say that continual supervision was not required. Everything will depend upon the facts of the case'*, CA/127/88, para 8. However, remember there is a close overlap between supervision and attention. Even if your need for help to avoid the risk of falls does not amount to a need for continual supervision, it is possible that that help could also count as attention – see 18.

15. What is 'watching over'?
'Watching over' has its ordinary English language meaning: so it includes needing to have someone else being awake and listening, as well as getting up and checking how you are.

Remember that the care component is based on what help or supervision you reasonably need to have from another person: not on what help or supervision you actually get. Your care needs must stem from physical or mental disablement, but you don't have to show that it is medically essential that you have that help or supervision: just that, given all the

G.4 Terminal illness

Automatic DLA
If you count as terminally ill, you don't have to serve the qualifying period in order to get DLA. Claims identified as being from terminally ill people are given high priority. If you are claiming under what the DSS call the 'Special Rules', the DSS hope to achieve a 10 working day turnaround between claim and notice of an award.

You will qualify automatically for higher rate care component if your death *'can reasonably be expected'* within the next six months. If you pass the 'terminal illness' test, you are treated as satisfying the conditions for the higher rate for the remainder of your life – even if at the time of the claim you don't need nursing-type help from another person. However, to get the mobility component you must pass one of the disability tests – see 20.

Living with a terminal illness, particularly with the shock on first diagnosis, is distressing. Claiming benefits and sorting out any financial problems tends to be the last thing on your mind. In part, claiming DLA is an acknowledgement, if not acceptance, of what is happening to you: and you may not yet be ready to fully face up to that. Unfortunately DLA cannot be backdated to before the day you actually claimed it. There is no extension of the time limit for claiming to allow time to adjust. All we can advise is to claim as soon as you feel able.

Do note that even though you are suffering from a terminal illness, you will fail the test if at the time you first claim, your death cannot reasonably be expected within the next 6 months. Discuss things with your doctors to make sure a claim is submitted quickly. If you are turned down, check with your doctor and ask for a review of that decision, or simply make a fresh claim when your situation changes.

How do you claim?
Claim in the normal way – see 25. The claim pack explains which bits of the DLA1 you need to fill in. If you are claiming under the 'Special Rules', you are asked to send a factual statement, a DS1500 report, from your doctor or consultant to the DSS along with your claim form. Your doctor should have a supply of factual statement forms available.

The person who is terminally ill does not have to sign the claim form. Another person, including their doctor, can claim benefit on their behalf, for example where the terminally ill person is not up to completing the form, or has not yet been told the full nature of their condition. In this box we refer to the terminally ill person as the 'claimant' even though s/he may not physically make the claim, or even know about the claim.

However, payment will be made direct to the claimant. In some cases where a doctor has claimed for you, no-one in your family may know about that claim until you are sent an order book for DLA!

Harmful medical information – If the claimant has not been told about specific medical evidence or advice about their condition or prognosis, you or your doctor should give details on a separate letter attached to the claim form or factual statement. If the Adjudication Officer (AO) considers that disclosure of that medical advice or evidence to the claimant *'would be harmful to his [or her] health'*, it won't be included in any papers sent to the claimant. In your letter, ask how the AO intends to exercise discretion under reg 8, Social Security (Adjudication) Regulations 1995/1801.

Hospital – If you are in hospital when you first claim DLA, it cannot be paid until the first day you leave hospital. If you are in 'special accommodation', you can claim and be paid the mobility component as normal, and in some circumstances you may get the care component. See 9 and 10 for more details.

What happens once you claim?
Once you have claimed, an Adjudication Officer (AO) decides if you satisfy the test of terminal illness. Decisions are based on the evidence about your clinical condition, diagnosis and treatment which your doctor or consultant gives in the factual statement. The DS1500 report does not ask about prognosis (ie about your life expectancy). However, the AO may refer your case to a doctor for expert advice. That doctor may phone your doctor to clarify any matters. In some cases your doctor may not feel ready to complete the DS1500 – for example, where the diagnosis and future treatment are not yet fully confirmed because one or two other possibilities, with different implications for treatment, have yet to be ruled out. Your doctor can complete the statement based on what is currently known about your condition, and forward complete details when they are available.

If you satisfy the 'terminal illness' test at this first stage, you will be awarded higher rate care component for the remainder of your life.

If the AO considers that you don't satisfy the 'terminal illness' test, based on the information from you and your doctor, a medical examination may be arranged. A doctor, usually a GP, working on a fee basis for the DSS, will examine you and complete a report. The AO will then decide your claim under the terminal illness provisions. If you don't satisfy that test, the AO will go on to consider your claim under the ordinary disability tests. If the AO's decision on part, or all, of your claim is negative, you can ask for a review of that decision – see below.

What if you already get DLA?
In some cases, you will already be getting a lower or middle rate care component. You don't have to make a separate claim under the terminal illness provisions. Instead, you just write to ask for a review on the basis that you now count as 'terminally ill'. You don't have to send in a completed factual statement from your doctor along with your review letter, but it will speed

circumstances, the help is reasonably required. Nor do you have to require that level of help on every night in the week. It all depends on the normal pattern of your needs – 3 nights a week may well be sufficient, perhaps less if the dangers would be very grave.

A *'prolonged period'* is at least 20 minutes. It is arguable whether or not this includes the time before and after the time during which you actually need someone *'watching over'* you. (The night attention test does take this extra time into account: ie the time a carer would take to get out of bed and back to bed after attending to your needs.)

'Frequent intervals' means at least 3 times: but it's worth trying if you require watching over twice a night.

Tackle the test in the following way.
- If you need any 'active' help at night (eg soothing back to sleep, rearranging bedding), state that your night-time care needs are both attention and supervision needs – you might pass the attention test more easily.
- Show that your disability or medical condition is such that it may give rise to substantial danger – as in 14.

up the decision-making process if you can do so.

If you are successful on this review, the increase in your care component can be backdated to one month before the day your request for a review reached the Disability Benefits Unit.

The legal definition of terminal illness
S.66(2)(a) of the SSCBA provides that you count as being 'terminally ill' at any time *'if at that time [you have] a progressive disease and [your] death in consequence of that disease can reasonably be expected within 6 months'*.

The diagnosis question should be straightforward. Are you suffering from a disease which is a progressive one? Is the disease one which, by its nature, develops and gets worse, perhaps in identifiable stages. Multiple sclerosis, for example, is a progressive disease, even though some people may have long periods of remission, or may never develop the final range of symptoms. Similarly, although AIDS is a syndrome, it counts as a progressive disease as it involves a progressive breakdown of the body's immune system.

It is easily possible to satisfy the diagnosis part of the terminal illness test. What is crucial for qualifying for DLA automatically is the question of prognosis. To pass the prognosis part of the test, the AO has to agree that your *'death in consequence of that disease can reasonably be expected within 6 months'*.

There are two aspects to the prognosis test. Firstly, the connection between the disease and the expected death. Secondly, that your death can reasonably be expected within 6 months.

The disease alone doesn't have to be solely responsible for your death. Industrial death benefit, which was abolished in April 1988, had a similar test: death had to be *'as a result of'* an industrial accident or disease. Case law established that so long as death was 'materially accelerated' by the industrial accident or disease, the widow qualified for industrial death benefit even though the immediate cause of death was, for example, pneumonia.

The DLA prognosis test looks forward, rather than backwards as did the industrial death benefit test. It may be that given your progressive disease alone your death could not reasonably be expected within 6 months: but your age or general physical condition may, for example, make respiratory infections more likely. You may be more prone to complications associated with, but not part of, your progressive disease. So long as the progressive disease plays the key role in whether your death can reasonably be expected within 6 months, you should succeed in your claim for automatic DLA. With diseases such as AIDS or motor neurone disease, the progress and nature of the disease itself makes you more vulnerable to other conditions – the connection between the disease and those other conditions is clear.

Note that we keep using the actual words from the Act. It is important not to translate them into different words as a different form of wording may imply a different test. The statutory test of terminal illness is not a matter of what is possible, or of what is or is not hoped for. Instead, it focuses on expectations of death: if, on all the evidence, your death could reasonably be expected within 6 months, you are entitled to succeed. It is a test of what can reasonably be expected on the evidence, rather than certainty.

This test does not put an upper limit on life expectancy: it is not a matter of what is the longest period you can reasonably be expected to live. Clearly no-one can predict death 6 months ahead to the day, nor even to the month. It is quite possible that your death could reasonably be expected at any time within a period of 5 to 10 months ahead. In this case, the upper limit of your reasonable life expectancy would be 10 months ahead, with death at that stage pretty certain; while 5 months ahead would be the start of the period during which your death could reasonably be expected, rather than being a possibility. Once DLA is awarded you should normally keep it for the remainder of your life even though this may be more than 6 months.

Reviews
Decisions on whether or not you satisfy the terminal illness test can be reviewed in the normal way. An existing award can also be reviewed – although the DSS have said they don't intend, for example, to review terminal illness awards just because you have lived for over 6 months.

Review within 3 months – If you ask for a review within 3 months of the date the AO's decision was sent to you, it can be reviewed for any reason at all.

Review at any time – If it has been over 3 months since you were sent the AO's decision, that decision can still be reviewed, but only for certain reasons.

A decision on the 'terminal illness' test can be reviewed at any time if:
- it was made in ignorance of any material fact; or
- it was based on a mistake about the material facts; or
- there has been a relevant change of circumstances since the decision was made.

More importantly, the Act provides that a decision on the 'terminal illness' test can also be reviewed if:
- *'there has been a change in medical opinion with respect to [your] condition or [your] reasonable expectations of life'*.

This allows a decision to be reviewed easily even if nothing has changed and the AO had full details about your condition when that decision was first made. For example, if the final decision on review is negative, the AO's written statement of reasons may make clear how and why s/he came to that decision. If your consultant disagrees with that opinion on prognosis because some factors haven't been highlighted sufficiently, a further medical report to that effect could lead to the AO reviewing the original decision.

- ❏ Outline the nature of the danger(s) – explain the basis for all your fears of the risk of danger; refer to anything which supports your fears, eg the previous pattern and course of 'attacks', wandering at night, falls etc.
- ❏ Think about 'simpler methods' (see 16 below) which may bypass the need to have another person watching over you. Explain fully how and why they haven't worked, or don't or would not work. Are they 'reasonable'?
- ❏ Explain why you cannot avoid the substantial danger without help from another person: eg mental disorder; inability to administer medication, oxygen etc during an 'attack', etc.
- ❏ Relate the danger(s) to the need to have another person awake and watching over you. Do the dangers warrant having another person watching over you for 20 minutes, or longer? Or to have another person wake up to listen out for you, or to get up to check on you 2, 3, or more times in the night? On how many nights a week?

Remember the test is based on what you 'reasonably require', not on what is actually done for you. If you've had a fair number of 'accidents' or incidents at night (or even just one bad accident), that may well suggest that you need more 'watching over' than you've been getting. If you've had few 'accidents' etc, the chances are that the 'watching over' you get is also the 'watching over' you need.

16. Simpler methods?

It is important to explain why you need particular types of attention or supervision. There may be simpler, practical ways of meeting your needs. This could mean you don't reasonably (or medically) need as much attention or supervision from another person as you are currently getting. So the AO might ignore part of the help you are actually getting. If you can show that you have tried the simpler methods (whatever they may be) and fully explain why they are not suitable for your particular circumstances, the AO should take the actual help you get into account. In R(A)1/87, the Commissioners said the decision maker should *'explain how his suggestion is practical and compatible with the evidence of [the disabled person's abilities and] agility and with anything resembling normal domestic arrangements...'*. It is clear that a simpler method must also be 'reasonable'.

A typical 'simpler method' is the use of a commode or portable urinal. If you could use one without help, it is often said that you don't reasonably require the help you need with trips to the toilet. Although the DLA1 asks about this, you may not realise it is an issue. Doctors often write that you can use a commode without thinking about all the practical issues involved – securing privacy, washing your hands etc – and without thinking about the effect on your morale, or on your general health if trips to the toilet are your only regular exercise. AOs must properly consider the practical issues arising from the suggested use of a commode, particularly during the day [cf CA/156/88].

Sometimes you won't realise the AO has taken a 'simpler method' into account until you get the written reasons for a review decision. If it's not a practical method for you, ask for a further review and consider appealing – see 27.

17. Keeping a diary?

Most people won't need to keep a detailed diary of daily events to support their claims. But for some people it could mean the difference between success or failure, or between the different rates. If you think it might help you to keep a diary, do ask for advice – you don't want to spend hours writing up a diary unnecessarily!

If your need for attention is unpredictable, or changes from day to day, a diary can show exactly how much help had to be given, and why.

If your condition is getting slowly worse, a diary can help pinpoint the date you began to qualify for a higher rate. It can also help you remember things you would otherwise forget as they are so much a part of your everyday life.

A detailed diary only needs to be kept for long enough to show the normal pattern of your attention and/or supervision needs. You may just need to concentrate on one or two aspects of those needs.

For example, if your needs at the beginning and end of a day aren't really in doubt, you might just need to keep a note of the help you need during the middle of the day. Remember you have to show that you need 'frequent attention' or 'continual supervision' throughout the day.

At night you might just have to keep a note of the time(s) your carer had to get up to look after (or watch over) you (and why) and the time(s) they were able to get back to bed. This is so you can show that the attention you need has to be 'prolonged' or 'repeated' or comes 'at frequent intervals'.

If you need continual supervision or watching over to prevent substantial danger to yourself, or others, a diary can show exactly what happened – or what could have happened if someone hadn't been there to stop it. If you have had no major accidents, that may just be because you have always had someone on hand.

18. Attention or supervision?

There is often a very close overlap between attention and supervision and it can be difficult to distinguish between the two. Sometimes both can be given at the same time: eg if you are deaf and don't have much traffic sense someone walking beside you could be supervising you (waiting to grab you to stop you walking) and giving attention in connection with walking ('telling' you what you need to know in order to continue walking in safety) – CA/86/87.

Similarly, if you are unsteady on your feet and liable to fall, you might need both supervision and attention when walking. The supervision could be a matter of looking out for any unexpected objects in the way, and being on hand to catch you if you fell. The attention might involve telling you about what is in front of you; or it could be a hand on your arm to steady you.

There are many other possibilities where the help you need can amount to both attention and supervision. It is sensible not to divide the help you need into watertight 'attention' and 'supervision' compartments. A 24 hour diary which lists all your needs throughout a typical day should help you think about the types of help which could count as both.

The difference between attention and supervision is important. *'The vital contrast is between activity and a state of passivity coupled with a readiness to intervene'* (*Mallinson v Secretary of State for Social Security*). With supervision, much of the help is passive, with active supervision (or attention) coming at varying intervals. The object of supervision is to avoid the risk of substantial danger. Depending on how great that risk is, and the nature of the danger, the actual situations of potential danger could be quite infrequent. For example, the chance of being run over by a bus may be small – but it takes only one incident to kill you. On the other hand, the attention condition is based only on whether you reasonably need attention in connection with your bodily functions. Instead of showing that the object of that help is to avoid the risk of substantial danger, you simply have to show that your needs are 'frequent' throughout the day, or 'prolonged' or 'repeated' at night.

If the AO does not look at the same needs under both the attention and supervision conditions, you might find that you fail both the day attention and supervision conditions. A long gap during the middle of the day might mean that the pattern of help you need does not amount to *'frequent . . . throughout the day'*. Under the supervision condition, the risk of danger and the situations of potential danger may not be great or frequent enough to warrant 'continual' supervision. Yet if some of the needs which were considered only under the supervision condition could also be taken into account under the attention condition, the combination of needs could well amount to frequent attention throughout the day (and give you the middle rate rather than the lower rate). All depends on the facts of the case. This argument only works where some of the supervision also amounts to active attention in connection with any of your bodily functions.

To summarise, attention tends to be active help, while supervision is more passive. In practice, don't worry about this. Just explain the what, why, where, and how of all your needs for help from another person. Think broadly: for example, help with maintaining or developing communication or speech skills for a deaf person can also count as 'attention'.

Try to use the DLA1 form to explain about all your care needs. If you are unsuccessful, or are awarded a lower rate than you think you should get, you can ask for a review – see 27. In your review letter, ask the AO to consider all your needs under both conditions. If you can, list the needs which could count as both attention and supervision.

19. Renal dialysis

There are special rules for some kidney patients to help them qualify for the middle rate of care component. In general, the nature of haemodialysis and intermittent peritoneal dialysis means you need enough help to pass these rules. Depending on when and where you dialyse, you'll be treated as satisfying the disability tests for the day or for the night. You must show that:

- you undergo renal dialysis 2 or more times a week; and
- the dialysis is of a type which *'normally requires the attendance or supervision of another person during the period of the dialysis'*; or
- because of your particular circumstances, eg age, visual impairment or loss of manual dexterity, you *'in fact [require] another person, during the period of the dialysis'*, to supervise you in order to avoid substantial danger to yourself, or to give you some help with your bodily functions.

Hospital – If you are dialysing as an outpatient, getting help from hospital staff, that doesn't automatically satisfy the disability tests, but does help you pass both qualifying periods for DLA (3 months backward test and 6 months forward test – see 5). This is helpful if you alternate between outpatient dialysis and dialysis at home. You'll be treated as satisfying the disability tests for the period you dialyse at home (if this is at least twice a week and you need assistance) even if it is only a short period.

If the help you get as an outpatient is from someone who doesn't work for the hospital, this does pass the disability test. In-patient dialysis counts for both the qualifying period and the disability test – but payment of the care component is affected by a spell in hospital – see 9.

Other types of dialysis – Continuous ambulatory peritoneal dialysis (CAPD), continuous cycle peritoneal dialysis (CCPD) and peritoneal rapid overnight dialysis (PROD) are designed to be carried out without help. You can only be covered by these rules if your disabilities, or age, mean you actually need help during the dialysis.

D. THE MOBILITY COMPONENT

20. The disability tests

For anyone aged 5 and over, the disability tests are as follows.

Higher rate

To qualify for the £34.60 higher rate mobility component under the number 1 to number 3 disability tests, you must be *'suffering from physical disablement'*. But if it is accepted that your severe learning disabilities have a physical cause, you may also qualify. Your *'physical condition as a whole'* must be such that:

EITHER

1. you are unable to walk – see below;

or

2. you are virtually unable to walk – see 22;

or

3. the *'exertion required to walk would constitute a danger to [your] life or would be likely to lead to a serious deterioration in [your] health'* – see below;

S.73(1)(a) SSCBA; reg 12(1)(a) DLA Regs

or

4. you have no legs or feet (from birth or through amputation) – see below;

S.73(1)(b), (2)(b) SSCBA; reg 12(1)(b) DLA Regs

or

5. you are both deaf and blind – see below;

S.73(1)(b), (2)(a) SSCBA; reg 12(2),(3) DLA Regs

or

6. you are entitled to the higher rate care component and are severely mentally impaired with extremely disruptive and dangerous behavioural problems – see 23;

S.73(1)(c), (3) SSCBA; reg 12(5), (6) DLA Regs

or

7. you are switching from the pre-1976 invalid vehicle scheme and still meet those rules – see Chapter 20.

Lower rate

To qualify for the £13.15 lower rate mobility component, it doesn't matter that you are able to walk but you must be: *'so severely disabled physically or mentally that, disregarding any ability [you] may have to use routes which are familiar to [you] on [your] own, [you] cannot take advantage of the faculty out of doors without guidance or supervision from another person most of the time'* – see 24.

Children – There is an extra disability test for the lower rate only for a child under 16. S/he must show that either:

- s/he *'requires substantially more guidance or supervision from another person than persons of [her] age in normal physical and mental health would require'*; or
- people of her age *'in normal physical and mental health would not require such guidance or supervision'*.

S.73(4) SSCBA

Unable to walk?

Being 'unable to walk' means just that. You cannot take a step by putting one foot in front of the other. If you have one artificial leg it is your walking ability when using it that will be considered. You are unlikely to count as being 'unable to walk' but you may well qualify on the basis that you are 'virtually unable to walk'.

Effects of exertion

For the third way of qualifying for the mobility component remember that it is the exertion needed to walk that must cause the serious problem. How far you can actually walk is not relevant. The point is that medically you should not walk very far because of the effect of the effort of walking on your life or health. People with serious lung, chest or heart conditions, or blood disorders such as haemophilia, may qualify in this way.

The 'danger' or 'serious deterioration' does not have to be immediate, nor does any 'deterioration' have to be likely to last for 6 months. If you can only recover from the deterioration in your health by some kind of medical intervention (eg oxygen, drugs) you should explain this on the DLA1 form. Danger arising from other causes besides the effort needed to walk (eg being run over by a bus) cannot be taken into account.

No legs or feet?
If you have no legs or feet (for any reason), or both legs have been amputated at or above the ankle, you qualify automatically for higher rate mobility component. How you manage with artificial prostheses does not affect this.

Deaf and blind
You may qualify for the higher rate if you are blind and are also profoundly deaf. You must show that because of the effects of those conditions in combination with each other, you are *'unable, without the assistance of another person, to walk to any intended or required destination while out of doors'*.

Reg 12(2) defines blind as 100% disablement resulting from loss of vision. Deaf is defined as 80% disablement resulting from loss of hearing (where 100% is absolute deafness).

The definitions of degrees of disablement used for industrial injuries benefits have now been adopted for the mobility component (CDLA/192/94). Disablement of 100% means loss of vision so that you are unable to do any work for which eyesight is essential. For the hearing test, you will be referred to a DSS doctor to assess your hearing loss. An average hearing loss at 1, 2 and 3 kHz of at least 87dB in each ear counts as 80% disablement. The doctor will also advise on the degree of disablement from loss of vision.
Sch 2, SS (General Benefits) Regs 1982; Sch 3, Part II, SS (Industrial Injuries) (Prescribed Diseases) Regs 1985

21. Other factors
In a coma? – If your condition is such that you cannot *'benefit from enhanced facilities for locomotion'*, you won't be entitled to the mobility component. This really only excludes people who are in a coma, or whose medical condition means that it is not safe to move them. If you can get out from time to time, even if no-one has ever taken you out, you are not excluded from mobility component.
S.73(8) SSCBA

Personal circumstances – The first three disability tests for the higher rate ignore the effects of your personal circumstances on your mobility. Where you live (eg on a steep hill or

G.5 Learning disabilities

If you don't qualify for higher rate mobility component on the basis of 'severe mental impairment' (see 23), you are more than likely to pass the test for the lower rate – see 24. However, it is still possible for some people who are autistic, deaf/blind, or have a learning disability to qualify for higher rate mobility component on the basis of 'virtual inability to walk' – see 22.

Virtually unable to walk?
First the need for help to get from one point, A, to another point, B, is totally irrelevant to the 'virtually unable to walk' test. The purpose of walking is also wholly irrelevant. Instead this test is tied to physical limitations on a person's ability to put one foot in front of the other and to continue to make progress on foot. These physical limitations include behavioural problems where they are a 'reaction', a result, of the person's physical disablement such as genetic damage in the case of Downs Syndrome, or brain damage. This test looks at interruptions in the ability to make progress on foot. These interruptions have been referred to as *'temporary paralysis (as far as walking is concerned)'*. The interruptions must be accepted as physical in origin; as part and parcel of your accepted physical disablement, rather than under your direct and conscious control.

Thus being able to put one foot in front of the other does not stop you passing the 'virtual inability' test. You must, however, be able to show that any behavioural problems, which may sometimes include a failure to exercise your powers of walking, stem from a physical disability. And that your walking difficulties, including interruptions in your ability to make progress on foot, happen often enough so that your walking is *'so limited . . . that [you are] virtually unable to walk'*.

If you have had a history of behavioural problems since birth, the decision-maker *'should provide very clear reasons for attributing the behavioural problems in question to something other than brain damage'* [or Downs Syndrome etc], CM/98/89.

The R(M)3/86 test
Commissioner's decision, R(M)3/86, establishes that there are two parts to the 'virtually unable to walk' test. The first part is to look at all the facts of a particular case in the light of reg 12(1)(a)(ii) – quoted in 22. The adjudicator must consider separately the distance, the speed, the length of time, and the manner in which you can make progress on foot. Any walking which is possible only while suffering severe discomfort must be discounted.

If the adjudicator finds you 'virtually unable to walk', they must then decide whether that condition is attributable to some physical impairment such as brain damage, or, *'physical disability which prevents the co-ordination of mind and body'*.

What can you do?
❑ Provide evidence (from the GP, consultant etc) to show that:
■ the learning disabilities have a physical cause, such as brain damage;
■ all the behavioural problems which interrupt outdoor walking stem directly from that physical cause.
❑ If you wish, you can also provide evidence (from the GP etc) to show that it is not appropriate to talk of the person as being able to exercise deliberate and self-conscious choices in the sense of making a 'deliberate election' to walk or not to walk. The key thing is to get evidence to show that the interruptions in the ability to make progress on foot outdoors are simply 'reactions' to various stimuli. Those reactions are simply the result of the brain damage or the genetic damage which caused the learning disabilities and prevents or interferes with the normal co-ordination of mind and body.
❑ You need to be able to give the adjudicator a clear picture of the person's normal walking difficulties and the frequency of the interruptions in their ability to make independent

far from the nearest bus stop); your ability to use public transport; and the nature of your employment, are all ignored.
Reg 12(1)(a) DLA

Artificial aids – The first three disability tests for the higher rate take into account your walking abilities when using any suitable artificial aids or a prosthesis. If there is an artificial aid or prosthesis which is *'suitable in [your] case'*, and you wouldn't be unable or virtually unable to walk if you used it, you'll fail the test. A guide dog does not count as an 'artificial aid'. Nor do pain killers – but if you're taking the normal dosage of pain killers recommended by your doctor, it is your walking ability under that medication which will be taken into account. If you use crutches and can only swing through them rather than use them to walk, then you are unable to walk.
Reg 12(4) DLA

Terminal illness – Although you are treated as passing the qualifying period for mobility component, you must actually pass one of the disability tests in order to be paid mobility component from the time you claim it.

22. 'Virtually unable to walk'?

Regulation 12(l)(a)(ii) of the DLA Regulations spells out the factors to be taken into account in deciding whether you are *'virtually unable to walk'*. The factors are:
your *'ability to walk out of doors is so limited, as regards*
- the distance over which, or
- the speed at which, or
- the length of time for which, or
- the manner in which

[you] can make progress on foot without severe discomfort, that [you are] virtually unable to walk'.

Physical cause
The cause of your walking difficulties must be physical. If you are simply afraid of the idea of walking outdoors (and could walk if you overcame your fear) that fear cannot be taken into account as a physical cause of being virtually unable to walk.

Someone with a severe learning disability can meet this initial test if it is accepted that their disabilities (and any behavioural problems which interrupt their ability to make progress on foot) have a physical cause, if they are unable to meet the conditions outlined in 23 – see Box G.5.

Severe discomfort
If you start to suffer from 'severe discomfort' when walking outdoors, any extra distance that you can walk should be ignored.* For example, you may be capable of walking about 40 yards without too much pain or breathlessness, but this discomfort then begins to get worse and worse until eventually you are just forced to stop. By the time you stop you may well be in agony. The question is first: at what point do you start to suffer what can be called 'severe discomfort'? If it is at 60 yards, (or 70 yards), then any extra walking should be

---

progress on foot. The idea is to present an objective picture of how the person normally makes, or doesn't make, progress on foot outdoors using only artificial aids which are suitable for them, and without active help from another person.

Focus on walking difficulties
We suggest that you do this by trying to carry out a ten-minute outdoor walking test. Ask someone else for help to take notes if necessary. How far you take our suggestions is up to you. Don't go overboard. If you are in any doubt whether it is worth it, discuss your situation with an experienced adviser.

For each test:
❑ Describe the place where you carried out the test. Mark the starting point. Note the time.
❑ Let the person loose. Don't actively intervene to help them walk. A gentle hand on the shoulder or words to help them go in the right direction is OK (to help overcome any fear because they cannot see where they are going). But don't give any physical support or restraint which you wouldn't routinely expect to give to a non-disabled person of the same age (so you'll need to be sure that the test place you choose is a safe one).
❑ Describe exactly what happens. Did they move at all? If yes, then how do they walk, or run? What size steps; how do they lift their legs; speed of walking; changes in speed; in direction; what about balance; the effect of distractions? This all relates to the 'manner' in which a person walks, and the 'speed' at which a person walks.
❑ For each stop, or interruption in their walking: note the time; mark the place and measure the distance from the starting point (or from the previous stop).
❑ Describe exactly what happened. Why do you think they stopped? Note the time when they start to move on again. What made them move on? Or, why do you think they

moved on (give all your reasons)?
❑ At the end of the 10 minutes, mark the place they have reached. How far, in a straight line, is it from their starting point? If they didn't move in a straight line, also measure how far they walked or ran.

Note that if the person's walking ability is also limited by 'severe discomfort' do not continue with the test. As soon as they start to suffer what they, or you, consider to be severe discomfort, note the time and mark the place. Describe the 'severe discomfort' which made them stop. Are there any physical changes in their appearance from when they started walking? Any breathing problems? Any outward and visible signs of their discomfort?

Adapting the test
It is quite easy to adapt the 10 minute walking test for people who have a physical disability. But first check with your GP to make sure that it is safe for you.

Walk until you start to suffer 'severe discomfort', or for 10 minutes if that is longer. Besides the points mentioned above, you'll also be looking at all the other physical factors which affect your ability to make progress on foot outdoors.

The types of things you'll be looking at include the effects of: spasticity, tremor, rigidity, uncontrollable actions or reflexes, muscle spasms, 'freezing up', falls, fits, giddiness, vertigo, head spinning, severe pain, pressure sores, bad scarring, angina, asthma attack, coughing fit, breathlessness, and fatigue. Describe the what, where, when, how and why of each of the difficulties which affect your outdoor walking ability.

Don't go overboard with all this – the decision maker may just diagnose 'compensationitis'. But you should measure the exact distance you are normally able to walk without 'severe discomfort'. Put the exact distance in your DLA1 claim form and use the results of your test to help you fill in clear details about your walking difficulties.

discounted. The second question is whether or not the 60 (or 70) yards you are capable of walking *'without severe discomfort'* is *'so limited ... that [you are] virtually unable to walk'*.

'Severe discomfort' is something subjective – different people have different thresholds of pain; and will also show that pain in different ways. The Court of Appeal in *Cassinelli*** accepted that 'severe discomfort' does not mean 'severe pain or distress': *'discomfort is a lesser concomitant [of pain]'*. So 'severe discomfort' is less of a problem than 'severe pain', and is far from being 'excruciating agony' – which would cause the most stoic disabled person to stop walking.

The Commissioners (in R(M)1/83 have said that it includes 'pain' or 'breathlessness' – things that are brought on by the act of walking. But it does not include the screaming fits of an autistic child or other things which are the result of resistance to the very idea of walking.

* R(M) 1/81 and CM/267/93
** Cassinelli v Secretary of State for Social Services TLR 6.12.91. This overrules the opposite view taken in R(M)1/91.

Artificial aids
Unless both your legs are missing (see 20), when assessing your walking ability, the AO will take into account your abilities at walking with the help of any artificial aid, such as a calliper or orthopaedic shoes, or any prosthesis which you normally use or could use – see 21.

Distance, speed, time and manner
All four factors affect someone's ability to walk outdoors; and they will often be closely inter-related. There is no set walking distance which marks the difference between success and failure – if there were, there would be little point in the law requiring the decision-maker to look also at the speed, time and manner of walking. All of these factors must be considered – as well as the question of 'severe discomfort'.

If you need to appeal, it helps to do a 'time and motion' study on your outdoor walking ability, looking at these four points in turn. If you start to suffer from 'severe discomfort', put down what happens and when – see Box G.5 for more details. Note down how long it takes you to recover before you feel able to walk again without severe discomfort – this should also be taken into account (CDLA/805/94).

If an occupational therapist, or physiotherapist, has assessed you for equipment and adaptations to your home, or you have been getting therapy from one, you may find that s/he is willing to write a report on your outdoor walking ability – either for a Disability Appeal Tribunal (DAT), or when you first claim. You can ask her to fill in a statement at the end of your DLA1 claim form.

The easiest report to write is one where s/he just has to confirm that s/he has read your own 'time and motion' study and agrees that your results are consistent with his or her own view of the effects of your physical disabilities. It is useless to get a letter saying you 'need' mobility component. It gives no help in establishing the extent of your physical walking difficulties in terms of the legal criteria.

Intermittent walking ability
If your walking ability varies from day to day, you may have difficulty qualifying for mobility component. You must also be able to show that you are virtually unable to walk, have been so for the 3 months before your claim, and are likely to remain like that for at least six months after your claim.

It helps to keep an accurate diary. Even though you may be able to walk on some days this might not disqualify you. The question is whether or not the evidence about your walking abilities would allow an AO (or DAT) to consider that, looking at your physical condition as a whole, it would be true to say of you that you are virtually unable to walk and, had been so for the 3 months before your claim, and are likely to remain like that for at least 6 months after your claim.

23. Severe mental impairment
This way of qualifying for the higher rate mobility component is aimed at people with severe learning disabilities. If you don't pass this test, you may pass the 'virtual inability to walk' test. Box G.5 looks at how that test applies to people with learning disabilities. If you fail both tests, you are more than likely to pass the disability test for the lower rate – see 24.

To be entitled to higher rate mobility component on the basis of severe mental impairment, you must pass the following tests:
- you must be entitled to higher rate care component (even if it cannot be paid because you live in hospital or special accommodation);

S.73(3)(c) SSCBA

and
- you suffer from *'a state of arrested development or incomplete physical development of the brain, which results in severe impairment of intelligence and social functioning'*; and

---

G.6 For more information
In this chapter we refer to various legislation on DLA. Here we explain the abbreviations used in the chapter and suggest other sources of information.

The Acts
SSCBA = Social Security Contributions and Benefits Act 1992
SSAA = Social Security Administration Act 1992
S. or s. = section of an Act
ss. = subsection of an Act
Sch = schedule to an Act
para = paragraph in a schedule

The Regulations
DLA Regs = The Social Security (Disability Living Allowance) Regulations 1991
Intro = The Social Security (Introduction of Disability Living Allowance) Regulations 1991
C&P = The Social Security (Claims and Payments) Regulations 1987
Adj = The Social Security (Adjudication) Regulations 1995
reg = regulation

Case law
See Box O.6 in Chapter 52 for information about Commissioners' decisions.

Guidance
- *The Disability Handbook* – a handbook on the care needs and mobility requirements likely to arise from various disabilities and chronic illnesses, Benefits Agency, published by The Stationery Office Ltd.
- *Medical and Disability Appeal Tribunals: The Legislation*, commentary by Mark Rowland (Sweet & Maxwell).
- Action for Blind People produce a checklist, factsheets and helpful information, available from: Action for Blind People, 14-16 Verney Road, London, SE16 3DZ.
- Disability Alliance's advanced training notes on *DATs – Identifying Errors of Law* (1993).

- you *'exhibit disruptive behaviour'* which *'is extreme'*, and
- *'regularly requires another person to intervene and physically restrain [you] to prevent [you] causing physical injury to [yourself] or another, or damage to property'*, and
- *'is so unpredictable that [you require] another person to be present and watching over [you] whenever [you are] awake'*.

Reg 12(5), (6) DLA

The DSS will normally arrange for a specialist's opinion before awarding the higher rate on the basis of severe mental impairment.

'Arrested' development' means that the brain does not function properly, but there is no apparent physical deficiency. 'Incomplete physical development' means the brain has failed to grow properly and this can be seen physically. Arrested or incomplete development must take place before the brain is fully developed. In most cases this will be by the late twenties, and always before age 30. See CDLA/156/94.

This rules out anyone whose severe behavioural problems start later in life, eg because of a later head injury or a disease such as Alzheimer's. It also rules out those whose behavioural problems more than pass the test in the daytime, but who only get the middle rate care component because they sleep soundly and safely all night – if you are in this situation, see Box G.5.

If you think you satisfy each part of this disability test and are turned down at the first stage, or after a review, do get expert advice and help with an appeal to the Disability Appeal Tribunal – see Chapter 52.

24. The lower rate

To qualify for the lower rate mobility component, your mobility difficulties can be caused by mental disability as well as by physical disablement. It is aimed at people who can walk but cannot make real use of that ability when outdoors unless they have someone else on hand to guide them or to supervise them. People who are blind or have a learning disability are most likely to qualify. However, other conditions may also affect your ability to walk outdoors in an unfamiliar place without help: eg deafness if you haven't learned how to cope safely with traffic, or you need an interpreter to guide you if you get lost, confused or disorientated (CDLA/206/94). If you are under 16, see also 20.

If you need guidance or supervision whenever you walk outdoors, you'll pass the test for the new lower rate. For example, someone with epilepsy who passes the day supervision disability test for the care component, will almost certainly require supervision when walking outdoors just in case they have a fit. If you suffer from incontinence, you might qualify if you need supervision because of anxiety over having an attack while out of doors (CDLA/494/94).

In a case relating to a claim by a person with agoraphobia, CDLA/42/94 looks at what counts as 'guidance or supervision', eg monitoring your physical, mental or emotional state, looking out for obstacles, encouraging, persuading, distracting from alarming situations by conversation and reassurance.

Some people can manage to walk safely by themselves in areas they know well. However, this test ignores *'any ability [you] may have to use routes which are familiar to [you] on [your] own'*. The key question for this test is to consider what happens if, or when, you try to walk by yourself outdoors in an area you are not 'familiar' with, or do not know at all.

Can you *'take advantage of'* your ability to walk if you are in an unfamiliar area without another person to guide you or supervise you *'most of the time'*?

If you require supervision whenever you are outdoors, or in a strange place, you'll pass this test – even if you don't pass the day supervision test for the care component because you don't require *'continual'* supervision.

If visual impairment means you couldn't take advantage of your ability to walk in a strange area unless you had another person to guide you *'most of the time'*, you'll pass this test. Note that guidance also counts as 'attention' for the care component. If you have a guide dog, can you use the dog safely and effectively in an area unfamiliar to you or the dog, or would you also need another person to guide you 'most of the time'?

If you are awarded the lower rate, do double check to see if you might not pass one of the higher rate tests. Get advice and ask for a review, or appeal to a Disability Appeal Tribunal if necessary – see 27 below and Chapter 52.

E. CLAIMS, PAYMENTS & REVIEWS

25. How do you claim?

The claim pack

The claim for DLA is part of the DLA claim pack – the DLA1 (from April 1997 there is a special claim form for children, the DLA1 Child). This comes with two leaflets on DLA and two forms. The DLA1 claim form has two separate sections. Section 1 is the claim form. It asks for personal and general details for administrative purposes. In Section 1 you can tick a box if you would prefer to have a doctor visit you, rather than fill in Section 2. Section 2 is the 'self-assessment questionnaire' for the DLA disability tests. There is a page in Section 2 for your doctor, or another professional, to confirm your statements. Your doctor will not charge you for completing this page. There is also currently an extra part to fill in which goes along with Section 2. This is to take account of recent developments in case law – see 13 above.

Don't be put off by the length of the DLA1! There is a lot of space for your answers if you write on both the white and cream coloured parts of the pages. The questions themselves are pretty straightforward – some of them only need a tick for an answer. But it is important to give as much information as you can and not to underestimate the help you need. Think about the things you can't do or have trouble with, rather than the things you can do. If you don't fill in the form fully, or your answers don't give a clear picture of the effects of your disabilities, the DSS may ask a visiting officer to go through the form with you, or they may get a factual report from your GP, or ask a doctor to examine you.

Getting help – Anyone can help you fill in the DLA1 – but try and give accurate answers, rather than guesses. Although many people will get DLA just by ticking the boxes in the form and without writing much more about their care needs or mobility difficulties, adding extra details may be important. Where the form asks how long something takes, don't make a wild guess – time it. Where it asks how far you can walk, measure the distance – most people find it difficult to estimate distances with any accuracy. Whenever you tick a 'no help needed' box, think about whether you should add a note to explain what you mean. For example, if you don't use a commode, you will probably tick the 'no help' box. If you couldn't cope with using a commode without help, you can tick one of the other boxes. Or you can put down why a commode isn't a simple solution to your need to have help when you go to the toilet.

If you would like help from the DSS, you can make a free phone call to the Benefit Enquiry Line (BEL) on 0800 882200. BEL can answer any queries about the questions in the DLA1 – using Minicom if you are deaf, or by sending you the forms in braille or large print, if you are visually impaired. You can also ask BEL for the Forms Completion Service – on 0800 441144. Someone in your Disability Benefits Centre can complete the forms for you over the phone and then send them to you for checking, signing and returning. If necessary, they may arrange for a visiting officer to help you complete the forms.

Starting your claim
The best way to start your claim is to ask the DSS for the DLA claim pack – form DLA1. If you're claiming for a child under 16, ask for the special claim pack for children (DLA1 Child) available from April 1997. You can do this by phoning or calling in at any DSS office. Or you can make a free phone call to the Benefit Enquiry Line on 0800 882200. Or you can use the postage-paid coupon in the DLA information leaflet DS704.

If you cannot make the claim yourself, someone else can do it for you. If they sign the form for you, there is space for them to explain why, eg you are too ill to sign.

If you get the claim pack from the DSS, any DLA can be backdated to the date you asked for the pack – see below. Although Citizens Advice Bureaux (CABx) and some other advice agencies can give you the DLA claim pack, this method has a catch. If you use a claim pack given to you by a CAB etc, any DLA can only be backdated to the date your completed claim pack reaches the DSS – see below.

Renewal claims – If you have been awarded either DLA component for a fixed period, the Disability Benefits Unit will write to you before the award ends to invite you to reapply for the fixed period component(s).

Your 'date of claim'
If you write to the DSS, or send in the DS704 coupon, DLA can be backdated to the date your letter or coupon reached the DSS. If you phone or visit a DSS office, DLA can be backdated to the date of your call.

A DLA claim pack issued by the DSS is date stamped with the date you asked for the pack and the date, 6 weeks later, by which you should return the completed pack. The DSS will also give you a postage paid envelope addressed to the Disability Benefits Centre which will be handling your initial claim.

So long as you return the completed claim pack within 6 weeks, the date you asked for the pack counts as your 'date of claim'. If you take longer than 6 weeks to return the completed claim pack, explain why at the end of Section 2 of the claim pack. If your delay is reasonable, the Secretary of State can extend the time limit. If not, your date of claim is the day your completed pack reaches the DSS. If the DSS have failed to record the date you asked for a claim pack, your date of claim will be treated as being 6 weeks before your completed claim is received by the DSS.

Advice agencies – If you claim on a DLA1(A) given to you by a CAB or other advice agency, your 'date of claim' is the day your completed pack reaches the DSS. If you just return Section 1 of the DLA1(A), any DLA can be backdated to the day that section reaches the DSS – so long as you return your completed Section 2 within a month. Tick the box provided in Section 1 to show you're doing this – otherwise, the DSS will start other follow-up action unnecessarily. Remember to keep a note of the address on the envelope supplied with the claim pack.

Don't delay – As DLA can only start to be paid from the first payday on or after your date of claim, you might lose a week or more of benefit if you delay. The DLA payday is normally a Wednesday. If you ask for the claim pack on a Wednesday, you can be paid from your date of claim. If you ask for it on a Thursday, payment cannot start until the next Wednesday. The safest way to avoid these problems is to start off your claim with a free phone call to the Benefit Enquiry Line (BEL) on 0800 882200.

Backdating
DLA cannot be backdated to earlier than your 'date of claim'.
There are only limited situations in which DLA can be backdated:
- if industrial action has caused postal disruption, the day your claim would have been delivered to a DSS office is treated as your 'date of claim';
- if the Secretary of State uses his discretion to treat anything written as being sufficient in the circumstances to count as a valid claim, the date of that earlier document is treated as your 'date of claim' – see Chapter 52(1);
- if you make a renewal claim within 6 months of the end of your previous award of DLA, the component you had previously can be fully backdated. However this provision to link renewal claims will be removed from 1.9.97 – you should make sure you return your renewal claim before your current award expires otherwise you will lose benefit.

26. Who decides your claim?
Claims for DLA and attendance allowance are handled first of all by one of the regional Disability Benefits Centres. Decisions are made by Adjudication Officers (AOs), not by doctors.

To help the AOs make decisions, the DSS, together with the DLA Advisory Board, produced a guide called the *Disability Handbook*. This outlines the main care and mobility needs which are likely to arise in a number of different illnesses and disabling conditions. If your situation doesn't fit neatly within the picture painted by the *Disability Handbook* or if the Handbook emphasises the need for medical evidence, the AO may ask your own doctor, or an independent doctor, for a report. If you are claiming the higher rate of mobility component, the AO will ask for more information either from your doctor, or from a medical examination. They can also call upon advice from doctors working for the Benefits Agency Medical Services and upon the DLA Advisory Board.

Delays
From the day your DLA claim is received by the DSS, they aim to give you a decision within 53 working days (ie not including weekends or public holidays). If you are claiming under the 'Special Rules' (see Box G.4) you should get a decision within 10 working days. If you have to wait more than 7 months for payment of your benefit (or 2 months for a Special Rules claim) compensation may be payable. For renewal or current claims, compensation becomes payable if your benefit payments are interrupted for 3 months. See Chapter 52(6) for details of compensation schemes.

In any case, if your claim is taking too long, complain to the Customer Services Manager at the Disability Benefits Centre dealing with your claim.

27. What happens after you claim?

Initial claim
After the Adjudication Officer (AO) makes the decision on your initial claim, you'll be sent a short notification of that decision.

Length of your award – Your DLA award could be for life, or for a fixed period. You can have one component for life and one for a fixed period. If both components are for a fixed period, these will be set to end on the same day. The minimum length of award is 6 months.

From 27.12.93, separate awards of the care and mobility components were combined into a single DLA award consisting of two components. But if you had two separate fixed period awards set to end on different days, these would continue being separate awards until either one or both awards are given for life, or, on review or renewal, both are set to end on the same day. The intention is that combining the two awards of DLA into one award of both components should not jeopardise or cut short the longer award.

If you are not happy with the AO's decision on your claim – You have the right to ask for a review within 3 months of the date that decision was sent to you. Write to the Disability Benefits Centre which handled your claim. You can ask for a review for any reason at all – the length of the award, the rate of the award, the starting date for the award etc. This is called an 'any grounds' review. If the decision was over 3 months ago, you can ask for an 'any time' review but only if certain grounds are satisfied, eg your condition has become worse. You can only get to the appeal stage once you have had a decision from an 'any grounds' review. Normally benefit can only be backdated for one month from the date you ask for the review, so if you're not happy with a decision you should act quickly.

Warning – When you ask for a review, the AO may have power to review the whole of your DLA award. If you are happy with the decision on one of the two DLA components, say so in your review letter. If you already have one component and are making a 'top up' claim for the other component, your claim counts as a request for a review.

If you are happy with the decision on one component of the DLA, the AO 'need not' review the decision on that component. If you have been awarded that component for life, the AO can only review it if you specifically ask for it to be reviewed, or if the AO has information *'which gives [her] reasonable grounds for believing'* that the life award, or its rate *'ought not to continue'*. However, a change in the law is expected soon which will specifically permit the Secretary of State to supply information to the AO reviewing the life award.
S.32(2)–(4) SSAA for AOs; S.33(4)–(6) SSAA for tribunals

Any grounds reviews

If you ask for a review within 3 months of the decision on your DLA claim, the 'any grounds' review will be carried out by a different AO.

To help with the review, the DSS may call for more information, eg a factual report, or a medical examination, but they won't do this in all cases. They see the review procedure as giving a snappy second look at the initial decision on your claim. If some aspects of your claim are not clear, they are more likely to arrange for a short factual report (perhaps from your own doctor) which concentrates on just those aspects.

If you are unhappy with the reviewing AO's decision, you have the right to appeal to an independent tribunal within 3 months of the date the 'any grounds' review decision was sent to you. If your appeal is only about a non-disability question, it will be heard by a Social Security Appeal Tribunal. If your appeal is about a disability question, or about a mixture of the two, it will be heard by a Disability Appeal Tribunal – see Chapter 52 for more details.

Any time reviews

You can ask for a review at any time at all if you have certain specific reasons, eg:

- the original decision was made in ignorance of, or was based on a mistake about, a material fact; or
- an AO (not a tribunal or Commissioner) made an error of law in the decision; or
- there has been a change in your circumstances since the original decision was made.

If you are terminally ill, see Box G.4. For more about reviews in general, see Chapter 52.

If you are asking for an 'any time' review, write to the central Disability Benefits Unit. You need to show how you meet one of the grounds for review. For example, a change of circumstances might be that your condition has worsened and you now qualify for a higher rate of DLA or for another component. Or perhaps in your claim form you missed out details of your condition, or how it affects your need for care or your mobility, which might have made a difference to the Adjudication Officer's decision had they known. An AO at the Unit will make a decision on your review. If you are not happy with the result of the 'any time' review, you have the right to ask for an 'any grounds' review within 3 months. You cannot appeal directly to a tribunal from an 'any time' review. Once you have had a decision on an 'any grounds' review, you can appeal to an independent tribunal within 3 months of the date the decision on review was sent to you.

If the AO refuses to carry out an 'any time' review, you can ask for an 'any grounds' review of that AO's decision (not of the original decision). If the 'any grounds' AO confirms the 'any time' AO's decision (in effect refusing to review the decision at all), you have the right to appeal against that decision within 3 months. See Chapter 52.

The AO may carry out a review even though you have not requested one (technically on request from the Secretary of State). Usually this will be an 'anytime' review. You can ask for an 'any grounds' review of that decision, and can then appeal if you still disagree. A change in the law is expected soon which will specifically allow the Secretary of State to *'undertake investigations to obtain information and evidence'* for such a review.

Backdating

Arrears from an 'any grounds' or 'any time' review can only be backdated for one month. If your situation changes, a review on the grounds of a change of circumstances obviously cannot be backdated to earlier than the date of the change which made you entitled to benefit, or to a higher rate. If you haven't served the qualifying period for that rate on an earlier linked award, benefit can only be backdated to the end of the qualifying period (see 5) – subject to the overall one month limit on backdating. There are certain circumstances in which benefit can be fully backdated – see Chapter 52(10)(e).

The rules on backdating on review were more generous before the law changed on 7.4.97. If you requested a review before 7.4.97, the old rules still apply: arrears from an 'any grounds' review can be backdated to the date of claim; arrears from an 'any time' review can be backdated for up to 52 weeks if you have good cause for your delay, or 3 months if you don't.

When can you see your case papers?

You can ask for copies of your case papers at any stage. You aren't told you can ask for your case papers until you get the final decision on your 'any grounds' review. If you don't ask for your case papers, they won't be sent to you unless you appeal to a tribunal – and when you see them depends on when the Independent Tribunal Service sends them to you.

If you haven't kept a copy of your DLA claim form, or

haven't seen any of the other evidence used in your case, you may have missed some obvious mistakes or gaps in the evidence. Get evidence to correct those mistakes or plug the gaps and you can write a very clear initial review letter.

If you are happy with the decision on one component, you may risk that component by asking for the other component, or for a review or an appeal. In this situation, it is sensible to ask for a copy of your case papers on the basis that you need to be sure that award is 'safe' before you take action. The risk of losing what you already have is small, and the success rate on DLA reviews has been good (44%). An experienced adviser may be able to reassure you after looking through the case papers.

28. How are you paid?
DLA is usually paid once every 4 weeks. If you wish, it can be paid direct into your bank or building society account. If not, you'll usually be sent an order book which you can cash every fourth week, three weeks in arrears, one week in advance. Over the next 3 years, order books are due to be replaced by benefit payment cards which you take to the post office to collect your benefit.

Paydays – The normal payday for DLA is a Wednesday. However, if you switched to DLA from attendance allowance, you may keep your old payday (usually a Monday). The DSS will write to you to let you know if they are going to change your payday. If the DSS change your payday, they will pay you for the part of the week to bring you up to your new payday.

Weekly payments – If you are terminally ill, DLA is payable once a week. For other people, weekly payments are only possible if your DLA is paid in a combined weekly order book with another benefit, such as income support; or where you previously had attendance allowance and want to continue to have weekly payments.

Appointees – If you are unable to manage your own affairs, the DSS can appoint another person to act on your behalf – see Chapter 52(5). But DLA is your benefit, not your appointee's benefit. If you are under 16, the appointee is usually your mother. If you don't want to have someone else formally appointed to act for you, but cannot cash DLA yourself, you can arrange for them to cash your DLA orders.

29. What if your condition changes?

If your condition gets worse
If you already have DLA, you just ask for a review – see 27. A 'top up' claim for the component you don't already have counts as a review.

If you don't get DLA, or have been refused it in the past, just make another claim.

If your condition improves
If there is an improvement in your care needs or mobility difficulties, this could mean your rate of DLA should drop. Write to the Disability Benefits Unit to give them details. The AO will usually review your entitlement.

If your rate of DLA drops (or it ends), but you have a relapse within 2 years, you can regain your former rate of benefit. You don't have to re-serve the qualifying period for that rate.

If you are now over 65, do note that if your DLA ends altogether, you can only regain it if you make a renewal claim within 12 months of the end of your previous award. You don't have to re-serve the qualifying period for your former rate of DLA – see 4 and 5. If you leave it longer than 12 months you will have to claim attendance allowance.

18 Attendance allowance

1. What is attendance allowance?
Attendance allowance is a tax-free benefit for people over 65 who are severely disabled, physically or mentally, and who need help with personal care or need supervision. You do not actually have to be getting any help; what matters is the help you need. You can get attendance allowance even if you live alone – you do not need to have a carer. It is not means-tested and there are no National Insurance contribution tests.

In this chapter we just give an outline of attendance allowance. This is because the rules are almost exactly the same as disability living allowance (DLA) care component at the middle or higher rate. Chapter 17 deals fully with DLA. Below (see 7) we give the key differences from DLA and list the parts of Chapter 17 which are also relevant to attendance allowance.

2. Do you qualify?
You must meet the following conditions:
- you are aged 65 or over – see below; and
- you pass the residence and presence test – see Chapter 17(6); and
- you satisfy one of the 'disability tests' and have done so for the last six months – see below; or
- you are terminally ill – see Box G.4 in Chapter 17.

If your care needs started when you were under 65 and you are still under 66, you should claim DLA instead, but only if you are claiming before 6.10.97. If you claim on or after 6.10.97, you can only make a first claim for DLA up to the day before your 65th birthday. See 7 below.

The disability tests
To pass the disability tests, you must meet at least one of these four conditions.
You must be *'so severely disabled physically or mentally that . . . [you require] from another person'*
DURING THE DAY
- *'frequent attention throughout the day in connection with [your] bodily functions,* or
- *continual supervision throughout the day in order to avoid substantial danger to [yourself] or others'* or

DURING THE NIGHT
- *'[you require] from another person prolonged or repeated attention in connection with [your] bodily functions,* or
- *in order to avoid substantial danger to [yourself] or others [you require] another person to be awake for a prolonged period or at frequent intervals for the purpose of watching over [you]'*.

These disability tests are explained in detail in Chapter 17(11) to (18).

Lower or higher rate
The higher rate of £49.50 is for people who need help both day and night. So if you meet one of the day conditions and one of the night conditions, you will qualify for the higher rate allowance. If you meet either one of the day conditions or one of the night conditions, you will get the lower rate of £33.10.

Kidney patients
There are special rules for some kidney patients to help them qualify for attendance allowance at the lower rate – see Chapter 17(19).

Six month qualifying period

New claim – You must have been in need of care for six months before your award can begin. You can claim before the six months are up. It does not matter if these six months fall at a time when you could not receive attendance allowance in any case – say if you were in hospital. The six month qualifying period applies to both the lower and higher rates.

Terminal illness – If you are claiming under the terminal illness provisions, you can be paid from the date the AO accepts that you satisfy the legal test of terminal illness – see Box G.4. Payment will usually start from the Monday on or after the day your claim is received in a DSS office. You do not have to serve the six month qualifying period, or pass the 26 week presence test, if you count as terminally ill.

Current award – If you already have lower rate attendance allowance, you can qualify for the higher rate allowance after you have needed the greater level of attention or supervision for six months. Once again, you can ask for a review of your award before the six months are up.

Linked claim – If you previously received attendance allowance (or dropped to the lower rate) and have a relapse no more than 2 years after the end of your previous award, you don't have to re-serve the six month qualifying period to regain your former (or the lower) rate of benefit from the pay day on or after your linked claim reaches the DSS. For example, on your previous claim you received higher rate attendance allowance. This was reduced to the lower rate because your condition improved. You have a relapse within 2 years and ask for a review to get the higher rate. Your higher rate can be backdated for one month.

3. How much do you get?

Higher rate	£49.50
Lower rate	£33.10

4. Does anything affect what you get?

Attendance allowance can be paid in full in addition to almost any other benefit, such as retirement pension, income support and severe disablement allowance.

It is ignored as income for means-tested benefits, so does not reduce the amount of income support, housing benefit or council tax benefit. However, if you are in residential care and have 'preserved rights', attendance allowance is taken into account for income support – see Chapter 38. It may also be taken into account in the means test for charging for local authority services – see Chapter 32(6).

You cannot get attendance allowance if you are entitled to DLA. If you get constant attendance allowance with industrial disablement or war pension, this overlaps with attendance allowance and you'll be paid whichever is higher.

Check your benefits – Getting attendance allowance can trigger extra help with means-tested benefits. You might qualify for a higher pensioner premium or severe disability premium with your income support, housing benefit or council tax benefit. And if you have not been able to get these benefits before because your income was over the limit, you might qualify now. Contact your local DSS office and your local authority to make sure they know you are getting attendance allowance. See Box G.1 in Chapter 17 for other help available.

Hospital and other special accommodation – If you go into hospital or some types of residential care, your attendance allowance stops after 4 weeks – see Chapter 17(9) and (10) and Chapter 36(2).

5. How do you claim?

You can phone the Benefit Enquiry Line on 0800 882200 and ask for the attendance allowance claim pack (DS2). Your date of claim will usually be the day you phone (see Chapter 17(25)). They can also answer any queries you might have. Otherwise, if you write to the DSS, or use the coupon with the attendance allowance leaflet, your date of claim will usually be the day your letter or coupon reaches the DSS. You can also get a claim pack from a Citizens Advice Bureau or other advice centre, but, in this case, your date of claim is the date you get the completed form back to the DSS.

If you want help to fill in the form, you can phone the Forms Completion Service on 0800 441144. A DSS adviser will go through the questions with you and complete a form on your behalf. This form will be posted to you so you can check it and sign it.

Backdating

Attendance allowance cannot be backdated to earlier than the Monday payday on or after your date of claim. In some limited circumstances an earlier date can be treated as your date of claim – see Chapter 17(25).

Medical examination

Usually you will not see a DSS doctor at all. Section 2 of the claim pack is a lengthy self-assessment questionnaire, and includes a form for your own doctor or another professional involved in your care to complete. This may well give the Adjudication Officer enough information to make a decision. If not, the DSS may arrange for a short report from your doctor, or another medical person you've named on the form. If you would prefer to have a medical examination instead of filling in the questionnaire, there is a box to tick in Section 1 of the claim pack.

Length of award

Attendance allowance may be awarded for life or for a fixed period. If your award is for a fixed period, the Disability Benefits Unit will invite you to make a renewal claim about 4 months before the end of your current award.

How are you paid?

Attendance allowance is paid to you, not to a carer, and you can spend it how you please. It is usually payable on a Monday. You can choose to have it paid by a weekly order book to cash at the post office, or it can be paid direct into a bank or building society every four weeks in arrears. If you prefer an order book, it can be combined with certain other benefits such as income support and retirement pension. Over the next 3 years order books will be phased out and replaced by new benefit payment cards which you take to the post office to collect your benefit.

6. Reviews and appeals

If you are claiming attendance allowance for the first time, or after a break, an Adjudication Officer (AO) based at one of the regional Disability Benefits Centres will make the initial decision on every aspect of your claim. If you are making a renewal claim, an AO based at the central Disability Benefits Unit in Blackpool makes the initial decision on your claim.

If you are asking for a review within 3 months of the decision on your claim, a different AO based at the regional Disability Benefits Centre will deal with it. For later reviews, the central Disability Benefits Unit makes the review decision. The decision letter should make it clear who you should write to.

If you make a renewal claim, or have a review of the decision on your award, all the law and case law current at that time will be applied to the facts about your situation.

You have the right to ask for a review, for any reason at all, within 3 months of the day the DSS post you a notice of the AO's decision on your claim or renewal claim. This is referred to as an 'any grounds' review. A different AO will consider your claim completely afresh. S/he can confirm the initial decision, or increase or reduce the rate of your award, or the length of your award. In practice, the risk of losing what you have already been awarded is small – an experienced adviser can help you assess this risk in your particular situation.

If you ask for a review over 3 months after you received the initial decision on your current award, you must give reasons for your request. The DSS can also pass your case papers to the AO for a review. Chapter 17(27) explains the basis on which the AO can carry out an 'any time' review. For example, a change of circumstances such as an increase or decrease in your care needs, enables a review. So if your care needs improve, or you no longer need as much help from other people as before, you should write to the Unit.

If you are unhappy with the result of an 'any time' review, your next step is to ask for a further 'any grounds' review by an AO within 3 months. After that further review, you can appeal to the Disability Appeal Tribunal. You can't go straight to the Disability Appeal Tribunal after an 'any time review'.

Once an AO has made an 'any grounds' review decision, or has refused to review a decision, you have the right to appeal to an independent tribunal. In most cases, your appeal will involve the 'disability' tests, so it will be sent to the Disability Appeal Tribunal. If your appeal only concerns a non-disability matter, such as whether or not you are in special accommodation, it will be sent to the Social Security Appeal Tribunal.

Chapter 52 covers the general rules about claims, reviews and appeals. Chapter 17(25) to (27) and (29) look at these rules in the context of DLA. The basic rules are the same as for attendance allowance.

7. DLA or attendance allowance?

Until 5.10.97, if your care needs first started when you were under 65, you can claim the DLA care component (rather than attendance allowance) up to the day before your 66th birthday. You do not have to have served the DLA qualifying period before reaching 65. It is enough if on the day before your 65th birthday:
- you passed the residence and presence tests – see Chapter 17(6); and
- that day was the first day on which you satisfied any one of the disability tests in Chapter 17(11).

DLA care component would become payable once you had served the 'under-65' qualifying period of 3 months: ie when you were a day short of being aged 65 and 3 months.

From 6.10.97 the rules are changing, so that you can no longer claim DLA for the first time after you reach your 65th birthday. Once you reach the age of 65, you will have to claim attendance allowance.

If you already get DLA mobility component, you can claim DLA care component (at the middle or higher rate) rather than attendance allowance, even if you are aged, say 70. Because this type of claim is a review of your DLA award, it can be backdated for up to one month – see Chapter 52(10).

What are the differences?
Disability living allowance (DLA) began on 6.4.92. It was formed by taking the lower and higher rates of attendance allowance and turning them into the middle and higher rates of the new DLA care component, and adding on mobility allowance as the higher rate of the new DLA mobility component.

Each DLA component has a new lower rate which is not available for people who first started to qualify for that lower rate when they were already 65. Indeed, DLA itself is not available to people who first started to qualify for either component, at any rate, when they were aged 65 or older.

The DLA care component, apart from its £13.15 lower rate which has no equivalent in attendance allowance, is almost exactly the same as attendance allowance. The disability tests for the lower and higher rate of attendance allowance and for the middle and higher rate of DLA care component are exactly the same – as is the benefit payable. So Chapter 17 which gives full details of DLA is also relevant to attendance allowance. The relevant parts are Chapter 17(2), (4) to (6), (8) to (10), (11) – but only the No. 1, No. 2, No. 3 and No. 4 disability tests apply to attendance allowance – (13) to (19), (25) to (27), (29) and Box G.2, Box G.3 and Box G.4.

The main differences between attendance allowance and DLA care component are:
- attendance allowance has no £13.15 lower rate for part-time care needs;
- attendance allowance has a backwards qualifying period of 6 months in all cases;
- attendance allowance has no forwards qualifying period.

For someone already on DLA whose care needs start to change when they are aged 65 or older, the DLA rules for the care component are for all practical purposes the same as for attendance allowance. The qualifying period for changing from the lower rate up to the middle rate, or up to the higher rate, or for making a renewal claim, switches from 3 to 6 months. Although someone with a 'pre-65' lower rate care component can stay on the lower rate after reaching 65, and make renewal claims (including renewal claims made after a break in entitlement to the lower rate of up to a year), and move up to the middle or higher rate after a review, no-one getting the DLA care component can drop down to the lower rate from the middle or higher rate.

19 Invalid care allowance

1. What is invalid care allowance?

Invalid care allowance (ICA) is a benefit for people under 65 who regularly spend at least 35 hours a week caring for a severely disabled person. You don't have to be related to, or live with, the disabled person. You can get ICA even if you've never worked. You can get ICA even if you also get attendance allowance (AA) or disability living allowance (DLA) – but you must be caring for another person who gets AA or DLA care component at the middle or higher rate.

If you are paid ICA, or have claimed ICA on or after 1.10.90 and would have been paid it but for the fact that it overlaps with another benefit (eg incapacity benefit), a £13.35 carer premium will be included in the assessment of your applicable amount for income support, income-based jobseeker's allowance (JSA), housing benefit and/or council tax benefit – see Chapter 3(16). If you are actually paid ICA, the person you are caring for is excluded from the severe disability premium – see Chapter 3(13).

Invalid care allowance is not means-tested and does not depend on contributions; but it is taxable. ICA gives you Class 1 contribution credits – see Chapter 9.

2. Do you qualify?

- You must be spending at least 35 hours a week caring for a person who receives either:
  - DLA care component (at the middle or higher rate); or
  - attendance allowance (at either rate); or
  - constant attendance allowance (of £40.50 or more) paid with a war or industrial disablement pension, workmen's compensation or equivalent benefit.

If you are caring for more than one person, you can't add together the time you spend caring for each of them. You have to show that at least 35 hours are spent caring for one person.

If you meet the 35 hours test during part of the year (eg in school holidays and at weekends) you may qualify for ICA during that period. An ICA week runs from Sunday through to the following Saturday – so you would usually need the hours of caring from two consecutive weekends to pass the 35 hours test. On the day you collect or return the disabled person, you can also count the time you spend on any activity directly related to their presence with you over the weekend – see CG/12/91 and CG/6/90.

- You must be aged between 16 and 65 at the time of your claim (if you are 65 or over, see Chapter 43(4)).
- You must be living in the UK.
- If you have any restriction on your right to reside in the UK, you are not entitled unless you or a member of your family is an EEA national (see Chapter 41), or lawfully working and a national of Algeria, Morocco, Slovenia or Tunisia, or you have refugee status or exceptional leave to remain. If your ICA entitlement goes back to before 5.2.96, this test does not apply unless your ICA is reviewed.
- You must not be in full-time education. You are treated as being in full-time education if you attend a course for 21 hours or more a week. The 21 hours includes supervised study but does not include meal breaks or unsupervised study.
- If you work, you must not earn more than £50 a week once allowable expenses are deducted – see 5.

G.7 Caring away from your home

Seek legal advice
If you have to leave your own home in order to care for a disabled or elderly relative or friend, you must try and seek advice before you go. You may be able to get free legal advice under the Green Form scheme (see Chapter 53); otherwise a Citizens Advice Bureau or housing aid centre is the best starting point – you need a mix of benefits and legal advice. The consequences of not seeking effective advice can be distressing.

Housing benefit and council tax
You need advice about the effect of your absence from home on your right to housing benefit in respect of your own home. Your housing benefit position is outlined in Chapter 4(6). You remain liable for the housing costs for your own home, even though a continuous absence of 13 weeks may remove entitlement to housing benefit and income support (or jobseeker's allowance) housing costs. However, benefit may be paid for up to 52 weeks if the care you provide is 'medically approved'. So if you think your absence might be for longer than 13 weeks, you should get a letter from the doctor, or another professional involved in the care of the disabled person (eg a district nurse), to acknowledge that your care is 'approved'. Regular trips back to your own home (perhaps with the disabled person) may maintain enough presence to enable you to continue to get housing benefit beyond the limits. Keep a note of all trips back to your own home.

You also need to check your council tax liability. If there is no-one living in your home because you are living elsewhere in order to care for someone, your former home is exempt from council tax if your absence is permanent, or if you have already been away for a long time, say over 6 months. An absence can be permanent from the outset, for example if you intend to care for the disabled person in their own home until they die. It all depends on your intentions and on your situation. If your absence is only temporary, and your former home is unoccupied, you can get a 50% discount on that home. Council tax benefit may stop after an absence of 13 weeks (or 52 weeks if you provide 'medically approved' care) – see above.

If the disabled person's home is now your sole or main residence, you may be liable for council tax there. However, as long as the person you are caring for is not your child under 18 or your partner, if s/he gets higher rate attendance allowance, higher rate DLA care component, or the equivalent from the war or industrial injuries schemes, and you spend at least 35 hours a week caring for them, you get a status discount. This just means that the council tax for the home will be the same as if you were not resident there. See Chapter 5 for more details.

Security
You need advice about the best way to ensure your security in the disabled person's home, both in terms of housing tenure and the practicalities of running the home, given the following events:
- if the disabled person's mental competence deteriorates so that s/he can no longer act for herself (an enduring power of attorney [continuing power of attorney in Scotland] covers this problem);
- if the disabled person has to go temporarily, or permanently, into hospital or residential accommodation;
- if the disabled person dies.

You also need advice if you have to let your own home. If you have to sell your home, you need to be sure of your housing prospects if, or when, the disabled person dies, or goes permanently into a residential home. Does anyone else have a legal interest in the disabled person's home? Could the capital value of the disabled person's home affect the amount they would have to pay for a residential or nursing home?

Do not make assumptions about your housing rights. It is best to have an express agreement, ideally in writing; and ideally after expert legal advice on the effect of that agreement. You can, for example, have a licence to occupy the disabled person's home for the length of your life rather than his or her life: but if such an agreement is not express, and in writing, you are likely to find great difficulty in proving it. Even so, if the agreement is challenged, it will be up to the courts to decide on the true nature of the agreement. These are troubled waters, so do seek legal advice.

Even if you think that your situation will only be temporary, it is still sensible to seek advice. Things may change. At that time, it may no longer be possible to obtain the right sort of agreement, or to put your past agreement in writing. There is also the point that the physical and mental efforts involved in caring can make it very difficult to deal with other types of crises.

The disabled person will also need legal advice on these points. Your interests will not always be the same.

❑ If another person is getting ICA to look after the same disabled person, you cannot also get ICA to look after that person. But you can get Home Responsibilities Protection. You can decide which one of you should claim ICA. You can only get one award of ICA even if you care for more than one person.

3. How much do you get?
You get each week:
- **for yourself** £37.35
- **for an adult dependant** £22.35
- **for the first child** £9.90
  (plus child benefit of £11.05)
- **for each other child** £11.20
  (plus child benefit of £9.00)

4. How do you claim?
Claim on form DS 700. You can get this, and a free stamped envelope from a DSS office. Send your claim to the *Invalid Care Allowance Unit, Palatine House, Lancaster Road, Preston, PR1 1NS*. It is important to submit your claim form even if the disabled person is waiting to hear whether they have been awarded DLA or AA.

Backdating
If you were entitled to ICA before you actually claimed, and can show that you met all the qualifying conditions, ICA will be backdated for up to 3 months.

If the person you care for has claimed DLA or AA but is still waiting for the decision, don't delay making your ICA claim. Your ICA claim will be refused if there is no decision on the DLA or AA claim. But if you then make another ICA claim within 3 months of the DLA or AA decision, your ICA is backdated to the date of your original claim, or to the date of the DLA or AA award if that is later.

Before 7.4.97, the rules on backdating ICA claims were more generous. If you claimed before 7.4.97, your ICA would be backdated for 12 months so long as you met all the qualifying conditions in the earlier period.

What happens next?
You will be sent a written decision on your claim. If you are not satisfied with the decision you can appeal to a Social Security Appeal Tribunal – see Chapter 52.

You will be paid on an order book which you can cash at a post office. Over the next 3 years, order books will be phased out and replaced by new benefit payment cards.

5. How do earnings affect ICA?
You cannot get ICA if your net earnings are more than £50 a week (ie after deducting tax, NI contributions and half of any contribution towards an occupational or personal pension) and after any other allowable deductions. See Chapter 11(4), (look under 'Calculating earnings') – the rules are the same as those for incapacity benefit dependants' additions, except that for ICA there is a more generous disregard for care costs. If you pay someone other than a 'close relative', to look after the disabled person you care for, or to look after your child aged under 16, the payments are disregarded up to a maximum of half your net earnings. A 'close relative' is the parent, son, daughter, brother sister or partner of either yourself or the disabled person you care for.

If your partner earns more than £22.35, the increase for him or her will not be paid. If s/he earns £135 or more in any week, you will lose an addition for one child in the next week. For each extra £17 earned you lose another child addition.

Occupational and personal pensions count as earnings for adult and child dependant additions, but not for the basic invalid care allowance.

If you get a means-tested benefit, note that although earnings over £50 a week may not stop that benefit, they will stop your entitlement to ICA.

6. How do other benefits affect ICA?
You cannot be paid ICA while you are receiving the same amount or more from the following benefits:
- severe disablement allowance
- incapacity benefit
- contribution-based JSA
- state training allowance
- unemployability supplement
- retirement pension
- widows' benefits

But you can get ICA as well as DLA or attendance allowance. The addition for an adult dependant won't be paid if s/he gets personal benefits (other than attendance allowance or DLA) of £22.35 or more. Note that if the person you look after gets the severe disability premium, or an increase to their own benefit for you, both will stop once you get ICA. But if you cannot be paid ICA because of the overlapping benefit rules, the person you care for won't lose the severe disability premium.

7. ICA and income support
If you get ICA, you may be eligible for income support (IS) – see Box B.1 in Chapter 3. Income support is means tested so it is reduced by the amount of your ICA. Before a decision is made on your ICA claim, your full IS should be paid until you start to receive your ICA; the 'extra' IS paid is then deducted from arrears of ICA. The advantages of claiming ICA are outlined in 8. If you are paid ICA, the person you care for is excluded from the severe disability premium, but only once ICA is actually awarded; arrears of ICA do not affect entitlement to the premium – see Chapter 3(13).

8. Why claim ICA?
You might find that your household income is no greater after claiming ICA since it overlaps with other benefits. But there are advantages to claiming.

Carer premium – If you get ICA, a £13.35 a week carer premium is included in the assessments for IS, income-based JSA, housing benefit, council tax benefit and NHS benefits. A carer premium is included for each person who gets ICA (or who would be paid ICA if it didn't overlap with another benefit, such as incapacity benefit). If you haven't claimed ICA because you saw no advantages, and meet the qualifying conditions, it is worth making a formal claim (or re-claiming ICA on or after 1.10.90), so that the carer premium can be included. See Chapter 3(16). If you cannot be paid ICA because of the overlapping benefit rules, the person you are caring for won't lose a severe disability premium.

Credits – For each week of ICA, you get a Class 1 National Insurance contribution credit (so long as you have lost, given up, or never had the right to pay reduced-rate contributions). ICA Class 1 credits give you a better deal than other credits – see Chapter 9(2). If you had ICA for the 1994/96 tax years, (or would have got ICA or arrears but for the overlapping benefit rules, or clawback by IS/JSA), your Class 1 credits for those years mean:
- that if you fall sick in 1997, you'll have passed the second contribution condition for incapacity benefit;
- that each tax year with 52 credits is a 'qualifying year' for retirement pension (see Box M.1 in Chapter 44).

However, if you yourself get unemployment or incapacity credits, because you are signing on or are incapable of work, you cannot also get ICA credits for the same period.

Contribution conditions for JSA – If you stop being a carer and need to sign on for jobseeker's allowance, your National Insurance record before you claimed ICA may be used to decide entitlement to contribution-based JSA if this would help you pass the contribution conditions – see Chapter 9(3).

Christmas bonus – If you get ICA you may also get the £10 Christmas bonus.

Retirement – If you don't have enough contributions for full-rate retirement pension, your pension can be topped up to £37.35 with ICA. But you need to claim before you're 65. See Chapter 43(4) for more details.

9. Time off from caring

Once you have established your entitlement to ICA, you may have a total of 12 weeks 'off' in any six month period, without your benefit being affected. Up to 4 weeks of not caring for the disabled person are allowed, eg you or s/he are on holiday without each other. If you, or the disabled person have been in hospital, up to 12 weeks are allowed.

If you (or s/he) have been away from each other for 4 weeks in the last 6 months, you won't be entitled to ICA if you (or s/he) have another week apart during the same 6 month period. However, if you (or s/he) goes into hospital, this won't affect your right to ICA. In this situation, ICA can be paid for another 8 weeks.

However, your ICA depends on the disabled person getting AA or DLA care component. An AA or care component beneficiary aged 16 or over may spend 4 weeks in hospital (up to 12 weeks for a child). After that the AA or DLA care component (and therefore your ICA) will stop – see Chapter 17(9) and (10). But your ICA might stop sooner if you've used up most of your 12 weeks off in the past 26 weeks. The disabled person may be able to arrange a pattern of respite care in hospital or residential care that allows them to keep their attendance allowance or care component – see Box G.3 in Chapter 17.

You must immediately report any of these changes in writing, to the Invalid Care Allowance Unit.

If all this seems confusing, keep a diary. The golden rule is that you can be paid ICA for any week in which you are caring for the disabled person for 35 hours. If you (or s/he) are away from each other, the 12-weeks-off rule applies. If you have had more than 12 weeks off in the past 26 weeks, you cannot be paid ICA for any week in which you care for the disabled person for less than 35 hours. A week off is a week in which you cared for the disabled person for less than 35 hours: so odd days or weekends away are unlikely to affect things. A weekend straddles two ICA weeks: an ICA week runs from Sunday through to Saturday.

20 Help with mobility needs

1. Orange badge scheme

The Orange Badge Scheme of parking concessions is designed to help people with severe mobility problems (and blind people) by allowing them to park close to shops, public buildings and other places they may wish to visit. You should not be wheel clamped if you are displaying a current Orange Badge, although the police may remove your vehicle if it is causing an obstruction. The badge requires a photo; the section showing the name of the badge holder and the date of expiry must be legible from outside the vehicle, but there is no need for the photo to be visible from the outside.

The Scheme allows a vehicle displaying an Orange Badge in the correct place and driven by a disabled person, or with a disabled person as passenger, to park:
- without charge or time limit at parking meters;
- without time limit in streets where otherwise waiting is allowed for only limited periods;
- for a maximum of 3 hours in England and Wales or without any time limit in Scotland where parking restrictions indicated by yellow lines are in force.

This is provided that the disabled person leaves the vehicle, and:
- in England and Wales a special orange parking disc is also displayed showing the time of arrival, if parked on yellow lines or in a reserved parking place for badge holders which has a time limit;
- the vehicle is not parked in a bus lane or cycle lane during its hours of operation;
- the vehicle is not parked where there is a ban on loading or unloading; and
- all other parking regulations are observed.

Red routes in towns and cities are subject to special controls on stopping, but there is parking provision for badge holders – check signs.

If the disabled person is not, or has not, been in the vehicle, it is an offence to display an Orange Badge – unless the driver is on the way to collect the disabled person, or has just dropped them off.

The Scheme applies throughout England, Scotland and Wales with the exception of four areas in Central London: the City of London, Westminster, Kensington and Chelsea and part of Camden. In these areas there is limited recognition, including parking in designated disabled parking bays. Contact the *Greater London Association of Disabled People (GLAD), 336 Brixton Road, London, SW9 7AA (0171 346 5813)* for more details. You may also find that in your area there are variations from the national scheme.

In order to qualify for an Orange Badge you must be aged 2 or over and:
- receiving the higher rate mobility component of disability living allowance; or
- getting war pensioners' mobility supplement; or
- using a vehicle supplied by a government department or getting a grant towards running your own car; or
- be registered blind; or
- drive regularly, and have a severe disability in both arms so that you cannot turn a steering wheel by hand (even if the wheel is fitted with a turning knob); or
- have a *'permanent and substantial disability which causes inability to walk or very considerable difficulty in walking'*.

Local authorities have discretion to charge up to £2 to issue a Badge.

If your local authority refuses to issue an Orange Badge as they do not think you have 'very considerable difficulty in walking', you have no formal right of appeal. You could, however, see if your Councillor or local group or advice agency can help change their mind. You only have a formal right of appeal (to the Secretary of State for Transport) if you have been denied a Badge on grounds of misuse.

Orange Badge holders who visit certain countries, which provide parking concessions for their own disabled citizens, can take advantage of the concessions provided by the host country by displaying their Orange Badge. Concessions vary from one country to another but usually allow for an extension

G.8 Mobility Checklist

Besides the help covered in this chapter and in Chapter 17, there is a range of other help, some of it practical, some of it cash. All of this help is covered in a Department of Transport guide, called *Door to Door* – the 5th edition is available from The Stationery Office bookshops, price £5.99.

Information on choosing a car

It is important to choose the car and adaptations that are best suited to you. The Department of Transport has set up a Mobility Advice and Vehicle Information Service to offer practical advice. Information is free but they make a charge for other types of help. For details, write to them at: *TRL, Old Wokingham Road, Crowthorne, Berkshire RG45 6AU*. Otherwise, contact the Mobility Information Service, or Banstead Mobility Centre.

Motability

Motability is a voluntary organisation, set up on the initiative of the Government, and designed to help people with disabilities use their higher rate mobility component of disability living allowance (DLA) to buy or hire a car. It offers two types of scheme, a hiring scheme and a hire purchase scheme. Under the hire purchase scheme it is possible to buy an electric wheelchair or a good used car as well as a new car.

Anybody receiving the higher rate mobility component (including the parents of children who receive it), or war pensioners' mobility supplement, can apply to Motability for help. Trike drivers who think that one of Motability's schemes may help them, can also apply, provided they opt to change to mobility component.

Most people choose to hire a car rather than buy on hire purchase. To hire a car, your mobility component must be either a life award or a fixed period award with at least 3 years still to run. To buy on hire purchase, your mobility component must be either a life award, or have at least 2 years left to run if you buy a used car, or at least 4 years left to run if you buy a new car. The Disability Benefits Unit will pay your mobility component directly to Motability.

You can't renew a Motability agreement if you are in hospital, except under the wheelchair scheme. See Chapter 17(9) for more details.

Full details of these schemes are in the leaflets Motability Car Hiring and Hire Purchase Schemes and Used Car Hire Purchase Scheme. You can ask for these (and an application form) from *Motability, Goodman House, Station Approach, Harlow, Essex CM20 2ET. Telephone (01279) 635666*.

In some circumstances, Motability can help towards the cost of driving lessons. Write to Motability for details.

Hire purchase agreement on standard cars

There are no controls on hire purchase agreements (although there is consumer protection legislation). So it is entirely up to the individual finance house to come to an agreement on terms with the borrower.

Concessions on cars and wheelchairs

If you plan to buy a new car or wheelchair or to hire a car, you may get cash concessions if you get DLA mobility component, or, in some cases, help under the pre-1976 scheme. Some car companies offer discounts to any disabled person. Concessions range from discounts on retail prices of cars to an extension of the guarantee on electric wheelchairs. For details, contact: RADAR, the Disabled Living Foundation, or Disability Scotland.

The National Health Service still supplies free wheelchairs, and may provide a voucher towards the cost of a more expensive wheelchair of your choice – see Chapter 33.

Pre-1976 vehicle scheme

If you have a car or trike provided under the pre-1976 invalid vehicle scheme, you can switch to DLA higher rate mobility component, whatever your age, without any problems, so long as you are still eligible on medical grounds for help under the old scheme. You can transfer to mobility component temporarily if your vehicle is off the road (for example awaiting repairs after an accident – but not for repairs for normal wear and tear). To switch to mobility component, write for an application to:

England – *Invalid Vehicle Scheme, Warbreck House, Warbreck Hill, Blackpool, FY2 0YE.*
Wales – *Welsh ALAC, Rookwood Hospital, Llandaff, Cardiff, CF5 2YN.*
Scotland – *SHHD, Room 205, St Andrew's House, Edinburgh, EH1 3DE.*
Northern Ireland – *DLA Branch, Castle Court, Royal Avenue, Belfast, BT1 1TZ.*

For more information on the scheme see Chapter 20 in the 19th edition of the *Disability Rights Handbook* (send us a stamped, self-addressed envelope if you would like a photocopy).

Concessions on public transport

British Rail has a Railcard for people with disabilities. The scheme is for people getting DLA middle or higher rate care component or higher rate mobility component, attendance allowance, war pensioners' mobility supplement, SDA, or 80% or more war pension, or who are registered as visually impaired or deaf, or have recurrent attacks of epilepsy.

British Rail also offers some other fare concessions to disabled people. You can get a leaflet from your local station, giving information about the Railcard, fare concessions, access to stations and trains, and travel arrangements.

It is best to let British Rail know before your journey so that any necessary arrangements can be made.

Some local authorities offer concessions to disabled people on local buses. Your Social Services Department can give you details.

Help with travel to work – see Chapter 15.

Sources of information

Mobility Information Service
Unit 2a, Atcham Industrial Estate, Upton Magna, Shrewsbury SY4 4UG (01743 761889)

This voluntary organisation offers a wide range of information on cars, adaptations, costs, etc. It has a great deal of experience in mobility for disabled people. They issue a series of leaflets covering all aspects of choosing, buying and converting a car. Personal assessment may also be possible within a 100 mile radius of Shrewsbury.

Banstead Mobility Centre
Damson Way, Orchard Hill, Queen Mary's Avenue, Carshalton, Surrey, SM5 4NR (0181 770 1151)

The Centre is both an advisory information service on the different types of vehicles available for disabled people and a multi-discipline assessment service.

of the time limit where waiting is restricted, and an entitlement to use parking places reserved for disabled people. You can get full details of concessions and the participating countries from the Department of Transport.

2. Exemption from road tax (VED)

Who can get exemption?
All vehicles on the road are liable to Vehicle Excise Duty, better known as road tax. However, exemption from VED for one car only is given to the cars of three groups of disabled people:

Pre-1976 vehicle schemes – If you have an invalid tricycle, or a small car issued by the Department of Health or the Scottish Home and Health Department (SHHD), you are exempt.

Mobility component – If you get the higher rate mobility component of disability living allowance you, or your appointee or someone you choose to nominate in your place, may apply for exemption from VED. Long stay hospital patients affected by the July 1996 changes to mobility component can still get the exemption, but the Vehicle Licensing Agency will be reviewing this at the end of 1997.

Technically the vehicle is only exempt while it is being used solely by or for the purposes of the disabled person. What exactly this means has never been defined. The disabled person does not necessarily have to be in the car: instead, it could be being used to do their shopping or running errands; however, the use of an exempt car for purposes totally unconnected with the disabled person is technically illegal. The probability of being prosecuted is low and is only likely to occur where there is flagrant abuse of the exemption, for example where a non-disabled person uses the vehicle to drive to work. The DSS has implied that, where the car is used substantially for the purposes of the disabled person, there is nothing to worry about.

Anyone receiving higher rate mobility component (or war pensioners' mobility supplement) should automatically have been sent a VED exemption form by the DSS.

You can then use the certificate issued by the DSS (or SHHD) as proof of exemption when applying for a 'tax exempt disc' from the Vehicle Licensing Agency. If you are getting higher rate mobility component and have not been sent an application form, or want guidance on it, write to the Disability Benefits Unit (VED). If you are getting war pensioners' mobility supplement and have not been sent an exemption form write to the War Pensions Agency – you'll find the address in Chapter 22(7).

If there is a delay in your DLA claim, the exemption cannot be backdated.

Passengers getting DLA care component or attendance allowance – Road tax exemption for passengers getting DLA care component or attendance allowance was abolished on 12.10.93. So long as you were exempt before this date, or applied for help before 12.10.93, transitional arrangements mean you will continue to get help under the old scheme. For more details of the old scheme, see the 17th edition of our Handbook.

Nominating another person's vehicle
Someone getting the higher rate mobility component can nominate another person's vehicle to be exempt from road tax. This may also apply to a company car registered in the name of the company – the person receiving mobility component should nominate the company for exemption. In order to qualify for exemption, the vehicle should be used *'by or for the purposes of'* the disabled person.

The named person who gets the exemption may be changed at any time. For example, if you have nominated someone else for exemption and then get your own car, the exemption can be returned to you.

If you are refused exemption
Even if you have an exemption certificate from the DSS, it is within the discretion of the Vehicle Licensing Agency to refuse to grant exemption from road tax if they think that the vehicle will not be used 'solely by or for the purposes of' the disabled person. They are unlikely to do this unless your intended use of the vehicle would blatantly breach this condition.

If you are refused exemption, there is no formal procedure for appealing. However, you can write, giving full details of why you think you qualify for exemption, the purposes for which the vehicle will be used, etc, to: *Driver Vehicle and Licensing Agency, Vehicle Enquiry Unit Centre, Longview Road, Swansea SA99 1BL (telephone 01792 772134)*.

Special compensation schemes

This section of the Handbook looks at the following:

Industrial injuries scheme	Chapter 21
War disablement pension	Chapter 22
Criminal injuries compensation	Chapter 23
Vaccine damage payments	Chapter 24
Compensation recovery	Chapter 25

21 Industrial injuries scheme

1. Who is covered by the scheme?

The industrial injuries scheme provides benefit for an employee who *'suffers personal injury caused after 4.7.48 by accident arising out of and in the course of'* work, or who contracts a prescribed industrial disease or a prescribed injury while working.

S.94 SSCBA for accidents; s.108-110 for prescribed diseases

You are covered by the industrial injuries scheme if you are working for an employer. It does not matter if you do not earn enough to have to pay National Insurance contributions, or if you are too young or too old to pay them. Nor does it matter if the accident happens on your first day at work. What counts is that you are gainfully employed under a contract of service, or as an office holder with earnings that would be taxable under Schedule E. So if you are genuinely self-employed you will not be covered by the scheme unless the accident happens while you are doing specified types of voluntary work – such as working as a special constable.

You are covered by the industrial injuries scheme if your accident occurred outside the EC so long as your employer was paying NI contributions for you while you were working abroad; and if you are a voluntary service worker who continues to pay UK contributions.

Apprentices who are not 'gainfully employed' are covered by the scheme. If you are a trainee on a Youth Training Scheme or other government training programme, you are covered instead by a scheme run by the Department for Education and Employment. Benefits are equivalent to those paid under the industrial injuries scheme. For more information ring free on 0800 590395.

If there is any doubt over your status as an earner, your case will be referred to the Secretary of State, (in practice this means a DSS official acting on behalf of the Secretary of State). Note that it may be possible to show that you were an employee for benefit purposes – despite the tax and NI arrangements – if the real relationship between you and the contractor is that of an employee and employer. Seek expert advice. This applies in particular to building workers who are very often categorised as self-employed; the Secretary of State may well decide you are in fact an employed earner – contact your trade union for advice.

In most cases there is little difficulty in proving that an accident was 'industrial'. The main questions are over the extent of the disablement resulting from the industrial accident or prescribed industrial disease. However, Box H.1 looks at some of the problems that can arise when you are trying to prove that an accident was industrial.

If your accident occurred before 5 July 1948 see leaflet WS1 which gives details of the Workmen's Compensation Scheme.

2. What to do after an accident

As soon as possible after an accident at work you should report the details to your employer. Enter them in the accident book (one must be kept at any workplace where 10 or more people usually work). Do this even if things don't seem serious at first. A cut can turn septic. A pain in the stomach can turn out to be a hernia. If you think the accident might have some ill-effect in future, apply to the DSS for a declaration that you have had an industrial accident. You can get the application form, BI 95, from your local DSS office.

If you are in any doubt whether you are covered by the industrial injuries scheme just go ahead and apply for an 'accident declaration', or claim benefit if necessary. The case law is complex and without checking it in detail, and without knowing all of the facts of your case, it will be difficult for anyone to advise you.

3. Prescribed industrial diseases

At present, 67 different diseases are prescribed as being risks of particular occupations and not risks common to the general population.

For diseases contracted in work since 5 July 1948 see leaflet NI 2. This lists all of the diseases and the types of occupations you must have been working in, in order to qualify for benefit.
Leaflet NI 3 covers pneumoconiosis and byssinosis.
Leaflet NI 272 covers asbestos-related diseases.
Leaflet NI 207 covers occupational deafness – see 6 below.
Leaflet NI 237 covers occupational asthma – see 6.
Leaflet NI 7 covers chronic bronchitis and emphysema for coal miners – see 6.

If your disease was contracted in work before 5 July 1948 see leaflet PN 1 which gives details of the *Pneumoconiosis, Byssinosis and Miscellaneous Diseases Benefit Scheme*; leaflet WS1 gives details of the *Workmen's Compensation Scheme*.

The onus is on you to claim benefit for a prescribed disease. If you have any reason to suspect that your illness is related to your work, you must ask the DSS and your doctor for advice. If you do not, you may lose benefit. For example, few secretaries realise they are covered by prescribed disease A.4 if they suffer from cramp of the hand or forearm.

If your disability arises from a non-listed disease which was contracted at work, you may still be able to claim. Some cases have shown that the 'catching' of the disease can be claimed as an industrial accident.

4. Common law compensation

You may also have a civil claim for personal injury against your employer. Your union may be able to help you with this or you can consult a legal aid lawyer, or contact Accident Line – see Box H.3. For some industrial diseases there are no-fault compensation schemes which have been negotiated by unions and employers: contact your union for advice. The time limit for filing civil claims is 3 years from the date of the accident or from the date you became aware that your disease or condition was caused by work.

For information about the way in which benefits are affected by compensation payments, see Chapter 25 and Chapter 3(31).

For certain chest diseases such as pneumoconiosis, asbestosis and byssinosis, a lump sum payment can be claimed, under the Pneumoconiosis and Byssinosis (Workers Compensation) Act 1979, when a civil compensation claim is not possible, perhaps because the employer no longer exists. This scheme is now run by the Department of the Environment and has advantages over civil action as it is quicker, negligence need not be proved and payment is made in full without recovery of DSS benefits paid. Some chest diseases are only diagnosed at death so claims can also be made by dependants. Claim forms and more information are available from *Department of the Environment, HSFO, 23rd Floor, Portland House, Stag Place, London, SW1E 5DF (0171 890 4972)*.

5. What help can you get?

SSP or incapacity benefit
If you are employed but incapable of work, you should claim statutory sick pay from your employer (see Chapter 10). If you are not entitled to statutory sick pay, you can claim incapacity benefit if you have enough National Insurance contributions (see Chapter 11).

Incapacity benefit replaced sickness and invalidity benefit in April 1995 when the provision for claiming no-contribution sickness benefit on the grounds of industrial accident or disease was also abolished. If you claimed sickness benefit because of an industrial accident or disease before 13.4.95 and were turned down you should still be able to challenge this.

Disablement benefit
Disablement benefit is paid to compensate those who have suffered disablement from a *'loss of physical or mental faculty'* caused by an industrial accident or prescribed disease. The rules on payment vary depending on whether your claim was made before or after 1.10.86 – see 8.

It makes no difference whether or not you are incapable of work or have had any drop in earnings. If you suffer from disablement due to a loss of physical or mental faculty amounting to 14% or more, you will usually be entitled to disablement benefit from 15 weeks after the date of the accident or the onset of the disease. A loss of faculty may include disfigurement even if that does not trouble you. For some prescribed respiratory diseases you can get benefit if the assessment is from 1% to 13%. For occupational deafness you can only get benefit if your disablement is 20% or more.

If you are claiming for a prescribed disease, the date of onset should be the date the disease started not the date of claim. Some DSS administrative procedures have led to the wrong date being used. As benefit is only payable 15 weeks after this date, you should check this and challenge it if necessary. However, for occupational deafness, the law says that the date of onset must be the date a successful claim was made, and payment can start from that day. From April 1997 the 15 week waiting period is removed for people suffering from diffuse mesothelioma (PD D3).

Disablement benefit, REA and RA are all paid on top of any other non-means-tested benefit you may receive.

Reduced earnings allowance
Reduced earnings allowance (REA) replaced special hardship allowance from 1.10.86. Reduced earnings allowance itself was abolished on 1.10.90 but only for accidents or diseases occurring after this date. So if your accident, or the onset of a prescribed industrial disease (which must be listed before 10.10.94) was before 1.10.90, you can still claim REA. See 14 below for more details.

Retirement allowance
Retirement allowance (RA) replaces REA at pension age if you were getting at least £2 pw REA and are not in regular employment – see 15 for more details.

Industrial death benefit
Industrial death benefit is now only payable where the death occurred before 11.4.88. Instead, if you are widowed on or after 11.4.88 as a result of an industrial accident or prescribed disease, you will be entitled to ordinary widows' benefits, even if your late husband failed to satisfy the contribution conditions – see Chapter 46.

6. How do you claim disablement benefit?
You should get form BI 100A for an accident; BI 100(Pn) for pneumoconiosis, byssinosis, or an asbestos-related disease; BI 100(OD) for occupational deafness; BI 100(OA) for occupational asthma; BI 100C for chronic bronchitis and emphysema in underground coal miners; or BI 100B for any of the other prescribed industrial diseases. DSS leaflet NI 6 covers disablement benefit generally and NI 2 covers prescribed diseases. Both are available from your local DSS office.

Do not delay returning the completed form or you may lose some benefit. You have 3 months from the first day you were entitled to benefit (15 weeks after the accident/accepted date of onset of the disease) in which to make your claim. For claims made on or after 7.4.97, benefit cannot be backdated beyond 3 months even if you have a good reason for not claiming earlier.

If you claimed before 7.4.97, a weekly disablement pension will be **fully** backdated if you can show 'good cause' for claiming late and your eventual assessment covers the earlier period. As benefits under the industrial injuries scheme are arguably the least well-known and most complex of all benefits, the rules are often misunderstood by advisers, solicitors and DSS staff themselves, so many people will have good cause for not claiming earlier. There are special time limits for occupational deafness and occupational asthma – see below.

When you claim disablement benefit in respect of a particular industrial accident, you only ever make one claim. If the assessment of disablement on that claim is a provisional one for a set period – your disablement is just re-assessed from the expiry date. If your condition is taking time to stabilise, you may have a series of provisional assessments: all in respect of the same claim to disablement benefit.

Occupational deafness – To qualify, you must have worked in one or more of the listed jobs for a total of at least 10 years, and have suffered damage to the inner ear causing a hearing loss of at least 50db in each ear, due, in the case of at least one ear, to occupational noise. You will be paid from the date your claim is received in a DSS office – and that date must be within 5 years of the last day you worked in one of the jobs prescribed for occupational deafness. There is no backdating of claims even if you have 'good cause'. The Court of Appeal, in *McKiernon v Secretary of State* [1989], held that the five year time limit was not valid in law, however the law was changed to make the time limit valid retrospectively.

Occupational asthma – You cannot get disablement benefit for occupational asthma if you stopped working in the prescribed job more than 10 years before your date of claim. But

H.1 Principles of entitlement

Accident or process?
What an accident is may seem obvious and, in most cases, there will be little difficulty in proving that the injury was caused by an identifiable accident. However, problems arise where the injury developed relatively slowly through the normal course of work. This is called injury by 'process'.

If your injury developed as a result of a continuous process at work you will not be entitled to industrial injuries benefits, unless your injury is listed as one of the prescribed industrial diseases.

If your case is a borderline one it is always worth appealing. The Social Security Commissioners tend to recognise that an industrial accident has happened where an injury can be shown to be the cumulative result of a series of accidental injuries.

A series of small incidents, each of which are separate and identifiable, that were slightly out of the ordinary can be enough to count as 'accidents'. But each one must have led to some physiological or pathological change for the worse.

For example, in one case the claimant developed a psychoneurotic condition and skin disorder. He had been working near a machine that irregularly produced loud explosive reports. Any one of them could have been the start of a major explosion. It was held that each explosion was an 'accident' with a cumulative and aggravating effect on him.

If a process has only been going on for a short time, as you have just started a new job, or have had a change in working conditions, it is likely that you will be covered by the scheme. However, it is difficult to give clear guidelines on your chances. Each case will be a matter of fact and degree.

What about other causes of injury?
If you have a condition that predisposes you to certain injuries you can still be covered by the scheme. You must prove that if you had not had the accident at work you would not have suffered that particular injury.

For example, an asthma sufferer had an acute asthma attack due to fumes from a fire at work. He was covered as it was probable that he would not have had that attack if it had not been for the fire at work.

You would only fail if you could not prove that your predisposition to the injury was just one of the causes of the injury.

If, say, nothing out of the ordinary had happened at work but you had just had an asthma attack or a heart attack and suffered no other injury, then it would have just been chance that you had the attack at work. The point is that the industrial injuries scheme is there to insure you against the risks arising from work and not against the risks you would face ordinarily.

That even this point is not always clear cut is shown in R(I)6/82, where the Commissioner confirmed that, even if an accident happens out of the blue, it will count as an 'industrial' one if:
- the activity you are doing represents a special danger to you because of something in yourself; or
- you are also injured because of coming into contact with the employer's premises – eg by falling on to the floor.

Is it an 'industrial' accident?
To count as an 'industrial' accident, it must have arisen out of and in the course of employment. Once again this looks like a straightforward matter, and it often will be. However, the many borderline cases dealt with in Commissioners' decisions mean that it is always worth appealing.

You must show that your accident was due to the risks arising from your employment or from something reasonably incidental to it. You must also show that it occurred while you were in the course of your employment. If your accident happens during a short permitted break spent on the premises you would probably be covered – but if you had overstayed the break purely for your own purposes, you would have taken yourself outside the course of your employment.

Travelling to and from work
If you have an accident while travelling to or from work or during your work you may still be covered by the scheme if, given all the circumstances, your journey can be accepted as having formed part of the work you were employed to do – see R(1)7/85 and *Smith v Stages and Another* [1989] 2 WLR 529. One important (but not conclusive) factor is whether you were being paid for the time spent on the journey, or were able to claim overtime or time off in lieu for it. You may also be covered if you are in transport provided by your employer. You will not be covered if your journey is for your own purposes, unconnected with your work (unless it is reasonably incidental to it).

If the accident happens when you are on your employer's land you will usually be covered if you are there in order to get ready for work. If you get there early in order to have a game of snooker or a snack in the canteen you will not be covered as you are there purely for your own enjoyment. (But if the accident happens during a short permitted break you would be covered.)

'Emergencies'
If you have an accident while responding to an emergency, you will be covered if what you did was reasonably incidental to your normal duties and was a sensible reaction to the emergency. Besides the obvious emergencies of fire and flood, unexpected occurrences have also been counted as 'emergencies'.

In one case the 'emergency' was a concrete mixer which had been left on a site where bricks had to be stacked. The lorry driver delivering the bricks helped move the mixer and was injured. He was covered, even though that was not a normal part of his duties, for it was reasonably incidental to his work. If he had not helped shift the mixer, he would have been delayed on site, the task did not require great skill, and it was in his employer's interests for him to get back to work quickly.

Accidents treated as 'industrial'
Some accidents, which otherwise would be borderline cases, are treated as arising out of work. If you have broken any rules but what you have done is for the purposes of, and in connection with, your employer's business, you will be covered if you have an accident. You will have problems if what you have done is not part of your job. However, if there is evidence to show that your employer would not automatically have stopped you doing something that was not strictly part of your duties then you might succeed. You must also show that it furthered your employer's interests.

If you have an accident during work because of someone else's misconduct, negligence or skylarking, you will be covered if you can show that you did not contribute directly or indirectly to the accident. You will also be covered if, during the course of your work, you are struck by any object or by lightning.

this 10 year limit does not apply if you suffer from asthma because of an industrial accident and have been awarded disablement benefit for life or for a period which includes your date of claim.

Coal miners – Chronic bronchitis and emphysema were prescribed as industrial diseases for underground coal miners from 13.9.93. Because of the large number involved, claims were initially taken in two stages. Normal rules apply to claims made since 31.8.94.

To qualify you must have worked underground for a total of 20 years (from April 1997, this includes periods of sick absence). The condition that you must also have category 1 coal workers' pneumoconiosis has been removed from April 1997 and the requirement that your lung capacity must be at least 1 litre below the expected level for your age, height and sex has been modified for miners with naturally small lung functions. This means that if your claim was refused under the old stricter rules, you should now reapply.

Also from April 1997 the conditions for getting some asbestos-related diseases have been relaxed. Again if an earlier claim has been refused, you should get advice about reclaiming.

7. How is your claim decided?

Accident cases

The Adjudication Officer (AO) is responsible for deciding whether you have had an industrial accident and if so, whether the accident arose out of and in the course of your work. If the AO decides these questions in your favour, s/he will refer your case to an independent adjudicating medical authority.

The adjudicating medical authority can consist of one, or two or more, adjudicating medical practitioners. The adjudicating medical authority is responsible for deciding whether you have a loss of faculty as a result of the accident. If so, the adjudicating medical authority will assess the extent to which that loss of faculty leads to disablement and the period over which you are likely to experience that degree of disablement. The percentage assessment of your disablement can cover a past period as well as a forward one.

Prescribed industrial diseases

The Adjudication Officer (AO) is responsible for deciding whether you have worked in one of the occupations prescribed for your particular disease or injury and whether it was caused by that occupation. If s/he decides you don't satisfy these employment conditions, your claim will be refused. You have the right to appeal to a Social Security Appeal Tribunal within 3 months and should not give up without first seeking expert advice.

If the AO decides that you do satisfy the employment conditions, there is a special procedure. This is known as the diagnosis question. If you have claimed for pneumoconiosis, arrangements will be made to X-ray your chest. If the X-ray shows no trace of the disease, the AO will disallow your claim. You have 3 months in which to appeal to a special medical board or specially qualified adjudicating medical practitioner. If the X-ray shows that you have pneumoconiosis, or if you have claimed for one of the other respiratory diseases, you'll be examined by a special medical board or specially qualified medical practitioner.

If you are suffering from a non-respiratory disease, the Benefits Agency Medical Services (BAMS) will provide a report, sometimes after considering your hospital case notes or a report from your GP. If there is any doubt, they will refer you to a consultant. If the BAMS report is unfavourable and they consider that you are not suffering from a prescribed disease, the AO will disallow your claim. You have 3 months in which to appeal to an adjudicating medical authority. If the BAMS medical report is favourable, the AO will refer your case to an adjudicating medical authority who will examine you. If they decide you have the disease, they will assess the percentage and period of the disablement which results from it.

If you have had (or have) disablement benefit for the same disease, the adjudicating medical authority may need to decide whether or not you have contracted the disease afresh. This is known as the recrudescence question.

What happens?

The proceedings before an adjudicating medical authority are in private. You don't have the right to be represented, although they may permit this. They will assess the extent and likely duration of your disablement and must consider all of the disabilities suffered as a result of the accident or disease, including the worsening of pre-existing conditions. They will assess the disablement resulting from any 'loss of faculty' by comparing your condition with that of a healthy person of the same age and sex – for this purpose your job and other personal circumstances do not matter.

See Box H.2 for more details on the principles of assessment. An adjudicating medical authority can make a 'provisional' assessment or a 'final' assessment. A provisional assessment will be reviewed towards the end of the period. A 'final' assessment may be for life if they consider that your disablement will be permanent and unlikely to change appreciably. If you seem likely to make a full recovery, they may make a final assessment for a fixed and limited period.

Since 21.7.89, provisional assessments cannot be made if your disablement is less than 14% and it looks unlikely that the current assessment can be added to any other assessments to reach the 14% minimum for payment – see 8. Instead, the assessment will be a final one.

REA is payable to existing claimants during the period of a disablement assessment of at least 1%. If your assessment is a final one for a limited period, REA cannot be paid beyond that period. You can either appeal against the assessment to the Medical Appeal Tribunal (MAT); or you can wait until near the end of the assessment period and ask for an 'unforeseen aggravation' review (see 10). You can do both. But an appeal to the MAT could result in a nil assessment (see 9); and a final assessment made by a MAT can only be reviewed on the basis of unforeseen aggravation if the MAT give permission. An increased assessment as a result of unforeseen aggravation can only be backdated one month (3 months if you requested your review before 7.4.97).

8. How much do you get?

Weekly pension

You can usually get benefit only if your disablement is assessed at 14% or more. If it is assessed at 1% to 13%, you cannot get disablement benefit for that injury alone: unless you are suffering from pneumoconiosis, byssinosis, or diffuse mesothelioma.

Payment for assessments of 14% to 19% disablement are at the 20% rate: as a weekly pension. If you are suffering from pneumoconiosis, byssinosis, or diffuse mesothelioma, and are assessed at 1% to 10%, you'll be paid at the 10% rate. In these cases, assessments of 11% to 24% are paid at the 20% rate.

Note that if your disability is assessed at 24% (or 44% etc) it is rounded down and you will be paid at the 20% rate (or

40% etc). If it is assessed at 25% (or 45% etc) it is rounded up and you will be paid at the 30% rate (or 50% etc).

As disablement benefit is compensation for your injury, it is paid on top of any contributory benefit you are entitled to and on top of your earnings. You may also be entitled to increases in your basic disablement benefit – see 11.

Percentages and amounts

20%:	£20.22	50%:	£50.55	80%:	£80.88
30%:	£30.33	60%:	£60.66	90%:	£90.99
40%:	£40.44	70%:	£70.77	100%:	£101.10

Aggregation of assessments

Disablement assessments of 1% to 13% in respect of earlier industrial injuries can be added to the assessment of disablement for the current industrial injury if the assessment periods overlap – so helping you reach the minimum payment figure of 14% during a common core period. However, you cannot combine an earlier % disablement assessment with any later assessment if you have a final assessment for that earlier injury and were paid a disablement gratuity under the Social Security Act 1975 (now under Sch 7, SSCBA).

However, if you have a provisional assessment of disablement on a pre-1.10.86 claim, that can be added to assessments of disablement in respect of claims made on or after 1.10.86. The assessment periods must overlap, or cover a common core period. If the total of the assessments reaches 14%, you can be paid a pension during the common core period – but with the % for the pre-1.10.86 assessments being off-set until the expiry of that award.

For example, adding a 9% provisional assessment for a pre-1.10.86 claim to a 12% assessment for a post-1.10.86 claim, comes to 21%. You can't be paid a pension at the 20% rate (you'll already have had compensation for the pre-1.10.86 claim). Instead, you'll be paid a pension at 11% of the 100% rate (20% less 9%). This continues to the end of the common

---

H.2 Assessment of disablement

We have put most of the information on the assessment of disablement into Box E.9 in Chapter 13. Box E.10 repeats the schedule of prescribed degrees of disablement for the listed conditions.

Box E.9 is geared towards severe disablement allowance (SDA). But the test of 80% disablement used for SDA is based on the long-standing test of disablement (at any percentage) used for industrial disablement benefit.

When you read Box E.9, do remember that for industrial disablement benefit there is a complete scale of assessment – from 1% disablement up to 100% disablement.

Although the adjudicating medical authority will take into account all your disabilities, the disabilities that count towards a percentage assessment for industrial disablement benefit are those disabilities that are based on a loss of faculty which has been caused by an industrial accident or prescribed industrial disease.

A *'loss of faculty'* means a loss of power or function of an organ of the body. It is not itself a disability, but is a cause, actual or potential, of one or more disabilities. A *'disability'* is an inability, total or partial, to perform a normal bodily or mental process. 'Disablement' is the sum total of all the separate disabilities you might experience as a result of the accident.

The adjudicating medical authority will decide what degree and for what period your resulting disablement should be assessed. The assessment is done by comparing your condition after the accident with that of a person of the same age and sex whose physical and mental condition is 'normal'. If your condition differs from normal prior to the accident and means that the industrial injury is more disabling than it would otherwise be, the assessment may be increased to take account of this. For example, an adjudicating medical authority or MAT *'are entitled to increase the disablement percentage to take account of the fact that, when disaster struck, he was blind. They are not entitled to compensate him for the blindness itself, but they are entitled to take account of the fact that a particular happening to a blind man, or somebody suffering from some other disability, may be more serious of itself than it would be in the case of a man who suffered from no disability'* (R(I)3/84, pages 12/13).

If your disablement also has a mental element, CI/81/90, a starred decision, provides a useful summary of the ways in which that might affect the assessment of disablement.

R(I)13/75 discusses the differences between hysteria, malingering and functional overlay.

The medical report completed by the adjudicating medical authority provides a useful guide to the methods of assessment where there is more than one cause of the same disability and where the interaction of another condition causes greater disability.

Pre-existing condition

If your disability has some other cause you may have problems – eg where a previous back injury is followed by an industrial injury to your back. However, your percentage assessment should only be cut, or 'off-set', if there is evidence that a pre-existing condition would have led to a degree of disablement even if the accident had not happened. If there is no evidence for this, the 'off-set' should not be made. R(I)1/81 explains the concepts fully.

If an off-set is justified, the net assessment (ie after the off-set) should reflect any greater disablement because of the interaction between the two (or more) causes of the same disability. Note that a pre-existing condition may cause disablement later. Although the disablement you would have had from that pre-existing condition alone cannot be taken into account, its interaction with the effects of the industrial injury may lead to greater disablement. This could justify an unforeseen aggravation review.

Conditions arising afterwards

If a condition is 'directly attributable' to the industrial accident or disease, it is assessable in the normal way. If it is not 'directly attributable', but is also a cause of the same disability, then whether or not any greater disablement can be taken into account depends on the % assessment for the industrial accident or disease. If the disablement resulting from the industrial accident is assessed at 11% or more, that assessment can be increased to reflect the extent to which the industrial injury is worsened because of the later condition. This can be done at the time of the assessment, or later on an unforeseen aggravation review. Note that in reaching the 11% benchmark, account is taken of any greater disablement because of the interaction with a pre-existing condition which is also an effective cause of the disability.

The 11% rule does not apply where one is considering the interaction between two or more industrial accidents or diseases – see R(I)3/91(T).

core period. In this example, when your pre-1.10.86 claim is reassessed, the pension continues if you have another provisional or final assessment of 2% or more. Note that the off-set position in this case is different from the unforeseen aggravation case – see 10.

The possibility of combining percentage assessments of between 1% and 13% in respect of different industrial injuries to reach the 14% figure means that it is still worth claiming disablement benefit for two or more 'minor' injuries, such as the loss of the whole of a middle finger (12%). If you have had just one minor injury, make sure you apply for an accident declaration. If you have a second industrial accident, claim disablement benefit.

Lump sum gratuity – pre-1.10.86 claims
If you claimed disablement benefit before 1.10.86, the old rules about payment apply to your claim. Note that from 12.2.90, the special provision which allowed a post-1.10.86 claim to be treated as if it had been made beforehand, was abolished.

If you claimed before 1.10.86 and your disablement is assessed at less than 20% you will be paid a lump sum gratuity (unless you are suffering from pneumoconiosis, byssinosis or diffuse mesothelioma for which a pension is paid). You can no longer choose to have the disablement benefit paid as a weekly pension on top of reduced earnings allowance. But an existing pension in lieu of a gratuity can continue (if you remain entitled to a reduced earnings allowance) until the end of the period of your assessment.

Your gratuity depends on the rates for each percentage assessment current at the start of the period of assessment and on the duration of your assessment. So, if a fresh assessment started on or after 10 April 1996 and your disablement was assessed at 10% for life, you would receive £3,619. If it was only assessed at 10% for one year, you would receive one seventh of that amount. If your new assessment starts on or after 9 April 1997, the most you can receive for a 10% assessment is £3,696.

For assessments beginning on or after 9 April 1997, the amounts are: 1% – £672; 5% – £2,016; 13% – £4,704; 19% – £6,720.

9. How do you appeal?
If a decision was taken by an Adjudication Officer (AO) you have the right of appeal to a Social Security Appeal Tribunal. You have 3 months from the date the AO's decision was sent to you. To appeal, you should fill in the form in leaflet NI 246 *How to Appeal* from the DSS. You should give as much detail as possible as to why you disagree with the decision. As industrial injury benefits are complex, you may need expert advice – your trade union may help, or a local advice centre.

If you are dissatisfied with an adjudicating medical authority's decision you have three months in which to appeal to a Medical Appeal Tribunal (MAT). This applies even if you have just had a provisional assessment. Once again, fill in the form in leaflet NI 246 giving reasons for your appeal. Remember that the MAT looks at your case afresh and is not bound by an earlier decision. So they could reduce your assessment to nil, or reduce the period of assessment. The Secretary of State, or an Adjudication Officer, can also decide to refer your case to the MAT. If you are not sure about appealing, ask your local DSS office for a copy of the adjudicating medical authority's report to help you come to a sensible decision about appealing. You don't have to lodge an appeal in order to be sent a copy of the report. (See Chapter 52 for more details.)

10. Unforeseen aggravation and other reviews
If your disability increases because of a deterioration in your condition it is always possible to seek a review of a disablement assessment, even a final one, or of a nil assessment, by applying for a 'review on the grounds of unforeseen aggravation'. Your existing final assessment will be safe – it cannot be cut during this review. However, if the first review assessment is provisional, any later provisional or final assessment can be lower than your original final assessment. Note that if a MAT decided your case, they have to grant leave before it can be reviewed. There is no appeal if they refuse leave, but a detailed consultant's report supporting your case might help persuade the MAT to give you leave. NB there are special rules for prescribed industrial diseases.

If you want an adjudicating medical authority or MAT decision reviewed, write to your local DSS office. For other reviews, see Chapter 52(10)(c).

How to prove 'unforeseen aggravation'
To succeed on an unforeseen aggravation review, you have to pass each of the following tests.
- Has your condition worsened since the original decision was given? If yes:
- Is the worsening due to an aggravation of the results of the original injury, rather than being due to constitutional or other factors? An 'aggravation' can include greater disability resulting from the interaction of the industrial injury and a non-industrial injury, or congenital defect. Another injury, or disease, may make the original industrial injury more disabling (see Box H.2).
- If there has been aggravation, was it foreseen and sufficiently allowed for in the original assessment, or was it unforeseen and merited a higher assessment? There are two ways of looking at this:
- are the effects of the industrial injury worse than would have been expected at the time the original assessment was made, given your previous medical history and the usual progression of that injury; or
- does the original assessment sufficiently cover your current disablement arising from the industrial injury?

You can also ask for a review if you have 'fresh evidence' that an adjudicating medical authority or MAT decision was made in ignorance of, or based on a mistake about a material fact. Fresh evidence is something that you did not know about at the time of that decision, or something that you could not reasonably have been expected to produce. A consultant's report is not 'fresh evidence'; but a firm diagnosis of a previously unidentified condition would be.

Payment and aggregation of assessments
Since 1.1.87, if you are successful on an 'unforeseen aggravation' review of a final assessment of a pre-1.10.86 claim, and the new assessment is 19% or less, you cannot be paid a gratuity.

If the new assessment is below 14% and you cannot be paid a gratuity for the increase in that % assessment following an 'unforeseen aggravation' review, that increase can be aggregated with, or added to, assessments for post-1.10.86 claims, so helping you reach the minimum payment figure of 14%.

Where you are successful on an unforeseen aggravation review and the new % is 14% or more, you will get a pension: even if the actual increase in the assessment is only 1%. However, if you had been paid a gratuity for that injury in the past, the 20% pension is subject to an offset until the assessment period for the original gratuity has expired.

If you had a gratuity for a life assessment, the offset ends 7 years after the start of the gratuity's assessment period. (See R(I)11/67 and CI/522/93.) For example, someone was assessed at 10% for life from 1.1.85 and was paid a 10% gratuity. The 7 year period ended on 1.1.92. In 1987 an unforeseen aggravation review was successful: the % assessment was increased to 14%. That assessment was rounded up to 20% but because the 7 year period hadn't ended, an offset had to be made to take account of the gratuity s/he had already been paid. S/he was paid a 20% pension (at current rates) less the weekly equivalent of the 10% gratuity (at 84-85 benefit rates). This continued until 1.1.92 (the first disablement benefit payday after the end of the 7 year period). Since 1.1.92, s/he is paid a pension at the 20% rate.

However, the position is slightly different if you are currently getting a pension in lieu of a gratuity for the original assessment. In this case, your right to a pension in lieu will end and you'll receive the balance (if any) of the original gratuity, plus the appropriate gratuity for the increase in the % assessment or period. Or, if your disablement is assessed at 14% or more, you'll receive a pension at the appropriate rate.

11. Extra allowances

The following additional allowances can be paid:
- **constant attendance allowance:** Part-time: £20.25; Normal maximum: £40.50; Intermediate rate: £60.75; Exceptionally severe cases: £81.00
- **exceptionally severe disablement allowance:** £40.50
- **unemployability supplement:** £62.45 (earnings limit £2,418 pa). This is only payable to existing claimants. It was abolished from 6.4.87 for new claims.
- **reduced earnings allowance:** maximum £40.44
- **retirement allowance:** maximum £10.11

12. Constant attendance allowance

To qualify for constant attendance allowance, your disablement assessments must add up to 95% or more. You have to be so seriously disabled that you need care and attention as a result of the effects of an industrial accident or disease. This allowance is paid at four levels and was introduced before the general attendance allowance outlined in Chapter 18. It is automatically considered when disablement is assessed at 95% or more. Claim on form BI 104, which you can get from your DSS office. If you claim disability living allowance (DLA), the DLA care component will be reduced by the amount of your constant attendance allowance.

Your entitlement is a matter for the Secretary of State, although in practice a decision will be taken by a DSS officer acting on his behalf. There is no right of appeal against a refusal – but you can always ask for a review of the decision if you feel some facts weren't taken into account.

13. Exceptionally severe disablement allowance

If you qualify for one of the two higher rates of constant attendance allowance, you may also qualify for exceptionally severe disablement allowance. However, your need for that level of attendance must be likely to be permanent. This is paid on top of constant attendance allowance and continues even though you may be a patient in hospital. You do not have to apply separately for this allowance. Note that this is also a decision for the Secretary of State. (See leaflet NI 6 for more details.)

14. Reduced earnings allowance

Claiming REA
You can claim REA if:
- your accident happened before 1.10.90; or
- your disease started before 1.10.90, provided the disease (or the extension to the prescribed disease category) was added to the prescribed list before 10.10.94. REA will not be paid for newly prescribed diseases or extensions to those already listed.

REA can be backdated for up to 3 months from the date you send in your claim providing you request this. For claims made on or after 7.4.97 it is not possible to backdate benefit beyond the 3 months time limit even if you have a good reason for your delay.

The rules on backdating REA claims (and reviews) have changed twice since 1996. If you claimed (or asked for a review) before 7.4.97, benefit can be backdated for up to 12 months if you had 'good cause' for your delay. If you claimed (or asked for a review) before 24.3.96, REA could be fully backdated if you had 'good cause' for a delayed claim. As REA (like SHA before it) has always been one of the less well known and more complex of benefits there are often strong arguments to show 'good cause' (see CI/417/92).

You must claim REA separately from disablement benefit. Get claim form BI 103 from your DSS office. It is possible to have more than one award of REA if you have had more than one industrial accident or disease but you cannot be paid more than the equivalent of 140% disablement when your disablement benefit and REA are added together.

Once you have made a successful claim for REA, you can make renewal claims, subject to the usual rules, but if you were entitled to REA immediately before 1.10.90, a break in entitlement of just one day after this date, may mean you lose REA for good.

REA can now only be paid up to pension age, but not after unless you are still in regular employment. Once you reach pension age, you may transfer to retirement allowance, paid at a lower rate. It may be possible to challenge this – see 15.

Who qualifies for REA?
REA is payable if your disablement has been assessed as at least 1% and you have a current assessment in respect of an accident or disease which occurred before 1.10.90 – see above.

The key test for REA is that you must be unable to return to your regular occupation or to do work of an equivalent standard because of the effects of the disablement caused by your accident or disease. The broad aim is to make up the difference between what you are capable of earning, as a result of the injury or disease, in any suitable alternative employment and what you would have been likely to earn now in your regular job, if you had not had the accident, and were still in it. There are two ways of qualifying for REA.

H.3 For more information

Industrial injury
The best book on the industrial injuries scheme is still *Compensation for Industrial Injury* by R. Lewis (1987, published by Professional Books Ltd/Butterworths). This edition is now out of print but you may be able to find it in a library. As it is only up-to-date to the start of 1987, use it together with the latest editions of *Non-Means Tested Benefits: The Legislation* by Bonner et al (Sweet & Maxwell) and *The Law of Social Security* by Ogus, Barendt and Wikeley (Butterworths).

Accident Line – If you have been injured in an accident or have an industrial disease, you can arrange a free legal consultation with a local solicitor specialising in personal injury claims, by phoning The Accident Line on Freephone 0500 192939 (England and Wales).

Under the continuous condition – You must have been incapable of following both your *'regular occupation'* and any *'employment of an equivalent standard which is suitable in [your] case'* ever since 90 days after your accident happened, or your disease began.

Under the permanent condition – It is enough if you are now *'incapable, and likely to remain permanently incapable, of following [your] regular occupation'* and also incapable of any *'employment of an equivalent standard...'*

Sch 7, Part IV, p.11(1)(b) SSCBA

Earnings

On a first claim your pre and post-accident earnings are individually assessed. Thereafter on subsequent claims for the same accident or disease, depending on how the law applies to your situation, revisions may be linked to the general movement in earnings of broad occupational groups.

Broadly, if your post-accident earnings are less than your pre-accident earnings would now be, the difference is made up by REA, subject to the maximum payment of £40.44. This comparison may be totally hypothetical, say if your 'regular' job no longer exists, and if disabilities which cannot be taken into account in the REA assessment make you incapable of all work. If you are unable to do any work because of the accident or disease you should get the maximum amount of REA even if you are still being paid full wages from your employer.

Tackling appeals

The case law on special hardship allowance is complex and extensive. Much of this case law also applies to REA. For example, there may be arguments over what your 'regular' occupation is, particularly if your accident happened during lower paid 'stop gap' work; or you may argue that your reasonable prospects of advancement should be taken into account. If your claim is turned down, or you don't receive maximum REA, do not give up without first taking expert advice. The 3 month time limit for appeals gives you plenty of time. As well as depending on case law your claim may rest on a mass of detailed facts, as well as medical evidence. It is quite possible for the AO to have made a decision in ignorance of some of the relevant facts.

An Adjudication Officer is responsible for decisions on your entitlement to REA. So your right of appeal against the refusal of REA, or against the amount awarded, is to the Social Security Appeal Tribunal.

No percentage assessment?

To get REA, you must have a current disablement assessment of at least 1%. You also need to be sure that the loss of faculty identified by the adjudicating medical authority covers all the disabilities created by the industrial accident or disease and is sufficient to contribute materially to your being incapable of following your regular occupation.

The adjudicating medical authority advises the AO about their opinion on the link between the accepted loss of faculty and your inability to follow your regular occupation.

If you don't have a current % assessment, or the loss of faculty needs to be more broadly identified, you have to tackle that side of things first.

Put in an appeal against the decision on your claim for REA to safeguard your rights. Then consider the best way of tackling the adjudicating medical authority's decision on your disablement: either by appealing, or by establishing grounds for a review. An appeal to the MAT is the best bet if you need to broaden the loss of faculty. If you are out of time, make a late appeal – see Chapter 52(13)(c). In a separate letter, ask for a review. Check whether a 'fresh evidence' or an 'error of law' review is possible. If you can establish grounds for either type of review, your whole case can be looked at afresh. If not, ask for an unforeseen aggravation review: but note that an adjudicating medical authority's or MAT's powers on an unforeseen aggravation review are limited to revising the assessment of the extent of disablement; they cannot broaden the accepted loss of faculty.

15. Retirement allowance

Retirement allowance is a maximum of £10.11 a week; a minimum of 50p a week. It is the lesser of 10% of the maximum rate of disablement benefit; or 25% of the REA you received immediately before retiring. In practice, if you had maximum REA, your retirement allowance would be £10.11.

If you had already retired and claimed your retirement pension before 10.4.89, or your claim for retirement pension was backdated to before 10.4.89, you don't get retirement allowance. Instead, your REA is frozen for life.

Retirement allowance is payable for life. It is only payable if you are transferring from REA. If you want to stay on REA, you need to avoid meeting all of the tests for retirement allowance. This may not be possible. Retirement allowance replaces REA if:

- you are over pension age (60 for women, 65 for men); and
- you give up 'regular employment' – see below; and
- on the day before you give up that work your award (or awards) of REA add up to at least £2 a week; and
- you are not entitled to REA.

Giving up 'regular employment' – From 24.3.96, *'regular employment'* is defined as gainful employment under a contract of service which requires you to work for an average of at least 10 hours a week over any 5 week period (not counting any week of permitted absence such as leave or sickness), or gainful employment (which may be self-employment) which you undertake for an average of at least 10 hours a week over any 5 week period.

If you were not in 'regular employment' and were over pension age on 24.3.96, you will have been treated as having given up regular employment in that week and moved from REA to RA. If you are not in 'regular employment' and you reach pension age after 24.3.96, your REA will be replaced by RA in the week you reach pension age.

However, several cases challenging the March 1996 legislation are at Commissioners. The arguments are complex and are discussed in some detail in the Summer 1996 *Disability Rights Bulletin*. One argument which has yet to be tested in the Courts is on the grounds of sexual discrimination as women lose their REA at age 60, five years earlier than men.

If you have had your REA converted to RA under the March 1996 legislation, you should get advice quickly about a possible appeal, or review.

If your REA is replaced by RA, you may be able to reclaim REA if you should start 'regular employment' providing you were not getting REA immediately before 1.10.90 (see 14). There appears to be nothing in the regulations to prevent this, although the DSS are likely to challenge such a claim as it is not policy intention that this should be possible. You should get advice if your claim for REA is refused in these circumstances.

22 War disablement pension

1. The war pensions scheme

The war pensions scheme is separate from the social security system, despite being administered by the DSS War Pensions Agency. It is similar in many respects to the industrial injuries scheme, but is primarily intended to provide benefits for a disability caused or made worse by service in HM Armed Forces. It is much wider in scope than the industrial injuries scheme; there is no list of prescribed diseases, jobs or substances. You can claim for any medical condition whatsoever providing you can show a link between that condition and your service. You do not have to have been involved in a 'war' or even on active service when the injury or condition was caused or made worse. You could have been injured simply playing sport on the base, or suffered an illness at some time during service which has done some permanent damage (for example an ear infection which has caused some hearing loss).

While most pensions are paid for physical injuries, claims for mental and psychological conditions such as schizophrenia and post-traumatic stress disorder are now being accepted in the light of new medical opinion, as are conditions such as multiple sclerosis, Menière's Disease, Hodgkin's disease, diabetes mellitus, gastritis and peptic ulcers linked by helicobacter pylori and heart disease linked to lower limb amputation. So, if you have claimed for one of these conditions in the past and been refused, you should claim again now.

Civilians are covered by the scheme but only for certain physical injuries which are due to the second world war. Other groups are also included – see below.

2. Who can claim?

You can claim for a present disability resulting from:
- an injury or condition caused or made worse by service in HM Armed Forces at any time. This includes the Home Guard; Nursing and Auxiliary Services; the UDR from 31.3.70; the Territorial Army and Cadet Force Officers;
- a physical injury sustained as a civilian during the 1939 war either as a result of enemy action or action in combating the enemy;
- a physical injury sustained while carrying out your duties as a Civil Defence Volunteer during the 1939 war;
- an injury or condition caused or made worse by service during the 1939 war in the Polish Forces under British Command or while serving in the Polish Resettlement Forces;
- certain injuries or illnesses sustained while serving in the Naval Auxiliary Services, Coastguard or Merchant Navy during the 1914 or 1939 wars, or later conflicts in the Gulf, the Falklands, Suez or Korea; or while being held prisoner.

If you are a dependant of someone whose death has been caused or 'substantially hastened' by one of the above listed injuries you can also claim a war pension (see 8 below).

3. How much do you get?

War disablement pension

The basic disablement pension depends on the degree of your disability. Your disablement is assessed on a percentage basis, like in the industrial injuries scheme – see Box H.2 in Chapter 21. If your assessment is 20% or more, a weekly pension is payable. If it is less than 20%, a one-off lump sum gratuity is paid. However, if your claim is in respect of noise-induced sensorineural hearing loss and is assessed at less than 20%, a gratuity is no longer paid and no account will be taken of any related condition such as tinnitus. If your hearing loss alone is assessed as at least 20%, any additional disability or symptom will be added on to increase the percentage you get. To get 20% your average hearing loss must be 50dB or more in each ear.

A gratuity can still be paid for hearing loss due to other causes such as bomb blast, ear infections or the effects of ototoxic drugs used to treat other conditions linked with service.

War disablement pensions are tax-free. The maximum war disablement pension at the 100% rate is £107.20 a week – see WPA Leaflet 9 for the full range of rates payable.

Supplementary allowances

Tax-free supplementary allowances may be payable on top of a basic war disablement pension or gratuity. Each has its own qualifying rules. Some are paid automatically, others have to be claimed – see below.

4. Allowances that have to be claimed

War pensioners' mobility supplement: £38.55 pw

This is payable if your walking difficulty is caused wholly or mainly by your pensioned disablement – if that is assessed at 40% or more (20% for claims made before 7.4.97). The qualifying conditions are similar to those for disability living allowance (DLA) higher rate mobility component (see Chapter 17(20)) except there is no special category for severe mental impairment. It cannot be paid at the same time as DLA mobility component but it is paid at a higher rate and there is no upper age limit for claiming. When claiming you can choose whether to attend a medical examination or fill in a self-assessment claim pack. Your disability must be expected to last at least 6 months from the date an award is considered but unlike DLA you do not have to meet a 3 month qualifying period prior to this. Mobility supplement can be paid even if you go into hospital or go abroad.

Mobility supplement replaced the former war pensioners' vehicle scheme. No new or replacement cars can now be issued in the UK under the former vehicle scheme.

Constant attendance allowance: £20.25, £40.50, £60.75, £81.00 pw

This is paid where your pensionable disability is assessed at 80% or more and you need a lot of care and attention of a personal nature; or supervision, mainly because of your pensionable disablement. It is payable at different rates depending on the amount of attendance needed. If, because of your pensionable disablement, you are terminally ill, you'll get the highest rate. If you are an in-patient at an NHS hospital, your constant attendance allowance normally stops after 4 weeks.

You cannot get constant attendance allowance as well as ordinary attendance allowance or DLA care component, you will be paid whichever is higher. When claiming you can choose to have a medical examination or fill in a self-assessment claim pack.

Unemployability supplement: £66.25 pw plus £37.35 for an adult dependent plus £9.90 for the first child and £11.20 for each other child

This is paid if your pensioned disablement is at least 60% (20% if you claimed before 7.4.97) and means you are likely to be permanently unable to work, or to earn more than a small amount of therapeutic earnings, ie for 1997/98 up to £2,418 in a year. From 7.4.97, new claims are restricted to those aged under 65. There are additions for dependants and you may also be able to get an invalidity allowance, depending on your age when you first became permanently incapable of work.

As unemployability supplement is an income replacement benefit, you cannot get it at the same time as incapacity benefit or retirement pension, but it is normally paid at a higher rate and any earnings-related or graduated retirement pension is paid separately by the DSS on top. If you are an in-patient at an NHS hospital, your unemployability supplement will normally be reduced after 8 weeks in hospital – see Chapter 39.

Allowance for lowered standard of occupation: up to £40.44 pw
This is similar to reduced earnings allowance in the industrial injuries scheme. It is paid where your pensioned disablement means you are unable to follow your regular occupation or do work of an equivalent standard. Claims made on or after 7.4.97 are now restricted to those aged under 65 whose pensioned disablement is assessed as at least 40%. This allowance plus your basic war pension cannot add up to more than the 100% rate pension. You cannot get unemployability supplement at the same time but you can keep your retirement pension or incapacity benefit so this allowance could be a better option if you meet the conditions for both. You need to ask the War Pensions Agency to check this for you as they will normally only consider this allowance if you are not entitled to unemployability supplement. But bear in mind that retirement pension and incapacity benefit are both taxable.

Clothing allowance: £137 a year
This is payable where your pensioned disablement causes exceptional wear and tear to your clothing, eg because of incontinence or the use of an artificial limb.

Treatment allowance: current assessment increases to 100%
This is payable if you suffer actual loss of earnings due to having treatment at home or in hospital because of your pensioned disablement. Treatment allowance is paid to top up your current percentage, (whether you have a pension or gratuity), to the 100% rate of the basic pension.

5. Allowances that are paid automatically

Exceptionally severe disablement allowance: £40.50 pw
This is paid where constant attendance allowance is payable at either of the two highest rates and you are not gainfully employed.

Severe disablement occupational allowance: £20.25 pw
This may be paid if you get either of the two highest rates of constant attendance allowance but nevertheless you are normally in employment. You cannot get it as well as certain social security benefits such as retirement pension, incapacity benefit, severe disablement allowance and invalid care allowance.

Comforts allowance: £8.70 or £17.40 pw
This is payable if you get unemployability supplement and/or constant attendance allowance.

Age allowance: varying from £7.15 to £22.10 pw
Paid at age 65, if you are assessed as at least 40% disabled. How much you get depends on the degree of disablement.

6. Does anything affect what you get?
A war disablement pension is payable whether you are working or not. The basic pension does not affect your entitlement to any non-means-tested social security benefit, with the exception of industrial injuries disablement benefit which may be payable for the same disablement.

The supplementary allowances payable with the basic war disablement pension can affect the payment of similar benefits available under the ordinary social security scheme. For example, war pensioners' constant attendance allowance normally overlaps with ordinary attendance allowance and DLA care component. So you cannot get both in full. And if you get war pensioners' unemployability supplement or severe disablement occupational allowance, see above.

You cannot get full allowances for dependants payable with non-means-tested social security benefits as well as those payable with unemployability supplement. But the total paid will be the higher of the two.

For means-tested benefits, £10 a week of a war disablement pension is ignored as income. Certain supplementary allowances are ignored in full, these are: constant attendance allowance, exceptionally severe disablement allowance, severe disablement occupational allowance and war pensioners' mobility supplement. So it is important to give a breakdown of how your war pension is made up when claiming means-tested benefits. Your local council may ignore more than £10 for claims to housing and council tax benefit under a local scheme.

If you enter hospital, unemployability supplement and constant attendance allowance are normally affected after a period – see Chapter 39.

7. How do you claim?
You can get a claim form by calling the War Pensions Helpline on 01253 858858; or by writing to the *War Pensions Agency, Norcross, Blackpool FY5 3WP*; or by contacting your local War Pensioners' Welfare Office, addresses in WPA Leaflet 1. Make sure you complete and return the form within 3 months otherwise you could lose benefit. The War Pensions Agency will no longer be sending out reminders.

When to claim?
There is no time limit for making a claim to war disablement pension. However, any award is normally only paid from the date of your claim. Backdating is at the Secretary of State's discretion and from 7.4.97, will be restricted to a maximum of 3 years in a prescribed list of circumstances. These are: if you have been unable to claim earlier due to ill health or disability; if there has been a change in medical opinion; or if the Ministry of Defence has failed to forward papers to the War Pensions Agency where someone has been invalided out of or died in service. In cases of clear and unambiguous official misdirection or error, full backdating is still possible. There is no right of appeal if backdating is refused, so any progress would have to be made by way of judicial review.

It is in your interest to claim quickly. If your claim is made within 7 years of leaving the Forces it is easier to have it accepted as the onus is on the War Pensions Agency to prove that your disability is **not** linked to your service. After 7 years, the burden of proof shifts to you to prove your claim. So, for example, a person contracting multiple sclerosis within 7 years of discharge from the Forces, has been awarded a war disablement pension solely because the cause of this condition is unknown, and it is therefore impossible for the War Pensions Agency to prove that it is **not** linked to their service.

For civilian claims, the War Pensions Agency has recently taken a stricter line and decided to consider claims only where the claimant provides independent supporting evidence. The types of evidence they will accept are listed on the claim form. If your claim is refused because of this, you should get independent advice.

At whatever stage your claim is made, the regulations state that the benefit of any reasonable doubt should always be given to the claimant.

If you are invalided from the Forces or die in service, the Ministry of Defence should send the DSS your service medical records automatically, for a claim to war disablement or war widow's pension to be considered.

What happens?
The DSS will send for your service records, if appropriate, to decide if you come within the scope of the war pensions scheme. If you do, the cause and the degree of your disability will be decided by the DSS doctors, after a medical examination.

8. War widows and other dependants

A war widow's pension can be paid if your husband's death was due to, or substantially hastened by, an illness or injury for which he was either getting a war disablement pension or to which he would have been entitled had he claimed; or, if he was getting constant attendance allowance (at any rate) or would have been had he not been in hospital or, from 7.4.97, was getting unemployability supplement at the time of death and his pensionable disablement was at least 80%.

In some circumstances a woman living with the man at the time of his death and looking after his child can also qualify.

If your late husband was getting a war disablement pension when he died you will not be awarded a war widow's pension automatically – you have to apply. However, if he was getting constant attendance allowance or unemployability supplement prior to his death a temporary widow's allowance is paid automatically for the first 26 weeks. This allowance is normally paid at the same rate as that paid to the man before his death.

If you qualify for a war widow's pension you can also claim help with the funeral costs. There is no means-test but you must apply within 13 weeks of the date of the funeral.

You cannot be paid a war widow's pension as well as a National Insurance widow's pension but a war widow's pension is tax-free and normally paid at a higher rate. You can also get benefits based on your own National Insurance contributions such as retirement pension and incapacity benefit on top. If you go into hospital your war widow's pension is unaffected for the first 12 months and then reviewed. It can continue to be paid in full for a further 12 months before being reduced.

A 'special payment' of £52.80 a week is paid on top of a war widow's pension if your late husband's service ended before 31 March 1973. This amount is totally disregarded for means-tested benefits. There are also extra allowances that widows can claim.

H.4 For more information

War Pensions Helpline – 01253 858858
Call the Helpline if you have any query about your claim or the war pensions scheme. The Helpline can give advice and information and send out claim forms and leaflets.
WPA Leaflet 1 *Notes about war pensions and allowances*
WPA Leaflet 6 *Notes for war pensioners and war widows going abroad*
WPA Leaflet 7 *Notes for ex-Far East and Korean prisoners of war*
WPA Leaflet 9 *Rates of war pensions and allowances*
WPA Leaflet 10 *Notes about War Pension claims for deafness*

Entitlement to a war widow's pension automatically stops if you remarry or cohabit, but since 19.7.95 it can be reinstated if the new marriage has ended in divorce, legal separation or widowhood. From 7.4.97 your war widow's pension can also be restored if you stop co-habiting. If this applies to you contact the War Pensions Agency as soon as possible.

In some circumstances widowers and other dependants can claim a pension or help with funeral costs. More details can be found in WPA Leaflet 1.

9. Reviews

If your condition gets worse at any time since you last claimed you should contact the War Pensions Agency and ask for your claim to be reviewed on the grounds of deterioration. From 7.4.97, you need to show that you have grounds for seeking a review, eg by providing evidence that you have sought medical advice or treatment for your condition since your last assessment was made. But do not delay, as if you are successful any payment will normally only be made from the date of your request.

Once a decision has been made on your claim, and you are unhappy either with the DSS assessment of your disability or because your claim is refused you can ask for a review if you think there are some facts about your condition that the DSS do not know. You do not have to ask for a review, you can appeal straight away. In any case, when you appeal the DSS will carry out a review and could change their decision, making a tribunal hearing unnecessary.

It is important that you get help with an appeal or a review. Many ex-service organisations such as the Royal British Legion can help you prepare your case and provide a representative to speak on your behalf. Or you can contact an advice centre or your local War Pensions Committee (see below).

10. Appeals

1939 War and onwards
When the DSS send you their written decision on your entitlement to a pension, or on your percentage assessment, that letter will tell you how to appeal, and the time limit for appealing.

You can appeal to the Pensions Appeal Tribunal (PAT), an independent body set up by the Lord Chancellor's office and not part of the Independent Tribunal Service.

Entitlement appeals – The tribunal consists of a chairperson who is normally a lawyer, a doctor, and a service member who will normally have similar service experience to you. They will consider questions relating to your basic entitlement. There is no time limit for appealing in these cases but if you win, the date payment begins depends on when you put in your appeal.

Assessment appeals – These consider the extent of your disability and so the tribunal chairperson is a doctor and a medical examination is normally carried out. With assessment appeals you have three months to lodge the appeal (12 months if it is against a final assessment) although a late appeal can be accepted if you can show good reason for the delay.

Appeals to a PAT take considerably longer to be heard than is normal for other social security tribunals. It can be over 18 months before the papers, (which are known as a 'statement of case') are prepared and a date of hearing has been set.

Any further appeal against a decision of a PAT is only possible on a point of law to the High Court.

1914 war and supplementary allowances
You do not have a right of appeal against being refused a

supplementary allowance or if you are claiming for an injury arising out of the 1914 war. But you can ask your local War Pensions Committee to look into your case.

War Pensions Committees are independent of the DSS and are made up of people who are mainly ex-service or who work for voluntary organisations. They can discuss your case with you and make recommendations to the DSS on your behalf. Such recommendations are considered carefully by the DSS but not necessarily accepted. You can get details of your local War Pensions Committee from the War Pensioners' Welfare Office in your area.

11. Extra help you can get

If you get a war disablement pension (or have had a gratuity) for a disability, you can apply to the War Pensions Agency for any of the following services or appliances you need because of that disability. These are provided free and are not means-tested but you should apply before arranging any treatment or appliance, as refunds are not normally made unless prior approval has been given.

Hospital treatment expenses – Payment can be made for travel costs, and in some cases for subsistence or loss of earnings, incurred when attending for treatment at hospital or elsewhere, for example an artificial limb fitting centre.

Private treatment – Payment for approved treatment not available on the NHS.

Priority treatment – The War Pensions Agency can arrange for you to be seen or receive treatment earlier.

Chiropody – Fees can be paid if the local health authority cannot provide free treatment.

Appliances – Various items can be provided if not available through other agencies such as orthopaedic chairs, spectacles, corsets and dental treatment.

Home adaptation grant – Up to £750 can be allowed for small adaptations, for example a stair lift, when these cannot be provided by the local authority.

Nursing home fees (skilled nursing care) – If you need 24 hour nursing care because of your pensioned disability the War Pensions Agency can pay up to a maximum of £394 (£446 in London) a week nursing home fees; more if no other nursing home is suitable. The nursing home must be approved by the War Pensions Agency and a DSS doctor may visit you to assess your needs. Any fees are paid without any means-test, it does not matter how much savings or income you have. In these cases your basic war disablement pension will continue to be paid in full while you are in the nursing home but any constant attendance allowance stops after 4 weeks and some other extra allowances such as unemployability supplement are reduced or withdrawn after 8 weeks.

Short-term breaks (convalescence) – You can claim nursing home fees for up to a maximum of 4 weeks a year to enable you to have a holiday or short-term break. But if you are truly convalescing – for instance if you have recently been discharged from hospital and are recovering from an operation – the War Pensions Agency will not pay as they consider this a Health Service responsibility. As a rough guide you need to be assessed as at least 50% disabled to qualify to have your fees met but each case is looked at on its individual circumstances.

Respite breaks – These are designed to give **your carer** a break. Your carer has to provide medical evidence that a break is needed and your disability must be such that you would be unable to stay in a hotel or boarding house.

For all of the above services and appliances you can ask your local War Pensioners' Welfare Officer to visit to discuss things with you and help you apply.

23 Criminal injuries compensation

1. Do you qualify?

You can claim compensation from the Criminal Injuries Compensation Authority if you suffer personal injury directly resulting from a crime of violence in Great Britain, or on a British vessel, aircraft or hovercraft, or in a lighthouse off the coast of Great Britain, or within 500 metres of an installation in any part of the seas around Great Britain, over which Britain exercises control.

A crime of violence includes child abuse, and personal injury might include shock, or pregnancy or sexually transmitted diseases contracted as a result of rape. You can also claim compensation if you are injured when trying to stop someone from committing a crime, or trying to stop a suspected criminal, or helping the police to do so. In this case, if the injury is accidental, you must have been taking a justifiable, exceptional risk.

You can claim compensation even if your attacker is immune from prosecution under the law, for example because of insanity.

You can get compensation if you suffer nervous shock as a result of seeing a trespasser on a railway line die or commit suicide; or if you suffer any other injury directly attributable to an offence of trespass on a railway.

If the injury was caused by a traffic accident, it is only covered if the driver of the vehicle deliberately drove it at you in an attempt to injure you.

Compensation can be reduced or withheld unless the Criminal Injuries Compensation Authority is satisfied that:
- you took all reasonable steps to inform the police or, in limited circumstances, another appropriate authority, of the incident, and co-operated fully in their investigations;
- you have given the Authority all reasonable assistance, eg by providing information;
- your *'conduct . . . before, during or after the incident giving rise to the application'* does not make it *'inappropriate that a full award or any award at all be made'*. If you have a criminal record, or if you in any way contributed to the attack, compensation may be reduced or refused.

Violence within the family – If you and your attacker were living together as members of the same family, you can apply for compensation provided that:
- your attacker has been prosecuted (unless there are good reasons why this has not been done);
- you and your attacker have stopped living together, except in the case of child victims – though a full explanation will be required in this case, and the attacker must not be likely to benefit from a compensation award.

A man and woman, who aren't married, but are living together as husband and wife, are treated as members of the same family under this scheme.

Sexual offences – The Authority looks with particular care at all claims in respect of sexual or other offences which arise out of a sexual relationship, especially if there has been any delay in submitting the application. Compensation won't be payable unless the Authority is satisfied that the attacker will not benefit from the award.

2. Previous schemes

The Criminal Injuries Compensation Scheme was originally introduced in 1964, revised in 1969, in 1979, in 1990 and again in 1996. If you were injured before 1.4.96, your application is considered under the terms of the particular scheme in operation at the time of your injury, subject to any changes inserted by a later scheme. Details of these schemes are available from the Authority.

In 1994, a 'tariff' scheme was introduced; this was later withdrawn in 1995 and replaced in April 1996 by the current scheme. The 1994 tariff scheme was withdrawn after the House of Lords ruled that the scheme had been introduced unlawfully. Under the 1994 tariff scheme, flat rate payments were made depending on the type of injury, with no account taken of loss of earnings or other individual circumstances. Applications assessed under the tariff scheme since April 1994 are being reassessed under the 1990 scheme. This may result in increased awards. The Authority has written to all applicants affected. If your award is reassessed, make sure you supply any additional evidence of loss of earnings, or other financial loss, to the Authority.

New claims after 1 April 1996 are dealt with under the replacement tariff-based scheme outlined in this chapter.

3. How do you claim?

Get the appropriate claim form from the Criminal Injuries Compensation Authority – see Box H.5. Apply as soon as possible after the incident.

You can apply for compensation if your attacker is unknown or has not yet been arrested.

All applications must be made to the Authority within 2 years of the date of the injury, although they can accept late applications in exceptional circumstances if it is in the interests of justice to do so. The Authority is sympathetic to late claims made in respect of children and young people (under age 18) or people with learning difficulties, and may waive the time limit. Claims in respect of child abuse should therefore be made even if the injuries occurred over 2 years ago. Send a covering letter explaining the delay. Applications for children have to be made by a person with parental responsibility for the child.

H.5 For more information

The Criminal Injuries Compensation Authority publishes a guide to the Criminal Injuries Compensation Scheme called *Victims of Crimes of Violence*.

You can get this free from: *Criminal Injuries Compensation Authority, Tay House, 300 Bath Street, Glasgow G2 4JR (0141 331 2726)*.

Traffic accidents
If you are the victim of an uninsured or untraced motorist, there is a different scheme for compensation for personal injuries. This is run by the Motor Insurers' Bureau (MIB), a company established by motor insurers, which has agreements with the Government to provide that compensation. The MIB schemes cover damage of over £175 to property. They cover personal bodily injuries arising because of a traffic accident where the driver was not insured, or cannot be traced. Compensation is worked out in the same way as common law damages. You must report the accident to the police within 14 days or as soon as reasonably practicable. If the driver cannot be traced, you must apply to the MIB within 3 years of the accident, but generally you should act quickly. For details of the uninsured drivers' agreement and the untraced drivers' agreement, contact: *Motor Insurers' Bureau, 152 Silbury Boulevard, Milton Keynes MK9 1NB (01908 240000)*.

4. How much do you get?

Compensation is made up of several possible elements:
- **for the injury itself** – a lump sum payment assessed by reference to a fixed table. The Authority will obtain a medical report on you, and will decide where in the table your injury features; this 'tariff of injuries' is included in the guide available from the Authority – see Box H.5;
- **loss of earnings** – no compensation is paid for the first 28 weeks of lost earnings. Any loss of earnings beyond that will be compensated, subject to certain maximum limits. Loss of pension rights may also be compensated;
- **special expenses** – for example, care costs, or equipment such as a wheelchair, or towards expenses for medical, dental or optical treatment. To qualify, you must have suffered from the injury for at least 28 weeks but if so, the award will be backdated to the date of injury.

Compensation if the victim has died
If someone has died as a result of a criminal injury, an amount for funeral expenses will be paid, and compensation may be paid to their family.
Funeral expenses – The Authority only pays an amount they consider reasonable. The religious and cultural background of the victim and their family will be taken into account in deciding what is reasonable. Whoever has paid for the funeral of a victim of a crime of violence may claim.
Fatal injury award – A relative of someone who has died as a result of violence can claim a flat-rate fatal injury award of £10,000 for one claimant, or £5,000 each for two or more claimants.

The only people who can claim this award are the husband or wife; an unmarried partner who had been living with the deceased for at least 2 years; a parent; a child (this includes people of any age).
Dependency award – If a relative was financially dependant on the deceased for their living expenses, an award will be made to reflect the extent of financial dependency, subject to a maximum amount. Close relatives (parents, children and partners) can claim, as for the fatal injury award above, and also former husbands or wives if s/he was being financially supported by the deceased.
Loss of a parent – In the case of an application on behalf of a child under 18, a payment of £2,000 per year will be made to the child in respect of the death of their parent, to reflect the extent the child was dependent on the parent in ways other than financially, eg caring for the child.

Compensation recovery
Your award may be reduced in some cases to take account of other payments received.
Social security benefits and insurance payments – Benefits received or insurance payments for the same event are deducted in full from an award for loss of earnings, special expenses or a dependency award. Any award which is tariff-based is not affected (eg for the injury itself or a fatal injury award).
Occupational pensions – Any loss of earnings or dependency award will be reduced to take account of an occupational pension payable as a result of the injury or death. Pension rights from payments made only by the victim or dependant are disregarded.
Compensation from the courts – The full amount of any compensation payment for personal injury or damages made by a civil or criminal court in respect of the same injury is deducted from any award under the Criminal Injuries Compensation Scheme.

24 Vaccine damage payments

1. What is this scheme?
The scheme provides a tax-free lump sum of £30,000 for a person who is (or was immediately before death) severely disabled as a result of vaccination against specific diseases. It is described in leaflet HB3 *Vaccine damage payments*.

The £30,000 award is available only to people who make (or made) their very first claim for help under the scheme on or after 15.4.91. If your claim was made before 18.6.85, you are restricted to a payment of £10,000. For claims from 18.6.85 to 14.4.91, the payment is £20,000. In all cases, the date of the vaccination makes no difference to the level of payment.

2. Who qualifies?
Payments can be made to a person who has been severely disabled as a result of vaccination against diphtheria, tetanus, whooping cough, poliomyelitis, measles, rubella, mumps, tuberculosis or haemophilus influenzae type b (Hib). Those damaged before birth as a result of vaccinations given to their mothers are also included in the scheme, as are those who have contracted polio through contact with another person who was vaccinated against it using orally administered vaccine. The claimant must also satisfy these conditions:

- the vaccination must have been carried out in the UK or Isle of Man (except for serving members of the forces and their immediate families vaccinated outside the UK as part of service medical facilities, who are treated as if vaccinated in England);
- the vaccination must have been carried out either when the claimant was under 18 (except for rubella and poliomyelitis) or at a time of an outbreak of the disease within the UK or Isle of Man;
- the claimant must also be over the age of 2 on the date of the claim, or, if s/he has died, s/he must have died after 9 May 1978 and have been over the age of 2;
- the claim must be made within 6 years of the vaccination, or, where this is later, within 6 years of the disabled person's second birthday;
- in the case of someone who contracted polio through contact with another person who was vaccinated against it, you must have been *'in close physical contact'* with that person during the period of 60 days which began on the 4th day after the vaccination. She or he must also have been *'looking after'* or have been looked after jointly with the vaccinated person.

3. What is 'severe disablement'?
A person is considered to be severely disabled if the disablement due to vaccine damage is assessed at 80% or more (as for severe disablement allowance). This excludes many people who can prove they have been damaged by vaccination, but who are assessed at less than 80%.

4. How do you claim?
Get leaflet HB3 and a claim form by writing to the *Vaccine Damage Payments Unit, Palatine House, Lancaster Road, Preston PR1 1HB*.

Don't delay in claiming. If you can't enclose supporting medical evidence or all the information needed, send it on later. If the disabled person is under 18, the claim should be made by the parents or guardian. If you cannot obtain some evidence, tell the Unit. They can ask the hospital or doctor concerned for any available evidence.

5. What if you are refused?
If your claim is refused, you will be sent a written decision with reasons. If the refusal is on the basis that the claimant is not considered 80% disabled and/or that disablement is not as a result of vaccination, you can ask for a review of the decision by an independent vaccine damage tribunal. Claims refused for other reasons cannot be reviewed in this way, but you can ask the Secretary of State to reconsider the decision.

The tribunal is made up of three people, a chairman and two doctors. At the hearing you may be represented by another person, and you may call and question witnesses. Legal Aid is not available for representation but you can get legal advice under the Green Form scheme for the work leading up to the hearing. You will be able to study the evidence on which the refusal was based before the hearing.

The tribunal's decision and reasons for it will be sent to you in writing. If you are refused again, you can ask for the decision to be reconsidered by the Secretary of State only if there has been a material – ie relevant – change of circumstances or if the tribunal's decision was made in ignorance of,

5. How is your claim decided?
The Authority's staff will look at your claim to check that the information you have given is correct. On the claim form, you are asked to give them authority to contact the police, your doctor, employer, or anyone else relevant, to obtain confirmation of the incident, your injuries, loss of earnings, etc. They may ask you for other details. All these enquiries are made in strict confidence. In some cases, you might be asked to undergo a medical examination by a doctor chosen by the Authority.

After gathering this information, the Authority's staff will decide if you come within the scheme, and, if so, will assess the amount of compensation.

You will be sent a written decision. You must reply in writing and accept the decision before any payment is made. Where the award has been reduced or disallowed, you will be given reasons.

6. If you don't agree with the decision
If you are not happy with the decision, you can apply for a review. You must apply in writing within 90 days of the date of the letter notifying you of the decision. Your application must be supported by reasons, together with any additional evidence. If you haven't had help with your claim, it is important to get advice now to make sure you have included all the relevant information.

If you ask for an extension within the 90 days and can show good reason for applying late, or if it is in the interests of justice to do so, the 90 day time limit can be extended.

After the review, if you are still dissatisfied with the decision, you can appeal to an independent body, the Criminal Injuries Compensation Appeals Panel. You must appeal within 30 days of the date of the letter notifying you of the outcome of the review.

Your appeal will be screened by an adjudicator who may decide to refer your case to an oral hearing. You will get at least 21 days notice of the hearing. You can bring a friend or a legal adviser to represent you.

Both reviews and appeals involve a full reconsideration of eligibility and the amount of the award, and may result in loss of an award or a reduced award.

or based on a mistake about, some material fact. You must ask for a reconsideration within 6 years of the date you were notified of the decision.

The Secretary of State can reconsider payment at any time where he has reason to believe that there was a misrepresentation or non-disclosure of relevant information.

6. Does it affect other benefits?
The value of a vaccine damage payment held in a trust fund is ignored for the purposes of income support, income-based jobseeker's allowance, family credit, disability working allowance, council tax benefit and housing benefit. But any payments actually made from the trust will count in full as income or capital.

If the payment is not held in a trust fund, it will be taken into account when assessing eligibility for means-tested benefits. It makes no difference at all to non-means-tested benefits such as severe disablement allowance.

25 Compensation recovery

1. Compensation recovery
The rules on recovery of social security benefits from compensation awards are changing this year, probably from October 1997. The new rules apply to compensation payments made in pursuance of a court order or agreement made on or after the date the new rules come into force. We give an outline of the main changes in 5 below. First we look at the current rules.

If you get compensation of over £2,500 in respect of a personal injury, accident or disease, an amount equivalent to the total of certain benefits you have received up to the date of settlement or for the first 5 years, whichever is sooner, will be deducted from the compensation payment (unless the payment is exempt – see 3 below).

This applies to compensation for an accident or injury that happened on or after 1.1.89, or if you first claimed benefit on or after 1.1.89 in respect of a disease.

When the offer of payment is about to be made, the Compensation Recovery Unit sends you and the compensator, a 'certificate of total benefit', showing the amount which is to be deducted. It is valid for 8 weeks from the date of issue. The deduction is paid direct to the DSS by the compensator before you receive your payment.

Different rules apply if your accident or injury happened before 1.1.89. Your compensation may still be reduced, but the money will be kept by the compensator, not paid over to the DSS.

2. Benefits which can be recovered
Most benefits that are paid 'in respect of' the injury or disease can be recovered from your compensation. The period of recovery starts from the day following the accident, or the day you claim benefit for a disease, until the day compensation is paid, or for a maximum of five years.

Benefits which can be recovered are: attendance allowance, industrial injuries benefits, family credit, income support, incapacity benefit, sickness benefit, invalidity benefit, mobility allowance, SDA, statutory sick pay (up to 5.4.94), unemployment benefit, jobseeker's allowance, DLA (both components), DWA, and any dependency increases paid with these benefits.

If you were already on benefit before your injury, it is important that your solicitor is aware of the rules on benefit recovery; to avoid under-compensation, your claim for damages should include a claim for the loss of your existing benefit.

You can argue that benefit which is paid otherwise than 'in respect of' the injury should not be recovered (see the Court of Appeal decision in *Hassall and another v Secretary of State for Social Security*, 15.12.94).

3. Exempt payments
Some compensation payments are exempt from the recovery rules: payments of £2,500 or less; vaccine damage payments; Criminal Injuries Compensation Scheme; Macfarlane Trust; Eileen Trust; payments under the Fatal Accidents Act; redundancy payments; NHS industrial injuries scheme; payments by the criminal courts; certain trusts and contractual insurance payments.

4. Appeals
You can appeal against the 'certificate of total benefit' within 3 months of the compensation payment being made.
You can appeal on three grounds:
- whether benefits were paid in consequence of the incident;
- the amount of benefit recovered; and
- the period of recovery.

Appeals are heard by a SSAT, or by a MAT if it is a medical question (see Chapter 52).

5. Changes during 1997
The Social Security (Recovery of Benefits) Act 1997 replaces the previous scheme for recovery of benefits from compensation payments for any compensation payments made out of a court order or agreement made on or after the date the new rules come into force (including cases where the accident or injury happened before 1989). It is proposed that the changes should come into force from October 1997. The main changes are as follows.
- Benefits cannot be deducted from damages awarded for pain and suffering.
- There are three broad categories of compensation from which recovery can be made, and only certain benefits can be deducted from payments under each category:
  - loss of earnings – DWA, disablement pension, incapacity benefit, income support, invalidity benefit, JSA, reduced earnings allowance, SDA, sickness benefit, SSP (before 6.4.94), unemployment benefit, unemployability supplement;
  - cost of care – attendance allowance, DLA care component, constant attendance allowance, exceptionally severe disablement allowance;
  - loss of mobility – DLA mobility component, mobility allowance.

  In making an order for a compensation payment, the court must specify how much is to be awarded under each of these three categories. If you receive more in benefit than the amount of compensation awarded under the relevant category, that element of the compensation award will be reduced to nil. Any excess cannot be deducted, but must be met by the compensator.
- The small payments limit of £2,500 is abolished. The Act allows regulations to specify a new small payments limit.
- Appeals will be heard by a MAT in all cases.

6. For more information
Leaflets and information about the recovery scheme can be obtained from the DSS at *The Compensation Recovery Unit, Reyrolle Building, Hebburn, Tyne and Wear, NE31 1XB (0191 201 0500)*. In Northern Ireland contact the unit at *Castle Buildings, Stormont, Belfast, BT4 3RA (01232 520520)*.

Children and young people

This section of the Handbook looks at the following:

Maternity rights	Chapter **26**
Child benefit	Chapter **27**
Family credit	Chapter **28**
Children with disabilities	Chapter **29**
Young people with disabilities	Chapter **30**
Financing studies	Chapter **31**

26 Maternity rights

1. Help with health costs

As soon as you know you are pregnant you can qualify for free prescriptions and free dental treatment up until your baby is 12 months old. You can still get this if your baby is stillborn or dies.

If you get income support or income-based jobseeker's allowance (JSA), you will qualify for help with your fares to and from hospital; and for milk tokens for yourself (once you've told the DSS you're pregnant, these should come through automatically). You also qualify for free vitamins from your antenatal clinic while you are pregnant or breastfeeding. If you are on income support or income-based JSA, you continue to get milk tokens and vitamins for your child until s/he is five.

You may also qualify for hospital fares if you are on a low income or get family credit or disability working allowance – see Chapter 39.

2. Maternity leave

Every woman who is working while she is pregnant is entitled to 14 weeks maternity leave. Women who have worked for two years for the same employer by the end of the 12th week before the week the baby is due, qualify for an additional period of maternity absence (29 weeks from the actual week of childbirth). For both types of leave you must fulfil strict notification requirements. Check carefully for details.

Maternity Alliance produces a leaflet, *Pregnant at Work*, which describes your rights to maternity leave and time off for antenatal care, as well as health and safety rights at work for pregnant women – see Box I.1.

3. Statutory maternity pay

If you work for an employer and are pregnant, you may be able to get this weekly payment from your employer when you stop work to have your baby. You will not have to repay it if you do not return to work.

You qualify if:
- you have worked for the same employer for at least 26 weeks by the end of the 15th week before the week the baby is due; (a 'week' starts on Sunday and runs through to the end of the following Saturday. The DSS call this 15th week, the '*qualifying week*'); and
- you are still in your job in the qualifying week (it doesn't matter if you are off work sick or on holiday); and
- your average earnings are at least £62 a week; and
- you give your employer the right notice – see below.

How much do you get?
Statutory maternity pay (SMP) can last for a maximum of 18 weeks. For the first six weeks you get 90% of your average weekly pay. The average is calculated from your gross earnings in the eight weeks, if weekly paid, or two months, if monthly paid, before the end of the 15th week before the baby is due. After that you get the flat rate of SMP which is £55.70 per week for up to 12 weeks.

You may have to pay tax and National Insurance contributions out of your SMP. SMP is paid by your employer.

When is it paid?
The 11th week before the birth is the earliest you can get SMP. It is for you to decide when you want to stop work and start your maternity pay period. You can work right up until the week of childbirth. But see 5 below if you are off work with a pregnancy-related illness.

You should write to your employers at least 3 weeks before you plan to stop work, asking for SMP. You must also send them your maternity certificate, form MAT B1, which your doctor or midwife will give you when you are about six months pregnant.

If the baby is born early, tell your employers within 21 days or as soon as is reasonably practicable.

If you are not eligible for SMP, your employer will give you form SMP1, together with your form MAT B1. You may be eligible for maternity allowance (see 4 below).

SMP works in a similar way to statutory sick pay (see Chapter 10). So you have the right to ask your employer for a written statement about your SMP position. If you disagree, you can refer your case to an Adjudication Officer (AO) based in the DSS for a decision. Your employer cannot ask the AO for a decision. If the AO decides against you, you can appeal to a Social Security Appeal Tribunal within 3 months. Your employer can also appeal.

See Box I.1 for where to get more information on SMP.

4. Maternity allowance

If you can't get SMP, you may qualify for maternity allowance. You may get maternity allowance if you are self-employed or if you gave up work or changed jobs during your pregnancy. To qualify, you must have worked and paid Class 1 or Class 2 National Insurance contributions in at least 26 of the 66 weeks before the week in which the baby is due. Maternity allowance is paid by the DSS.

How much do you get?
There are two rates of maternity allowance. The lower rate of £48.35 per week is paid if you are self-employed or not employed in the 'qualifying week' (the 15th week before the week the baby is due). A higher rate of £55.70 per week is paid if you are employed in the qualifying week. Maternity allowance is tax-free.

It is paid for up to 18 weeks. The earliest it can start is 11 weeks before the expected week of childbirth. If you are employed or self-employed, you may delay the start of your maternity allowance up until the baby's birth (but see 5 below if you are off work with a pregnancy-related illness). However, if you are not employed, your maternity allowance must start in the 11th week before the expected week of childbirth.

How do you claim?
To claim, fill in form MA1 and send it to your local DSS together with your maternity certificate (MAT B1) and form SMP1 if you have it (an employer gives you this if you are not eligible for statutory maternity pay). You can get MA1 from the DSS or your antenatal clinic. Send in form MA1 as soon as you can after you are 26 weeks pregnant. Don't put off sending it in because you are waiting for MAT B1 or SMP1. You can send them later.

If you are not entitled to maternity allowance, the DSS should check to see if you can get incapacity benefit instead – see 5 below.

5. Unable to work due to sickness or disability?
If you are employed, you may be able to get statutory sick pay (SSP) – see Chapter 10. If you can't get SSP, you may be able to get incapacity benefit. Incapacity benefit is for people who are unable to work through sickness or disability and have paid enough National Insurance contributions. Chapters 8 and 11 look at when and how you can get incapacity benefit. Below we look at what happens if you are pregnant or have recently had a baby.

I.1 For more information

Working rights
For rights at work during pregnancy, for maternity pay and return to work after maternity leave, see the guide produced by the DSS and Department of Trade and Industry, *Maternity Rights – A Guide for Employers and Employees* (PL 958) available free from Jobcentres.

For more on maternity benefits, see DSS booklets: *A Guide to Maternity Benefits* (NI 17A); *Pregnancy Related Illness* (NI 200); and *Statutory Maternity Pay: Manual for Employers* (CA29).

General information
The Maternity Alliance can help with queries you may have on benefits, employment rights and on practical support from the social services and health services – you can contact them at *5th Floor, 45 Beech Street, London EC2P 2LX* (please send a stamped, self-addressed envelope).

If you are a disabled parent, contact ParentAbility, part of the National Childbirth Trust. If there is an organisation specialising in your own disability, try contacting that organisation. See our Address List at the back of this Handbook.

The DSS have a good leaflet called *Babies and Benefits* (FB8) which may help you. It includes an order form for other relevant DSS leaflets.

Education
See the ACE *Special Education Handbook* – £8.00 (plus £1 p&p) from the *Advisory Centre for Education, 1B Aberdeen Studios, 22 Highbury Grove, London N5 2EA*. The Department for Education and Employment produces a free guide, *Special Educational Needs: A Guide for Parents* (available in Braille and audio cassette) from *DFEE Publications Centre, PO Box 2193, London, E15 2EU*.

If you are entitled to SMP or maternity allowance
You can stay on SSP or lower rate short-term incapacity benefit (this is paid for the first 28 weeks of incapacity) up until the date of the baby's birth, or the date you are due to start your maternity leave. But if you have a pregnancy-related illness in the last 6 weeks before the week the baby is due, your SMP or maternity allowance starts automatically.

SMP – Once your SMP begins any SSP or lower rate short-term incapacity benefit stops. If you were getting higher rate short-term, or long-term incapacity benefit and went on to SMP, you can stay on incapacity benefit as well. The amount you get is reduced by the amount of SMP you receive, so it could be overlapped completely.

Maternity allowance – You can claim, or continue to receive incapacity benefit (at any rate) while you are on maternity allowance. But they overlap so you are paid whichever is higher. Unless you are on lower rate short-term incapacity benefit (£47.10 a week), you are normally better off staying on incapacity benefit. You don't have to pass any tests of incapacity to show you are incapable of work while you are entitled to maternity allowance.

The time you spend on maternity allowance counts towards working out when you are due to move to the next rate of incapacity benefit, so you could become entitled to higher rate short-term incapacity benefit if you were on the lower rate before your maternity allowance started.

If you are not entitled to SMP or maternity allowance
If you pass the National Insurance contribution conditions, you may be entitled to incapacity benefit from 6 weeks before the baby is due up to 2 weeks after the birth. You need your MAT B1 but you don't need any medical certificates, nor do you have to pass any incapacity tests.

You may be able to get incapacity benefit outside of these weeks. But in this case you must usually pass the 'own occupation' test or 'all work' test to prove you are unable to work, as well as all the usual conditions for benefit – see Chapters 8 and 11. You do not have to pass these tests at any time during your pregnancy if there is a serious risk to you or the baby because of pregnancy unless you stop work, or if you tried to work – see Chapter 8(4).

6. Maternity payment from the social fund
If you get income support, income-based JSA, disability working allowance or family credit, you may qualify for the £100 maternity payment from the social fund. See Chapter 6 for more details.

7. When can you claim other benefits and help?

From the birth
Claim child benefit – see Chapter 27. Claim an addition for your new child from your higher rate short-term or long-term incapacity benefit, SDA or ICA, etc. If your partner earns £135 a week or more, you may not get an addition – see Chapter 11(4).

A new baby may entitle you to family credit for the first time, but if you are already getting it, it will not be increased until your current award ends – see Chapter 28.

Ask for a review of your income support, income-based JSA, housing or council tax benefit. A new baby means you can get more help, or qualify for the first time.

Your baby automatically qualifies for free prescriptions.

You have 6 weeks to register your baby's birth. When you register the birth, the registrar will give you form FP58. You need to complete this and send it to your GP so that your baby can get a National Health Service card.

If your child is disabled, you can register him or her with the Social Services Department. You can also apply to your local education authority for an assessment of your child's special needs, but until your child reaches 2 this is discretionary. However, a local education authority should not turn down a request unreasonably.

You may be able to get help from the Family Fund with some of the extra costs arising from a child's disability – see Chapter 29. If your child is disabled, you may get help with adaptations – see Chapter 49.

You have 3 months from the date of birth (or adoption) in which to claim the social fund maternity payment – see Chapter 6. It may also be possible to get a grant or loan under the discretionary part of the social fund – see Chapter 7.

From 13 weeks
You can be paid the care component of disability living allowance (DLA) for your baby once s/he is 3 months old – claim any time beforehand. If your baby is terminally ill, s/he qualifies automatically for the higher rate care component and payment can begin just as soon as you claim DLA after the birth – see Chapter 17.

If your baby gets DLA care component at the middle or higher rate, you can get invalid care allowance – see Chapter 19.

From 30 weeks
If you get income support or income-based JSA you can continue to get milk tokens and free vitamins for your child. You can exchange your milk tokens for dried milk for a child under 1 year.

Your child will automatically qualify for free NHS dental treatment and vouchers for glasses as necessary.

From 2 years
You can now be paid or claim:
- vaccine damage payment – see Chapter 24;
- help under concessionary transport or fares schemes – see Chapter 20;
- an orange badge – see Chapter 20;
- a special educational needs assessment.

A local education authority in England and Wales has a duty to identify any child who may have special educational needs. You can ask them to assess your child. If they give you a statement of your child's special educational needs, this must be reviewed every year. See Box I.1 for where to find out more about education rights. In Scotland, there are similar provisions for children with special educational needs.

From 5 years
A disabled child can now be paid the mobility component of disability living allowance – see Chapter 17. Claim from 3 months beforehand.

Free milk will stop once the child reaches 5 years – but see Chapter 48 if your disabled child is not registered at school.

If you get income support or income-based JSA, you are entitled to free school meals for each child attending school. You may also be able to get a discretionary school clothing grant from the education authority. If your child has to travel more than 2 miles to school, the travel is free. If your child is disabled, you may get help even if s/he has to go less than 2 miles.

A DLA care component award for a Downs Syndrome child is often for a short period, so that it can be reviewed at this time. If you yourself need continual supervision to prevent the risk of danger to a young child, your award may end on their 5th birthday (if it didn't end on their 3rd birthday) so that your care needs can be reviewed when you put in a renewal claim – see Chapter 17. Treat this type of renewal claim as if it was a review.

From 8 years
If your child has to travel more than 3 miles to school, travel is free.

From 12 years
DLA care component for deaf children is often reviewed at this time – see Chapter 17.

If your child has a statement of special educational needs from the local education authority, from age 14 the annual review must include a Transition Plan.

From 16 years
At 16, your child can claim social security benefits in his or her own right – see Chapter 30.

27 Child benefit

1. Who gets it?

Child benefit is a tax-free benefit for each dependent child. You can get it whatever your income.

You can get child benefit for each child under the age of 16 and for children under 19 who are studying for more than 12 hours a week at school or college (excluding homework, private or unsupervised study or meal breaks), up to and including A level standard. You don't have to be the parent of the child, so long as you are responsible for him or her.

If your child has left school or college and is not entitled to SDA, income support (IS) or income-based jobseeker's allowance (JSA), you will continue to be entitled to child benefit for that child until the 'terminal date'. This is the first Monday after the end of the school holiday following his or her school leaving date (ie the first Monday in January, or the Monday after Easter Monday, or the first Monday in September). But benefit is not payable in any week in which your child works for 24 hours or more, or gets a YT allowance. Note that even though benefit is not payable in these circumstances, you remain entitled to child benefit. So, if your child stops work, or leaves the YT course during the holiday period up to the 'terminal date', and you pass the other tests, ask for a review and your child benefit will again be paid.

Once your child reaches the 'terminal date', you may continue to be entitled to child benefit during what is called the 'child benefit extension period' (CBEP). The CBEP starts from the 'terminal date' for your child. It lasts for 16 or 17 weeks for summer school or college leavers, and for 12 weeks for those who leave at Easter or Christmas.

To be entitled to child benefit during the CBEP you:
- must write asking for benefit to continue; and
- were entitled to child benefit before the CBEP began on the basis that your child was still in full-time education, or was in the holiday period up to the 'terminal date'; and

your child must be:
- under 18 and not in (or treated as being in) full-time education; and
- registered at a Careers Office for work or for training under YT; and
- not on a YT course; and

- not working for 24 hours or more a week; and
- not entitled to IS or income-based JSA.

If your child stops work, or leaves a YT course, during the CBEP, child benefit is again payable until the end of the CBEP if you and s/he pass the other tests.

Remember that many disabled 16 and 17 year olds are likely to be eligible for IS and/or SDA while they are still at school and during the CBEP. You cannot be paid child benefit for a child who receives IS or SDA.

Residence and presence
You (or your spouse) must be in Great Britain the week you claim, and have been here for 182 days or more in the 52 weeks before you claimed (with certain exceptions – see leaflet CH5). The child must also have been in Great Britain in the week you claim. You can get child benefit for 8 weeks if the child is temporarily absent abroad – see Chapter 41 for when it can be paid for longer.

From 7.10.96, you are not entitled to child benefit if you are subject to immigration control except in the following circumstances. You are entitled (if you also pass all the other conditions) if you have indefinite leave to remain in the UK or right of abode; or you have refugee status or exceptional leave to remain; or you or a member of your family are an EEA national or lawfully working in Britain and a national of Algeria, Morocco, Slovenia or Tunisia; or you came to the UK from Australia, Austria, Canada, Finland, Germany, Gibraltar, Guernsey, Isle of Man, Jersey, Mauritius, New Zealand, former Yugoslavia, or you are a national of Switzerland. If you were already being paid child benefit on 7.10.96, the new test does not apply until your child benefit is reviewed.

Other conditions
You can't get child benefit if the child is on an advanced course of education higher than A level, or sponsored by an employer or a TEC or LEC; or receiving SDA (see Chapter 13), IS or income-based JSA in his or her own right. Nor can you get it if you (or your partner) are exempt from paying UK income tax because you work in this country for a foreign government or international organisation.

Also, you may not be able to get child benefit if:
- your child is in local authority 'care' for more than 8 weeks, unless the child regularly stays with you for at least a day each week (midnight to midnight). But you can get child benefit if your child is home for seven consecutive days plus an extra one week's benefit if s/he is at home for at least a 'day' at the end of that 7 days;
- you are a foster parent to a child boarded out by a local authority or voluntary organisation and get an allowance.

I.2 For more information

You can get the following leaflets from a DSS office:
Child Benefit (CH 1)
Child Benefit for Children Away from Home (CH 4)
Social Security and Children in the Care of a Local Authority (CH 4A)
Child Benefit for People Entering Britain (CH 5)
Child Benefit for People Leaving Britain (CH 6)
Child Benefit for Children Aged 16 and Over (CH 7)
Guardian's Allowance (NI 14)
See Chapter 29 for information on services and benefits for children with disabilities.

2. How much do you get?
You get each week:
- **only/eldest qualifying child**
  higher rate   £11.05
  lone parent rate   £17.10
- **each other child**   £9.00

The lone parent rate was introduced in April 1997 and includes the former one parent benefit. It is payable for the eldest qualifying child if you do not have a married or unmarried partner living with you. If you have a partner living with you, the higher rate is payable for the eldest qualifying child.

Does anything affect what you get?
Child benefit is counted in full as income when your resources are calculated for entitlement to income support, income-based JSA, housing and council tax benefit, but is ignored when calculating entitlement to family credit and DWA.
Child dependants' additions – If you are entitled to a child dependant's addition with another benefit, such as incapacity benefit, the addition is reduced to £9.90 if you get the higher rate of child benefit for the same child. The extra amount in the lone parent rate of child benefit overlaps with child dependants' additions – you'll get £9.90 child dependant's addition for that child plus £11.05 child benefit (or for incapacity benefit and SDA, the addition will be reduced to £3.85 and child benefit will stay at £17.10).

3. Who should claim it?
The parent or other person responsible for the child must make the claim. This person must be living with the child or be contributing at least the rate of child benefit for the child's support.

If you are a married woman living with your husband, make the claim yourself. If your husband wishes to claim instead, he has to get a signed statement from you to confirm that you agree to him making the claim.

People who get child benefit are entitled to home responsibilities protection (see Chapter 45). This can protect the amount of retirement pension you may get when you retire. So if you are the parent whose National Insurance contribution record is affected because you are bringing up children, it is important that you are the parent who claims child benefit.

4. How do you claim?
Just after your baby is born, you should receive an information pack; inside will be a child benefit claim pack. If you don't receive one, you can get one by using the coupon in leaflet FB8 *Babies and Benefits* or asking at your local DSS office.

You will be asked to send the birth or adoption certificate of each child with the form, and your claim may be delayed if you don't send it. But, you only need do this for a child for whom you are claiming child benefit for the first time.

Send the claim form and the birth or adoption certificate, if required, to the *Child Benefit Centre, (Washington), Newcastle upon Tyne, NE88 1BR*.

Don't delay making your claim. It can only be backdated for 3 months from the date the DSS receives your claim. If you made your claim before 7.4.97, child benefit could be backdated for 6 months.

5. What happens after you claim?
The birth or adoption certificate will be returned to you within a short time, and you will be sent a written decision on your claim. If it is successful, you will be told that an order book or benefit payment card is being sent to the post office you have chosen. Collect the book or payment card right away, or you

may lose money. You have the choice of payment direct into a bank or building society account – but only on a 4-weekly basis. If the claim isn't successful, or is stopped at a later stage, you can appeal against the decision within 3 months of the refusal date.

Weekly or 4-weekly payments?
You are generally paid child benefit every four weeks in arrears. You may get weekly payments if:
- you were receiving child benefit on 15.3.82 and chose to stick to weekly payments; or
- you are entitled to the lone parent rate of child benefit; or
- you are getting income support, income-based JSA, family credit or disability working allowance; or
- 4-weekly payments are causing you hardship.

You need to write to the DSS to say you prefer weekly payments.

28 Family credit

1. What is family credit?
Family credit is a means-tested benefit for working people on low wages who have children. Family credit is paid in addition to the family's normal weekly income and each award normally lasts for 26 weeks. For couples, the woman makes the claim and is paid any family credit for the family. DSS leaflet NI 261 *A Guide to Family Credit* gives full details. If you have any queries, call the Family Credit Helpline 01253 500050.

Family credit is a gateway to some other types of help, such as free prescriptions, dental treatment, fares to hospital and vouchers for glasses.

Disability working allowance – If you are eligible for disability working allowance (DWA), depending on your circumstances, you could get up to £50.85 a week more on DWA than on family credit. If you've claimed family credit and had a decision to award you benefit, you can't normally switch to DWA until the end of your family credit award – see Chapter 16.

2. Do you qualify?
There are 5 key qualifying conditions for family credit. At the time you claim:
- you, or your partner, must normally be working for 16 or more hours a week;
- you, or your partner, must be responsible for a child who lives with you;
- you must be in Great Britain without restrictions on your right to remain (but see below), and your partner ordinarily resident in the UK;
- you and your partner must not have savings or capital of over £8,000;
- your income must be within a set limit, which varies according to your family circumstances.

All of the rules outlined below depend on your circumstances at the time you make a claim for family credit.

Working 16 or more hours a week
Either you or your partner if you have one, must normally work as an employee or self-employed person for an average of 16 or more hours a week. You (or your partner) must have worked for at least 16 hours in the week you claim, or in either of the two previous weeks. If you have just started work, you can qualify if you are expected to work 16 or more hours in the week after your week of claim.

You'll be treated as being 'normally engaged' in that work if, in the week in which your claim reaches the DSS, you are engaged in that work and are likely to work for 5 or more weeks. If you take a casual job for less than 5 weeks, you may be excluded from both income support and family credit.

Work that you do on a training scheme while getting a training allowance does not count. Nor does it count if you are paid by a health authority, local authority or voluntary organisation to provide respite care in your own home for someone who does not normally live with you.

Some disabled workers can choose between claiming family credit or income support – you must be working for 16 or more hours a week but not count as being in remunerative work for income support purposes – see Chapter 3(6).

Responsible for a child
A child is someone aged under 16; or under 19 if s/he is still in full-time, non-advanced education. If a child normally lives with you, you'll be treated as responsible for the child even if s/he is elsewhere at the time of claim. If s/he has been in hospital or residential accommodation during the 12 weeks before your claim, you must still be in regular contact with him or her.

If there is a question about which household a child normally lives in, s/he is treated as living with the person who has claimed or gets child benefit for him or her. If no-one has claimed or gets child benefit, then s/he is treated as living with the person who has 'primary responsibility' for him or her.

Generally, you don't count as being responsible for a child who has been placed with you by social services or certain other organisations acting under the powers in a number of Acts listed in the Family Credit Regulations: eg where you are fostering a child. If in doubt, ask the Family Credit Helpline to run through these rules.

In Great Britain
You must be both present and ordinarily resident in GB (England, Wales and Scotland). If you have a partner, s/he must be ordinarily resident in the UK (GB and Northern Ireland). Your (or your partner's) earnings must at least in part come from work in the UK. If one of you works in an EEA country, there are special rules – see Box L.3 in Chapter 41.

Family credit in Northern Ireland comes under separate legislation. The rules are the same except the claimant must be ordinarily resident in NI; any partner must be ordinarily resident in the UK; and earnings must come from work in the UK or the Republic of Ireland.

If you have any restrictions on your right to reside in GB, you are not entitled unless you or a member of your family is an EEA national (see Chapter 41) or lawfully working and a national of Algeria, Morocco, Slovenia or Tunisia, or you have refugee status or exceptional leave to remain.

Capital
If you (or your partner) have capital of over £8,000, you won't be entitled to family credit. A child's capital is not added to your own. However, if a child has over £3,000 capital, s/he won't be included in the assessment; but s/he will still be regarded as part of the family in order to satisfy the rule that you must be responsible for a child.

If your capital is from £3,000.01 to £8,000, it is treated as producing a 'tariff' income (see Chapter 3(29)).

Your capital is worked out in the same way as for income support: some types of capital don't count (eg business assets or the home you live in). Chapter 3(30) and (31) give details. There are two main differences from income support. If you have sold any business asset, and intend to reinvest the proceeds in your business within 13 weeks of the sale (or a longer period, if that is reasonable) those proceeds will also be ignored as capital. If a relative is living in other premises which you own, the value of those premises will be ignored only if s/he has been incapacitated throughout the 13 weeks immediately before you claim family credit; or if s/he is aged 60 or over. Also, a Back to Work Bonus and a Child Maintenance Bonus is ignored for 52 weeks from the date it's paid.

Income
Your earnings are taken into account net of tax, National Insurance contributions and half of any contributions to an occupational or personal pension scheme. Income is worked out in broadly the same way as for income support: eg disability living allowance is ignored as income. Chapter 3(24) to (28) gives full details.

However there are a number of differences in the way in which your earnings and other income are treated for family credit purposes. We have listed the important ones below. If you are not sure how an item of income is treated for family credit purposes, ask the Family Credit Helpline for details.

- Your normal weekly earnings are assessed, using a fixed formula, by looking at the 6 weeks (weekly paid) or 3 months (monthly paid) before the week your claim reaches the DSS. But if the AO thinks you have chosen to work less hours in this period than you normally would, they can look at the 6 weeks or 3 months earlier instead, unless you can show your intention was not to gain more family credit.
- If you are self-employed, the AO will usually look at 6 out of the last 7 calendar months or at your last year's set of accounts, if they cover a 6–15 month period and the accounting period ended during the year before your claim.
- A child's earnings are ignored completely.
- Statutory sick pay counts as earnings. Statutory maternity pay is completely ignored in the assessment.
- If you have a boarder, what s/he pays you counts as earnings only if those payments form a 'major part' of your total income which is taken into account in the family credit assessment. Otherwise, those payments will be treated as 'other income' and £20 plus half of the rest of each payment from a boarder will be ignored in the family credit assessment.
- **Childcare costs:** up to £60 a week childcare costs can be deducted from your earnings. You can have childcare costs deducted if:
  - you are a lone parent; or
  - you **and** your partner are both working 16 or more hours a week; or
  - you **or** your partner are working and the other is 'incapacitated'.

  The disregard only applies to charges paid for care of children under 11 by a registered childminder, or nursery or playscheme, or for children aged 8 to 10 attending a scheme such as an after school club or holiday playscheme. See Chapter 16(3) for more details. From 7.10.97, help with childcare costs is extended. If you claim family credit before the first Tuesday in September following your child's 11th birthday, you will still be eligible for the childcare disregard.
- Child benefit, guardian's allowance, income support, income-based JSA, maternity allowance, housing and council tax benefit are all ignored as income.
- If a child's own income (but not a maintenance payment made to that child) is higher than the appropriate maximum credit for that child, the extra is ignored.
- Maintenance payments are taken into account in family credit but the first £15 you receive each week is ignored when benefit is calculated.

If you get regular maintenance payments, the amount actually received is taken into account. If maintenance isn't paid regularly, or the amounts are not regular, the average payment over the previous 13 weeks is taken into account. If maintenance has been assessed by the Child Support Agency, the amount taken into account will never be more than that assessment (less the £15 disregard).

3. How is family credit worked out?
If your net income is below or equal to a prescribed limit, called the 'applicable amount', you'll be entitled to the maximum family credit for your family circumstances.

If your net income is higher than the applicable amount, 70% of your extra net income is deducted from the maximum family credit for your family circumstances.

Applicable amount
There is just one figure: £77.15 a week.

If your income is over £77.15 a week, work out 70% of your extra income. Now add up the maximum family credit for your family. The credits for children depend on their ages. Add one '30 hours credit' if you and/or your partner work 30 hours or more each week. You deduct 70% of your extra income from the maximum family credit for your family – this gives your family credit entitlement.

Maximum family credit

Lone parent or couple	£47.65
Child * aged 18	£34.70
aged 16 or 17	£24.80
aged 11 to 15	£19.95
aged 0 to 10	£12.05
30 hours credit	£10.55

Example – You have two children aged 10 and 12, and your partner works 35 hours a week earning £177.15. Earnings are £100 higher than the applicable amount of £77.15. Maximum family credit is £90.20. Take 70% of the difference between earnings and applicable amount: 70% of £100 is £70. Deducting £70 from the maximum family credit of £90.20 leaves £20.20. You get £20.20 family credit a week.

Minimum payment – The smallest payment of family credit is 50p per week.

* **Changes from 7.10.97** – Currently the amount included for your child depends on whether they have reached their 11th, 16th or 18th birthday by the beginning of your family credit claim. From 7.10.97, the amount will depend on whether you claim before or after the first Tuesday in September following their 11th or 16th birthday. The age 18 band is abolished. Instead, the age 16 to 17 age band is extended up to the day before the child's 19th birthday. For example if your child's 11th birthday is on 31.10.97, you'll get £12.05 included for them if you claim before 1.9.98. The amount will go up to £19.95 if you claim or renew your claim on or after 1.9.98. But if your child is already aged 11, 16 or 18 before 7.10.97, the amounts are assessed under the old rules on any renewal claim made before 1.9.98.

4. How do you claim?
Claims are made by post. You can get a family credit claim pack by phoning the Family Credit Helpline on 01253 500050, or by contacting the local DSS office. You can also get a claim pack from post offices although this may delay your claim. In

Britain, send it to: *DSS, Family Credit Unit, Government Buildings, 1 Cop Lane, Penwortham, Preston, PR1 0SN.* In Northern Ireland, send it to: *Family Credit Branch, DSS, Castle Court, Royal Avenue, Belfast BT1 1DF.*

You can have your claim and payment dealt with more quickly if you're just about to start work or started in the last 5 weeks. Contact a Client Adviser at the Jobcentre if you've been signing on, otherwise ask at your local DSS about fast track family credit.

Don't delay returning the form or you may lose some benefit. So long as you send in all of the information asked for on the claim form (such as payslips) within one month, your claim should be backdated to the day you first contacted the DSS – see Chapter 52(2) for details. You can either send in payslips or ask your employer to fill in form FCS500 (enclosed in the claim pack). If you do neither, the DSS will write to your employer asking for details about your earnings. If you are self-employed and cannot send in your accounts straightaway, the DSS will write to you for more information.

If you qualify for some family credit, it will be paid at the same rate, normally for 26 weeks, whether or not your family circumstances or the benefit rates change during that time. However, it will end sooner if:
- there is only one young person in the family aged 16 or over who is included in the family credit award and that person leaves full-time, non-advanced education;
- a reduced benefit direction from the Child Support Agency is given, ends or is suspended – see Chapter 50;
- someone else claims income support, income-based JSA or family credit in respect of a child who was included in your award of family credit;
- if the claimant dies: unless s/he is survived by his or her partner who can continue to receive the family credit until the end of the award;
- you get DWA awarded for a period beginning before the start of the family credit award.

Payment – You can choose to be paid by an order book or by direct credit transfer straight into a bank or other account. Orders can be cashed weekly in arrears at a post office. Credit transfer payments are credited to your account every 4 weeks in arrears. Awards of £4 a week or less will be payable in a lump sum.

Appeals – You can appeal to a Social Security Appeal Tribunal against any decision made by an Adjudication Officer about anything to do with your family credit. The letter giving you the decision will outline your rights of appeal. See Chapter 52 for more details.

Reviews – Reviews are also possible under the normal rules (see Chapter 52). However, you cannot get a review just because your circumstances have changed. Instead, you have to show that the Adjudication Officer didn't have full or accurate details about your circumstances at the time of claim, or applied the law wrongly.

29 Children with disabilities

A. THE FAMILY FUND

The Family Fund is run by the Joseph Rowntree Foundation and is financed by the Government. Its job is to help families caring for a severely disabled child under the age of 16, by giving a lump sum grant for specific items which arise from the care of the child.

1. Do you qualify?
Any family caring for a child under the age of 16 with a severe physical or learning disability, sensory impairment or chronic condition, and living at home with them may apply for help from the Family Fund. The Fund is discretionary but works within general guidelines agreed upon with the Government. New applicants are asked to complete a simple form about income and savings. You cannot get help for a foster child in the care of a local authority.

2. What kind of help is there?
The Fund's purpose is to relieve stress arising from the day to day care of a disabled child. It is not to replace the help available from your health or local authority but to complement it, though occasionally help will be given with items that local authorities could provide. There is no set list to choose from: **ask for whatever you most need**. The most common choices are for help with laundry equipment for a child who causes extra washing; clothing, bedding and footwear if these get worn out quickly; a holiday for the whole family; recreation equipment for a child who is difficult to amuse; outings; and help with transport if your child is difficult to take out but doesn't qualify for the higher rate of DLA mobility component. But the choice is yours and anything you feel would make life easier for your family will be considered.

If you want a clear idea about the ways in which the Family Fund might help, further details are available from the Fund. The Fund also produces a series of information sheets, eg for families with a deaf or a hyperactive child, notes about transport, holidays, bedding, benefits, etc.

3. Applying to the Family Fund
You can get an application form from the *Family Fund, PO Box 50, York YO1 2ZX.*

After they get your application, the Family Fund will ask one of their visitors to arrange to see you if it is the first time you've applied. The visitor will discuss your application with you in greater detail. You will be notified as soon as possible about the outcome of your application.

If your application is refused, you may appeal by reapplying to the Fund, giving as much information and evidence as possible as to why your application is justified. This will be re-examined with any new evidence or changes in your circumstances which you can put forward. If you still do not agree with their decision, you can take it to the Management Board of the Fund.

B. BENEFITS FOR DEPENDENT CHILDREN

If your child is disabled, you may be entitled to some or all of the benefits or services described in other chapters in this Handbook. Your right to some benefits or services will depend only on the effect of your child's disability. Your right to others will depend on your own financial, or other, circumstances. The benefits checklist at the front of the Handbook is a quick guide to the sort of help available. In this chapter we highlight some of the specific help for disabled children.

Many parents mistakenly fail to claim all the cash or practical help that they, or their disabled child, are entitled to. If you read about something in this Handbook and think you might qualify – go ahead and make a claim. If you are turned down and disagree with the decision – go ahead and appeal. Your local Citizens Advice Bureau may be able to help you with this.

4. Income support, JSA, housing benefit

If your child is under 16, s/he is dependent on you and cannot claim income support (IS) or SDA in his or her own right. However, if your income is less than your 'applicable amount' (a set amount representing your family's weekly living needs), you may as a family be entitled to income support, or income-based jobseeker's allowance (JSA) if you are required to sign on for work. Your savings must be no more than £8,000, and if you work, that must be less than 16 hours a week. If you have a partner, s/he must not be working 24 hours a week or more. You are not required to sign on as available for work if you are a lone parent or your child gets the middle or higher rate of disability living allowance care component (see Box B.1 in Chapter 3).

If you don't qualify for IS or income-based JSA, perhaps because your income is higher than your 'applicable amount', you may still qualify for housing or council tax benefit whether or not you are working. Your savings must be no more than £16,000.

Your resources and needs are assessed in much the same way in these schemes. Chapter 3 covers income support, Chapter 14 covers JSA while Chapter 4 deals with the housing and council tax benefit assessments, highlighting any differences from income support.

A disabled child premium is included in the assessment for each child who is registered as blind or gets disability living allowance (DLA). If you or your partner are entitled to invalid care allowance, a carer premium is included in the assessment. These are included on top of the family premium.

A child's own capital is ignored totally when working out your savings for the capital limits. But if s/he has savings of over £3,000, your assessment won't include the personal allowance or disabled child premium for that child. But neither will it include any of that child's income (other than maintenance payments) – see Chapter 3(24). Some types of capital are ignored – see Chapter 3(31).

If a child's own income (apart from maintenance payments) is higher than his or her personal allowance (and any disabled child premium), the extra income is ignored.

Income support and income-based JSA can include help with mortgage interest payments. You can also have included in your assessment, interest on a loan used to adapt your home for the special needs of your disabled child. If you need adaptations in the home, check first to see if you can get help from social services (Chapter 32) or a disabled facilities grant from your local housing authority (Chapter 49).

> **I.3 For more information**
>
> The DSS produce helpful leaflets: *Babies and benefits* (FB8); *Bringing up children?* (FB27); *Caring for someone?* (FB31).
>
> If your child is coming up to 16, you may also find a free booklet called *After Age 16 – What Next?* written by the Family Fund, very useful. It is full of practical advice on education and training opportunities as well as information on benefits and services. Available from the *Family Fund, PO Box 50, York, YO1 2ZX*. Another publication called *The Next Step* was written with a group of young disabled people for anyone reaching school-leaving age – available from the same address.
>
> Some local Social Services Departments publish their own guide to facilities for disabled children in the area.

5. Social fund

If you get income support or income-based JSA, you may be able to get a community care grant from the social fund – see Chapter 7. Often the needs of disabled children are given a high priority.

6. DWA and family credit

If you are disabled and working for 16 or more hours a week, you may qualify for disability working allowance (DWA). Your savings must be no more than £16,000. An allowance for a disabled child is included in the assessment if your child is registered blind or gets DLA. See Chapter 16.

If you or your partner are working 16 or more hours a week, you may qualify for family credit – see Chapter 28. Your savings must be no more than £8,000.

For both DWA and family credit, the amount you get depends on the level of your earnings. You may have up to £60 a week disregarded from earnings for childcare costs for children under age 11 – see Chapter 16(3).

7. Invalid care allowance

If your child gets the middle or higher rate of DLA care component, you can get invalid care allowance (ICA) for looking after her or him. ICA is not means tested but if you are working, you must not earn more than £50 a week. See Chapter 19.

8. Disability living allowance

DLA provides help with the extra costs of bringing up a disabled child. It is paid on top of any other income you may have, and also gives you access to other kinds of help.

DLA care component

This is payable from 3 months old, if your child needs far more help than a non-disabled child of the same age (or from birth if s/he is terminally ill). Chapter 17 deals with the main rules for DLA. We look at how these apply to under 2 year olds below.

Under 2s – *The Disability Handbook* (see Box G.6 in Chapter 17) gives guidance to DSS doctors about the care needs of under 2 year olds. It points out that all young babies require extensive care and that mobility inevitably leads to increased supervision needs. Thus even though your child may have had a specific disability or condition diagnosed, that does not necessarily mean that s/he will also qualify for DLA care component at that stage. Ironically, if your child is not mobile that reduces his/her supervision needs – but it may increase other needs, or lead to other needs at a later stage. For example, if you routinely have to carry your 1–2 year old from room to room. Remember that what counts for the care component is the practical effect of that disability in terms of the child's needs for personal care, supervision or watching over. For a child under 16, such requirements must also be substantially in excess of what is *'normally required'* by a child of the same age.

The guidance in the *Disability Handbook* essentially rests on the incidence of non-standard interventions or actions which the child requires because of his or her disability. For example, all babies require feeding, but if your baby has severe feeding problems or requires feeding parenterally or by gastrointestinal tube, s/he would be likely to qualify for the care component.

Babies with disabilities which involve or require the following types of actions or interventions are also likely to qualify: frequent losses of consciousness; fits which are secondary to asphyxia at birth or to a rare metabolic disease; breathing difficulties or airways problems: regular mechanical suction, regular administration of oxygen, tracheotomy; dealing with a gastrostomy, ileostomy, jejunostomy, colostomy, or nephrostomy; stimulating severely hearing or vision-impaired babies; caring for babies with severe multiple disabilities.

Further examples are given of children whose care needs may increase from age 1. Children with brittle bones or haemophilia at risk of fractures or haemorrhage from bumps and falls; mobile children with hearing or visual problems who cannot respond to a warning shout or see a potential danger; children with cerebral palsy with impeded mobility who need their parents to change their position frequently to reduce the risk of postural deformity; children with severe learning disabilities who need extra stimulation to maximise their potential, or who eat undesirable substances or mutilate themselves.

The guidance stresses that this is not an exhaustive list. For example, it does not mention the care needs created by severe eczema/ichthyosiform erythroderma and similar skin conditions. These can often involve a substantial amount of extra care, eg frequent bathing, nappy changing, applying preparations and dressings, comforting a child whose sleep is disturbed.

If your child qualifies for the care component and it seems that the condition(s) giving rise to a need for help are likely to continue, the Adjudication Officer at the DSS may well make an award until the 6th birthday. This is to avoid undue stress on parents and to enable the child's care needs to be reassessed after the end of the first year at school. An award for a very severely disabled child with considerable and lasting care needs can be for life.

Refused DLA care component? – If your child is refused the care component, or awarded only the lower rate, seek advice and ask for a review. Even if you are not successful on review, or on a later appeal, you will get written reasons for that decision. These reasons may give you a clear picture of why the current claim failed. The reasons may also give you some idea of the type of changes which might lead to entitlement in the future. If s/he does not qualify now, s/he may well qualify at a later stage in childhood. The borderline between entitlement and non-entitlement, and between the different rates, is always difficult to assess, so, if s/he has not been awarded the care component, it is sensible to seek expert advice, make regular claims, and if the claim is again unsuccessful, ask for a review.

DLA mobility component
This can be paid from the age of 5 years. The lower rate mobility component has an extra disability test for children under 16 – see Chapter 17(20).

30 Young people with disabilities

1. Becoming a claimant
Once your child reaches 16, s/he can claim income maintenance benefits in her or his own right, even though s/he may still be at school. Most 16 and 17 year olds cannot get income support (IS); but many severely disabled 16 and 17 year olds do qualify for IS. Read Chapter 3 – this chapter just gives a brief sketch of the IS rules.

Appointee or agent?
Disability living allowance (DLA) is a personal benefit. Although someone will have acted as the appointee, your child was the DLA claimant. At 16, the need for an appointee will be reviewed. If s/he is able to act for him or herself, your appointment to act for your child will end. If s/he is mentally capable of handling her own affairs, but is physically unable to manage them, s/he can nominate someone to act as agent in order to collect benefit payments. Ask the DSS for details.

If s/he continues to need an appointee, that appointment will now be for all social security benefits, rather than restricted to DLA.

Disability living allowance
DLA may be awarded for any period: from 6 months to life. It should only stop at the 16th birthday if the Adjudication Officer thought a renewal claim would be necessary to review the care and/or mobility needs.

DLA care component and the lower rate mobility component each have an extra test for children under 16. This ends on the 16th birthday – your child no longer has to show that his or her care, supervision, and/or guidance needs are much greater than those of a non-disabled person.

If your child has to make a renewal claim at 16, be careful. Some people have lost benefit even though the disability tests become easier at 16. Don't assume that s/he will automatically continue to get the same rate as before. Read Chapter 17 again before you fill in the claim form.

Late claims
If you, or your child, miss claiming severe disablement allowance (SDA) or income support (IS) from her 16th birthday, you may be able to recover arrears of benefit. A claim for SDA, can be backdated automatically for 3 months. To get up to 3 months arrears of IS, your child has to have 'special reasons' for a delayed claim – see Chapter 52(4).

2. Severe disablement allowance (SDA)
If your child is approaching 16 years of age and is unlikely to be able to work because of illness or disability, s/he can claim SDA. This is an income, as of right, to people who have not been able to work and build up an entitlement to incapacity benefit through the National Insurance system. SDA can be paid from your child's 16th birthday. Chapter 13 gives full details.

SDA is currently £37.75 a week, with an extra age allowance of £13.15 a week if the current period of incapacity began before the age of 40. Getting SDA is one way of qualifying for the disability premium. SDA is less than the IS personal allowance for a 16–17 year old who qualifies for the disability premium, so s/he should always claim IS as well.

3. 'Normal' schooling and SDA
If your child is under 19 and still at school or undergoing full-time education, her (or his) entitlement to SDA also depends on the type and hours of schooling received.

S/he still has to meet the basic condition of entitlement. To show that s/he is 'incapable of work' s/he will have to pass the 'all work' test of incapacity, unless s/he is exempt. People with severe learning difficulties are exempt. For more details of the all work test and who is exempt, see Chapter 8. (This test was introduced in 1995 and does not apply to people whose SDA has been paid since before 13.4.95.)

S/he can get SDA so long as s/he attends classes or periods of supervised study adding up to less than 21 hours a week. Lunch breaks, breaks between lessons, free periods, and periods of private (unsupervised) study or homework do not count.

If s/he attends classes for less then 21 hours, the type of education s/he receives and the school s/he attends make no difference to SDA.

If s/he attends classes for 21 hours or more each week, s/he may still qualify for SDA if the extra hours of classes would not be *'suitable for persons of the same age and sex who do not suffer from a physical or mental disability'*.

A Commissioner's decision, R(S)2/87, looks at this definition: it establishes that the methods of teaching may make a course unsuitable for a non-disabled person. This is a key decision for deaf or blind teenagers, as well as those who have other verbal or written communication difficulties.

When adding up the hours of instruction, you ignore the time spent on any course that would not routinely be followed by a non-disabled person of the same age or sex. You are looking at both what is taught, and at how it is taught. If special teaching (eg speech practice) or special methods (eg use of braille texts) are integrated into all lessons, you don't have to quantify the 'non-suitable' hours precisely. It is enough if the 'balance of probabilities' shows that any 'suitable' hours are less than 21 a week.

For a teenager with learning disabilities whose mental age is well below their physical age, the whole of their course would not be suitable for a non-disabled person of the same age. In other cases (and where a teenager is in an integrated class with non-disabled pupils of the same age), you may have to look more closely at the nature of the course.

For example, if s/he is deaf and has to receive extra hours of English and Mathematics, those extra hours are only necessary because of her deafness – so they should be ignored. The point is that you wouldn't expect to find a non-disabled 16 year old of the same general intelligence doing all those extra hours of English and Maths.

The fact that s/he may be following a GCSE course does not automatically mean that the course is 'suitable' for a non-disabled teenager. The methods of teaching may make it unsuitable. Or the particular course may be spread over, say, 2 or 3 years, whereas normally it would take 1 or 2 years, or would normally be taught, in that way, to a slightly younger age group.

Even though your child may not be able to qualify for SDA, s/he could well meet the easier qualifying test for income support – see below.

4. Income support (IS)

At 16 a disabled child can claim IS in her or his own right, whether she or he is at home, still at school or attending a training centre – see Chapter 3(4) and (5) for full details. Even though 16-17 year olds are generally excluded from IS, many disabled teenagers should still qualify.

If s/he is still at school, s/he just has to show that because of her mental or physical disability, s/he would be unlikely to get a job within the next year, if s/he left school now and signed on for work. S/he does not have to prove s/he is 'incapable of work'. The IS test is wider – it looks at your current job prospects given your disability.

However, if s/he has left school, s/he does have to show that s/he is incapable of work. This is assessed under the own occupation test, or all work test of incapacity unless s/he is exempt – see Chapter 8.

At 16 a child living with you in your home, or at a boarding school, will usually qualify for an IS personal allowance of £29.60. However, if s/he qualifies for the disability premium of £20.95, s/he will be entitled to a higher personal allowance of £38.90. This brings his or her IS 'applicable amount' up to £59.85 pw – £8.95 a week higher than SDA.

Capital
Once your child reaches 16 the rules about capital change if s/he makes a claim for IS in her or his own right. If s/he has over £3,000, a 'tariff' income is assumed. However, capital in a trust fund, set up from a payment made because of a personal or criminal injury to the child, is disregarded indefinitely. See Chapter 3(31). The capital limits are higher for people living in a residential care home – see Chapter 36(5).

5. IS or SDA; or both?
Some people won't have this choice in the first place. If your child's capital is above the IS limit of £8,000, s/he can only claim SDA. If your child is still at school, the hours and type of education s/he receives may rule out SDA, even though it makes no difference to his or her IS entitlement.

The best advice is simple: claim both IS and SDA when your child is 16. If the IS assessment includes the £20.95 disability premium, s/he can get £8.95 a week from IS to top-up the £50.90 from SDA.

6. Child benefit
If a child between the age of 16 and 19 is receiving SDA or IS, you cannot claim child benefit as well, even though s/he may still be at school. When your child is awarded SDA or IS, the arrears will be reduced to take account of any child benefit you have received for your child for the same period.

31 Financing studies

1. Student grants
Grants may be available from your local education authority (LEA), or the equivalent in Scotland and Northern Ireland, for courses such as GCSE and A levels, diplomas and first degrees. There are two types of student grant – mandatory awards and discretionary awards. Post-graduate courses throughout the UK are covered by the British Academy or Research Councils. For a free booklet giving details of student grants see Box I.5.

Mandatory awards
Mandatory awards can only be given for designated courses. Designated courses are those full-time courses, including sandwich courses and certain part-time courses of initial teacher training (ITT), provided by a UK university or other publicly funded UK college leading to a first degree, Diploma in Higher Education, a Higher National Diploma or a Post-Graduate Certificate of Education (PGCE) or other post-graduate course of ITT. Your college can advise you if the course you wish to attend is a designated course. You are automatically entitled to a mandatory award if you are attending a designated course and meet certain basic qualifying conditions. However, the amount you get is subject to a means test.

In England and Wales apply to the LEA in the area you live in before you start the course. In Northern Ireland most student grants are the responsibility of the five Local Education and Library Boards. Mandatory awards are calculated the same way as for England and Wales. If you live in Scotland, the Student Awards Agency for Scotland administers student allowances which are similar to mandatory awards. The main difference in Scotland is that travel expenses in excess of the fixed travel component (see Box I.4) can be reclaimed annually on a form available from colleges in December.

If you take time out (intercalate) from your course, for

example, due to illness, your grant will normally stop. However, the LEA has discretion to continue to pay your grant during your absence although few do. Your grant will not usually be paid if you have to repeat part of your course, for example, due to exam failure. However, your grant can be paid for a repeat period which is due to illness or disability.

Calculating mandatory awards – Mandatory awards are made up of two parts, tuition fees which are always paid, and a subsistence allowance which is means tested. The means-tested part means that a contribution towards your grant may be assessed from your parents if you are under 25, or from your spouse (but not from an unmarried partner).

Your own income is also taken into account subject to a basic disregard of £800 a year. However some social security benefits, but not all, are ignored in the calculation. Benefits ignored include income support, housing benefit, disability living allowance, severe disablement allowance, incapacity benefit and child benefit. Any earnings you have during your course are ignored.

The subsistence allowance of a mandatory award is made up of: a basic rate including a set amount for rent, travel, books and equipment (see Box I.4); an extra week's allowance if the term time at your college is more than 30 weeks and 3 days in the academic year (25 weeks and 3 days at Oxford and Cambridge); a dependant's addition for any children, partner or other adult financially dependent on you.

Disabled students' allowance – Disabled students who receive a mandatory award (or Scottish student allowance) can claim this special allowance. However, if you have a discretionary award, the LEA does not have to pay it (unless you are attending a designated course) but it is worth claiming as some LEAs do. Ask for advice – see Box I.5.

The disabled students' allowance comes on top of the normal grant up to a maximum which depends on the type of cost. It is for any additional disability-related costs of study. It is up to local authorities to decide whether the particular cost is necessarily incurred, but go ahead and claim if in doubt. For rates, see Box I.4.

LEAs have in the past met claims for typewriters, microcomputers, tape-recorders and other special equipment, extra heating and dietary needs, and help with readers, note takers, other paid helpers, and extra aids. If you need something because of both your disability and your course, claim it, but some authorities are more generous than others.

The disabled students' allowance is not intended to cover extra travel costs. Some disabled students have heavy travelling costs because of their disability and, where they have a mandatory award and the costs have been necessarily incurred for a course, the LEA must meet the travel costs above the travel element in the basic maintenance grant.

Discretionary awards
If the course you attend is not a designated course, or if it is but you do not meet the basic qualifying conditions for a mandatory award, you can only claim a discretionary award. These range from a full award (ie the same as a mandatory grant) to a small payment for fees only. Discretionary awards can be very difficult to get. Contact your LEA for details. LEAs must consider each individual request on its merits. LEAs are often sympathetic towards disabled students so give full details of your disability and any special needs in your grant application. Organisations like SKILL and RADAR can give useful advice and may be able to help with your application (see Box I.5 and our address list). In Northern Ireland, discretionary awards are the responsibility of the Local Education and Library Boards. In Scotland, LEAs administer student bursaries which are similar to discretionary awards.

If you want to take a further education course and have special needs, contact either the LEA Specialist Careers Officer or the college's Student Services Officer. Each of them can outline any grants or financial and practical help which may be available for the course you hope to take.

The Further Education Funding Councils (England and Wales) and the Further Education Funding Unit (part of the Scottish Office Education and Industry Department) have power to fund a wide range of activities and facilities to support students with learning disabilities.

2. Student loans

State-funded loans are available to students in full-time higher education, but not to students starting courses after their 50th birthday nor for post-graduate courses, apart from the PGCE. The loans are not means-tested.

Applications are made via the college once you have started the course. The loans are administered by the Student Loans Company Ltd (SLC) and normally paid by credit transfer.

For maximum loans, see Box I.4. For further details of student loans, contact the *Student Loans Company Ltd, 100 Bothwell Street, Glasgow, G2 7JD (Helpline 0800 405010)* or consult the booklet published by the relevant government education department: addresses in Box I.5. Your college or student union can also advise.

Loans become repayable in April after the end of the course or when you abandon it. Repayments are normally made in 60 monthly instalments (or 84, if your course was for 5 or more years). If you receive a disability-related benefit, the SLC has discretion to give you longer to repay a loan, or to defer the start of your repayments. You can defer repayments for at least 12 months once the SLC is satisfied that your gross monthly income is not over 85% of average gross national earnings. Disability-related benefits are not counted as income. The SLC will consider deducting disability-related costs when working out your gross monthly income. However, interest continues to accrue during any period of deferment.

For vocational courses in Great Britain, the Government has established the Career Development Loans scheme. These loans are offered by several high street banks. There is no equivalent scheme in Northern Ireland. The DfEE pays the interest on loans during the course. Loans are usually for a maximum of two years, and of between £200 and £8,000. More information is available by telephone on Freeline 0800 585 505 or in writing from *Career Development Loans, Freepost, Newcastle upon Tyne X, NE85 1BR*.

3. Access and hardship funds

The government has created access funds to provide additional emergency financial help but only to full-time students attending publicly-funded colleges. There are separate funds for post-graduate, undergraduate and further education (which has a minimum age of 19) students. The access funds are administered by colleges who are allocated a fixed sum by government each year. Each college has its own rules on how it allocates access funds. So ask your student union, personal tutor or welfare office for help in making a claim.

Colleges may also have their own hardship funds in addition to the government access funds. Ask for information at your college.

4. Income support

Chapter 3 deals with the main rules for income support. Chapter 30 looks at the position of disabled teenagers under 19 who are at school or doing non-advanced courses. Here we look at the position of disabled students who are under 19 but on an advanced course, or over 19 and in full-time education (advanced or non-advanced). We also look at the separate provisions for unemployed people doing part-time study – see 5 below. For full details, ask your student union or an advice centre. If you are one of a couple and your partner is not also a student, s/he may be eligible for benefit in the normal way.

Full-time courses
Most students attending a full-time course are excluded from income support (IS) until the end of their course – during the long vacations as well as the rest of the time. The exclusion stops once the course finally ends (or until you abandon it or are dismissed from it). However it can be difficult to determine if a particular course (especially if it is 'modular') can be described as full time for benefit purposes. Additional problems can arise if you transfer from full-time to part-time attendance on the same course or take time out (intercalate) from the course. If you are in this position, seek specialist advice.

However, lone parents (including lone foster parents), disabled students, students who are entitled to a disabled students' allowance because of deafness, pensioners, people getting a state training allowance, refugees on a course learning English, and certain people from abroad who have a temporary problem in getting funds from their usual source are eligible for IS during term time and all vacations. Student couples with a child can get IS in the long vacations.

You will count as a disabled student if your applicable amount includes a disability premium or severe disability premium. For students claiming a disability premium who don't have a qualifying benefit (such as DLA or SDA) you have to be incapable of work for 52 weeks before the premium is paid. But after 28 weeks of incapacity for work you will count as a disabled student and thus be eligible for income support. Chapter 8 has details about how incapacity for work is assessed.

If you are a deaf student, you should claim the disabled students' allowance even if you know that the grants means-test will result in no award. So long as you have an underlying entitlement to the disabled students' allowance, you will be eligible for IS while a student.

Income – Where the parents or spouse of a disabled student are unable or unwilling to meet their contribution to a grant in full, only the actual contribution is taken into account.

The following parts of the grant are ignored as income: extra expenditure because of your disability; travel costs; books and non-specialist equipment (unless a higher or lower amount is earmarked for this purpose in your grant); tuition or exam fees; a 'two homes grant'; and a grant to cover extra costs because you are on a term-time residential course away from your normal college (etc). The following maximum disregards apply to students' other weekly income:
- £5 – covenant income above the level of the standard maintenance grant;
- £10 – student loan treated as income if the student could obtain it, whether or not they have done so;
- £20 – regular voluntary or charitable payments but this £20 maximum takes into account any covenant or loan income disregarded.

For example, if you are entitled to a student loan of up to £1,000, you'll be assumed to have a weekly income of £19.23 (over 52 weeks), no matter how much, if anything, you have borrowed. £10 can be disregarded but £9.23 will be cut from your benefit. As it uses up your £10 disregard, any charitable payment over £10 a week will count as income.

The maximum student loan for your situation is taken into account as income over 52/53 weeks, unless it is a one-year course, or you are in the final year of a course, when the loan is taken into account over the period from the start of the academic year to the end of the course. Repaying the loan does not enable a review of your past benefit entitlement. Note that student loans are treated differently for health benefits – see Chapter 48.

Once you've completed the course, any grant, loan or covenant income is disregarded. If you cease to be a student before the end of your course, any grant or loan which has to be repaid continues to be taken into account as income until you've repaid it or until the end of the term or vacation when you left the course.

Career Development Loans are disregarded for IS (and other means-tested benefits), except for any amount loaned for specified living expenses (eg rent, food, fuel, clothing, council tax) which is taken into account as income over the period of your studies covered by the loan.

Payments from the access fund are taken into account as part of your income.

Part-time study
If you are not required to sign on for work, for example because you are assessed as incapable of work, you can do a part-time course and get IS. See Box B.1 in Chapter 3 for the situations in which you are not required to sign on.

If you do have to sign on for work you may be able to claim jobseeker's allowance – see 5 below.

5. Other benefits

Housing benefit
This section looks briefly at a student's housing benefit (HB) position: for full details ask your student union or local authority.

Most students attending a full-time course are excluded from HB throughout the year(s) until the course finally ends. If you are one of a couple and your partner is not a student, s/he can claim HB (the student rules will apply to your eligible rent and income). Student couples who have a dependent child will be eligible for HB throughout the course (not just in the long vacations as for jobseeker's allowance and IS).

If you get IS as a full-time student, you will also be eligible for HB. You will also be eligible for HB if you are a disabled student, a student who is entitled to a disabled students' allowance addition to a student grant because of deafness (but not for any other disability), a lone parent or a pensioner. You count as a disabled student if you qualify for a disability premium or severe disability premium. If you don't qualify for a disability premium because you don't get a qualifying benefit (such as DLA or SDA), you are still eligible for HB if you are accepted as incapable of work for 28 weeks, even though your disability premium won't start until 52 weeks of incapacity. Chapter 8 has details of how your incapacity for work is assessed. If you are under 19 and a full-time student but not in higher education, you will also be eligible for HB.

Students on IS – If you are on IS, occupying your dwelling as your home, and liable to pay rent for it, your housing benefit is worked out in the normal way – see Chapter 4. But you won't get HB if you pay rent to your educational establishment, or if you are living in a hall of residence (except during the summer vacation if you have to stay in hall). And during summer vacations you won't get HB if you are away from your term-time home for a full HB benefit week – unless you are in hospital; or where your term-time home is also your normal home and not just your home because you are on the course.

Other students – If you don't get IS, your HB is worked out normally (as above), but is also subject to special rules for the treatment of grant income, covenant income, a student loan, and eligible rent. The treatment of income is much the same as under IS (but all students, including disabled students, are assumed to receive the full assessed parental contribution towards their grant). During the period of study (terms and short vacations) your eligible rent is cut by a weekly deduction – see Box I.4. But that cut won't be made if your income is less than your HB applicable amount plus the rent deduction, and your HB assessment includes the disability premium (or you have been accepted as incapable of work for 28 weeks) or lone parent rate of family premium or you have a partner who is not also a full-time student.

If you have a partner and have to live in two separate homes while you are on the course, you can get HB for both homes only if you are eligible for HB as a student.

Council tax benefit
If the only adult residents in your home are students (including students temporarily absent, intercalating from their course), you will not be liable to pay council tax at all, your home is an exempt dwelling – see Chapter 5. If you're not liable to pay council tax, you cannot get council tax benefit in any case. Even if you are liable to pay council tax, you may not qualify for council tax benefit. Only some full-time students are eligible for main council tax benefit (CTB). If you would be eligible for HB as a student – see above – you will also be eligible for CTB. Your income is worked out in the same way as for HB.
Second adult rebate – Students who are liable to pay council tax can claim second adult rebate even if they are excluded from main CTB. It is worked out in the standard way – see Chapter 4(26).
Non-dependant deductions – If you are a full-time student, living in someone else's home as a non-dependant, no deduction is made from the householder's CTB during your whole period of study, including the summer vacation. For CTB purposes, there is no deduction even if you get a job during the long vacation. However, for HB, if you get a job (for 16 or more hours a week) during the summer vacation, a non-dependant deduction will be applied.

Jobseeker's allowance (JSA)
JSA has replaced unemployment benefit and income support for people who sign on for work – see Chapter 14. Students attending a full-time course are excluded from JSA until the end of their course or until you abandon it or are dismissed from it. However, if you have a partner who is also a student, and you have a dependent child, you can get JSA during the long vacation, as long as you are available for work.
Part-time study – You may be able to study part-time and still get income-based or contribution-based JSA. Generally you must be available immediately to take up work of at least 40 hours a week. The times you are available for work are usually recorded in your jobseeker's agreement. If the hours you are studying are outside these times, part-time study does not affect your JSA. But if the course overlaps with the hours you must be available for work, you can still get JSA if:
- you are a part-time student – see below; and
- you are willing and able to rearrange the hours of your course immediately to take up employment; and
- for the whole 3 months before you started the course you were on a Youth Training course, or getting JSA, incapacity benefit, statutory sick pay or getting IS on the grounds of incapacity for work; or
- in the 6 months before you started the course you met the

above condition for a total of 3 months, so long as for the rest of the time you were in full-time work, or earning too much to get any of those benefits.

If you meet these conditions, your studies are ignored when deciding if you are available for work. If you don't meet these conditions, you can still study part-time if the employment officer at the Jobcentre accepts that you are genuinely available for work despite your studies.

Whether your course is full or part-time usually depends on how it is classed by the college. However, if your course is funded by the Further Education Funding Council (in England and Wales), it is full-time if it involves more than 16 'guided learning hours' per week. In Scotland, if the course is funded by the Further Education Unit, it is full-time if there are more than 16 hours a week of classroom or workshop-based learning under the guidance of a teacher; or up to 16 hours a week of guided learning and additional hours using structured learning packages supported by teachers where the total hours are more than 21 a week.

If you were getting income support on 31.7.96 and you were treated as available for work and you were part-way through a part-time course on that date (even if you were not attending

---

I.4 Rates of grants and loans (97/98)

Student grants
Basic rates are shown for mandatory awards in England, Wales and Northern Ireland (EWNI) in one column and for allowances in Scotland in the other.

Place of residence	EWNI	Scotland
Parental home	£1,435	£1,290
London	£2,160	£2,085
Elsewhere	£1,755	£1,685

The travel component in Scottish student allowances is £70.

Disabled students' allowance
The figures shown are the maximum in each case for non-travel disability related costs of study.

Any cost	£1,275 per year
Non-medical personal helper	£5,100 per year
Major items of specialist equipment	£3,840 per course

Student loans

Place of residence	Final year	Other
Parental home	£945	£1,290
London	£1,520	£2,085
Elsewhere	£1,230	£1,685

Housing benefit
The weekly eligible rent deduction for a full-time student during each week of the 'period of study' for 1996/97 is:

Place of residence	
London	£25.20
Elsewhere	£17.45

Books and equipment disregard
The standard disregard for the books and equipment element in a student grant for 1996/97 is £280.

I.5 For more information

Careers help
❑ If you are still at school, you should make sure you have an interview with the special needs careers adviser in your area. Ask about all courses which interest you. Do not assume you cannot go on studying if you want to, just because you will be leaving school.
❑ If you have already left school, contact the nearest further education college (address from your library), and ask for an interview with the college co-ordinator for special needs, to discuss the courses on offer and how the college might help if you have particular needs (eg access, special equipment, tutorial help, etc).
❑ If you left school some time ago, or have become disabled since leaving school, you should talk to the Placement, Assessment and Counselling Team's Disability Employment Adviser (who can be contacted at the Jobcentre) about further education and training.

Information for students with disabilities
Skill publishes a range of information sheets, including (£2 each):
■ *Financial Assistance for Students with Disabilities in Further Education and Training*;
■ *Financial Assistance for Students with Disabilities in Higher Education*.
Skill also provides a telephone information service, 2–5 pm, Monday to Friday. Contact *Skill, National Bureau for Students with Disabilities, 336 Brixton Road, London, SW9 7AA (0171 274 0565)*.

The RNIB can offer advice and assistance to visually impaired students. Contact *RNIB Student Support Service, PO Box 49, Loughborough, Leicestershire, LE11 3DG*.

Student grants
There are three government guides to student grants.
■ England and Wales: *Student Grants and Loans – A Brief Guide for Higher Education Students*. Available from local education authorities, or from *Publications Centre, DfEE, PO Box 2193, London, E15 2EU*.
■ Scotland: *Student Grants in Scotland – A Guide to Undergraduate Allowances*. Available from *Student Awards Agency for Scotland, Gyleview House, 3 Redheughs Rigg, Edinburgh, EH12 9HH*.
■ Northern Ireland: *Grants and Loans to Students – A Brief Guide*. Available from *Student Support Branch, Department of Education for Northern Ireland, Rathgael House, Balloo Road, Bangor, Co Down, BT19 7PR*.

Charities and trusts
There are a number of reference books, which should be available through public libraries. The list below is only a selection.
■ *Charities Digest* published by Family Welfare Association
■ *Directory of Grant Making Trusts* (Charities Aid Foundation)
■ *Educational Grants Directory* (Directory of Social Change)
■ *The Grants Register* (Macmillan)

The Students Awards Agency for Scotland maintains a Register of Educational Endowments covering all education trusts set up in Scotland. Only students who have been refused an allowance may apply for a search, by contacting the Agency at the same address as above.

due to the summer vacation), you can continue to study on the same course (but not a different course) under the old 21 hour rule.

Incapacity benefit and SDA
Incapacity benefit and SDA are payable during term-time as well as vacations. For SDA, if you are under 19 you may also be caught by the full-time education exclusion – see Chapter 30(3). To qualify for these benefits you must be accepted as incapable of work. This is assessed under the 'all work' test of incapacity unless you are in an exempt group – see Chapter 8 for more details. Your incapacity benefit or SDA is ignored in the student grant means test.

Disability living allowance (DLA)
This can be paid over and above your grant and/or income support. If your college provides care and assistance for you, the college authorities may claim some or all of the DLA care component from you to help defray their costs. Otherwise you can put the allowance towards the cost of employing a personal care helper, or any other service you may need. See Chapter 17 for details. Do note that if you are living in a residential college, your care component will stop for the time you are there if it counts as 'special accommodation' (see Chapter 17(10)).

Students entitled to a student grant requiring help with personal care can claim a disabled students' allowance to cover the cost of non-medical helpers – see Box I.4. It is sensible to reserve your disabled students' allowance for academic helpers without whom you would be unable to follow the course. For your basic personal care needs (which arise whether or not you are on the course), you should apply for financial assistance from the Social Services Department in your home area and use, eg a Community Service Volunteer. In some cases, the local authority will take into account the parents' or student's income and whether the student receives DLA care component. District nursing help should be available in the normal way – see Chapter 33.

The DLA mobility component is paid over and above your grant and/or income support/HB/CTB – see Chapter 17.

6. Charities and trusts
Few trusts can offer substantial financial aid. It is unlikely you could finance a course lasting more than one year entirely from charitable sources. Trusts will not usually provide you with your main source of finance for a full-time course, but they may give you a top-up or pay for a special need.

Some trusts give small grants or loans to students with disabilities who are in particular difficulty. Trusts usually expect you to have approached your local education authority first and to have claimed the disabled students' allowance.

There are numerous small local trusts, and you should consult your local education authority, public library or local churches for any information they may have.

Some universities and colleges may have funds available to assist students in special needs – separate from any access funds. Some student unions offer loans to students in special cases – ask the President or welfare officer.

This section of the Handbook looks at the following:

Care services	Chapter **32**
Help with equipment	Chapter **33**
Help with buying your own care	Chapter **34**

Practical help at home

32 Care services

In this chapter we look at:	
What is Community Care?	see 1
Where do you go for help?	see 2
Getting an assessment of your needs	see 3
Checklist of care services	see Box J.1
How can you register as disabled?	see 4
What help can be provided?	see 5
The law and community care	see Box J.2
Do you have to pay for your care?	see 6
If you are not satisfied with your care services	see 7
Housing	see 8
For more information	see Box J.3

1. What is Community Care?

Community care is defined in the Government White Paper, *Caring for People*, as *'providing the right level of intervention and support to enable people to achieve maximum independence and control over their own lives'*. To achieve this, money which had been used by the DSS to pay for people in residential care was passed over in 1993 to Social Services Departments, so they could provide more help for people in their own homes. Chapters 35 to 38 look at what happens if you need residential care on a respite or permanent basis. The object was that fewer would need to go into residential care, and the local authority would act as a gatekeeper for such care.

Assessment of a person's needs is seen as fundamental as this triggers the provision of service either directly from the local authority or arranged by them from the independent sector, at home or in residential or nursing homes (called collectively, residential care). Local authorities have the lead role in this, but both health authorities and housing departments are recognised as key players in helping someone remain at home. There is a duty on local authorities to invite these agencies to assist in the assessment where there is a health or housing need.

Because there is no obvious dividing line between what is a social care need and what is a health need, it is often an area of dispute. More so as most health care is free at the point of delivery, whereas people are increasingly being charged for social care. In 1995, guidance was issued (HSG 95/8 and LAC 95/5 – see Box K.1 in Chapter 35) to clarify the NHS responsibilities for meeting continuing care needs. It was left to health authorities to agree their policy and eligibility criteria with the local authority. Since April 1996 these have been in place and publicly available. What is provided by the health authority and therefore free will vary from area to area. The local criteria may be reviewed for 1997 and so may change.

Likewise, since the new system started in 1993, each local authority has to publish its community care plans, and from April 1996 must have a Community Care Charter publicly available which sets out their standards of service.

There is no single piece of legislation which covers community care, but a complex web of Acts, Regulations, directions and guidance going back to the National Assistance Act 1948. Box J.2 gives relevant sections of some of the law as a starting point. Services for children come under the Children Act 1989. Broadly, children should be able to obtain similar services and have similar systems for appeal as adults.

2. Where do you go for help?

Go to the local area office of the Social Services Department. In Scotland, it is the Social Work Department. For help with housing you may be passed on to your local housing department. The Social Services Department has the lead responsibility for assessing your needs and ensuring that services are provided to meet the assessed needs. Social Services should involve the housing department and the health authority where there is a need for their services.

In some parts of the country the health authority may undertake the community care assessment at the request of Social Services. But in general the Social Services Department is the place to start.

If you already have a social worker, discuss your needs with them. Otherwise, look up the address of your nearest office in the phone book under the name of your local authority. For example, look up 'Essex County Council' and find the heading 'Social Services Department, Area Office'.

If you outline the type of help you want, they can put you through to the right section. Your health visitor or occupational therapist may also be able to help arrange for the services you need.

See also Chapter 34 for the help available to buy your own care at home.

3. Getting an assessment of your needs

Basically, if you have difficulty managing at home because of your age, illness or disability, you can ask for an assessment. If it is apparent to the local authority that you might have a need for services, then you do not have to ask for it. However it is not only disabled people who can get an assessment from the local authority. We look at the law covering assessments in Box J.2.

The assessment should look at the whole range of community care services, your capacities and incapacities, your preferences and aspirations, what support you have available and other sources of help.

In order to decide whether an individual's need for service is sufficiently substantial for him or her to actually receive it, authorities draw up a general list of 'eligibility criteria', ie the criteria which must be present in any particular case before a person is considered eligible for services. Local authorities produce information about their assessment procedures and their 'eligibility criteria', and it may be useful for you to refer to this.

Guidance states that you should be informed in writing of

the result of your assessment. If you are not given a written result you should ask for a copy. If your needs are urgent, services can be provided before an assessment takes place. It should then be carried out as soon as possible.

If you are refused an assessment, or there is a delay in carrying it out you can use the complaints procedure or seek legal advice if it is very urgent – see 7 below.

Carers – Some of the legislation mentions carers, and it is stressed in much of the guidance that the contribution of carers should be formally recognised in any assessment. The Carers (Recognition and Services) Act 1995 (see Box J.2) has strengthened this and carers can request that an assessment of their own abilities to provide and to continue to provide care be carried out at the same time as the person for whom they are caring is assessed for services. The assessment of the carer should be taken into consideration in the decisions made as a result of the disabled person's assessment.

4. How can you register as disabled?

Anyone whose disability is *'substantial and permanent'* can register with their local authority. **But you don't have to register in order to qualify for an assessment or for services.** The requirement to keep registers only applies to England and Wales. This section does not apply to Scotland.

If you want to register, contact the area office of your local Social Services Department. They will arrange for someone, usually a social worker or occupational therapist, to visit you and complete a registration form. Registering may not have any immediate benefit, but it is a useful thing to do. The more accurately the register reflects the number of disabled people in the community, the better services can be tailored to meet their needs.

Some local authorities may automatically register you when you apply for help from them. In some cases, the authority will send you a card confirming your registration and all should give you information on the services available to disabled people. Other authorities give no written confirmation of your registration.

5. What help can be provided?

Local authorities have various duties and powers to provide services. Certain services **must** be provided by the local authority. There is a legal duty to do so. Other services **may** be provided but there is no requirement to do so. The list in Box J.1 gives an idea of the type of services that may be available. Although all these services may not be available in your local authority area, neither is the list exhaustive.

J.1 Checklist of care services

Where can you get help from?
Practical help with caring is available from a number of sources:
- relatives;
- friends and neighbours;
- private organisations or individuals;
- voluntary organisations;
- local authorities; and
- the National Health Service.

To find out what help is available in your area, first contact your area Social Services (in Scotland, Social Work) Department. If they do not provide a particular service, they should, at least, be able to put you in touch with the right organisation. Don't be surprised if your area does not have all the services listed below!

Getting services into the home
Where there is more information in other chapters, we will refer you to the right place in the Handbook.
Adaptations – see Chapter 49.
Alarm system
Benefits – see the Benefits Checklist at beginning of the Handbook.
Care attendant scheme – voluntary schemes, with trained helpers, aimed at helping disabled and elderly people stay in the community. There may be a local scheme. If not, contact Crossroads – see the Address List at the back of this Handbook.
DIAL – see our Address List for the nearest Disablement Information and Advice Line (DIAL) group and other sources of telephone advice. If you have (and can use) a phone, they may be able to give you the advice you need. If not, they can put you in touch with the right organisation.
Direct payments – by Social Services Departments – see Chapter 34.
District nurses – may provide nursing care at home, or in a care home, if you need it. Or they can arrange to supply equipment to help with nursing care, as well as incontinence aids.
Equipment – see Chapter 33.

Good neighbour scheme – less formal than the Care Attendant Scheme and volunteers don't need to be specially trained.
GPs – your general practitioner is the key person in ensuring that you get, or are referred to, the services you need. So, if you are really dissatisfied with your GP you should seriously consider transferring to another doctor.
Health visitors – can provide information and advice on services available locally, and act as a liaison or referral point between disabled people and Social Services Departments. Health visitors automatically visit families where there are any children under the age of five. They also offer practical advice and support. If you are not already in touch with a health visitor, contact one through your local GP, health centre or child health clinic.
Home helps or carers – can provide a range of practical help in the home. It could be help with domestic tasks, including shopping and cashing your order book, or more personal care tasks. Social Services can provide help with these if they have assessed you as needing this service – see Chapter 32(5).
Home visits – it is possible to arrange a home visit from a chiropodist, dentist, doctor, hairdresser, occupational therapist, optician or a physiotherapist. A Citizens Advice Bureau worker will try to visit you at home if you are housebound and it is not possible to advise you over the phone or by letter.
Homemaker scheme – a volunteer can take over when your carer is ill, so you can stay at home and be properly looked after.
Incontinence – see Chapter 33(4).
Independent Living Funds – see Chapter 34.
Laundry service – see Chapter 33.
Library – if you are housebound, you can get home visits from the library service. Check our Address List for organisations, such as The National Library for the Blind.
Macfarlane Trusts – if you have haemophilia and have HIV – see our Address List.
Meals on wheels – are usually provided from central kitchens and delivered to your home by voluntary helpers.
Occupational therapists – can help you learn or relearn the

What are your rights to services?

If you are disabled and you are assessed as needing one of the services listed in Section 2 of the Chronically Sick and Disabled Persons Act 1970, your local authority has a duty to make arrangements for the provision of the service. These services are:

- practical help in the home, eg a home help;
- providing or help in getting a radio, television, library or similar recreational facilities;
- lectures, games, outings, or other recreational facilities outside your home and any help needed to take advantage of educational facilities;
- help with travelling to any of these or similar activities;
- any adaptations, such as a ramp or lift or special equipment needed in the home *'for greater safety, comfort or convenience'*; this can even include building an extra room on the ground floor;
- holidays;
- meals, either in the home or a local centre;
- a telephone, and any special equipment necessary to use the phone, eg Minicom.

See Box J.2 for the definition of disability and the legal provisions to provide services.

Your needs and local authority resources

Local authorities are finding it increasingly difficult to budget their finite resources against the needs of people in their area. This has led to the withdrawal of services previously provided, or for them to draw up very tight eligibility criteria to decide who gets help.

This has led to challenges about whether local authorities could take the lack of resources into account when deciding whether to provide services. The House of Lords has now ruled (*R v Gloucester County Council ex p Barry*, 20.3.97) that it is lawful for a local authority to take their resources into account when deciding whether a person needs services under section 2 of the Chronically Sick and Disabled Persons Act. They could thus decide to revise their eligibility criteria. The local authority can also take its own resources into account when deciding **how** it will meet that need. However, local authorities can only reduce or withdraw services provided under section 2 if they have first assessed or reassessed the person's needs in the light of the revised eligibility criteria.

6. Do you have to pay for your care?

A local authority may charge for domiciliary services (ie services provided at home) and other services in the community (eg day centres) which it either provides or arranges for you.

---

skills of independent self care and personal management in all aspects of everyday life. They can also offer advice on, or arrange the provision of, any necessary equipment or adaptations to your home.

Odd Job Scheme – this could come under a variety of names. The schemes give practical help with tasks you cannot manage yourself – decorating, gardening, etc.

Physiotherapists – provide treatment and advice to relieve pain and help restore and maintain mobility. This includes advice about equipment (perhaps designed by REMAP – see our Address List).

Recreational facilities – radio, TV etc.

Rehabilitation – most District General Hospitals have well-equipped rehabilitation departments which can provide a variety of services and techniques to help patients develop their maximum ability. Treatment may also be provided at Health Centres, at home, or at other suitable centres.

Self-help and socialising – check our Address List. You could, for example, join a PHAB club.

Sitting In Service – allows your carer time off and may help you get a wider network of friends who can also help.

Sleeping In Service – allows your carer a night away, or a weekend away.

Social workers – play a key role in getting services into your home. Sometimes just talking things over can help.

Social Fund – discretionary help may be available – see Chapter 7.

Speech and language therapists – cover all forms of communication disorders.

Support for the carer – contact the Carers National Association – see our Address List.

Telephone – if you can't handle and/or read a printed phone book, register for free use of Directory Enquiries. Call 0800 919195 for details and an application form.

Services away from the home

Adult education

Advice – contact your Town Hall for a list of local advice centres.

Day centres – are provided by the local authority (or in some cases by voluntary organisations) as places where elderly people or those with disabilities can meet. Meals, chiropody, diversional therapy are usually available. If necessary, you can get transport to and from the centre.

Day hospital care – it is possible to arrange to stay in hospital during the day but be in your own home at night. This can be done on a regular basis or just in emergencies.

Education work centres – contact Social Services for more information.

Emergency overnight stay – in a hospital or residential care home.

Employment schemes – contact Social Services and/or the Disability Employment Adviser (via the Jobcentre).

Holiday/Short-term care – a 'foster' scheme with volunteer families.

Housebound Association – volunteer scheme to transport people with disabilities who are housebound to regular meetings and social activities (eg Contact the Elderly – see our Address List).

Medical Escort Service – if you cannot travel to hospital etc on your own. The British Red Cross offer this service.

Respite or Short-Stay Care – can be in a hospital or residential care home. Allows carers a break or holiday and may help you to remain at home longer – see Chapters 17, 36 and 39 for the benefit implications.

Residential care – can be provided by local authorities, the NHS, private and voluntary organisations. You can get more information on the availability and conditions of entry to homes in your area from your GP, Social Services, or Social Work Department – see Chapters 35 to 37.

Sheltered housing – see Chapter 32(8).

Transport – most Social Services Departments arrange transport to clubs, day centres and workshops for people with disabilities who are unable to use public transport. In some areas there are voluntary schemes, such as Dial-a-Ride. Local authority travel-pass schemes may allow you to travel free or at a reduced rate if you are elderly or disabled.

You cannot be charged for services provided by the NHS, such as district nurses. Many local authorities are introducing new or increased charges. Each local authority's charging policy for domiciliary and day care is different, so what follows will be general principles. The system for charging for respite, or permanent residential care is explained in Chapter 37.

The local authority has the power to charge a reasonable amount for its services. However it has a responsibility to consider each person's case individually. They should provide you with written details of how much you will be charged and a breakdown of how this has been worked out, together with details of what to do if you think you cannot afford the charge.

In deciding how much to charge you, the local authority should take into account the amount you spend on meeting your everyday needs as well as any extra costs you may have as a result of your disability. For example, you may have extra costs for laundry, extra fuel costs, transport, special diet, specially made shoes, extra or warmer clothing and bedding, cleaning materials, painkillers; maybe you pay for gardening or walking the dog. They should make sure you have enough money for these things if you are charged for services.

DLA mobility component should not be taken into account in assessing your income (s.73(14) Social Security Contributions and Benefits Act).

The local authority cannot charge:
- anyone (family, carer or friend) other than the person using the service; they can only take into account the income and capital of the service user when deciding how much you should pay;
- the parent or guardian for children's services if the child is under 16 and the parent or guardian is on income support, family credit or disability working allowance;
- a young person aged between 16 and 18, on income support or income-based JSA;
- for services provided under section 117 of the Mental Health Act 1983.

J.2 The law and community care

The duties and powers of the statutory authorities, such as local authority Social Services Departments, come under a range of different legislation. As well as the law, in Acts, Regulations and Orders, your local authority must also act in accordance with any directions issued by the Secretary of State for Health, and act on any guidance issued by the Secretary of State. Details about the law for provision of residential care are in Chapter 35. But the law on assessment in this box applies equally if you want an assessment of your need for residential care.

Although you don't need to know anything about the law in order to get the practical help you need from Social Services, it does help if you know your rights. In this box we outline the main provisions in the various Acts.

Most of the provisions in Scotland come under different legislation, but they are broadly equivalent to the law in England and Wales (as described below).

Assessments
The following legislation covers assessments.

NHS and Community Care Act 1990
Section 47(1) and (2)
'(1) . . . where it appears to a local authority that any person for whom they may provide or arrange for the provision of community care services may be in need of any such services, the authority
(a) shall carry out an assessment of his needs for those services; and
(b) having regard to the results of that assessment, shall decide whether his needs call for the provision of such services.
(2) If at any time during the assessment . . . it appears to a local authority that he is a disabled person, the authority –
(a) shall proceed to make such a decision as to the services he requires as is mentioned in section 4 of the Disabled Persons (Services, Consultation and Representation) Act without him requesting them to do so under that section; and
(b) shall inform him that they will be doing so and of his rights under that Act.'

Disabled Persons (Services, Consultation and Representation) Act 1986
Section 4(a) and (c)
'When requested to do so by –
(a) a disabled person
(c) any person who provides care for him . . .
a local authority shall decide whether the needs of the disabled person call for the provision by the authority of any services in accordance with section 2 of the Chronically Sick and Disabled Persons Act 1970.'

Carers (Recognition and Services) Act 1995
Section 1(1)
' . . . in any case where –
(a) a local authority carry out an assessment under section 47(1)(a) of the NHS and Community Care Act 1990 of the needs of a person for community care services, and
(b) an individual (carer) provides or intends to provide a substantial amount of care on a regular basis for the . . . person,
the carer may request the local authority, before they make their decision as to whether the needs of the . . . person call for the provision of any services, to carry out an assessment of his ability to provide and to continue to provide care for the . . . person; and if he makes such a request, the local authority shall carry out such an assessment and shall take into account the results of that assessment in making that decision.'

Providing services
Following an assessment, the local authority must decide how it will meet identified needs of the following people:
- *'persons aged 18 or over who are blind, deaf or dumb or who suffer from mental disorder of any description, and other persons aged 18 or over who are substantially and permanently handicapped by illness, injury, or congenital deformity or such other disabilities as may be prescribed'* – Section 29, National Assistance Act 1948 gives a general provision to promote the welfare of the above people including workshops, suitable work in their own homes or elsewhere, recreational facilities and to give information about services, and keeping a register.
- those above (to whom Section 29, National Assistance Act applies) who are *'ordinarily resident in their area'* – The local authority has a duty, under Section 2, Chronically Sick and Disabled Persons Act 1970, to make arrangements for the provision of a range of services. Chapter 32(5) lists these services.
- *old people* – A general provision, under Section 45, Health Services and Public Health Act 1968, to promote welfare.

If you cannot afford to pay the charge, the local authority has a duty to decide how much you can afford to pay and reduce the charge or not charge you at all. A council may not however say – if you do not pay we will not provide the service. It also may not withdraw a service because someone has failed to pay the charge. This is because the decision to meet a need is separate from and comes before the decision whether to charge for the service.

However, they can use debt enforcement proceedings, such as taking the individual to court, for the recovery of arrears. Although many people are willing (indeed, prefer) to pay a reasonable amount if they are able to, some councils are exacting charges from people living on income support or equally low incomes. Also some councils have higher charges if you get AA or DLA care component. You may be able to show you already use this money for other essential spending. If you cannot afford the charge, ask for it to be reduced or waived. For more information on charging, see the *Coalition on Charging Campaign Guide* available from Mencap (see our Address List), free to individuals – send a large SAE.

You can complain about the amount you are being charged and have your case heard by a review panel. Some local authorities have a separate charges complaints procedure which is shorter than the standard complaints procedure described in 7 below.

7. If you are not satisfied with your care services

Wherever possible problems should be resolved locally, perhaps with the aid of a local councillor. Social Services Departments must have a complaints procedure; most publish an explanatory leaflet. Information regarding the action you can take if you are unhappy about the assessment, or the services to be provided, should be given at the time of the care assessment and again when you are informed of any charge. A Social Services complaints officer can provide a copy of the complaints leaflet but it should be easily available from your local office.

- '*a person who is suffering from illness, lying in, an expectant mother, aged, handicapped as a result of having suffered an illness or by congenital deformity*' – Local authorities have a duty, under Schedule 8, National Health Service Act 1977, to provide adequate home help and may provide laundry services for households when such help is required owing to the presence of the above. This Schedule also places a duty to provide day and training centres for those with a 'mental disorder'.
- *persons who are detained or admitted to hospital under Sections 3, 37, 47 or 48 of the Mental Health Act 1983* – Section 117, Mental Health Act 1983 places a duty to provide after-care services.
- *children* – Section 17(1), Children Act 1989 gives local authorities the general duty to safeguard and promote the welfare of children in need. Children in need are defined in the same words as Section 29, National Assistance Act defines disabled person (see above); it just leaves out the 'aged 18 or over'. All services for children, including disabled children, are provided under the Children Act.

Charges

A local authority can charge for domiciliary services. They '*may recover such charge (if any) for it as they consider reasonable*'. If you satisfy your local authority that your '*means are insufficient for it to be reasonably practicable for [you] to pay*' what they have asked, they '*shall not require [you] to pay more for it than it appears to them that it is reasonably practicable for [you] to pay*' (Section 17(3), Health and Social Services and Social Security Adjudication Act 1983). See Chapter 32(6). **Note those whose services are provided under Section 117, Mental Health Act cannot be charged.**

Information

Various pieces of legislation lay a duty on authorities to publish information.
- NHS and Community Care Act 1990, Section 46(1)(a) and (c) 'Each local authority
  (a) shall . . . prepare and publish a plan for the provision of community care services in their area.
  (c) shall, at such intervals as the Secretary of State may direct, prepare and publish modifications to the current plan, or if the case requires, a new plan.'
- Chronically Sick and Disabled Persons Act 1970, Section 1 '(1) It shall be the duty of every local authority . . . to inform themselves of the number of persons (to whom Section 29, National Assistance Act) applies within their area and of the need for the making by the authority of arrangements under that section for such persons.
  (2) Every such authority
  (a) shall cause to be published from time to time . . . general information as to the services provided . . . under Section 29, which are for the time being available in their area; and
  (b) shall ensure that any person . . . who uses any other services provided by the authority (whether under such arrangements or not) is informed of any other of those services which in the opinion of the authority is relevant to his needs (and of any service by any other authority or organisation which in the opinion of the authority is so relevant and of which particulars are in the authority's possession.'

Complaints

Section 7, Local Authority Social Services Act 1970 and the Local Authority Social Services (Complaints Procedure) Order 1990/2244 and directions established the complaints procedures.

Local authorities have to give publicity, as they consider appropriate, to any procedure established. See Chapter 32(7).

Section 7 gives the Secretary of State for Health powers to hold an inquiry into a local authority's exercise of its social services functions, including any breach of its statutory duties. It also gives the Secretary of State 'default powers' to enforce action on a local authority.

As well as the specific provisions outlined above, you may also complain to the Local Government Ombudsman – see Chapter 54. Judicial review of local authority decisions is also a possibility.

This box only gives the basic provisions. If you are challenging a decision about the help you get or need at home you may find the following useful.
- *Community Care Assessments – A Practical Legal Framework*, by Richard Gordon (Longmans)
- *Challenging Community Care Decisions*, a briefing by the Public Law Project, 17 Russell Square, London WC1B 5DR
- *Community Care and the Law*, by Luke Clements (Legal Action Group)
- *The Care Maze – The Law and Your Rights to Community Care In Scotland*, by Colin McKay and Hilary Patrick (ENABLE)

Complaints

The procedure has three stages: informal problem solving, formal registration, and review.

Informal problem solving – At this stage you should contact the social worker, occupational therapist, home carer or person who is working with you. Talk through the problem and try to have it put right. If you are still unhappy, go on to the next stage.

Formal complaint – Write to the Director of Social Services, setting out exactly what your complaint is and ask for this to be registered as a formal complaint. If you need help to write the letter, the social worker can help you, or any member of Social Services or a friend, relative or neighbour.

At this stage the Director of Social Services will appoint an officer of the department to investigate the complaint. The officer will be somebody who has not had contact with you before. If a complaint is made on behalf of a child, an independent person must also be appointed by Social Services to assist in the investigation of the complaint. You must get a reply within 28 days of the authority's receipt of your registered complaint. If this is not the full response to your complaint, you should get an explanation of the current position with a full response within 3 months.

Review – If you cannot resolve a complaint informally or are unhappy with the authority's full response to your registered complaint, you can ask for the complaint to be heard by a review panel. You must ask for a review within 28 days of the date the local authority tells you the result of their consideration of your complaint.

The review panel consists of 3 people; at least one person, the chairperson, must be independent of the authority (ie not an elected member or an employee). Its hearing must take place within 28 days of the date the local authority received your request for a review. You should be given at least 10 days notice, in writing, of the time and place of the hearing. You can be accompanied by someone who may speak on your behalf – this person should not be a lawyer acting in his or her professional capacity.

The review panel must record its recommendations within 24 hours of the hearing and notify you in writing. Their letter should explain the reasons for their recommendations.

Your local authority then has 28 days to decide what action, if any, to take in the light of the review panel's recommendations. The authority's reply should also give reasons for decisions taken. This is particularly important if the decisions differ from the review panel's recommendations. A High Court decision (*Avon County Council v ex parte M*) stated that your local authority can't overrule the Panel's decision without *'substantial reason and without having given (the Panel's) recommendation the weight it required'*.

Your next step? – If, after going through this complaints procedure, the authority continues in your opinion to be acting unlawfully, or wholly unreasonably, it is possible to ask the Secretary of State for Health to consider exercising his default powers. However, such a course of action is not an alternative remedy to judicial review. Contact RADAR for help (address in Box J.3). You may be able to take legal proceedings in a judicial review, or pursue other legal action. You must act quickly. Contact your local law centre, a legal aid solicitor, or the Disability Law Service (see the Address List at the back of this Handbook). Or you may wish to contact the Local Government Ombudsman – see Chapter 54.

8. Housing

Housing departments are required to consider the needs of disabled people in new housing schemes.

They may provide the following.

Wheelchair housing – This is designed to give people who need to use a wheelchair all the time access to all principal rooms including the bathroom and lavatory, and to allow them to operate freely in them.

Mobility housing – This is designed for disabled people who have problems moving around inside and may sometimes use a wheelchair. The entrance should be level or ramped and the entrance, corridors and doors of principal rooms (though not bathroom or lavatory) should be wide enough for a normal wheelchair. The bathroom, lavatory and at least one bedroom should be on the same level as the entrance. The advantage of mobility housing is that it should be little or no more expensive than ordinary housing and is just as suitable for non-disabled tenants.

Sheltered housing – These are groups of flats with a warden and are mainly intended for elderly people. Sheltered housing schemes which are provided both by local authorities and housing associations may include both wheelchair and mobility housing. A very few sheltered housing schemes for younger disabled people exist. For more information contact RADAR – see Box J.3.

Lifetime homes – A few councils and housing associations build these homes to be adjustable to people's changing physical needs.

Many people, especially young disabled people seeking a first home of their own, may prefer to move to a purpose-designed house rather than to have their present home adapted. It is important that housing departments should know the needs of disabled people in the area. For example, if you have a disabled child, even if your home is perfectly adequate it may be wise to ask the housing department to record the fact that, in a few years' time, a specially designed home may be needed.

If you need adaptations to your home, see Chapter 49 which covers home renovation grants and disabled facilities grants.

33 Help with equipment

1. Items for daily living

Under the Chronically Sick and Disabled Persons Act 1970, local authorities have a statutory responsibility to arrange for the provision of equipment and adaptations to the individual's home that will help people to maintain their independence and secure their greater safety, comfort or convenience. If you live in a residential home, you may also get help. Any equipment and adaptations will be provided on the basis of a professional assessment of your needs. This assessment won't just look at your possible need for equipment – see Chapter 32(3).

Suitably adapted or specialised equipment is a key factor in enabling someone to live as independently as possible. The range of items is large – so don't buy anything without getting expert advice and, if possible, using the equipment on a trial basis to see if it really will work for you. If the occupational therapist recommends an item of equipment, ask if there is a centre where you can see the equipment – see Box J.3. Equipment provided by local authorities or by the NHS is generally considered to be on long term loan.

Items for daily living include items to make it easier to use the toilet, to wash, dress, use cooking facilities, etc: for example, handrails next to the bath and toilet, raised toilet seats, widened doorways, a bathroom on the ground floor, etc.

An occupational therapist in your Social Services Department may be the best person to turn to initially for advice and help. However, all personal and health care professionals may be able to give help and advice – eg a social worker, district nurse, health visitor, GP, or a child's school.

If you need any adaptations to your house, see Chapter 49.

2. Nursing equipment

Health authorities, including NHS trusts, as part of their community health services, may provide nursing equipment such as special beds, commodes, urinals, incontinence pads, etc. Some items may serve a dual purpose: for nursing care and for daily living. So some health and social service authorities have a jointly agreed procedure to determine who supplies which particular item.

In the first instance, apply for any item via your doctor, district nurse, health visitor, continence advisor, occupational therapist or social worker. If you have difficulty in getting the supplies you need, your local Community Health Council (in Scotland, Local Health Council, and in Northern Ireland, Health and Social Services Council) may be able to help you.

3. Appliances and devices

General Practitioners may prescribe only the equipment which is included in an approved list (ie the schedule of appliances and devices in the Drug Tariff). These include catheters, elastic hosiery, trusses, etc.

A hospital consultant may prescribe surgical footwear, leg appliances, artificial breasts, wigs and fabric supports etc. An NHS consultant may prescribe any piece of equipment which s/he considers is necessary as part of a patient's treatment. Hearing aids are supplied either on the prescription of a consultant Ear Nose & Throat surgeon or consultant in audiological medicine, or patients can be referred direct by their GP to the audiology department. They are supplied on free loan from NHS Hearing Aid Centres. Low vision aids, including hand magnifiers and more complex appliances, can be prescribed under the NHS through the Hospital Eye Service. Artificial eyes and orbital prostheses can be supplied on the recommendation of a hospital ophthalmologist.

4. Services to help with incontinence

Many disabled people have trouble either occasionally or regularly with incontinence, which can be costly besides causing a lot of extra work. The help available and how it is administered will vary from one area to another. It is important that you first seek the advice of a GP, practice nurse or physiotherapist to check whether there is treatment that might help. The need for further assistance should be taken into account during a community care assessment.

There are several types of provision:
- treatment (eg drugs, physiotherapy, surgery, etc);
- supplies and equipment;
- laundry services;
- disposal of waste.

How can you get help?

Health authorities have powers to supply, free of charge, aids and equipment to help in nursing sick or disabled people at home and in residential care. These may include the loan of a commode and bed linen, the supply of incontinence pads, protective pants, inter-liners, disposable drawsheets and bedpans, nappy rolls, etc. It is up to the health authority to decide on the quantity of items, such as pads, and some, indeed, decide not to supply any at all. If this happens, you may want to complain to your Community Health Council.

Protective pants and pads are not available on GP prescription (except in Scotland). If you cannot get an item through the health authority, you can buy it privately either from chemists (a limited range) or more generally through specialist mail order firms. Body worn urinary appliances can be prescribed by GPs: but take the prescription to a chemist or surgical supplier providing a skilled fitting service.

For more information on aids and equipment, as well as guidance on general management, contact the Disabled Living Foundation for details of their publications (see Box J.3) or the Continence Foundation (helpline 0191 213 0050).

How can you obtain a laundry service?

If a laundry service is available in your area, it will normally be run by the local Social Services Department, probably attached to the home help service. However, in some areas the laundry service is run by the health authority, and in others there is no laundry service as such, although extra practical help may be given through the home help service.

A laundry service may collect soiled sheets, bedding, clothes or nappies and return them laundered. It should be available to those too ill or disabled to manage laundry, as well as to people who are incontinent. Ask your Social Services Department or the health authority for details. If you find that the receptionist does not know whether a laundry service exists or not, ask to speak to the Information Officer or duty social worker.

For very severely disabled children, the Family Fund can provide washing machines and/or dryers – see Chapter 29. If you can't cope with the practical and care problems arising because of incontinence, you may find you qualify for either the

---

J.3 For more information

Equipment
Contact the Disabled Living Foundation for general information and advice about all types of equipment: *380 – 384 Harrow Road, London W9 2HU; telephone 0171 289 6111.*

Disabled Living Centres and Communication Aids Centres – have a wide range of equipment on show. You can usually try out equipment for yourself, as well as get advice about what might help you best. Contact the Disabled Living Centres Council for a list of local centres – see our Address List.

Ask your doctor, social worker, or health visitor for advice as well. See Department of Health booklet HB6: *A Practical Guide for Disabled People. Where to Find Information, Services and Equipment.*

Contact Disability Alliance's Rights Service for advice on social security matters only! Our Rights Workers are not experts on equipment for people with disabilities.

See also *Finding help at home*, Age Concern Factsheet 6 – see our Address List.

Social services
Contact RADAR for advice on the Disabled Persons (Services, Consultation and Representation) Act. Also where you think that your local authority Social Services Department has failed in its duty to you under the Chronically Sick and Disabled Persons Act and you haven't been able to resolve the problem locally. *RADAR, 12 City Forum, 250 City Road, London EC1V 8AF; telephone 0171 250 3222.*

disability living allowance care component or attendance allowance – see Chapters 17 and 18.

How can you dispose of waste?
The local authority refuse disposal service should collect soiled incontinence pads, dressings and other nursing waste which cannot be disposed of normally and which arises from the care of a sick or disabled person at home. This service can sometimes be arranged through the health authority, but is generally provided by your local authority Environmental Health Department.

5. Environmental control systems and communication aids

These enable people with severe disabilities to operate appliances and equipment from a central control, with switching mechanisms adapted to meet the person's needs. You should contact an occupational therapist or your doctor. A medical consultant will assess whether the equipment will help and if so arrangements for installation will be made. The equipment is provided on loan and serviced free of charge.

People with severe difficulties speaking or writing can be helped by a range of communication aids – from charts with pictures to specially adapted computers and electronic voice output devices. These can be provided by the local education authority, schools, Employment Service, as well as the NHS, and GP fundholders (up to the value of £6,000). If necessary local professionals will refer you to a communication aids centre for advice on the most suitable aids.

6. Wheelchairs

Under the National Health Service, wheelchairs (including powered wheelchairs) and hand and pedal propelled tricycles are supplied and maintained free of charge to a disabled person whose need for such a chair is permanent.

Any wheelchair on the market may be supplied by NHS Wheelchair Service Centres but it is a matter for local decision what will be provided bearing in mind the circumstances of the individual and the resources available.

Since 1.4.96, powered indoor/outdoor wheelchairs can be provided to severely disabled people by the NHS, if it is assessed that you need one because you are unable to walk or propel an ordinary wheelchair. Each health authority decides their own local eligibility criteria, but this should be within the broad national framework – that as well as being unable to propel a manual wheelchair, you should be able to benefit from an improved quality of life, and be able to handle the chair safely. If you move to another area and do not meet the new local criteria, your wheelchair should not be withdrawn unless there is a good clinical reason for doing so.

Attendant controlled wheelchairs are also issued where it would be difficult for the disabled person to be pushed out of doors, eg where the person is heavy, the attendant is aged, or the district is hilly.

Since 1.7.96, legislation allows NHS trusts to supply, at the request of the user, a wheelchair which is more expensive than the type clinically necessary. In these cases, the difference in costs can be recovered by the NHS from the user.

A new voucher scheme will be phased in over the next 2 years. This will provide financial aid from the NHS if you choose to buy a wheelchair from the private sector. The voucher will enable you to pay the difference between a wheelchair prescribed by the NHS as meeting your needs and a more expensive wheelchair of your choice. You cannot get a voucher for a powered indoor/outdoor wheelchair or a scooter.

You may also use the Motability scheme to buy an electric wheelchair on hire purchase – see Chapter 20.

Anybody who thinks they might need a wheelchair should be referred to their local Wheelchair Service Centre for assessment. Your GP, local health centre, physiotherapist or occupational therapy department can tell you where your local wheelchair service is; or you can phone the Health Information Service free on 0800 665544.

34 Help with buying your own care

In this chapter we look at:	
Introduction	see 1
Independent Living (Extension) Fund	see 2
Independent Living (1993) Fund	see 3
Social Services direct payments	see 4

1. Introduction

Under Community Care, local authorities have the main responsibility for directly providing or arranging services for disabled people and others who are assessed as needing them. Chapter 32 looks at the type of help they can provide, or arrange via private or voluntary home care providers. From April 1997 local authorities can give you the money to buy your own care – see 4 below.

There are social security benefits that may help you with the costs of care. Chapter 17 looks at disability living allowance care component for people under 65 who need help with personal care. If you are over 65, you may be able to get attendance allowance for help with care needs. Carers who spend at least 35 hours a week caring for a severely disabled person may be able to get invalid care allowance – see Chapter 19.

The two Independent Living Funds (see 2 and 3 below) make cash payments directly to you, which you can use to pay for care to help you live independently in your own home.

Their forerunner, the Independent Living Fund (ILF) was set up by the government in 1988 as there was concern that some severely disabled people had lost out in the reforms to social security. The old ILF was intended to be an interim measure until community care was introduced. Accordingly, the Fund was wound up with effect from 31.3.93.

Two new funds were established from 1.4.93. They are the Independent Living (Extension) Fund and the Independent Living (1993) Fund. Both are government funded but independent and discretionary trust funds, governed by a Board of Trustees. A legally binding trust deed sets out the powers and procedures of the Trustees and the eligibility criteria for help from the Funds. We look at the funds in detail below.

2. Independent Living (Extension) Fund

The role of the Extension Fund is to maintain the payments that were previously being made by the Independent Living Fund, so you can only get help from it if you were getting help under the old arrangements. No new applications are accepted.

The Extension Fund makes cash payments directly to you, which you can use to pay for personal care to help you continue to live independently in the community.

Payments are made four weekly in arrears and are normally paid directly into your bank account. Money from the Extension Fund is wholly ignored when means-tested benefits are being calculated.

See 3 below for the address of the ILF and how to appeal if there is a problem.

Carers' details
The Fund requires you to provide the name, address and National Insurance number of your carers. It also needs to know how much you pay each carer. The Fund's trust deed requires them to supply this information, on request, to the Secretary of State. If you have any difficulty providing this information you could contact the Fund to discuss the problem.

Tax and National Insurance contributions
Because the Extension Fund is a charity, the payments you receive are not liable for tax or National Insurance contributions.

Employment issues
It is important to check the status of the carers who work with you. Each individual case varies and is judged on its merits by the Inland Revenue and/or the Contributions Agency, but there will be cases where carers are treated as employees. **This also applies to the Independent Living (1993) Fund.** This means you will be treated as an employer, with all the responsibilities such as paying employers' National Insurance contributions, etc that being an employer involves. The Inland Revenue does have a simplified way of collecting tax in these situations. If the decision causes any difficulty, you could discuss it with the local tax office. In addition, the Funds have a Helpline for clients for general advice on tax and National Insurance which you can contact through the ILF's main phone number. You may find it helpful to read *Recruiting and Employing a Personal Care Worker*, published by the Disablement Income Group (see the Address List at the back of this Handbook).

Increases in awards
The Fund may consider increases for people who have *'experienced a significant change in their circumstances'*. For example, where total care needs have increased. In these circumstances, the Fund may contact your local authority to ask them to review their contribution as the statutory authority.

All requests for an increase in the amount payable from the Fund will be considered on their merits. The Fund has the discretion to increase payments but it must also keep within the funding given to it by the government.

Going into hospital or respite care
If you are admitted to hospital or another type of residential or institutional care, your payments from the Extension Fund will be suspended. If you return to live independently in the community within 26 weeks, your payments will be reinstated. As with any significant change in your circumstances, it is important that you inform the Fund of the details as soon as possible.

3. Independent Living (1993) Fund
Under Community Care, local authorities have primary statutory responsibility for the care of all disabled people. The 1993 Fund works in partnership with local authorities to devise 'joint care packages' that are a combination of services from the local authority and cash from the Fund.

As with the Extension Fund, payments are made four weekly in arrears and are normally paid directly into your bank account. See also 2 above for employment issues.

Money from the 1993 Fund is wholly ignored when means-tested benefits are being calculated.

Who can get help?
It is important to remember that the 1993 Fund is a discretionary body, but there are some basic guidelines to which the Trustees must have regard.

To qualify for help from the 1993 Fund, you should normally fulfil **all** of the following conditions. You must:
- be severely disabled to the extent that extensive help with personal care or household duties is needed to maintain an independent life in the community;
- be at least 16 and under 66 years of age;
- be receiving disability living allowance higher rate care component;
- be receiving (or it is planned that you will receive) services to a value of, currently, at least £200 a week from your local authority;
- have care needs whose total cost to the local authority and the 1993 Fund is no more, currently, than £500 a week;
- be receiving income support or income-based JSA OR have an income at or about income support level after an assessed contribution is made towards care costs (see below for how much you have to contribute);
- have less than £8,000 savings;
- be living alone or with people who are unable to fully meet your care needs;
- have care needs that are generally stable and will be met by the joint care package for the following six months.

(This means that some people who are terminally ill may not be eligible, but each application to the Fund will be looked at on its own merits, according to the criteria. There is no 'banned list' of conditions or diseases.)

How to apply for help
If you think you may be eligible for help from the 1993 Fund, you should do the following.
- Contact your local authority Social Services Department and ask for a social worker to carry out an assessment of your needs. Tell them you want to apply to the 1993 Fund.
- If the social worker decides that the care package you need will involve at least £200 worth of services from the local authority, but will not cost more than £500 a week in total, they will support your application to the 1993 Fund.
- Once your application has been accepted by the Fund, they will arrange for one of their Visiting Social Workers to organise a joint visit with you and the local authority social worker. At this visit your care needs can be discussed by all three parties and an agreement reached about the amount and type of care you need.
- The Fund's social worker will then send in a written report that makes recommendations about the care package needed.
- If your application is successful, the Trustees will make you a cash award of, currently, up to £300 a week. This amount will be put into payment once the staff at the Fund have received details from you of who your carers will be. You must supply the names, addresses and National Insurance numbers of your carers.

How much will you have to contribute?
You will not get help if your capital is over £8000. The financial assessment is based on income support rules (see Chapter 3) – so if you are one of a couple then your capital and income will be counted jointly.

If you get income support or income-based JSA which includes the severe disability premium, you will be expected to put all of this premium to the cost of your care. You will also be expected to put half of your disability living allowance care component towards the cost of your care.

If you are not on income support or income-based JSA, then all your income in excess of the amount you would get if you were on income support (excluding the severe disability premium) will have to be contributed towards the cost of your care.

Some of the allowances are more generous than income support or income-based JSA. For instance there is a £30 disregard on earnings, and all mortgage payments and endowments are taken into account.

If you are being charged by your local authority at the time of application for the care they are providing, this will be deducted from the amount the ILF will expect you to contribute.

What if your care needs change?
If your care needs increase and you need more money, you can apply for an increase in your payments. However, since the care arrangements are meant to be sufficient to look after your care requirements for at least 6 months, the Fund does not expect to receive requests for increases shortly after payments have started. The Fund may also approach your local authority to ask if they are able to increase their contribution. In considering your case, the Trustees must have regard to their budget, to the level of services provided by the local authority and the extent to which they consider the local authority to be fulfilling its statutory obligations under the community care legislation. If once you have been accepted as a client of the Fund your care costs increase to more than £500 a week, the Fund will not withdraw its commitment. If appropriate, the Fund will offer you a payment of the maximum amount (£300 a week). Currently, there are no circumstances in which the Fund can pay more than £300 a week.

Going into hospital or respite care
The guidelines about being admitted to hospital or another type of residential care are the same as for the Extension Fund – see 2 above.

Appeals
Under the community care arrangements, all local authorities are required to operate complaints procedures to protect the interests of individuals. If you have a complaint about Social Services that cannot be resolved informally, you should send it in writing so that it is registered. For more details, see Chapter 32(7).

If you are dissatisfied with any aspect of the way in which the Funds have dealt with your application, you should set out your reasons in writing and send them to the Director of the Funds at the address below. He will review the case and may then refer it to a subcommittee of the Board of Trustees for a decision. In exceptional circumstances, an appeal will be considered by the whole Board of Trustees.

Both Independent Living Funds are based at *PO Box 183, Nottingham, NG8 3RD. Telephone (0115) 9428191 or (0115) 9428192.*

4. Social Services direct payments
The Community Care (Direct Payments) Act 1996 has made it possible for Social Services Departments to pay money to you if you are willing and able to buy in your own care services for meeting your assessed needs rather than Social Services providing the care direct. Or you can have a combination of some services arranged or provided by Social Services and others by direct payments. It came into force in April 1997. There are various limitations.

- The Act does not require local authorities to make direct payments but simply allows them to do so. Some authorities may not run a scheme. If you want a direct payment and there is no scheme in your area you can use the complaints procedure – see Chapter 32(7).
- Regulations limit direct payments to particular categories of people, and at present only include disabled people under 65 years, although if you were getting a direct payment before 65 years it will continue. There is a commitment to review this in April 1998.
- Certain other people cannot receive direct payments, in particular those who have a mental illness and are still subject to conditions under the Mental Health Act (ie on leave of absence or supervision after discharge).
- The level of payment may be linked to your local authority's discretionary charging policy (see Chapter 32(6)) and paid net of any charge.
- It can only be used for care at home, or short periods in respite care up to a maximum of 4 weeks in any one year. Separate periods in respite care of less than 4 weeks are added together towards the maximum only if you are at home for 28 days or less in between.
- Direct payments cannot be used to pay for services from a spouse or partner, or a close relative living in the same household or elsewhere (except in exceptional circumstances).

If the money is not spent on the care that the local authority has assessed you as needing (ie what they would have been prepared to provide) – then they may ask for it to be paid back. How it will work in practice will vary from area to area.

The local authorities have been given a monitoring task to ensure both that the services you buy meet your assessed needs and for audit purposes to ensure the money is actually spent on the care. How this will work in practice will vary from area to area.

Guidance suggests that local authorities discuss with people at an early stage whether they wish to have a direct payment. There is a discretion to refuse direct payments to anyone they judge would not be able to manage, although they are told to avoid blanket assumptions. The person can have assistance in managing but has the final responsibility of how the money is spent.

The Act requires local authorities to make direct payments at the rate which would be equal to their estimate of the reasonable cost of the service.

If you are dissatisfied with any aspect of the direct payment, including being refused a payment, you should use the complaints procedure – see Chapter 32(7).

Residential care

This section of the Handbook looks at the following:

Help with residential care	Chapter **35**
Benefits in care – since April 1993	Chapter **36**
Charging for residential care	Chapter **37**
Benefits in care – before April 1993	Chapter **38**

35 Help with residential care

In this chapter we look at:

Who can get help with residential care?	see 1
Different types of residential care	see 2
How can you get residential care?	see 3
Choice of home	see 4
For more information	see Box K.1

1. Who can get help with residential care?

The system of community care arrangements introduced in April 1993 under the NHS and Community Care Act 1990 only affects you if you enter a residential care home or a nursing home on or after 1.4.93 and need financial help with the cost of your place. Most people now need to turn to local authority Social Services (or Social Work) Departments for help with residential care or nursing home fees. This help will be provided only on the basis of a professional assessment of your needs (see Chapter 32 and Box J.2). How much you pay depends on an assessment of your means (see Chapter 37).

As far as the local authority is concerned, the system of needs assessments and charging assessments is the same whether your accommodation is provided in a home managed or owned by a local authority, or in a home managed or owned by a voluntary or private organisation (sometimes described as the independent sector). All come under Part III of the National Assistance Act 1948 if the local authority has provided or arranged the place. This distinction is only important when it comes to claiming some benefits (see Chapter 36).

If you enter a residential home and don't want or need help with the fees, the current system won't affect you, unless in the future, your savings are likely to drop below £16,000. If your capital is only marginally above £16,000 and you know you will soon need help from the local authority, it may be best to discuss with them whether the type of home you plan to go in is suitable for your needs, and whether, once your capital is below £16,000, they will agree to help with the funding, or whether they think it is more expensive than they would be prepared to pay (but see 3 below, 'Important news').

If you were already living permanently in a private or voluntary residential care or nursing home on 31.3.93, you may have a 'preserved right' to help under the old system of higher rates of income support (or income-based JSA) from the DSS. You may also have a preserved right if you were only temporarily absent from the home on this date. What this usually means is that you need to apply to the DSS for financial help through the higher levels of income support to help meet the cost of the fees. For more information, turn to Chapter 38. Chapters 36 and 37 cover all those in local authority homes regardless of when they moved in.

Residential care for children under 18 is provided under the Children Act 1989.

In the rest of this chapter we only cover the different types of residential care, the local authority's duties and the choice you have in deciding on a home. This chapter does not cover social security benefits in residential care, or how the local authority assesses your charge – see Chapters 36 and 37.

2. Different types of residential care

Residential care is offered by a range of different providers, and local authorities are able to arrange accommodation in the type of home that most suits your needs. Health authorities as well as local authorities can arrange care in nursing homes. We use the term residential care when talking about any of the types of homes listed below (except hospices).

Local authority residential homes
These are homes which are owned or managed by local authorities. Mostly they are for elderly people, but local authorities also provide hostels for people with learning disabilities and for those with, or recovering from, a mental illness. All these local authority homes and hostels are now provided under Part III of the National Assistance Act 1948. Some local authority hostels, which tend to be for younger people, do not provide board as they want to help encourage independence. In this case you will count as a '*less dependent resident*'. It may mean a difference to the benefits you receive (see Chapter 36) and the way you are charged (see Chapter 37).

Although local authority homes do not need to be registered, they are regularly inspected by the local authority Inspection Unit.

Independent residential homes
These can be provided by private or voluntary organisations or private individuals. All independent residential care homes must be inspected by and registered with the local authority Inspection Unit, unless the home is exempt from registration. Small homes (with less than 4 residents) which provide both board and personal care now also have to be registered, although the conditions about services and facilities are less demanding than for larger homes.

Nursing homes
These may be provided by health authorities, NHS trusts, or by independent organisations. Independent nursing homes must be inspected by and registered with the health authority. If just one resident in an independent residential care home requires nursing care which is beyond the scope of a good carer with help from the community nursing services, the care home must apply for 'dual registration', ie it must also register as a nursing home.

Continuing nursing care – Both local authorities and health authorities can arrange places in nursing homes. If the NHS makes arrangements, it is free but your benefits will be affected in the same way as if you were in hospital. If the local authority has responsibility, it is subject to the means test. Much of the provision of non-acute nursing care has been transferred to the local authority. Guidance has been issued (HSG 95/8 and LAC 95/5) aiming to clarify where continuing nursing care is the responsibility of the NHS. Some major points are as follows.

- ❑ Local policies have been drawn up by health authorities regarding who is eligible for continuing NHS care. The first policies were published in April 1996, and there may be changes to the criteria in 1997/98.
- ❑ Patients being discharged from hospital should be given details about future care options and the likely costs.
- ❑ Patients have the right to refuse discharge to nursing homes or residential care and alternative options should be explored.
- ❑ Patients have the right to request a review of the decision about their eligibility for continuing nursing care provided by the NHS.

Local policies mean that who gets continuing nursing care varies around the country. The guidance also covers the type of health care you can get in your own home, or that should be provided to those in residential care.

Hospices

Health authorities are responsible for funding and arranging care for people with a terminal illness. Places may be provided in health authority or NHS trust hospices, or in independently run hospices, or the health authority may arrange for hospice type care in an independent nursing home.

Although local authorities are not excluded from arranging hospice care, they have to get the health authority's consent before arranging a placement in any registered nursing home, including hospices. The Department of Health considers that local authority placements in hospices will be unlikely.

So if you need a place in a hospice, this will usually be arranged via your GP through your health authority. Hospice care is free at the point of use. The local authority charging assessment does not apply to hospices. Obviously, the local authority assessment of your needs may well indicate a need for hospice care. In that case, the assessment would be done in conjunction with the health authority.

3. How can you get residential care?

The local authority's duty

In England and Wales, under s.21(1)(a) of Part III of the National Assistance Act 1948 (NAA), as amended by the NHS and Community Care Act 1990, local authorities have a duty to provide residential care for all those who *'by reason of age, illness, disability, or any other circumstances are in need of care and attention which is not otherwise available to them'*. Local authorities can meet this duty by:

- providing a place in a home which is owned or managed by themselves, or by another local authority – s.21 NAA;
- arranging a place in a residential care home in the independent sector – s.26 NAA;
- arranging a place in a nursing home (with the consent of the relevant health authority) – s.26 NAA.

In Scotland, the duty to provide residential care is to be found in the Social Work (Scotland) Act 1968. The wording is slightly different in that the powers to provide accommodation are wider.

The 1993 Community Care changes mean that most places in residential care are now provided or arranged under Part III. The only distinction is whether the place is provided in a home owned and/or managed by a local authority, or arranged in an independent sector home. This becomes crucial when you consider the effect on income support or income-based JSA, disability living allowance and attendance allowance – see Chapter 36.

The local authority must also exercise its powers and duties in accordance with any directions, and take account of any guidance, issued by the Secretary of State for Health. If you are in any doubt about a local authority's powers or duties, do consult the directions and guidance. Your local authority is expected to give *'support and encouragement'* to people making representations or complaints. So they should be ready to tell you about, or let you see, any relevant directions or guidance. See Box K.1 for more details.

Deciding if you need residential care

If you think you might need residential care, perhaps just on a respite care basis or on a permanent basis, ask your local authority for an assessment – see Box J.2 and Chapter 32 for details about the needs assessment. Funding will only be given if the local authority thinks that your needs can be best met in residential care. Recently there has been controversy over the fact that some local authorities now have a shortfall of funds and are more reluctant to provide expensive 'packages of care' for people to remain in their own homes. It is often cheaper, by the time the local authority has financially assessed you for your contribution, for them to arrange for you to go into residential care. In a recent case it was decided that it was lawful to provide care in a residential home rather than meet the 24 hour needs at home (*R v Lancashire County Council ex parte Ingham*). See Chapter 32(7) for details of what to do if you disagree with the local authority.

Important news – In a recent High Court case, *R v Sefton Metropolitan Borough Council ex p Help the Aged*, it was ruled that it was lawful for a local authority to take into account its own resources and the resources of the individual in deciding whether there is a duty to provide residential care. Because of its lack of resources, Sefton Council was only agreeing to make arrangements for, and fund, residential care when the individual's resources were down to £1,500 (rather than the £16,000 capital limit set by regulation).

This ruling means that when someone who has less than £16,000 in capital approaches the local authority for help with funding residential care, there can be no guarantee that the local authority will agree to make the arrangements for the care. If they do so, either in the independent sector or in one of their own homes, then all the charging rules outlined in Chapter 37 will apply. But until the local authority actually arranges the care, the charging rules do not apply. A local authority could set its own capital limits in order to meet the most pressing needs in its area within its resources.

It has always been the intention of Parliament that the capital rules laid down by regulation (originally £8,000, but since 1996 increased to £16,000) would trigger help with funding by the local authority as long as the person was assessed as needing the residential care. It is understood that there is a commitment to restore this intention as soon as possible. It is also likely that this ruling will be appealed. At present, it is not known whether other local authorities will start to refuse help to people even if their capital is below £16,000.

If it is agreed that you need residential care, and that you need help with the funding because you cannot afford the fees, the local authority will make the contract with the home and is liable for the full costs. They will recover from you any contribution you are assessed as having to pay according to national rules – see Chapter 37. If the local authority hasn't agreed to arrange a place in residential care, it is not responsible for paying the home – you will be (unless the authority has an agreement with the home to allow 'direct access' to people in urgent need; or where it retrospectively accepts responsibility).

Urgent cases
If your need is urgent, the local authority can arrange for residential care without carrying out a formal needs assessment. The assessment would be done as soon as possible. If you need to go into a nursing home urgently, the local authority does not have to get the health authority's consent beforehand, but should do so as soon as possible.

Contact your Social Services (or Social Work) Department; explain your crisis, and ask for a social worker to visit you urgently. Ask your GP for help if necessary when contacting the Social Services Department.

You are in residential care and your capital is now at £16,000
If you moved into residential care since 1993, but you have not needed help because your capital was above £16,000, you will need to contact your Social Services Department when your capital nears this figure. They will then assess whether you actually need residential care, and whether they will meet the cost in that particular home. At the same time you should also apply for help from income support or income-based JSA. The help you receive should start from the time your capital reaches £16,000 (but see above, 'Important news').

Note for couples with joint capital – If you have a joint account in excess of £32,000 it may be worth splitting your account so that you do not have to wait until your joint account is down to this figure. For example if you have £40,000 in a joint account, your partner will only get help after £8,000 has been paid in fees and your account is down to £32,000. If you split the account so you each have £20,000, help will be available after spending only £4,000 in fees (but see above, 'Important news').

4. Choice of home
If the local authority decides, after the needs assessment, to offer you a permanent, or respite, place in residential care, it will suggest a particular home, or give you advice on homes to choose from. In all cases where a local authority is making the arrangements, you have the right to choose your own residential home or nursing home ('preferred accommodation') – see below. However, if a health authority places you in a nursing home and is paying the full fee, you do not have the same right to choose a particular nursing home. But nor will you be liable to meet any of that home's charges. Although your health authority must consent to a local authority placing you in a nursing home, the health authority *'would be expected not to interfere with an individual's choice of nursing home'* (HSG 92/54 – see Box K.1).

Preferred accommodation
If you tell your local authority that you want to enter a particular residential home or nursing home, that home is called 'preferred accommodation'. The Secretary of State's directions are intended to ensure that you can *'exercise a genuine choice over where [you] live'* (LAC 92/27 – see Box K.1).

If you have preferred accommodation, the local authority must arrange for care in that accommodation, so long as:
- it is suitable in relation to your assessed needs;
- it is available;
- the person in charge of the home is willing to provide a place subject to the authority's usual terms and conditions for such accommodation;
- the accommodation would not cost the authority more than it would usually expect to pay for accommodation for someone with your assessed needs; and
- your authority has legal power to make such a placement.

More expensive homes
If you have chosen a home which costs more than your local authority would usually expect to pay for someone with your needs, your local authority will nevertheless arrange for your preferred accommodation (given that it satisfies the other conditions above) if a third party is able and willing to meet the shortfall, and to continue doing so for as long as you are likely to be in residential care. These are sometimes referred to as 'third party' contributions. You should not be expected to use your personal expenses allowance of £14.10 to help pay for a more expensive home (LAC 94/1 – see Box K.1). Neither can you use your own capital below £10,000 or disregarded income to top up the fees. This may change in the future but will require an Act of Parliament. If you wish to pay for 'extras' which are outside of the care package then this is permissable according to the Department of Health. As long as you do not feel pressured by the home owner or the local authority, there is no reason why a resident should not enter into a contract with the home owner for these extra services.

Note that a 'liable relative' (spouse or former spouse) can only act as a third party, paying the difference, if s/he can afford to pay both any maintenance contribution that may have been requested under s.42, NAA, and the contribution for the extra cost of more expensive accommodation.

The local authority cannot use the direction on the Choice of Accommodation to set arbitrary ceilings on the amount it will contribute towards residential care and to require third parties routinely to make up the difference. The authority must be able to justify its usual cost, and show that it is enough to buy a reasonable level of service – without contributions from third parties. If the local authority itself decides to place you in more expensive accommodation, perhaps because there are no vacancies in 'usual cost' homes, a third party cannot be required to contribute. Neither should you or your relatives be expected to find a place at usual cost when none exists, or where dependency, psychological or other needs clearly indicate a need for a more expensive place. This could be because of language, culture, religion or the need to be near family so that regular visits can be made.

Points to note – The local authority remains responsible for the home's full fees, even though a third party is making a contribution.
- Third party payments are treated as your own income in the charging assessment (even if they are made direct to the home).
- These contributions are disregarded as income for income support and income-based JSA purposes.
- If the third party stops making a contribution you will usually have to move to another home.
- The local authority will not automatically pay an equal share of any increase in the home's fees.
- An increase in your income won't necessarily lessen the need for a third party contribution; it depends on the result of the charging assessment.
- If the home doesn't keep to its contractual obligations, the local authority may terminate the contract.

What sort of home?
Most local authority owned homes are for elderly people, and for physically disabled people. Increasingly, local authorities are meeting their duties by arranging places in homes in the independent sector. All independent homes have to be

registered, and also those with 4 or more residents will be inspected regularly. But although certain standards have to be met, the services and facilities you'll be offered may vary greatly from home to home.

Ask your social worker or GP what things you should be looking out for, and what questions you should ask, when choosing a place in residential care. They may give you a checklist of questions. Don't take anything for granted. For example, how often will it be possible for you to have a bath? Can you take your favourite armchair with you?

You should go and see the home beforehand to make sure you will be comfortable there and get on well with the staff and other residents. You might want to enter the home for a short stay before committing yourself to a permanent stay. Make sure you are clear about the terms for your stay in the home. This is especially important if you are making your own arrangements with the home. If the local authority has made the contract it is still useful for you to know exactly what is covered. Do not let yourself be rushed into things. Try the Address List at the back of this Handbook for organisations that can support you and see Box K.1.

Complaints

If you have a complaint about a home owned or managed by a local authority, you can use the local authority complaints procedure – see Chapter 32(7). All independent residential care homes must have a complaints procedure. If your local authority has placed you in a care home, you can also use the local authority's complaints procedure.

Nursing homes don't have to have a complaints procedure, but many do. If you cannot resolve a problem with your nursing home, contact the authority which placed you in that home. If your local authority placed you in a nursing home, you can use their complaints procedure. Your Community Health Council (in Scotland, Local Health Council, and in Northern Ireland, Health and Social Services Council) may also be able to help. If not, complain to the Health Authority Inspection Unit.

36 Benefits in care – since April 1993

1. What benefits are you entitled to?

If you have moved into residential care (either temporarily or permanently), the only social security benefits which may be affected are:
- disability living allowance (DLA) care component;
- attendance allowance (AA);
- income support (IS) and income-based jobseeker's allowance (JSA);
- housing benefit (HB);
- council tax benefit (CTB);
- special help for war pensioners.

All other social security benefits can be claimed and paid in the normal way, subject to the standard rules outlined in the rest of this Handbook. It makes no difference whether the home you are in is owned or managed by a local authority, or by a private or voluntary organisation. However, the distinction between local authority homes and (registered) independent sector homes is important for DLA care component, attendance allowance and income support or income-based JSA.

Chapter 38 covers people with 'preserved rights' ie who were living in private or voluntary residential or nursing homes before 1.4.93. Only if for any reason you lose your preserved rights will you need to read this chapter. Those in local authority homes who moved in either before or after 1993 need to read this chapter and Chapter 37.

K.1 For more information

The law
- Health and Social Services and Social Security Adjudication Act 1983 (HASSASSA)
- Income Support General Regulations 1987 (ISG)
- Jobseeker's Allowance Regulations 1996 (JSA Regs)
- Mental Health Act 1983
- National Assistance Act 1948 (NAA)
- National Assistance (Assessment of Resources) Regulations 1992 (AOR)
- National Assistance (Sums for Personal Requirements) Regulations
- National Health Service Act 1977 (NHSA)
- National Health Service and Community Care Act 1990 (NHSCCA)
- Residential Accommodation (Relevant Premises, Ordinary Residence and Exemptions) Regulations 1993 (RPORE)
- Social Security Administration Act 1992 (SSAA)

Guidance and circulars
These are issued by the Department of Health and have to be followed by local authorities and health authorities.
- HSG = Health Service Guidance
- HC = Health Circular
- LAC = Local Authority Circular

They should be available from your health or local authority.

If you are challenging any decisions about residential care, you may find the following particularly useful:
- AOG = *Adjudication Officers' Guide* (issued by the DSS for DSS staff)
- *Charging for Residential Accommodation Guide* (CRAG); and
- LACs 92/19, 93/14, 94/1, 94/15, 94/21 are to be found at Annex H of CRAG. LAC 95/7, 95/21, 96/9, 96/9 (addendum) and 97/5 should be with CRAG. These explain the Assessment of Resources Regulations.
- LAC 93/6: deals with local authority powers to make arrangements for people who were in independent sector residential care and nursing homes on 31.3.93
- LAC 93/7: ordinary residence
- LAC 92/27: Choice of Accommodation Directive
- HSG 95/8, LAC 95/5 and EL 96/8: NHS responsibilities for meeting continuing care needs

Further reading
- *A Guide to Community Care Services for Older People*, Counsel and Care, Fact Sheet 18
- *Local Authority Charging Procedures for Residential and Nursing Home Care*, Age Concern, Fact Sheet 10
- *Financial Support for People in Residential and Nursing Homes Prior to 1 April 1993*, Age Concern, Fact Sheet 11
- *Finding Residential and Nursing Home Accommodation*, Age Concern, Fact Sheet 29
- *Moving into a Care Home? Things you need to know*, Department of Health

2. Attendance allowance and DLA care component

Chapter 17(10) covers the effect of a stay in 'special accommodation' on DLA care component and attendance allowance (AA). Read that section, and Box G.3, as well as this one. The mobility component is only affected if your stay is in hospital or a similar institution. Your mobility component is not affected in residential care, even if you are funded by the local authority. See Chapter 17(10).

Independent sector homes (registered)

It was the intention that AA or DLA care component should not be payable to you after the first 4 weeks in a residential care or nursing home unless you are paying the full cost yourself without any help from IS or income-based JSA, housing benefit or any funding from the local authority. But even if you are claiming IS or income-based JSA, in some circumstances you will be able to claim and receive AA or DLA care component.

The 'may be borne' provision – A flaw in the way the law was drafted means that you can still receive AA or DLA care component in a home at the same time as receiving IS or income-based JSA as long as you do not actually get financial help from the local authority. This loophole arises because the law says that AA and DLA care component are not payable where the cost 'may be borne' by the local authority. But it has been shown that this regulation has no real function in England and Wales. This is because if you have made your own arrangements, the local authority has no power to intervene unless the home is not suitable for your needs. Provided the local authority has no current contract for your care in the home, you can continue to receive AA or DLA care component, even if you receive IS or income-based JSA. It is only if the local authority has a contract with the home for the funding of your care that your AA or DLA care component will be affected.

However, depending on the level of the fee for the home, there is still likely to be a shortfall between the fee and the total amount you receive in IS or income-based JSA and AA or DLA care component. But the option may be attractive to you if your local authority has not agreed to fund your care or if you have a property to sell and can meet the shortfall until it is sold. Once your house is sold any IS or income-based JSA and AA or DLA care component is not clawed back by the DSS. If you were funded by the local authority, you would lose your AA or DLA care component, and you would have to refund to the local authority all the money they have paid once you have sold your home (see Box K.3 for an example of this).

It is very important that people who wish to use this provision should seek up to date advice; the law may be changed, or you may find that your benefit is stopped while the DSS make enquiries to be sure that you are not funded by the Social Services Department. You may prefer to have the security of the local authority arranging your stay in residential care (but see Chapter 35(3) 'Important news').

Please note that the rules are different in Scotland, as the powers to provide accommodation are wider. It is understood that a case is to be heard on this question in the near future so the situation in Scotland may change.

New residents in independent residential care homes who are funded by the local authority will lose their AA or DLA care component after 4 weeks (or earlier); see Chapter 17(10).

If you later start paying the full fee yourself, perhaps because you have received the capital from the sale of your house, you will be able to get AA or DLA care component again from the time the local authority no longer has to fund the placement. Remember you will need to tell the DSS when you start paying full fees in order to get your AA or DLA care component paid again. As long as you do not still get IS or income-based JSA, it does not matter if the local authority still has a contract with the home, as you are paying the full costs.

It had been argued that technically, because the full cost has to be refunded to the local authority once they have sold their house, people with houses to sell are self-funders. However, there have now been three cases which have looked at this question. Two have found that AA and DLA care component **cannot** be paid retrospectively for the period during which the local authority was helping with the fees and that money has now been repaid (CA/7126/95 and CA/11185/95). One case has found the opposite (CA/4723/95). It is important to be aware of all these cases if considering an appeal. You may wish to write to your MP if you think it is unfair that AA or DLA care component cannot be paid even though you have had to pay the local authority the full cost of the home.

Direct payments – From April 1997, local authorities can give you direct payments for you to arrange your own care at home (see Chapter 34(4)). You can also use the money to buy up to 4 weeks respite care in any one year. AA and DLA care component therefore will not normally be affected. But if you need another period of care or hospital treatment within the linking period (see Chapter 17(9) and (10)) your AA or DLA care component could be affected. For example, you use your direct payment to buy 4 weeks residential care. Two weeks later your carer falls ill, so you return to residential care. This time your stay is funded by the local authority under a contract with the home. Your AA or DLA care component is affected immediately as it links with a period when your care was being funded by local authority money because you were using the payment from the local authority to buy your respite care.

Local authority accommodation

If you are living in local authority owned or managed residential accommodation you will not be entitled to AA or DLA care component after the first 4 weeks. This is the case even if you are paying the full cost yourself. If you know you will be able to pay the full cost, you may be better off choosing an independent home so that you can get your AA or DLA care component paid once you are self-funding (but see Chapter 35(3) 'Important news').

3. Housing benefit

Independent sector homes (registered)

You cannot get housing benefit for the costs of a registered care or nursing home. See below for help with meeting the costs of your own home.

Local authority accommodation

You are excluded from housing benefit for the cost of local authority owned or managed residential accommodation which provides board (see below for help with meeting the costs of your own home).

If you live in a hostel that does not provide board you will be able to receive housing benefit to help meet the cost of your rent. Board means where meals are part of the charge. Even if the hostel provides meals, if you pay for them separately then this doesn't count as 'board'. From April 1996, only capital over £10,000 is counted as tariff income.

Help with meeting the costs of your own home

If you go into residential care for a temporary stay or for respite care, you can continue to receive HB (or IS/income-based JSA mortgage interest) for up to 52 weeks as long as it is clear that your stay is not likely to last longer than this and you intend to return to your own home.

However if you go into residential care for a 'trial period' with a view to a permanent admission, HB (or IS/income-based JSA mortgage interest) is only paid for up to 13 weeks (see Chapter 4(6)). Most people like to keep their options open and have time to decide whether residential care is for them before giving up their home. If you think there is any possibility of your being able to return to your home, you should describe your stay as temporary. Remember, if you get IS or income-based JSA only while in residential care, you need to reclaim HB on your return home.

4. Council tax benefit

You can get CTB only if you are liable to pay council tax. Your former home is exempt from council tax if it is unoccupied and you are now solely or mainly resident in any type of residential care or nursing home. If your own home has been left empty, but the residential accommodation is not yet your 'sole or main' home, you will get a 50% status discount. See Chapter 5. The rules for getting CTB during a temporary stay or trial period in residential care are the same as in HB – see above. Remember, if you get IS or income-based JSA only while in residential care, you need to reclaim CTB on your return home.

5. Income support and income-based JSA

Capital limits in residential care

For all types of residential care homes in this section of the Handbook, and also Abbeyfield and Royal Charter Homes, you can claim income support or income-based JSA if your capital is £16,000 or less, if you are a permanent resident. Tariff income (see Chapter 3(29)) only starts at £10,000. If you know you want to stay in residential care, your admission can be permanent from the start. Most local authorities, though, prefer you to have a trial period to see if you like it. The trial period should count as temporary until you decide to stay permanently. During a temporary period, the income support and income-based JSA capital limit is £8,000 and only goes up to £16,000 when your stay is permanent. You are still considered to be a permanent resident if you are temporarily absent for up to 52 weeks if you are over pension age, or 13 weeks in all other cases.

Note that you can still get help from the local authority if your capital is no more than £16,000 regardless of whether your stay is temporary or permanent.

Independent sector homes (registered)

For income support and income-based JSA the system for people who have moved in since 31.3.93 is very simple.

If you 'reside in' a residential care home or a nursing home which is run on a commercial basis (but not in a hospice), are aged 16 or more, and housing benefit does not meet any part of the charge, your IS or income-based JSA is worked out in the standard way by adding together:
- your personal allowance;
- any premiums to which you are entitled (which can include severe disability premium while AA or DLA care component is payable);
- a residential allowance.

The residential allowance is £62 a week in the Greater London area, and £56 a week elsewhere, and is paid whether your stay is temporary or permanent.

This will mean that even if you are not entitled to IS or income-based JSA in your own home, you may be entitled when you go into residential care. The person who assesses you from the local authority should be able to advise you.

For permanent residents, for whom the care home has become the main residence, the residential allowance stops once you have been absent from a residential care or nursing home unless:
- you intend to return to the home; and
- you have been absent for less than 6 weeks because you are a patient in hospital; or
- you have been absent for less than 3 weeks (for any other reason).

Periods of absence because you've gone into hospital that are separated by less than 28 days are linked together and treated as one long period of absence.

If you are absent for any other reason, then each period of absence is treated separately and there are no linking rules.

Temporary admission – So long as you enter or are expected to enter a home for a period of no more than 8 weeks, your IS or income-based JSA (which will now include the residential allowance) can be paid from the day of admission. If your stay is expected to be more than 8 weeks, your IS or income-based JSA can only be altered from the start of your benefit week (see Box B.3 in Chapter 3). The local authority charge should be based on what you actually receive, so if there are a few days when you receive less money, you should be charged less.

Temporary admission (couple) – If one of you goes into residential care for a temporary period, for IS or income-based JSA purposes you will still be assessed as a couple, but you will each get the appropriate single person rate. So the person at home will get his/her personal allowance, premiums and any housing costs, and the person in care will get a personal allowance, premiums plus the residential allowance. These are then added together, and your combined income is then taken from this figure to give the amount of income support or income-based JSA to be paid to the claimant. See Box K.3 for an example.

If you both go together into the same residential care home, then you will receive the couple rate of IS or income-based JSA, and will each receive a residential allowance.

HB/CTB will continue to be paid for your costs at home.

Severe disability premium and temporary admissions – There is still considerable confusion about the payment of the severe disability premium (SDP) for temporary admissions. The new *Adjudication Officers' Guide* (AOG, Vol 4, 28231-33) complicates the situation and narrows the payment of the SDP to where couples are joint owners or joint tenants in a property, or the partner at home is registered blind or gets AA or DLA middle or higher rate care component. This is a less generous interpretation than under the old AOG. If ICA is paid to a carer then the SDP will not be paid. In practice the SDP is often left out of the calculation for both temporary and permanent admissions, and if you are being assessed by the local authority you do not see any benefit from the extra money. The main thing you need to check is that the local authority is not assuming that you are getting the SDP and charging you even if you are not being paid it!

Permanent admission – Once your stay is permanent you can't get HB or IS/income-based JSA housing costs on your former home – see 3 above for the rules about help with housing costs for trial periods. If you still have housing costs after your stay becomes permanent, eg you have to give a month's notice,

you can ask the local authority to vary your personal expenses allowance to help meet the costs – see Chapter 37(5).
Permanent admission (couple) – Once one of a couple is permanently in residential care, each of you will be treated as separate claimants. So any jointly owned capital will be split and the IS or income-based JSA assessment should be based solely on each of your individual capital and income. If you both enter the same home you may still be assessed as a couple. See Chapter 35(3) for information about joint capital.

If the DSS regards you as a permanent resident when the local authority is still regarding you as temporary (eg during a trial period), seek advice.

Local authority accommodation (providing board)
The amount of IS or income-based JSA you get while in local authority residential accommodation depends on whether you go there temporarily or permanently and whether or not you are single or part of a couple. The amounts you get paid are much lower than in independent sector homes.
Temporary admission – Temporary admission into local authority accommodation can mean that you stop being entitled to IS or income-based JSA during the time you are in the home. You might then need to make a new claim for IS or income-based JSA and HB when you return to your own home. See Example 6 in Box K.3.
Single – Your IS or income-based JSA allowance will be £62.45 of which £14.10 is for personal expenses, plus any IS/income-based JSA housing costs.
Couple – If one of a couple is temporarily in residential accommodation, you will get the single person rate for the person remaining at home, plus £62.45 for the person in care. If both of you are temporarily in local authority residential accommodation, you will get two lots of £62.45 plus any housing costs.
Single parent – Your IS or income-based JSA allowance will be £62.45 plus the personal allowance for each child for whom you were receiving benefit before going into the home, plus the family premium (lone parent rate) and any housing costs.
Permanent admission (single and single parent) – Your IS or income-based JSA allowance will be £62.45.
Permanent admission (couple) – If one of you is in residential care permanently, you will be treated as separate claimants. The person in residential accommodation will get £62.45 and the other partner will be assessed as a single person or single parent. If you are both in residential accommodation, you will receive double £62.45.

Local authority accommodation (not providing board)
If you go into local authority accommodation which does not provide board, you will receive IS or income-based JSA at your normal rate. If you are one of a couple and only one of you goes into residential care then the same rules as above apply regarding whether you are assessed as a couple or individual claimants.

6. IS/income-based JSA and maintenance
A husband and wife are each liable to maintain the other. S.106 Social Security Administration Act gives the Secretary of State power to attempt recovery of expenditure on IS or income-based JSA from a person liable for maintenance. So normally any payment that is made to you is taken into account as income. But take note: if you are receiving a payment to help meet the costs of more expensive 'preferred' accommodation (see Chapter 35(4)), IS and income-based JSA ignores these payments.

The actions the DSS can take are described more fully in Chapter 38(10).

7. Special help for war pensioners.
Some war pensioners may qualify for help in getting their fees paid by the War Pensions Agency. It can cover nursing home fees and respite breaks. The help from war pensions is not means tested. For more information see Chapter 22(11).

37 Charging for residential care

In this chapter we look at:	
The legal basis of the financial assessment	see 1
Key points	see 2
Capital and income	see Box K.2
Less dependent residents	see 3
Couples and maintenance	see 4
The personal expenses allowance	see 5
Treating your home as capital	see 6
Meeting the costs of your own home	see 7
What happens when you move out?	see 8
Interaction of benefits and charges	see Box K.3

1. The legal basis of the financial assessment
Section 22(1) of the National Assistance Act 1948 (NAA), as amended by the NHS and Community Care Act 1990, provides for the local authority to charge you for the accommodation they provide, whether that is in a home owned by a local authority, or in an independent home (but see Chapter 35(3) 'Important news').

The local authority has to fix a standard rate for the accommodation. The standard rate for local authority homes is the full cost to the authority of providing your place in that accommodation. The standard rate for independent homes is the gross cost to the local authority of providing or paying for your place in that accommodation under a contract with the independent home.

If you cannot pay the standard rate, the local authority must assess your ability to pay and calculate what lower amount to charge you.

The basis of that assessment is in the National Assistance (Assessment of Resources) Regulations 1992 (AOR), as amended. These regulations are explained in various circulars which are at Annex H in the *Charging for Residential Accommodation Guide* (CRAG). Local authorities must take account of the CRAG because it is statutory guidance issued by the Secretary of State. It is updated and amended and circulars are issued with each amendment – see Box K.1.

The amount you can keep for your personal expenses depends on the National Assistance (Sums for Personal Requirements) Regulations which set a rate each year. Section 22(4), NAA, also gives the local authority discretion to pay a higher amount.

Capital
If you are in residential care (whether your stay is permanent or temporary) and your savings are over £16,000 you will have to pay the standard rate for your accommodation until your capital drops to £16,000 or less. Some items of capital are ignored, or disregarded, in the assessment. These are listed in Schedule 4 of the Assessment of Resources Regulations – see Box K.2 and 6 below for details. If you own capital jointly with someone else, the law treats you as having an equal share of that capital, even if your actual share is different.

If you have capital of over £10,000, a tariff income is assumed – Chapter 3(29).

See Box K.2 and 6 below for information about how your house is treated.

Income
In general, assume all income counts unless it, or a part of it, is specifically ignored under Schedule 2 or Schedule 3 of the Assessment of Resources Regulations – see Box K.2 for details. The 'income disregards' are very similar to income support – see Chapter 3(24) to (28). Half of your occupational pension, personal pension and payment from a retirement annuity contract has to be disregarded if you pay at least half to your spouse at home. The income support (and income-based JSA) rules do not have a similar disregard, unless you have preserved rights (see Chapter 38(6)). Note that income support or income-based JSA itself is taken into account as income by the local authority (except for IS housing costs).

2. Key points
Before explaining the charging assessment in more detail, do note a number of key points.

- The local authority does not have to carry out a charging assessment for the first 8 weeks in care; they can charge what is reasonable.
- If you count as a 'less dependent resident', the local authority can ignore the whole of the charging assessment if that is reasonable in your situation – see 3 below.
- If you are a temporary resident in the home, the charging assessment is slightly different in order to allow for your costs at home – see 7 below.
- If you are one of a couple, the law does not allow a joint charging assessment; only the resident's own income and capital affects the assessment.
- Whatever your source(s) of income, you'll generally be left with no less than £14.10 a week – except for any income which is ignored in the assessment, the rest of your income goes towards meeting the standard rate for your accommodation.
- If your accommodation is provided as part of your aftercare package under Section 117 of the Mental Health Act, then you cannot be charged for your accommodation. You will still be entitled to all your benefits.
- Any difference between what you pay and the standard rate

K.2 Capital and income

General
The assessment of capital and income under the National Assistance (Assessment of Resources) Regulations 1992 (AOR) is closely based on the assessment for income support. You will get a reasonable idea of the local authority assessment if you look at Chapter 3(24) to (31). However, there are some differences. We note the key differences below. All abbreviations can be found in Box K.1.

Capital
Limits – These are £16,000 (£10,000 for tariff income) in cases of both temporary and permanent stays. (Income support capital limits for temporary residents are £8,000, and £3,000 for tariff income.)
Your home – See also Chapter 37(6). If you are a 'temporary resident', the value of 'one dwelling' is ignored if:
- you intend to return to live in it as your home; and
- it is still available to you; or
- your property is up for sale and you intend to use the proceeds to buy a more suitable property for you to return to.

You count as a **temporary resident** if your stay is unlikely to last for more than 52 weeks, or *'in exceptional circumstances [is] unlikely substantially to exceed that period'*. If you are not sure of your long-term plans, it's best to say that you intend to return to your own home.

The local authority has discretion, not found in income support, to disregard the value *'of any premises occupied in whole or in part by a third party where the local authority considers it would be reasonable to disregard the value of those premises'* [para 18, Sch 4 AOR]. Examples are given where a carer has given up his/her own home in order to care, or the person remaining is an elderly companion of the resident [CRAG para 7.007]; these examples are not exhaustive!

While your home is up for sale – If you are a permanent resident, one important difference is the way your home is treated. Unlike income support, when your old home is up for sale, the local authority does not ignore the value for 26 weeks. It counts as capital immediately and although the local authority may help towards your care fees while it is up for sale, you will have to pay back the full amount once your old home is sold.

If you jointly own property – Unlike income support, it is only *your* interest which is to be valued. It is recognised that it might be hard to find a willing buyer for a part share in a property [CRAG 7.012]. Seek advice if you disagree with how your share is valued. If you jointly own a property with a spouse who decides to sell in order to move to eg a smaller house, then you can give him/her some of your share of the proceeds to help buy the new home. The local authority shouldn't consider this as deprivation of your capital [CRAG 6.063].

Personal possessions – The value of these are ignored unless you acquired them with the intention of reducing your capital in order to satisfy a local authority that you were unable to pay for your accommodation at the standard rate or to reduce the rate at which you would otherwise be liable to pay for your accommodation [para 8, Sch 4 AOR].

Jointly owned capital – If you jointly own capital it will be divided in equal shares regardless of whether you are temporary or permanent. This is different from the DSS rules which count your capital together as a couple until you become a permanent resident, when they divide your capital.

Deprivation of capital
The notional capital rules described in Chapter 3(24) are not mandatory for local authorities. They have discretion not to apply reg 25(1) of the AOR Regs. If they do apply reg 25(1), the rules are similar to the income support rules. However, the local authority 'diminishing notional capital' rule reduces your notional capital on a weekly basis. It is reduced by the difference between the charge you are currently paying, and the charge you would have paid if the local authority had not taken 'notional capital' into account [reg 26 AOR].

The six month rule
Section 21, HASSASSA, is the source of the '6 month rule'. It is separate from the 'deprivation of capital' rule in reg 25, AOR Regs. Even if s.21, HASSASSA does not apply, the local authority may nevertheless take the value of the transferred asset into account under reg 25.

is met by the local authority which is liable for the full cost of the fees.
- If the application of the law affects you unfairly, urge the local authority to use its discretion in s.22(4) NAA to correct that unfairness – by letting you keep more than £14.10 pw of your income for your personal requirements – see 5 below.
- The assessment is based on the income support rules, but there are some important differences and in addition the local authority has some more discretion – see Box K.2.

See Box K.1 for some further useful reading.

3. Less dependent residents

If you count as a 'less dependent resident' (see Chapter 35(2)), the local authority has complete discretion to ignore the whole of the charging assessment if that is *'reasonable in the circumstances'*. This is because it has been recognised that to live as independently as possible you will need to be left with more than the personal expenses allowance [CRAG para 2.007].

4. Couples and maintenance

The local authority has no power under the National Assistance Act (NAA) to assess couples jointly. The financial assessment should be of the income and assets of the resident only (including any entitlement to income support or income-based JSA). The spouse remaining at home has no obligation to fill in the section of the assessment form asking for income and assets of your 'spouse/partner'; indeed LAC 94/1 para 8 (see Box K.1) underlines this and states *'the use of a joint assessment form when requesting financial details from the resident is not appropriate'*. What the local authority can do is to approach the spouse (not an unmarried partner, who has no liability) and inform them of their duty as a 'liable relative' under s.42 of the NAA to maintain their spouse.

The spouse can voluntarily agree a 'reasonable' amount to pay in support of the resident in the home. There are no guidelines as to what counts as 'reasonable'. But ultimately it is only a court which can set an amount (if any) a liable relative should pay. Seek advice if you are in this position.

The DSS have similar rules about liable relatives – see Chapter 38(10).

Section 21 of HASSASSA may be applied if:
- you transferred cash or any other asset, which would have affected the charging assessment, to someone else; and
- you did this *'knowingly and with the intention of avoiding charges for the accommodation'*; and either
- you transferred the asset 6 months or less before the day the local authority has arranged a placement in residential accommodation; or
- you transferred the asset while you were being funded by the local authority in residential accommodation; and either
- you were not paid anything, or given anything, in return for the transfer; or
- you were paid, or given something, less than the value of the asset in return for the transfer.

The six month rule does not apply where a resident is self-funding in an independent sector home, has not been assessed, nor had their placement arranged by a local authority (CRAG, Annex D(2.1) and LAC 97/5).

If s.21, HASSASSA applies, the person to whom you transferred the asset is *'liable to pay ... the difference between the amount assessed as due to be paid for the [residential] accommodation ... and the amount [which you are paying]'*. In this case, the local authority has a choice. It may either:
- use reg 25 to base the charging assessment on the amount of 'notional capital' you gave away, as well as on your actual capital and income; or
- if you cannot pay the assessed charge, it may use s.21 of HASSASSA to transfer the liability for the part of the charges assessed as a result of the notional capital from you to the person(s) to whom you transferred the asset, up to the value of the transferred asset.

Some people mistakenly think that it cannot affect the amount they would have to pay for residential care if they have given away assets more than 6 months before entering a residential home. However, if a significant purpose of giving away an asset was to get help, or more help, from the local authority with the cost of residential care, the deprivation of capital rule may be applied – even if the transfer took place over 6 months ago. Obviously, if you have given away something which would not have affected the charging assessment at all, the deprivation of capital rule cannot apply, nor can s.21 of HASSASSA.

Charitable and third party payments

These are described in Chapter 3(27) and (28). Regs 42 and 51, ISG apply to the local authority's charging assessment. However, such a payment, of income or of capital, will be taken into account if it is for *'any item which was taken into account when the standard rate was fixed for the accommodation provided'* [regs 17 and 25, Sch 3, para 10(2), AOR]. If a third party is making a payment to meet the shortfall for more expensive residential accommodation, that payment is always taken fully into account as your income by the local authority, but not by the DSS for social security benefits.

Income

- Attendance allowance and DLA care component are only disregarded if you are a 'temporary resident' – see above [Sch 3 para 6 AOR].
- Income support and income-based JSA are taken fully into account. However IS payments made towards housing costs, eg payments toward mortgage interest are disregarded [Sch 3 AOR].
- Housing benefit and council tax benefit which is being paid in relation to your usual home will be ignored.
- Housing costs – the local authority can disregard any payments you are making towards your housing costs as a temporary resident – see 7.
- Contributory benefits dependants' additions – if you get a child or adult dependant's addition, eg as part of your incapacity benefit or retirement pension, it is disregarded if it is paid to the person for whom it is intended [Sch 3 para 28B AOR].
- Child support maintenance payments and child benefit are disregarded (unless the child is in the accommodation with you).
- If you have a spouse with whom you are not residing, half your personal or occupational pension or payment from a retirement annuity contract will be disregarded if you pass at least this amount to your spouse. If you pass nothing or less than half, there is no disregard. The disregard is for both temporary and permanent residents.

5. The personal expenses allowance

You will get the same £14.10 personal expenses allowance whether you are in a local authority home or an independent sector home.

In the past, people in local authority homes received a lower personal expenses allowance, but were not expected to meet expenditure on clothing, shoes or other big items out of that allowance. This *'expectation ... will no longer normally apply. However, in special circumstances where replacement clothing is required, such as where a resident has unusually high or high cost clothing requirements because of their special needs or because of an emergency such as a fire or theft, the local authority can provide clothing'* [para 8, LAC 92/19 – see Box K.1].

If you aren't able to manage your personal allowance because of ill-health, the local authority may (subject to your agreement, or that of your personal representative) deposit it in a bank account on your behalf, and use it to provide for your smaller needs. Any money that is unspent on your death will form part of your estate.

Increasing the personal expenses allowance

The local authority has discretion, under s.22(4), NAA, to award more than £14.10 in *'special circumstances'*. This discretion can be used if you need to keep more of your income in order to lead a more independent life or to pursue a hobby that is important to you. Guidance (LAC 97/5) also reminds local authorities that where a resident is temporarily absent there is the discretion to vary the personal expenses allowance to enable the resident to have more money while staying with family or friends. The personal expenses allowance may be

---

K.3 Interaction of benefits and charges

Here we give examples showing some of the problems caused by the different rules for the DSS and the local authority. Sometimes local authorities calculate a charge based on an assumed level of benefit which might be different when the DSS have worked out your entitlement. Mistakes are easily made so check carefully your benefits and your assessed charge. The amounts would be higher if the homes were in the London area. The first five examples all relate to independent residential care homes and assume no savings unless otherwise stated.

Example 1: Single – permanently in care

Mrs White, 74, goes into residential care on a permanent basis. This costs £230, £15 above the level the local authority will pay. Her son agrees to make a third party payment. She gets AA of £33.10, retirement and occupational pensions totalling £150.20 pw. IS will be paid from the first payday after she moves in.

First 4 weeks

IS applicable amount	£
Personal allowance	49.15
Higher pensioner premium	26.55
Severe disability premium	37.15
Residential allowance	56.00
Total	**168.85**
Income from pensions	150.20
Income support paid	**= £18.65**

Note, the DSS ignore the son's contribution.

The income counted by the local authority is £168.85+£33.10 (AA)+£15 (son's contribution) = £216.95. Personal expenses of £14.10 are allowed, so Mrs White's contribution is £202.85. The local authority pays £230 less £202.85 = £27.15.

After 4 weeks

IS applicable amount	£
Personal allowance	49.15
Pensioner premium	19.65
Residential allowance	56.00
Total	**124.80**
Income from pensions	150.20

Mrs White's income is now above IS level. Because AA stops after 4 weeks, she loses her higher pensioner premium and severe disability premium. The income counted by the local authority is £150.20 +£15 (son's contribution) = £165.20. Personal expenses of £14.10 are allowed so Mrs White's contribution is £151.10. The local authority pays £230 less £151.10 = £78.90.

Example 2: Single – temporarily in care

Mr King, 75, is going into a nursing home, giving his daughter a 3-week break. She gets ICA. He gets AA of £49.50; retirement and works pension come to £91.20 pw. He gets some HB and CTB to help with rent and council tax. His local authority assesses from the first day in care. IS will be paid from the first day as his stay is less than 8 weeks.

IS applicable amount	£
Personal allowance	49.15
Higher pensioner premium	26.55
Residential allowance	56.00
Total	**131.70**
Income from pensions	91.20
Income support paid	**= £40.50**

The income counted by the local authority is £131.70 less any disregards they allow for home commitments (see Box K.2). (AA is not counted for a temporary stay.) He should keep £14.10 (personal expenses) + £49.50 (AA) + any amount allowed for home commitments.

From the Monday following his admission, he will get full HB and CTB as he is now on IS. When he leaves, HB and CTB will stop the Monday after IS stops, so he will need to make a new claim.

Note that some local authorities do not assess during the first 8 weeks, but charge a 'reasonable' amount. Regardless of the charge, the DSS still pays the residential allowance. Even when local authorities do not assess, it is financially advantageous to claim IS during temporary care.

Example 3: Single – permanently in care (house to sell)

Mrs Green, 79, gets IS, and moved a year ago into residential care, costing £240 pw. After a 4-week trial period she put her house up for sale. Her AA had been paid at the higher rate. She has £2,500 in the bank.

After the trial period, the value of her house is included as capital by the local authority but, as she doesn't have this capital, the charge is based on her total income from pensions

increased so that the resident can help support the partner at home perhaps because you are not married and so cannot have half of your personal or occupational pension disregarded (CRAG 5.005). Basically the local authority should not require a charge that would leave your partner without enough money to live on; however, the local authority could consider being on IS as 'having enough to live on'.

6. Treating your home as capital

If you own your home and are a temporary resident in a residential or nursing home, the value of your house will be ignored when the local authority assesses your resources – see Box K.2.

If you own your home and have entered residential care permanently, the local authority must ignore its value if:

- your spouse/partner still lives there; or
- the house is occupied by a relative aged 60 or over; or
- the house is occupied by a relative who is under 60 and 'incapacitated'; or
- a child under 16 whom you are liable to maintain still lives there.

A relative is a parent, parent-in-law, son, daughter, son/daughter-in-law, step-parent, step-son/daughter, brother, sister, or the partner of any of the above, grandparent, grandchild, uncle, aunt, nephew, niece. 'Incapacitated' is not defined but guidance says you count as incapacitated if you get incapacity benefit, SDA, DLA, attendance allowance or constant attendance allowance, or you would satisfy incapacity conditions for any of these.

The local authority also has discretion to ignore the value

---

and IS of **£127.00**. After allowing £14.10 for personal expenses, her share is £112.90 pw. The local authority pay the home the difference of **£127.10**. After 50 weeks she sells her house, realising £80,000, out of which she is billed by the local authority for all the money they paid on her behalf since she became permanent – **£6,355**.

If she made her own arrangements with the home, she would have continued to receive AA at £49.50 pw, and thus get the severe disability premium in her IS. In total her IS and AA would be **£218.35**. This means she would still need to meet a shortfall of £21.65 pw (or £35.75 if she allowed herself the £14.10 personal expenses). Thus the amount she would have needed to find over the 50 weeks totals **£1,082.50** (or **£1,787.50**) compared to the £6,355 she now has to pay back to the local authority. She could have met it out of her savings.

See Chapter 36(2) for more details. It is important to seek careful advice in this situation. The law may change.

Example 4: Couple – one temporarily in care

Joe and Jean Brown are 68 and 57. He gets AA of £49.50 and a retirement pension of £99.80 which includes a £37.35 adult dependant's addition for his wife. They get IS to bring their income up to the 'applicable amount' for a couple in their circumstances of £115.15. (AA is ignored as income.) Jean is the appointee for Joe's pension, and the IS claimant. They jointly own their home. Joe goes into residential care for 2 weeks. Jean has never claimed ICA.

While Joe is in residential care, each will get a single person's applicable amount and their combined resources will be taken from this to give the amount of IS.

Jean	£	Joe	£
Personal allowance	49.15	Personal allowance	49.15
		Higher pensioner premium	26.55
		Severe disability premium	37.15
		Residential allowance	56.00
		Total	168.85
Combined applicable amount		= £218.00	
Less Joe's pension		£99.80	
IS paid		= £118.20	

IS is paid to Jean since she is the claimant. Even though Joe does not get the severe disability premium at home, he gets the premium while in residential care because he is counted as a single person, and Jean is not a non-dependant as they jointly own the property.

The income counted by the local authority is £99.80 (pension) less £37.35 (disregard of adult dependant's addition) = £62.45. (AA is not counted for a temporary stay.) Joe should be charged based on income of **£62.45**, less a disregard for home expenses, and £14.10 for personal expenses. The local authority may ask Jean to contribute as a liable relative. CRAG suggests for a temporary resident in this situation, a contribution of up to the level of Joe's 'applicable amount'.

If Joe had been the IS claimant, it would count as his income in the charging assessment. The local authority would need to vary the personal expenses allowance to allow him to pay over enough for his wife to live on.

Note that some local authorities do not assess for a stay of under 8 weeks, instead they charge a 'reasonable amount'.

Example 5: Couple – one temporarily in care (capital over £8,000)

Mr and Mrs Patel are aged 70. Mrs Patel needs temporary care. She has a pension of £37.35. As they have jointly owned capital of £10,200, they get no IS.

The income counted by the local authority is £37.35 (pension). The local authority disregard her half share of the capital (£5,100) since this is below £10,000.

The local authority has discretion to disregard any ongoing home expenditure and allow £14.10 personal expenses. These are taken from £37.35 to calculate the charge.

The local authority may ask Mr Patel for a contribution if they believe it is reasonable to do so under the liable relative rule.

Note – if her stay was permanent then Mrs Patel could have claimed income support and all her capital would have been disregarded as it is below £10,000.

Example 6: Single – temporarily in local authority care

Mr Edjvet, 73, goes into local authority care for a 5-week stay. He gets AA, HB and CTB. He gets IS at home to top up his pension of £73.50 to his applicable amount of £112.85. While in care his IS stops (because it is based on the allowance of £62.45). His charge is based on £73.50, less any disregard for home expenses, and £14.10 for personal expenses.

His HB and CTB stop the Monday after he goes into care because IS has stopped. He should make a new HB/CTB claim to cover his rent during his stay. His AA stops after 4 weeks. When he returns home he will need to reclaim IS and ask for AA to be paid again.

of the property if hardship would arise for someone else who has been sharing your home on a permanent basis, such as an adult son or daughter, long-term carer or a lesbian or gay partner. Box K.2 gives the legal basis for this discretion.

If your home is taken into account, its value will be based on the current selling price, less any debts (such as a mortgage) charged on it, and less 10% in recognition of the expenses involved in selling it. Its value will be reassessed periodically. The capital value of your home, assessed in this way, will be added to any other capital you may have, although the local authority may help towards your fees while it is being sold. Seek advice if you are refused help with funding if the local authority has assessed you as needing residential care.

The local authority can't make you sell your home to pay the assessed charge for your accommodation. But s.22, HASSASSA 1983 (see Box K.1), allows the authority to place a legal charge on the property so that it can recover any outstanding debts when the property is eventually sold. S.24, HASSASSA, enables the authority to charge reasonable interest on the sum owed after the day of death. Many local authorities place a legal charge on properties automatically while they are up for sale so they will know when they have been sold. You should check to see if your local authority does this and also if you have to incur the cost of them placing the legal charge on it. Recent advice (LAC 97/5) is for the local authority to place a caution against jointly owned property rather than a charge.

You may not be allowed to escape paying a charge based on the value of your former home indefinitely if you want to be able to hand your home on to someone else eventually. The local authority may take action to recover any arrears due, as an ordinary debt in the county court. Take legal advice if this happens.

However, if you are not sure whether you want to stay permanently in a residential home, you should not feel obliged to sell your home until you are ready to do so. If you might return home, or if you hope to sell your property and buy something more suitable, your stay should be treated as 'temporary' for up to 52 weeks, or longer in 'exceptional circumstances'.

Deprivation of capital
If you have given any assets away, such as your former home, or sold them for less than they are worth, the local authority may take their value into account in the charging assessment – see Box K.2 for more details.

7. Meeting the costs of your own home
If your partner, children or relatives continue to live in your home, the help they can receive for their housing costs depends on their circumstances. If they are paying the housing costs, even though you are the person liable for them, they can claim housing benefit instead of you.

If you are a 'temporary resident' (see Box K.2), the local authority can disregard payments you are making towards 'any housing costs... including any fuel charges, which are included in the rent of a dwelling to which (you) intend to return, ... to the extent that the local authority considers it reasonable in the circumstances to do so' [Sch 3 para 27 AOR].

CRAG gives a list of examples including service charges, insurance premiums, water rates, standard charges for fuel and any rent or mortgage payments not covered by HB, IS or income-based JSA [CRAG para 3.011 and para 3.012].

If no-one is left living in your home and you have entered residential accommodation for a short period, see Chapter 4(6); Chapter 5 covers the council tax. See also Chapter 36(3) and (4).

After 52 weeks, or 13 weeks in the case of a trial period, and as soon as it is clear that your stay in the home is permanent, you will be excluded from housing benefit and IS/JSA housing costs. Yet your liability to pay rent and/or a mortgage in respect of your former home continues until you have terminated your tenancy, or sold your home. In this case, you may be able to ask your local authority to vary your personal expenses allowance to help you meet these ongoing costs now you are a permanent resident. If your former home is vacant, you shouldn't have to pay council tax if you are now a permanent resident.

8. What happens when you move out?
When you move out, you will be entitled to social security benefits in the usual way.

If you are entitled to income support, or income-based JSA once you move from a residential home into unfurnished or partly furnished accommodation, you may get a social fund community care grant – see Chapter 7.

Your local Social Services Department will be able to advise you on local authority benefits and services that are available in your area; see Chapters 32 and 33 for details.

If you go away from your residential home on a temporary basis, your local authority can use its discretion to vary the personal expenses allowance to enable you to have more money while away. You may also be able to claim DLA care component or attendance allowance for periods away from the home. Chapters 36 and 38 cover the effect on benefits of stays in, and absences from, residential accommodation.

38 Benefits in care – before April 1993

In this chapter we look at:	
A. Preserved rights	
Help under the old system	see 1
Who has preserved rights to IS and JSA?	see 2
Protection for other benefits	see 3
B. Income support and JSA	
Getting higher levels of IS or JSA	see 4
Who cannot get higher levels of IS or JSA?	see 5
How is your IS or JSA worked out?	see 6
Personal expenses allowance	see 7
National limits	see 8
Payments to help meet any shortfall	see 9
IS, JSA and maintenance	see 10
Key points	see 11

A. PRESERVED RIGHTS

1. Help under the old system
The NHS and Community Care Act 1990 introduced radical changes to the public funding of places in residential accommodation from April 1993. If you were already in a local authority residential home on 31.3.93, until April 1996 you were protected from any financial loss by the Transitional Provisions in the Assessment of Resources Regulations (AOR). Since then you are charged the same way as if you had moved into a local authority residential care home after 1993 – see Chapter 37.

If you were in an independent residential care or nursing

home on 31.3.93, you will be protected from these changes if you have 'preserved rights' – see 2 below.

Note that even if you have preserved rights because you were in an independent care home, local authorities have some very limited powers to help you under the new system – see 9.

The new system for residential care will apply to you if you lose your preserved rights because of the length of your absence from a residential home.

Chapter 36 covers the effect on social security benefits of a stay in residential care for people who move in after 31.3.93 or those who have lost their preserved rights.

All abbreviations are listed in Box K.1 or at the back of the Handbook.

2. Who has preserved rights to IS and JSA?

Independent registered residential care & nursing homes

You will have a preserved right to higher levels of income support (IS) or income-based jobseeker's allowance (JSA) to help meet the cost of the fees for a residential care home or a nursing home, if you come within any of the following groups of people [reg 19 ISG, reg 86 JSA Regs].

You were getting the higher rates of IS on 31.3.93 – You have preserved rights if:
- you were living in, or only 'temporarily absent' from, a residential care home or in a nursing home on 31.3.93 (see below for 'small homes'); and
- you were entitled to IS up to the appropriate residential care/nursing home limit.

You count as being **temporarily absent** if you would have been living in a residential care home or nursing home on 31.3.93, but were temporarily absent in the following ways:
- you were a patient in hospital throughout the period of absence, and it was for no more than 52 weeks; or
- the absence was for no more than 4 weeks, if you were a temporary resident in the home beforehand; or
- the absence was for no more than 13 weeks, if you were a permanent resident in the home beforehand.

Once you have acquired preserved rights, a subsequent temporary absence for no more than the appropriate period above for your situation from a residential care or nursing home will not remove those rights.

Your preserved rights will also apply if you move to a new home, or even to a different type of home (eg from a residential care home to a nursing home). You will be paid at the rate for the type of care you receive in the new home.

You were paying the fees yourself – If you were paying the fees yourself, but now want to claim IS or income-based JSA because your capital is less than £16,000, you will have a preserved right to the higher rates of IS or JSA if you were living in, or only temporarily absent from, a residential care home or nursing home on 31.3.93; this provision does not apply to people living in small homes on 31.3.93 – see below.

If you were residing with your partner on 31.3.93 and your partner had a preserved right, but now you need to claim IS or income-based JSA yourself, you now have the preserved right.

Small homes (England and Wales only)

Small homes, ie those with fewer than 4 residents, were required to register with the local authority from 1.4.93 in England and Wales. Such homes had already had to register in Scotland. Higher rates of IS or income-based JSA normally can't be paid unless the home is registered. You will only have preserved rights to the higher rates if:
- on 31.3.93, you lived in such a home; or
- were 'temporarily absent' (see above); and
- were in receipt of the higher rates of IS on that date; and
- the home was either registered or in the process of being so; or
- you were resident on 31.3.93 in a small home which was exempt from registration because one or more residents are treated as close relatives for registration purposes; and
- you were continuously resident (ie not absent for a period of more than 13 weeks) between 1.4.93 and 4.10.93.

If you were paying the fees yourself without IS, you would not have a preserved right.

Homes owned by close relatives

You cannot receive the higher rates of IS or income-based JSA if you were living with, or later move to a home that is provided by a 'close relative'. However if the ownership changes, or you move to a new home where this does not apply, you just pick up the higher rates of IS or JSA again. Your preserved rights resume. A 'close relative' means a parent, parent-in-law, step-parent, son, daughter, son/daughter-in-law, step-son/daughter, sister, brother or the (married or unmarried) partner of any of those.

Abbeyfield Homes

From April 1996 new rules allow residents with preserved rights in unregistered (very sheltered) Abbeyfield Homes to give up preserved rights if they have to buy in care over and above that provided by Abbeyfield. They can then claim ordinary IS, or income-based JSA, and HB. Preserved rights are reinstated if the situation changes. Seek advice from your Abbeyfield society.

3. Protection for other benefits

DLA care component and attendance allowance

In general, (but there are a few exceptions – see Chapter 17(10)) if you have a preserved right to the higher levels of IS or income-based JSA, you also have a right to payment of DLA care component or attendance allowance (AA) under the old rules. But DLA care component and AA will be treated as income for IS or income-based JSA purposes.

You may have been living in or have been temporarily absent (see 2 above) from sheltered lodgings (adult placement scheme) and receiving normal levels of IS. If the placement was then required to register because it provided both board and personal care, you will keep the right to payment of DLA care component or AA under the old rules, and they are paid on top of your IS or income-based JSA.

Housing benefit

Some people may still be receiving protected housing benefit (HB) in an independent home. This continues only if you were receiving, or entitled to, protected HB on 31.3.93. If you have preserved rights to IS or income-based JSA, and then eventually claim the higher rates of IS, your housing benefit will stop permanently after 4 weeks.

If you were entitled to HB in a registered home on 29.10.90, you retain a lifelong eligibility (unless you claim higher rates of IS or income-based JSA – see above). You have more limited protection if you are in registered accommodation and are in remunerative work, or a home run by a close relative or are in a home which was not required to be registered (less than 4 people) until 1.4.93. In these cases, protection only remains while you live (or are temporarily absent for up to 52 weeks) at the same address.

If you are in a home of less than 4 people (often they are

known as sheltered lodgings or adult placements) which has now had to register, if your landlord/lady moves to a different address and you move with them, you will not be able to keep your protected HB, but will need to apply for help with the fees under the system explained in Chapters 36 and 37.

Note also that, although you have protected rights to HB, the level at which you are paid is not protected. If you get HB because you are in one of these groups (or an unregistered Abbeyfield Home) then tariff income will only start at £10,000.

B. INCOME SUPPORT AND JSA

4. Getting higher levels of IS or JSA

To get income support (IS) or income-based jobseeker's allowance (JSA) under preserved rights, you must be receiving personal care because of old age or disability and the nursing or residential care home must be registered, deemed as registered, or exempt from registration. Remember, you can only receive the higher rates of IS or income-based JSA while in an independent sector registered care home.

Respite care – The rules about temporary absence in 2 above, mean that you may well lose your preserved rights to the higher levels of IS or JSA before very long. To keep your preserved rights, each respite care stay would have to be no more than 4 weeks apart. But you are not restricted to your original 31.3.93 respite care home. So long as the stays are no more than 4 weeks apart, your respite care stay may be in any independent sector home.

In general, if you enter an independent home and have preserved rights, your IS or income-based JSA will increase to reflect the home's charges (up to the appropriate national limit). You'll also be eligible for any IS/JSA housing costs toward mortgage interest payments or housing benefit toward rent payments for costs incurred on your house.

If you are getting a special transitional addition under the old supplementary benefit rules, this addition will be protected by the usual linking rules during a spell of respite care; see Box B.2 in Chapter 3.

5. Who cannot get the higher levels of IS or JSA?

Even if you were living in a residential care or nursing home on 31.3.93 (or were temporarily absent), you won't be paid IS or income-based JSA at the higher rates if:
- the home is not registered (unless it is a 'small home' which falls as exempt in the very limited circumstances in 2 above); or
- it is not on a commercial basis; or
- your place in a voluntary or private residential home was already sponsored by a local authority under Part III NAA, before April 1993 and you were only receiving the Part III rates; or
- you move permanently to residential accommodation which is owned or managed by a local authority; this includes homes or hostels for the care of people who are or have been ill, and for mothers and young children but only where some board is available. If no board is available, you'll be eligible for IS/JSA/HB in the normal way while in the hostel (see Chapter 36(5)); or
- you were living in a local authority care home which, while you were living there, has been transferred to become an independent residential care home (if this was after 12.8.91). Note that the law was changed in November 1996 as a result of *CAO v Harris (Quinn) & Gibbon* (TLR 8.8.96) which said that once the home was transferred to the private sector the duty of the local authority ended. The change was to get back to the original policy intention; or
- you were living in a local authority owned or managed home on 31.3.93 and now want to move to an independent home. You will continue to get the Part III rates only; or
- the home is run (wholly or partly) by a 'close relative'. See 2 above for the meaning of 'close relative' and an outline of your preserved rights; or
- you have entered the home for the purpose of receiving an amount of IS or income-based JSA to which you would not otherwise be entitled.

Remember, you only lose your existing preserved rights if you are absent from a residential care home or nursing home and that absence exceeds a period of:
- 52 weeks if you were a hospital patient throughout the period; or
- 4 weeks (temporary residents); or
- 13 weeks (permanent residents).

6. How is your IS or JSA worked out?

The general rules about who is entitled to IS and income-based JSA and the way your resources are calculated, cover people with preserved rights in residential care and nursing homes like anyone else (see Chapter 3 and Chapter 14). However, from April 1996 there were two changes affecting those with preserved rights.
- ❑ The capital limit was increased to £16,000 so you can claim IS or income-based JSA once your capital is down to that level. Tariff income only starts at £10,000. You can continue to use these more generous capital rules if you are absent for up to 52 weeks if you are over pension age (or have protection given to those in small homes from 1987), and up to 13 weeks in other cases.
- ❑ If you have a spouse who is not living with you and you are giving them at least 50% of your occupational pension or (since April 1997) personal pension or payment from a retirement annuity contract, then half your pension is disregarded.

If you are in a residential care, or nursing home, and have a preserved right, your IS or income-based JSA 'applicable amount' is worked out differently.

7. Personal expenses allowance

Instead of the IS or income-based JSA personal allowance and premiums, you get an allowance for personal expenses while living in a residential care or nursing home.

		£ pw
Single person		£14.10
Couple		£28.20
Dependent child	aged 18+	£14.10
	aged 16–17	£9.80
	aged 11–15	£8.45
	aged 0–10	£5.80

8. National limits

The national limits for each type of home and category of resident are set out below. In all categories, the limit for a nursing home in the Greater London area is £46 higher; for a residential care home it is £41 higher. If you are away from the home for over a week, a retaining fee of up to 80% of the amount normally allowed towards the charge can be met for up to 4 weeks. If you are absent from the home because you are in hospital or temporarily admitted to local authority accommodation, the retaining fee can be paid for up to 52 weeks. If you are away for less than a week no alteration is made to the amount paid. If IS or income-based JSA does pay a retainer to the home, the DSS can also pay IS or income-based JSA for you in your current situation. There are two conflicting Commissioners' decisions on whether the DSS will pay for both if you have gone into another form of residential care, ie gone into a nursing home temporarily and you normally live in a residential care home (CSIS/833/95 and CIS 5415/95). Seek advice if you are in that situation.

Registered category	Residential care home	Nursing home
Mental disorder (but not mental handicap)	£220	£312
Drug or alcohol dependence	£220	£312
Mental handicap	£250	£318
Physical disablement	£285	£352
Terminal illness	–	£311
Very dependent or blind elderly	£240	–
Any other category (including homes for the elderly)	£208	£311

Physical disablement – This limit can only apply if you became disabled before reaching pension age. You must have been *'blind, deaf or dumb or substantially and permanently handicapped by illness, injury or congenital deformity'* [Section 20(1) Registered Homes Act 1984]. This is similar to the test for registration as disabled with a Social Services Department.

Very dependent or blind elderly – To come into this category, you must be blind, or be entitled to the higher rate of either DLA care component or attendance allowance, or any rate of war or industrial constant attendance allowance. If you become entitled to the higher rate while in the home, it is important to check that your IS now reflects the very dependent rate.

Where a home is dually registered, or registered for two or more categories of care, you'll receive the amount for the type of care you are receiving in the home. You have a right of appeal against an Adjudication Officer's decision on the category of care which you come into. A nursing home is not registered for particular categories of care. However, a residential care home must be so registered. If the home is not registered for the category of care you are receiving, seek advice. Basically, the home should notify the registration authority to make sure the records match the type of care being provided. If just one person in a residential care home requires nursing care beyond the scope of the community nursing services and a good carer, the home must also register as a nursing home.

9. Payments to meet any shortfall

It may be the case that the amount you receive from IS or income-based JSA does not meet the full fees of the home. You may need help from other sources (relatives, charities etc); in limited circumstances the local authority can help.

The legal basis for payments from local authorities

Section 26A(1) of the National Assistance Act 1948 (NAA)* prevents a local authority from helping fund a place in an independent home for a person with a preserved right, unless they can fund that person under the Residential Accommodation (Relevant Premises, Ordinary Residence and Exemptions) Regulations 1993/477 (RPORE).*

* S.86A(1) of the Social Work (Scotland) Act 1968, does the same for Scotland. These regulations are made under s.26A and s.86A.

If you can show that there is no suitable alternative accommodation within the national limits, the local authority can make extra payments to help people with preserved rights in the following circumstances:
- if you were already receiving a 'topping up' payment from the local authority on 31.3.93;
- if you are under pension age in either a residential care or nursing home;
- if you are over pension age in a residential care home only and you face eviction or the home is about to close;
- if you don't have preserved rights or have lost them.

If you are faced with eviction, the local authority can only place you in a home which is not owned or managed by the person or organisation which owns or manages your current home.

The very limited powers of the local authority to intervene are causing problems for people who cannot meet the shortfall and have preserved rights. It is particularly difficult if your care needs are such that you need to move to a nursing home and you are over pension age (note that under pension age, local authorities can help support people in nursing homes), or if you are already in a nursing home and cannot afford the fees any longer. In these circumstances the health authority may be able to help, but there is no guarantee. All the above is explained more fully in circular LAC 93/6 – see Box K.1.

The effect of local authority payments

When local authorities help toward the cost of the fees above the national limits these payments used to be called 'topping up payments'. There is now no such thing. What happens now is that the local authority takes on all the arrangements and becomes responsible for the full fee, rather than just the top up. However, IS or income-based JSA is still paid at the higher rates from which the local authority assesses your charge, leaving you with the personal expenses allowance of £14.10.

Other contributions to meet the shortfall

Other types of payments are possible. They must be specifically intended and used for the amount of a residential care or nursing home charge above the national limit. See Chapter 3(28).

If you were previously funding yourself and have been living in a residential care or nursing home since immediately before 29.4.85 (apart from any temporary absences of no more than 52 weeks for any reason), and now have to claim IS or income-based JSA because you are no longer able to pay the charges yourself, the Secretary of State has discretion to give you extra help. A key condition for this is that the local authority must not have accepted responsibility for funding, or part-funding, your place in the home at any time since 29.4.85.

10. IS, JSA and maintenance

The income and capital of the non-resident spouse cannot be taken into account in determining a permanent resident's claim to IS or income-based JSA. However, the non-resident may be required to pay maintenance. In this case, the non-resident should not feel pressured into paying more than s/he can reasonably afford given his or her actual resources and expenses. Unless the DSS obtain a court order, payment is voluntary. Seek advice. What follows is a sketch, largely from the viewpoint of the resident.

If the couple are not (and have never been) married to each other, the non-resident partner cannot be required to pay maintenance*, and any payments actually made by the non-resident partner are considered under the normal rules – they cannot count as 'liable relative payments'.

* unless you are a sponsored immigrant and the non-resident is liable to maintain you under s.78(6)(c) SSAA.

Although a former spouse cannot be required to maintain you, reg 54 ISG (reg 117 JSA Regs) defines a former spouse as a liable relative. Thus any payments from your divorced spouse are considered under the special rules for liable relative payments.

A husband and wife are each liable to maintain the other. S.106 Social Security Administration Act (SSAA) gives the Secretary of State power to attempt recovery of expenditure on IS or income-based JSA from a person liable for maintenance. This is by means of making a complaint against the liable person to a magistrates court (in Scotland, to the sheriff) for an order under s.106 SSAA. In practice, legal proceedings are rarely undertaken. Instead, the DSS may put pressure on the non-resident spouse to make 'voluntary' maintenance payments. Such payments are considered only under the special rules for liable relative payments.

Any maintenance actually paid by the non-resident spouse is, of course, taken into account as income when working out the resident's entitlement to IS or income-based JSA. The AO cannot assume a 'notional' income based on what the non-resident might pay. Instead, *'payments which* **would be** ... *made ... upon application being made by the claimant'* [our emphasis] are taken into account as income under reg 54 ISG (reg 117 JSA Regs). If the non-resident is paying some maintenance, or says that s/he cannot or will not pay maintenance, there is no legal justification for delaying making a decision on the resident's IS or JSA claim. It is then for the Secretary of State to decide whether to take action under s.106 SSAA.

If the residential care or nursing home's charges are above the appropriate IS or income-based JSA limit for the type of care you are receiving, you have a problem. If someone other than your non-resident spouse (or ex-spouse) helps you pay the part of the home's charge above the IS or income-based JSA limit, that payment is ignored as income – see Chapter 3(28). However, liable relative payments are usually taken fully into account. Reg 54 ISG (reg 117 JSA Regs) also gives the exceptions to this standard rule. The only way in which a non-resident spouse can give equivalent help with the part of the home's charge above the IS or income-based JSA limit is discretionary. If a payment is made to a third party (eg direct to the care home), it may be disregarded *'where having regard to the purpose of the payment, the terms under which it is made and its amount it is unreasonable to take it into account'* – reg 54(e) ISG and see R(SB)6/88: other relevant factors may also be considered, either by the AO or on appeal, by the Social Security Appeal Tribunal.

11. Key points

Maximum IS or income-based JSA
It is not possible to get more from IS or income-based JSA than the appropriate rate for the type of home you are living in and the category of care you are receiving plus the personal expenses allowance unless you are getting a transitional addition (see Box B.2 in Chapter 3), or were previously funding yourself and have been living in the same home since before 1985 (see 9 above). If you have lived in the home for over 12 months and have been funding yourself and now need to claim IS or income-based JSA, it is only possible to get above the limit for 13 weeks while you look for suitable alternative accommodation.

If both of a couple are living in the care home, you'll get two personal expenses allowances plus up to the appropriate limit for the type of home you are living in and the type of care each of you is receiving. If you have a dependent child living with you, seek advice.

Attendance allowance and DLA care component are fully taken into account as income.

Additional requirements are no longer payable. But if you were getting these additions before 13.4.87, they would have been included in the assessment of your transitional addition – see Box B.2.

Meals allowance
If your care or nursing home charge does not cover all your meals, you will get:
- the actual cost of the meals if you can obtain the meals within the establishment; or
- £1.10 for breakfast,
  £1.55 for midday meals,
  £1.55 for evening meals; or
- if you normally pay less, you'll just get enough to cover your meals.

But you can't get more than the appropriate limit for the type of accommodation you are in.

Eviction
Your status within the home is likely to be that of a licensee. If your licence is terminated, you count as homeless. The local authority has a duty to you under the homeless persons legislation. They may also be able to make new arrangements for payments to help you enter another residential care home – see 9 above. Most licensees cannot be evicted without a court order. Seek expert advice quickly.

Hospital and abroad

This section of the Handbook looks at the following:

Going into hospital	Chapter 39
Hospital – one year on	Chapter 40
Going abroad	Chapter 41

39 Going into hospital

1. What should you do beforehand?

Your benefits may change if you go into hospital, so let your DSS office know if you or a dependant are to be admitted. If you get invalid care allowance, you should also tell the DSS if the person you are looking after is admitted. If you get housing or council tax benefit, a spell in hospital may affect the amount you get so you may need to tell the local authority as well.

Write to the office(s) dealing with your benefits, to let them know the date you expect to be admitted to hospital and how long you are likely to stay. You should still report your actual admission, or tell the office(s) if this is cancelled or postponed. It is sensible to do this beforehand, but do not worry if you have been unable to. Just do it as soon as you can.

Medical certificates – If you need sick notes to get benefit when in hospital, you just have to ask the sister or charge nurse for one.

Private patients – If you are a private patient paying the whole cost of accommodation and non-medical services in hospital, only invalid care allowance is affected by your stay. All other benefits remain payable, subject to the usual conditions – ask your local social security office for advice.

2. Hospital fares

You may be able to get help with fares or other travel expenses for yourself (and for someone who has to go with you if you are incapable of getting to the hospital on your own), if:
- you are getting income support, income-based jobseeker's allowance (JSA), family credit or disability working allowance; or
- you live in a residential care or nursing home and the local authority helps with the care home fees; or
- you are covered by the low-income scheme. See Chapter 48(5). If your income is above your low-income level but would fall below it if you paid the fares, you may still be eligible for help with part of the cost.

Parents – If your child has to go into hospital or attend on a regular basis, you can claim help with travel expenses to accompany your child to and from the hospital if you fall within one of the groups listed above.

In-patients sent home on short leave – The hospital may pay travel expenses for you, and anyone who has to go with you, if you are within one of the groups above.

If you are sent home as part of your treatment, or for the hospital's convenience, your fares are regarded as part of your treatment costs and should be met by the hospital and not under the hospital travel expenses means-tested scheme.

If you are sent home on short leave for any reason, you will also get your full benefit entitlement (including disability living allowance and attendance allowance) so long as you notify the DSS. This is worked out on a daily basis – see 10 below.

How to claim the cost of fares

Most hospitals have a hospital fares office. If not, ask the receptionist which person in the hospital deals with fares. The hospital will refund your fares if you produce proof of your entitlement. If you get income support, income-based JSA, family credit, or disability working allowance, show your award letter or order book.

If you have already claimed on low-income grounds, show your HC2 certificate (full entitlement); or your HC3 certificate (partial entitlement) – these were previously called AG2 and AG3 certificates.

If you haven't yet claimed on low-income grounds, ask the hospital (or DSS) for form HC5 (to claim a refund) and form HC1 (to establish your entitlement to full or partial help with the cost of hospital fares etc), or form HC1(RC) if you are claiming on the grounds that you live in residential care. Ask the hospital to fill in their part of the HC5, then fill in the rest of the HC5 and the HC1 and send both forms off to the address given in the forms. Don't wait to return the form HC5; it must be returned within 3 months of paying your fares.

What travel expenses can be covered?

The law allows *'the cost of travelling by the cheapest means of transport available'*. Normally this means that the cost of second-class public transport by whichever method you use is covered. If public transport is available but you go by car, your petrol costs can be covered up to the amount of the second-class fare. If public transport is not available and you go by car, your full petrol costs can be covered.

Taxi fares can be covered if you are unable to use public transport because of a physical disability or no public transport is available for that particular journey. If public transport is available and you are not physically disabled, just the cost of second-class public transport for that journey will be covered.

Partial help with fares – The amount shown on an HC3 certificate for partial help is the amount you are expected to be able to pay for travel expenses in any one week (from Sunday to the following Saturday). If your actual hospital travel expenses in any particular week covered by that HC3 certificate are higher, the excess is refunded. This helps people who have to travel long distances to hospital – so long as your capital is no more than £8,000, your income could be well above your 'requirements', yet it would still be worthwhile claiming help. For example, if your excess income figure shown on the HC3 certificate is £34, but your travel expenses to and from hospital in a particular week are £54, you would be entitled to have £20 of your expenses refunded.

The 'expenses within one week' rule also helps those who have to make several visits to the same, or to different, hospitals within the same week.

For example, if the excess income figure shown on your HC3 certificate is £3.50 and your return fare to hospital is £2.50, you have to pay for the first visit, and £1 of the fares for your second visit in the week, but the rest of your hospital visiting fares in that same week (Sunday through to the following Saturday) would be refunded. Ask the hospital fares office for details of the arrangements for dealing with several visits within the same week.

Visitors' hospital fares
If you are on income support or income-based JSA, you may get a community care grant from the social fund – see Chapter 7.

If you are not on income support or income-based JSA, you might be able to get help from another source – see below.

War pensioners
If you attend hospital for treatment for your war disablement, you can get a wider range of expenses regardless of your income. Write to *War Pensions Agency, Norcross, Blackpool, FY5 3WP*.

Other sources of help
Other possible sources of help with travel expenses for patients and visitors include – hospital endowment funds, education departments, Social Services Departments, the Family Fund (see Chapter 29) and various charities. For advice about these, contact a hospital social worker, or an advice centre.

3. What happens to your income support?
If you go into hospital, part of your needs will be met by the NHS. So, your income support 'applicable amount' changes to take account of this. In some cases the change is immediate; in others it will be delayed. Box L.1 gives details. What happens depends on who is in hospital and whether s/he has been in hospital in the past 28 days.

4. What happens to your jobseeker's allowance
If you go into hospital, JSA can continue for up to 2 weeks, as long as you haven't received JSA through two previous spells of ill health or disability in the same jobseeking period, or in the last year if you've been signing on for over a year.

If your partner goes into hospital, the income-based JSA personal allowance is cut by £12.50 after 6 weeks. If a child is in hospital, the allowance for that child is cut to £12.50 after 12 weeks.

When your JSA stops, you should claim incapacity benefit and income support.

5. What happens to your housing benefit?
If you get housing benefit (HB), or council tax benefit (CTB), the 'applicable amount' may change during a spell in hospital. The rules are similar to the income support rules – see Box L.1.

6. What about family credit or DWA?
Family credit and disability working allowance are not affected by a stay in hospital until the award runs out. If you are in hospital when you renew your claim there are no special rules but you may not be able to pass the 16 hours a week work rule – see Chapters 16 and 28.

If a child is in hospital during the 12 weeks before you claim, s/he will be included in your claim as long as you are in regular contact. But if s/he has been in hospital for 52 weeks or more at the start of your claim, s/he no longer counts as living with you, so you won't get an allowance or credit for your child.

7. What about SSP and SMP?
Going into hospital does not affect entitlement to either SSP or SMP.

8. What happens to non-means-tested benefits?
Some benefits are reduced or withdrawn after a period in hospital. Incapacity benefit and SDA are reduced from the first day after the set period. Other benefits are reduced from the appropriate pay day after you have been in hospital for the set period. They can only be adjusted from a non-pay day if the conditions for payment at a daily rate are satisfied – see 10 for more details.

Below we look at what happens if you or a dependant are in hospital.

Up to four weeks
There is normally no change, except in the following cases.
❑ To decide when the reduction or withdrawal of benefit should start, separate periods in hospital which are no more than 28 days apart are added together and count as one continuous stay. So your benefit could be reduced or withdrawn as soon as you go back to hospital depending on how long you were in hospital in your earlier stay. To count the days in between hospital stays, start with the day after you leave hospital and end with the day you are readmitted. If this is 28 days or less, the two spells in hospital are added together. For DLA and attendance allowance you start counting the days between hospital stays from the actual day you leave hospital – but there may be a change in the law soon to bring this into line with other benefits.
❑ War disablement pension can often be increased when you go into hospital, if the treatment is for the war injury. See War Pensions Agency leaflet WPA 1.

After four weeks
Attendance allowance and disability living allowance (DLA) care component for adults, and war or industrial injuries constant attendance allowance, stop. DLA mobility component for adults also stops after 4 weeks except for those who have a car or wheelchair through Motability or long-stay patients covered by transitional protection – see Chapter 17(9).

Invalid care allowance (ICA) will stop if the person you are caring for has been in hospital for 4 weeks and attendance allowance or DLA care component has stopped.

Attendance allowance or DLA care component and your carer's ICA will stop before the 4 weeks is up, if you had been in hospital or any other 'special' accommodation in the 28 days before you were admitted to hospital. DLA mobility component will stop before the end of 4 weeks, only if you'd been in hospital in the 28 days before this hospital stay. If you are admitted to hospital from residential care, you keep the mobility component for the full 4 weeks.

For more details of the way DLA is affected by a stay in hospital or residential care, see Chapter 17(9) and (10).

After six weeks
If you or your partner have been in hospital for 6 weeks, your benefit will be reduced if you're on:
- incapacity benefit
- widows' benefits
- unemployability supplement
- severe disablement allowance
- retirement pension

If you don't have an adult or child dependant, your benefit will be cut by £25 (but you won't be left with less than £12.50). Do note that the reassessment of housing benefit may mean that, after you have paid your housing costs, you are left with less than £12.50 in your pocket – see Box L.1 for how to get extra HB/CTB.

If you have an adult or child dependant, your benefit is cut by £12.50.

If you have underlying entitlement to ICA, you may find that the reduction of your overlapping benefit means that some ICA is now payable.

War pensioners' unemployability supplement is reduced after eight weeks in hospital.

Twelve weeks to one year
Child in hospital – After 12 weeks, you can continue to get child benefit for a child in hospital only if you are regularly spending money on the child's behalf, eg on fares to visit the child, clothing, pocket money, magazines etc. If you continue to get child benefit, you will also continue to get a child dependant's addition payable with other benefits.

DLA care component and mobility component for a child under 16 stop after 12 weeks in hospital. But for DLA care component, because spells in hospital link with spells in 'special' accommodation, it may have stopped sooner – see Chapter 17(9) for more details.
If you or your partner are in hospital – Child benefit normally continues to be paid.

Invalid care allowance will stop after you, the carer, have been in hospital for 12 weeks (but it may stop sooner – see Chapter 19(9)).

The basic industrial or war disablement pension continues to be paid, along with any reduced earnings allowance, or exceptionally severe disablement allowance. War pensioners' mobility supplement continues to be paid in hospital.

Chapter 40 covers the benefits position after one year in hospital.

9. What extra help can you get?
We have already mentioned possible increases for war pensioners. But there are other possible extra benefits.

If you are in hospital, you may still have expenses outside – rent to pay, dependants to look after. Your income may not be enough. Are you getting income support to help you cover these costs? If not, should you be? See Box L.1 and Chapter 3. Note that the 'hospital down-rating' for income support, HB and CTB is different from non-means-tested benefits.

When your income is reduced during a spell in hospital, you may become eligible for means-tested housing and/or council tax benefit – see Box L.1 and Chapter 4.

10. What about when you leave hospital?
Whether or not any benefit has been changed or stopped while you or a dependant have been in hospital, make sure you let your DSS office (and your local authority, if you are getting housing benefit, or council tax benefit) know as soon as you know the date you, or your dependant, are coming home. You should still report your actual discharge, or tell the office if this is cancelled or postponed.

Temporary absence from hospital
If you or a dependant spend a few days at home – perhaps for a 'trial run', or if you are in and out of hospital on a regular pattern, tell your local DSS office and ask them to pay the full amount of benefit for the days at home. Get a note from the hospital or say how many days at home you have.

The day you leave hospital does not count as a day at home, so you won't be paid for that day. The day you go back into hospital does count as a day at home, so you are paid for that day. For DLA and attendance allowance, it is slightly different. Currently both the day you go into hospital and the day you leave count as days at home, so you can be paid DLA or AA for both days. But there may be a change in the law soon to bring this into line with other benefits (see our *Disability Rights Bulletin*). See Chapter 40(8) for more details.
Can your carer get ICA? – If you go home regularly each weekend and receive attendance allowance or DLA care component (at the middle or higher rate), your carer might qualify for the full rate of invalid care allowance. This is because ICA is a 'weekly' benefit and is never paid on a daily basis. See Chapter 19(2) to check whether your carer can meet the 35 hours a week caring test.
Income support – If you leave hospital for a break of less than a week you will get your full pro-rata IS entitlement for those days. If you are discharged for longer than a week, or for good the date your IS is changed depends on whether you are paid in advance or in arrears – see Box L.1.
HB and CTB – The 'benefit week' rules for housing and council tax benefit mean that a single short break away from hospital is unlikely to lead to an increased amount of benefit. However, it is worth writing to your CTB/HB section at the local council if you have regular short breaks in your own home, eg you go home at weekends, as downrating will stop. If your absence from hospital spans two 'benefit weeks' (eg two weekends in a row), your benefit will be increased in the second week (starting on the Monday). A change of circumstances can only be taken into account from the start of the next benefit week. This also means that if you are discharged from hospital on a Monday (the start of the benefit week), full benefit can only resume from the start of the next benefit week.
Incapacity benefit and SDA – These are paid again in full from the day after you go out of hospital. You get one seventh of your weekly benefit (including any dependant's addition) for each day at home.
Retirement and widows' pensions – Normally for retirement and widows' pensions, the full weekly benefit is paid from the first pay day after you leave hospital. But benefit can be adjusted on a daily basis if, on the day you leave hospital, you are expected to return to hospital within 28 days (see below). So you can get full benefit for each day that you are not in hospital. However, additions for dependants cannot be adjusted on a daily basis.
DLA and attendance allowance (AA) – These are adjusted on a daily basis where you are expected to return to hospital within 28 days (or for AA and DLA care component but not the mobility component, you are expected to return to a residential care or nursing home within 28 days) – see below.

If you are not expected to return to hospital within the appropriate time limit, and when you are finally discharged from hospital, full benefit resumes from the first pay day.
Are you expected to return within 28 days? – Payment at a daily rate depends on what is expected on the day you are discharged from hospital. What happens after you leave does not affect what was originally expected. These daily rate provisions apply to DLA, AA and 'weekly' benefits like retirement pension and widow's pension. They do not apply to incapacity benefit or SDA which are always paid from the first day that you are not in hospital, whether or not you expect to return.

The daily rate provisions do not apply if, on the day of discharge, you were not expected to return to hospital within 28 days. Nor can they apply even if you return to hospital within that period.

If you have been out of hospital for 28 days or less, your current spell in hospital 'links' with the previous spell. When you go back to hospital you'll have the remainder of your 4 weeks (for AA or DLA) or 6 weeks (for other benefits) or 12

L.1 What happens to income support, council tax benefit and housing benefit?

If you, or anyone in your income support (IS) family go into hospital, the effect on your income support can be pretty complicated. The effect on your benefit depends on who is in hospital and whether s/he has been in hospital in the past 28 days.

Who is in hospital?
The effect on your benefit will depend on whether or not the patient is:
- a dependent child;
- a single person, without a partner or dependent children;
- a lone parent;
- one of a couple;
- one of a couple with the partner also in hospital and no dependent children;
- normally living in a residential care or nursing home.

A child will be treated as a dependant if:
- you still get child benefit for him or her; and
- s/he has been a patient for a continuous (or linked) period of up to 12 weeks; or
- s/he has been a patient continuously for over 12 weeks and you are in regular contact with him or her.

The 28 day linking rule
Different spells in hospital will be linked together and treated as one continuous spell if you have been readmitted after spending only 28 days (or less) in your own home. The day you enter hospital counts as a day in your own home. The day you leave hospital counts as a day spent in hospital.

So, if you have been in hospital in the past 28 days, you may find your IS applicable amount is reduced, or downrated, right away.

This 28 day linking rule applies to all social security benefits. It also applies to housing benefit and to council tax benefit; but not to family credit or disability working allowance. (For DLA and attendance allowance the linking rule also applies, but currently both the day you enter and the day you leave hospital count as days at home – see Chapter 39(8)).

Changes in income support
The date from which your income support is changed depends on whether you are paid IS in arrears or in advance.

If you are paid in advance, the first 'downrating', or change, is put into effect from the first pay day after you have been in hospital for 6 weeks (42 days, not counting the day of admission to hospital). So you could gain up to 6 days full benefit. If your 43rd day in hospital is a pay day, the change will usually be put into effect from that day.

If you are paid in arrears, the change is put into effect from the first day of the benefit week in which you'll have been in hospital for 6 weeks (42 days, not counting the day of admission to hospital). So you could lose up to 6 days full benefit.

However, if you leave hospital for a break of less than a week you will get your full pro-rata IS entitlement for those days. If you are discharged for longer than a week, or for good, the 'normal' rules come into play.

Housing benefit
If you still get IS, a spell in hospital does not affect your housing benefit (HB), or council tax benefit (CTB) (but see Chapter 40). However, if you cease to get IS during a spell in hospital, you can claim these separately. If you get CTB/HB but you are not getting IS, the amount of benefit is affected.

Once you have been in hospital for 6 weeks, your CTB/HB applicable amount is reduced, or downrated. If a non-dependant has been in hospital for 6 weeks (linked, or in one spell), the deduction for him or her will not be made. These changes are put into effect from the start of the benefit week after you have been 6 weeks in hospital (42 days, not counting the day of admission). Even if your 43rd day in hospital is the start of the CTB/HB benefit week, the change is only put into effect from the start of the next benefit week. So you could gain up to 7 days benefit.

Even though your CTB/HB applicable amount is reduced, your income is also likely to be lower. You might become entitled to income support (and so would be 'passported' to CTB/HB during the spell in hospital). If your housing benefit is cut while you are in hospital, see Chapter 4(17): the local authority has discretion to pay extra housing and/or council tax benefit if the *'circumstances are exceptional'*.

Stage 1 – from the 1st day
There is normally no cut in your IS or CTB/HB applicable amounts during your first 4 weeks in hospital. If you don't get a severe disability premium, you won't see a cut until you've been in hospital for 6 weeks.

However, if you have been readmitted to hospital after spending 28 days (or less) in your own home (not counting the day you left hospital), the two spells 'link' together, and count as a continuous spell.

If you are a single claimant and are normally resident in special accommodation *'owned or managed by [a] local authority'* your IS applicable amount is reduced to £14.10 from the first day.

Extra benefit
IS does not increase if any of your IS family goes into lodgings to be near to the member of your family who is in hospital. Instead, you may have to look to the social fund for help – see Chapter 7.

You may qualify for the severe disability premium temporarily while your carer or another non-dependant is in hospital. See Chapter 3(13).

Stage 2 – from the 29th day
After 4 weeks in hospital, attendance allowance, DLA care component and (in most cases) DLA mobility component for an adult are withdrawn. If you had been in hospital (or for the care component, other 'special' accommodation) during the 28 days before your current spell in hospital, attendance allowance or DLA would have been withdrawn sooner. See Chapter 17(9) for more details.

Once attendance allowance or DLA care component stops, a severe disability premium is withdrawn. Although if you have a partner and one or both of you go into hospital, you keep the severe disability premium even after the attendance allowance or DLA care component stops (provided both of you had been getting attendance allowance or DLA care component) but it will only be paid at the rate of £37.15.

A carer premium may be withdrawn at stages 2, 3 or 4 depending on your situation. In general, it is withdrawn 8 weeks after ICA goes, or, if your ICA is overlapped by another benefit, after attendance allowance or DLA care component stops – see Chapter 19(9). However, a disability premium, or higher pensioner premium which is based solely on attendance allowance or DLA is not withdrawn until Stage 3. A disabled child premium, based solely on DLA, is not withdrawn until the child ceases to count as a dependant.

If you are entitled to an amount of IS only because of the inclusion of a severe disability premium in your applicable amount, the withdrawal of the severe disability premium at the 4 week stage means the loss of IS. You would have to make a fresh claim for housing benefit and council tax benefit on a means-tested basis. Apply directly to the local authority.

At the 6 week stage when your incapacity benefit, SDA, retirement pension, widow's benefit or unemployability supplement is downrated (see 8), you may again become entitled to an amount of IS (and thus to maximum help with eligible rent and/or council tax), or your HB and/or CTB would have to be recalculated.

Stage 3 – from the 43rd day

After 6 weeks in hospital income support, housing benefit and council tax benefit are generally downrated.

Single claimant
Your IS/CTB/HB personal allowance is cut to £15.60 pw. All premiums are withdrawn. IS housing costs, housing and council tax benefit continue.

Lone parent
Your IS/CTB/HB personal allowance is cut to £15.60. But you'll still qualify for allowances for dependent children, the family premium and disabled child premiums. If you've been getting a disability premium or any pensioner premium, these will stop but your family premium will switch from the ordinary rate to the higher lone parent rate. IS housing costs, housing and council tax benefit continue.

Couples
If only one of a couple has been in hospital for 6 weeks, your IS/CTB/HB personal allowance is cut by (not to) £12.50. So long as you still qualify for any of the premiums, they will still be included in the assessment. IS housing costs, housing and council tax benefit continue.

If both of a couple have been in hospital for 6 weeks, your IS/CTB/HB personal allowance is cut to £31.20. But you'll still qualify for allowances for dependent children, the family premium, and disabled child premiums. All other premiums are withdrawn. IS housing costs, housing and council tax benefit continue.

Child
If a child is in hospital, there is no cut until Stage 4.

Residential care
If you enter hospital from a residential care or nursing home, your IS applicable amount will not include a residential allowance once you have been absent from that home for 6 weeks. If you have a 'preserved right' (see Chapter 38), and have to pay the home, you can get up to the full RCH/NH rates for 6 weeks, followed by up to an 80% retaining fee for up to 52 weeks.

Stage 4 – from the 85th day

After 12 weeks in hospital, there is a change if the patient is a child. This affects IS only. After 12 weeks, a dependent child's IS allowance is cut to £12.50. There is no change to the CTB/HB allowance for that child.

If the patient is one of a couple (with the partner not also in hospital) his or her ICA is withdrawn after s/he has been in hospital for a total of 12 weeks out of the previous 26 weeks. The carer premium in this case continues for 8 weeks after ICA is withdrawn.

Stage 5 – after 52 weeks

Linking rule
This does not apply to the questions of whether or not you can still be treated as occupying your 'home', or whether or not you still count as members of the same household. A day at 'home' means that the rules have to be applied afresh once you return to hospital – see Chapter 4(6).

Couples
If you are one of a couple and you, or your partner, have been in hospital for over 52 weeks, you will be treated as separate claimants. This may have happened sooner if it had become clear that you, or your partner, would not be able to return home, or would be in hospital for substantially longer than 52 weeks.

Once you are treated as separate claimants, the patient's IS personal allowance will be cut to £12.50 (if s/he has been a patient for 52 weeks), or £15.60 (if s/he has been a patient from between 6 to 52 weeks). Whichever of you is still at home can then qualify for benefit in the normal way, but as a single claimant or lone parent.

If you are both in hospital, one of you can still get benefit for any dependent children and IS housing costs. The same would apply to a lone parent.

Housing costs
Once you have been away from your own home for 52 weeks, you can no longer be treated as occupying it as your home. IS housing costs will stop if you count as a single claimant. Your housing benefit entitlement will also stop. But they may have stopped earlier if it had become clear that you would never be able to return home, or that your stay in hospital would last for a substantially longer time than 52 weeks.

Child
Once a child has been in hospital for 52 weeks you continue to have the £12.50 allowance included in your IS assessment for as long as you keep visiting him or her. But s/he will be excluded from the HB assessment.

Council tax benefit
You are eligible for council tax benefit for up to 52 weeks, so long as you are liable to pay council tax. Your home is exempt from council tax if it is unoccupied and you are *'solely or mainly'* a patient resident in a hospital. Depending on the circumstances, this could happen at any stage: but you must apply for exemption. If your partner or another adult is living in your home, once you become solely or mainly resident in hospital, s/he may qualify for a council tax discount. Chapters 4 and 5 have more details on council tax benefit and council tax.

Before April 1995 the rules were more generous. If your stay in hospital began before 3.4.95, you continue to be eligible for council tax benefit without time limit, for so long as you remain liable to pay council tax.

weeks (for DLA for a child) at full-rate benefit. If your benefit had been adjusted (downrated or withdrawn) during the previous spell in hospital, it will be adjusted again. However, as the daily rate provisions do not apply, your benefit can be adjusted only from the first pay day after the day you were readmitted to hospital.

If you have had 29 or more days out of hospital (or out of other 'special' accommodation for attendance allowance and DLA care component) the separate spells are not linked together. So your benefit won't be adjusted until the pay day after 4 weeks (for attendance allowance etc) or after 6 weeks (for other benefits) or after 12 weeks (for DLA for a child).

If the daily rate provisions do apply, or if you receive a benefit payable at a daily rate (such as incapacity benefit or SDA), your benefit can be adjusted (upwards or downwards as appropriate) from the first day that you are not in hospital or from the day after you are admitted or readmitted to hospital.

The daily rate provisions cease to apply once you have been out of hospital for 28 days, or for AA and DLA care component if you've been out of hospital or other 'special' accommodation for 28 days.

The interaction of the various provisions can be complex. See: reg 4A (payment of 'weekly' benefits at a daily rate) and reg 17(4) (28 day linking rule) of the SS (Hospital In-Patients) Regs 1975/555; regs 6 and 8 (28 day linking rule for attendance allowance) of the SS (Attendance Allowance) Regs 1991/2740; regs 8 and 10 (28 day linking rule for DLA care component) and regs 12A to 12C (for DLA mobility component) of the SS (DLA) Regs 1991/2890; reg 16 (the pay day rule) and reg 25 (attendance allowance at a daily rate) of the SS (Claims & Payments) Regs 1987/1968.

11. Comments, suggestions or complaints
Most problems can be sorted out with the staff looking after you. If you want to take further any comments, suggestions, or complaints about the way you are (or were) being looked after in hospital, tell the administrator of the hospital concerned. If you would like help with this, contact your local Community Health Council, or in Scotland the Local Health Council. Community Health Councils are there to represent the interests of patients and the public in general over hospitals and health services. You can find out where your local health council is from your local council or advice centre or look it up in the telephone book.

Patients who are detained in hospitals or nursing homes under the Mental Health Act can contact The Mental Health Act Commission who will look into complaints. In Scotland, contact the Mental Welfare Commission for Scotland. See the Address List at the back of the Handbook.

Discharged before you're ready?
If acute nursing care in hospital is no longer essential for you, the hospital will clearly wish to discharge you. It may be impossible for you to return home without support services in place. In some cases you may even count as homeless. Get advice. Before being discharged, your care needs should have been assessed. However, don't agree to a discharge unless you are happy with the arrangements for continuing care and support as set out in your care plan. Don't agree to move to a nursing home unless you are absolutely clear about how, and for how long, the full cost will be met. See Chapters 32 to 38 for more details about Care in the Community.

40 Hospital – one year on

1. Single people
After one year in hospital, the amount of benefit paid to you will be reduced to £12.50 a week.

Once you have been in hospital for 52 weeks, you can no longer be treated as occupying your own home – so housing benefit and council tax benefit end (see 6).

2. Which benefits are affected?
All the following:
- income support (IS);
- incapacity benefit and severe disablement allowance;
- widow's benefits;
- retirement pension and non-contributory retirement pension for people over 80;
- industrial injuries unemployability supplement.

Not the following:
- war disablement pensions – which are not reduced at all from their normal rate; but extra allowances may be;
- war widow's pensions – are paid at the full rate for the first 52 weeks of a hospital stay and are then reduced;
- industrial injuries exceptionally severe disablement allowance.

3. Who cannot get the £12.50 allowance?
You can be paid less than £12.50 or nothing at all, if you have been in hospital for more than 52 weeks and:
- you cannot act for yourself; and your benefit is paid to the hospital authorities (either as the appointee or on the appointee's request); and
- the medical officer in charge of you certifies that you are unable to use part or all of the allowance which is intended to provide for personal comfort or enjoyment. The medical officer must state the amount (if any) which can be used by you or on your behalf. The medical officer has absolute discretion over how much money you get – or whether you get any at all, either directly or in the form of comforts. However, for IS alone, the AO (or SSAT) can award benefit if s/he considers it reasonable *'having regard to the views of the hospital staff and the patient's relatives if available as to the amount necessary for [the patient's] personal use'.*

Do note that the reduction cannot apply on any day that does not count as a day in hospital – you will be entitled to full pro-rata benefit for days of absence on leave (see 8).

4. People with dependants
If you have a dependent partner, or child, your local DSS office will send you a form shortly before you have been in hospital for a year, and you will be able to decide how you want your non-means-tested benefit (eg SDA, retirement pension, incapacity benefit) to be paid in future.

There is only one sensible decision to make. You'll be paid

L.2 For more information

The following leaflets are free from local DSS offices:
NI 9 *Going into Hospital?*
HC 11 *Help With Health Costs*
NI 6 *Industrial Injuries Disablement Benefit.*
And from your local War Pensioners' Welfare Office:
WPA 1 *Notes about War Pensions and Allowances*
The hospital linking rule is explained in Box L.1 but, if you get attendance allowance or DLA read Chapter 39(8), Chapter 17(9) and Box G.3 in Chapter 17.

£12.50 for yourself and the rest of your benefit (less £25) will be paid to your dependant. If you don't agree to have the rest of your benefit paid over, you'll lose it completely.

5. Dependants in hospital
If you have a dependent wife or husband in hospital, the weekly rate of incapacity benefit, SDA or retirement pension paid to you for her or him is reduced by £12.50 after s/he has been in hospital for 6 weeks. Once s/he has been in hospital for 52 weeks, the addition will be reduced to £12.50 a week. (See 6 below if you are one of a couple on IS.)

If you have an adult dependant, other than a spouse, in hospital, the benefit paid will usually have stopped as soon as they go into hospital.

If you have a dependent child in hospital, you can receive dependant's benefit for him or her if you are regularly spending on visits, gifts or comforts, or sending money.

6. IS, housing and council tax benefit
If you have no dependants living in your home: once you have been in hospital for 52 weeks, you can no longer receive IS housing costs. Nor can you get housing benefit or council tax benefit – but see Box L.1. 52 weeks is the maximum period of absence in one stretch during which IS housing costs and/or housing benefit can be paid.

If you have dependants, or other people living in your home, their right to benefit depends on their own circumstances. If you are one of a couple and have been in hospital for 52 weeks you and your partner are treated as separate claimants. This happens earlier if the AO and/or HB/CTB section considers that your stay in hospital is likely to be for substantially longer than 52 weeks.

7. DLA mobility component
For most people DLA mobility component stops after 4 weeks in hospital (12 weeks for children) unless you have a Motability agreement. Before 31.7.96 the law allowed you to keep your mobility component no matter how long your stay. There is transitional protection for those who had already been in hospital for a year or more when the rules changed on 31.7.96 and had been getting mobility component throughout. If you are covered by transitional protection your mobility component is not stopped completely but is only paid at an amount equal to the lower rate of £13.15 a week. See Chapter 17(9) for more details.

8. Days out of hospital
If you are discharged from hospital for a short break at home or are in and out on a regular pattern, you will receive your full benefit entitlement – worked out on a daily basis.

Note that if you have been receiving SDA at the personal expenses rate (or lower), you should also claim income support to top-up your SDA for any day of absence from hospital. See Chapter 39(10) for how the daily rates are worked out.

What days can you claim for?
You can get full benefit paid on a daily basis for each whole day spent out of hospital. If you stay in hospital as an in-patient throughout a complete 24 hour period, for benefit purposes you count as being in hospital on that day unless you are paying a charge which is designed to cover the whole cost of your accommodation or non-treatment services. The regulations don't spell out whether or not you count as being in hospital if you are only there for part of the day, and the case law is conflicting.

The day you leave or return to hospital – A Commissioner (CIS/571/94) decided that the day you are admitted or return to hospital is not counted as a day in hospital. But the day you are discharged or leave hospital is counted as a day in hospital. However, while this principle applies to all other benefits, it does not extend to DLA or attendance allowance. For DLA and attendance allowance the previous case law approach currently still applies: that is neither the days of entry or discharge from hospital count as days in hospital. So you can get full DLA or attendance allowance for those days. However, there is likely to be a change in the law soon which may bring DLA and attendance allowance into line with other benefits – see our *Disability Rights Bulletin*.

Absence during the day – One decision, R(S)4/84, (which was not considered by the Commissioner in CIS/571/94) held that a claimant who slept at hospital at night but had her meals at college during the day, could not be counted as an in-patient – only a complete 24 hour period of hospital in-patient treatment could count as a day in hospital. So if you return to sleep at night in hospital but are absent in the daytime, you might be entitled to full benefit for that day.

There are a number of relevant decisions including CIS/192/91, CS/249/89, R(S)1/66, R(S)8/51, R(S)9/52.

What if you have missed out on benefit?
If you have missed claiming benefits for short absences away from hospital, you may be able to recover arrears.

For most benefits, you have 3 months in which to claim. But for income support you must have special reasons if there is any delay in your claim, eg you didn't have help to make your claim earlier – see Chapter 52(4).

If you've been getting the personal expenses rate of any benefit, you must ask for the earlier decisions to be reviewed. For most benefits, arrears on review are restricted to one month.

Chapter 52 explains the rules for backdating benefits. Note that a claim for attendance allowance or DLA cannot be backdated.

9. Benefits when you leave hospital
In general, you should get the benefit you were getting before you went to hospital at the normal rate – which will usually be higher than it was when you went in, since benefits are increased each year. If you go from hospital into a residential care or nursing home, see Chapters 35 to 38 for details.

If you did not draw any benefit before you went into hospital and have no entitlement to contributory benefits, look at the chapters on SDA and IS. Once you leave hospital, all the normal rules for these benefits will apply to you. Chapter 7 covers the discretionary social fund. You are likely to get a community care grant to help re-establish yourself in the community. Your local Citizens Advice Bureau can advise you further.

41 Going abroad

1. Introduction
If you are planning a trip abroad or planning to live abroad, you may still be able to receive your benefit while you are away. Some benefits, such as retirement and widows' pensions, can be paid no matter how long you are away. For other benefits the conditions are more complex.

There are different rules depending on which country you are going to. The European Community (EC) rules are the most favourable. There are also various reciprocal agreements with European Economic Area (EEA) countries (see below) which can assist if you are not covered by EC rules, as well as reciprocal agreements with some non-EEA countries. If none of these can help, the general rules on payment of benefits abroad apply.

In this chapter we look at the general rules and indicate which benefits are payable in EC countries. But the EC rules and reciprocal agreements are too varied and complex to cover here. Generally it is best to write to your local DSS office (or to the Jobcentre if they pay your benefit), or to the Benefits Agency Pensions and Overseas Benefits Directorate (see Box L.3), for advice well before you go. Keep a copy of the letter. List the benefits you are getting; give your full name, date of birth, and National Insurance number (or pension number). Explain the purpose of your visit; where you are going to, and how long you plan to be away.

If you are going to an EC country – You may come under more favourable EC social security rules. The EC countries are Austria, Belgium, Denmark, Finland, France, Germany, Greece, Italy, Luxembourg, Netherlands, Portugal, Republic of Ireland, Spain, Sweden, UK (including Gibraltar, but not the Channel Islands or Isle of Man). **EC rules also apply to Iceland, Norway and Liechtenstein which joined with the EC to form the European Economic Area (EEA).**

The EC rules apply to EEA nationals, refugees and stateless people habitually resident in an EEA country, who are, or were, employed or self-employed, and to their families. Generally you count as employed or self-employed if you have paid contributions under the UK National Insurance scheme or are insured under a social security scheme of another EEA country.

See below for an indication of whether a particular benefit can be paid in another EC country, but note that we don't cover the details of the EC rules in this chapter.

Reciprocal agreements – The UK has reciprocal social security agreements with some countries (including all EEA countries except Greece and Liechtenstein – the reciprocal agreement applies where you are not covered by EC rules) which may help you be paid benefit abroad. Non-EEA countries covered by reciprocal agreements are Australia, Barbados, Bermuda, Canada, Cyprus, Isle of Man, Israel, Jamaica, Jersey & Guernsey, Malta, Mauritius, New Zealand, Philippines, Switzerland, Turkey, USA, former Yugoslavia.

L.3 For more information

There is a series of DSS leaflets available which may be helpful.
NI 38 *Social Security Abroad*
SA 29 *Your Social Security Insurance, Benefits and Health Care Rights in the European Community*
T 5 *Health Advice for Travellers*
CH 6 *Child Benefit for People leaving Britain*
NI 106 *Pensioners or Widows Going Abroad*
FB 5 *Service Families Abroad (and at home)*
WPA 6 *Notes for War Pensioners and War Widows Going Abroad*
There are also separate leaflets for each country covered by a reciprocal agreement with the UK.

Copies of these leaflets are available from your local DSS office, or from: *Benefits Agency Overseas Benefits Directorate, Tyneview Park, Whitley Road, Benton, Newcastle upon Tyne, NE98 1BA (0191 218 7777)*. If you live in Northern Ireland contact *Overseas Branch, Social Security Agency, Commonwealth House, Castle Street, Belfast BT1 1DX*.

---

2. Incapacity and maternity benefits

General rules – If you go to a country with which there are no reciprocal arrangements and get incapacity benefit, maternity allowance or severe disablement allowance (SDA), and have been incapable of work for a continuous period of at least 6 months, you should normally be able to receive your benefit for up to 26 weeks if your absence is temporary. In deciding whether your absence is temporary, the Adjudication Officer should consider your intentions, the purpose of your absence and the length of the absence – an indefinite absence can still count as temporary (*CAO and Secretary of State v Ahmed and Others*).

You can go abroad for any reason – including a holiday. However, as the Secretary of State must agree that it is reasonable for you to get benefit while you are abroad, there is no right of appeal if you are refused; your only recourse is judicial review. If the Secretary of State agrees payment but the AO decides that your absence is not temporary, you do have a right of appeal.

If you have been incapable of work for less than 6 months, you can only get benefit for up to 26 weeks if you have gone abroad temporarily for the specific purpose of being treated for an illness or disability that began before you left.

You can appeal against a refusal under the provision *'for the specific purpose of being treated'*. The treatment does not need to be the only reason you have for going abroad. However, going abroad to convalesce or for a change of air – even on your doctor's advice – is not enough. *'Being treated'* must involve some activity by another person. It does not matter whether the treatment is available in the UK or not. In some cases the claimants did not even receive any treatment – but they did go abroad specifically in order to try and get it.

People who are members of the family of a serving member of the armed forces who is abroad, and those in receipt of attendance or disability living allowance are exempted from the 26 week restriction as long as they are abroad to receive treatment, or they had been incapable of work for six months before the absence began.

If you are abroad because you are living with a serving member of the forces who is a close relative, you are treated as passing the 6 months presence condition for SDA and can get SDA while you are abroad.

EC – Generally, if you go to live in another EEA country, or you return to the EEA country where you ordinarily live, or you are authorised by the Overseas Benefits Directorate to go to an EEA country specifically for medical treatment, you may be able to get short-term incapacity benefit or maternity allowance there. You must obtain agreement from the DSS that your benefit can be paid there before you go. Long-term incapacity benefit can be paid to you in another EEA country.

3. Income support

Four week rule – You can be paid income support (IS) for the first 4 weeks of a temporary absence abroad. The absence must be unlikely to last for over 52 weeks. You must be entitled to benefit immediately before you leave and continue to meet the conditions while you are away (apart from the fact that you are out of Great Britain).

If you are entitled to IS on the grounds that you are incapable of work (including SSP entitlement), appealing against an incapacity for work decision, at school or full-time non-advanced education, a person from abroad, or involved in a trade dispute (see Box B.1 in Chapter 3) you can only get IS for the first 4 weeks abroad if:

- you are in Northern Ireland; or
- you and your partner are both abroad and a disability premium, severe disability premium or any pensioner premium is applicable for the partner who is not the claimant; or
- you have been continuously incapable of work during the 364 days before the day you leave GB, or 196 days if you are 'terminally ill' or entitled to DLA higher rate care component (two or more periods of incapacity are treated as continuous if the break between is not more than 56 days each time); or
- you are incapable of work and your absence is *'for the sole purpose of receiving treatment from an appropriately qualified person for the incapacity by reason of which'* you are eligible for IS.

8 week rule – You can get IS for the first 8 weeks abroad if you are taking your dependent child abroad for medical treatment, physiotherapy, or similar treatment, by an appropriately qualified person. The absence should be unlikely to be more than 52 weeks. You must continue to satisfy the IS conditions of entitlement. If the IS claimant stays in Britain his or her IS will include benefit for the first 8 weeks for members of his or her IS family who are abroad in these circumstances.

4. Jobseeker's allowance (JSA)

General rules – You can continue to be paid income-based or contribution-based JSA for a limited period if your absence is unlikely to exceed 52 weeks and you continue to satisfy the conditions of entitlement while you are away.

- You can be paid **for the first 4 weeks** if: you are in Northern Ireland; or both of a couple are abroad and a disability premium, severe disability premium or any pensioner premium is payable in respect of the claimant's partner; or you receive a government training allowance (but not for a YT course).
- You can be paid **for the first 8 weeks** if you are taking your dependent child abroad for medical treatment, physiotherapy or similar treatment by an appropriately qualified person.
- If you go abroad for **a job interview** and are away for no more than 7 consecutive days, you can be paid for your days abroad provided you give written notice in advance to the Jobcentre and on your return you satisfy the employment officer that you did attend the interview.

EC – For contribution-based JSA, if you are going to an EEA country, to look for work, then, provided you have been registered with the Jobcentre for, normally, 4 weeks, and getting contribution-based JSA up to the date you leave the UK, you can usually get benefit in the EEA country for up to 3 months. You must comply with the procedures in the state where you are seeking work.

Income-based jobseeker's allowance, like income support, is not covered by EC rules.

5. Attendance allowance and DLA

General rules – Attendance allowance (AA) and disability living allowance (DLA) will continue to be paid for the first 26 weeks of a temporary absence abroad. If you are away for longer, the Secretary of State may agree to pay you for the extra time abroad. However, to get an extension, your absence from the UK must be temporary and for the specific purpose of being treated for a medical condition that began before you left the UK.

If you are living with a close relative who is a serving member of the forces, you are treated as if you were present in the UK – so AA and DLA are payable.

EC – If your AA/DLA entitlement began after 1.6.92, you cannot continue to be paid if you go to live in another EC country (other than under the rules above for a temporary absence).

If your entitlement to AA or DLA began before 1.6.92, you can be paid your benefit without time limit in another EC country so long as you continue to satisfy all the other conditions of entitlement other than the residence and presence conditions. To be covered by this provision you must either be working currently in the UK, or else have worked in the UK in the past and at the time you apply to have your AA/DLA paid abroad you are also entitled to a contributory benefit such as incapacity benefit or retirement pension based on past National Insurance contributions. If this applies, you can make a renewal claim while you are abroad without having to satisfy the residence and presence conditions, but there must be no break in entitlement between the end of an award and entitlement under the renewal claim.

6. Invalid care allowance

General rules – This will be paid for the first 4 weeks of a temporary absence abroad if you go without the person you are caring for.

If you go abroad temporarily, specifically in order to care for that person, you will receive ICA for as long as they receive AA or DLA. Remember you must still show that you are caring for them for 35 hours a week.

If you are living with a close relative who is a serving member of the forces, you are treated as if you were present in the UK.

EC – If you go to live in another EC country, you can only continue to be paid your ICA if you were entitled to ICA before 1.6.92, you continue to satisfy all the other conditions of entitlement (other than the residence and presence conditions) and either you are currently working in the UK, or else you have worked in the UK in the past and at the time you apply to have ICA paid abroad you are also entitled to a contributory benefit such as retirement pension or incapacity benefit based on past NI contributions.

7. Child benefit

Child benefit can be paid for the first 8 weeks of a temporary absence abroad. It may be paid for longer if you stay in GB, but your child goes abroad:

- for the specific purpose of being treated for an illness or disability that began before s/he left the UK; or
- solely in order to receive full-time education up to a limit of 3 years continuous absence.

Special rules enable child benefit to be paid for the child of a civil servant posted overseas; of a serving member of the forces; and of someone employed overseas if half their income is liable to UK income tax (eg a VSO volunteer). Guardian's allowance can be paid abroad for the same period as child benefit.

8. Disablement benefit

A basic disablement pension and retirement allowance are both payable while you are abroad. However, there are time limits for other industrial injuries benefits.

Reduced earnings allowance – This is payable for the first three months of a temporary absence abroad so long as you were getting it before you left, and your absence is not connected with work. It may be paid for longer if the Secretary of State agrees. Note that if you lose REA for one day, you may lose it for good.

Constant attendance allowance and exceptionally severe disablement allowance – These are payable for the first six months of a temporary absence abroad. They can be paid for longer if the Secretary of State agrees.
EC – If you are already getting any industrial injuries benefit (including those above) before you leave, they are payable without time limit in an EEA country.

9. Retirement and widows' benefits
These are payable no matter how long you are away. If you intend to go for longer than 6 months, let your DSS office know so that they can make arrangements for paying your pension abroad. If you are living abroad permanently in a country outside the EEA you can only receive the annual up-rating increases if that country has a reciprocal agreement with the UK which covers the payment of annual increases.
EC – If you are living in an EEA country, you will get the annual benefit increases as if you were in the UK.

10. Statutory sick pay and statutory maternity pay
General rules – You can receive SSP while abroad (outside the EEA) if your employer is liable for Class 1 contributions for you on the first day of your period of incapacity, or would be if your earnings were high enough.

You can receive SMP if you go abroad.
EC – If you are in an EEA country you can be paid SSP or SMP subject to the normal conditions.

11. Family credit and DWA
Once you qualify for family credit or disability working allowance, you can be paid the remainder of the 26 week award while you are abroad.

12. The Secretary of State's discretion
Although it is the Secretary of State who must decide whether or not to extend payment or even, in some cases, to pay you in the first place, this decision will normally be taken in the local DSS office.

In most cases, there will be few problems over a short holiday abroad if you have been continuously incapable of work for the past six months. If you plan to go for an extended holiday, the DSS will look more closely at your case. Make sure that you tell them well in advance and in writing about all the factors that make it reasonable and necessary for you to go abroad.

There is no formal right of appeal from a decision taken by the Secretary of State. However, you can attempt to get a decision reversed – a letter from your MP, or from your doctor, social worker or health visitor could all help.

This section of the Handbook looks at the following:

Early retirement	Chapter 42
Benefits in retirement	Chapter 43
Retirement pensions	Chapter 44
Home responsibilities protection	Chapter 45

Retirement

42 Early retirement

For some people with disabilities, the prospect of working into their fifties and sixties may not be a realistic one. Those with progressive disabilities or illnesses may be unable to continue working or may not be able to continue in their normal job. For others, the efforts involved in going to work may get more difficult as they become older. Consequently, some people have to retire early and it is important to know what financial help they can receive.

1. Still able to work

If you are not incapable of work, you may be regarded as unemployed for benefit purposes should you give up work before state pension age. This may arise where your firm has a 'compulsory' retirement age below pension age. Or, you may feel that the job you are doing is just too much for you and you are not able to find one nearer home or easier to cope with. In both cases, you may be able to claim jobseeker's allowance (JSA). Read Chapter 14, and note the following points.
- You must be available for and 'actively seeking' work and have entered into a jobseeker's agreement.
- Benefit is not payable for up to 26 weeks if you leave your job voluntarily and *'without just cause'*. Those who are compulsorily retired or who have taken voluntary redundancy cannot be sanctioned. However, voluntary early retirement may lead to non-payment of benefit for up to 26 weeks – unless health problems were your main reason for taking, or asking for, early retirement.
- It is crucial to:
■ seek advice before taking early retirement; and
■ appeal against the benefit sanction itself; and
■ appeal against the length of the sanction.

26 weeks is the maximum length of time for which benefit is not payable. Even if a benefit sanction is applied, Social Security Appeal Tribunals can decide on a shorter period – the minimum for jobseeker's allowance is one week.

Contribution-based JSA, which is paid for up to 6 months, is £49.15 a week (for people aged 25 or over). If you have an occupational or personal pension of more than £50 a week, your JSA will be reduced by the amount your pension exceeds £50. Contribution-based JSA is paid at a slightly higher rate than the lower rate of short-term incapacity benefit. However JSA is taxable whereas the lower rate of short-term incapacity benefit is not. See Chapter 11 for more information about incapacity benefit.

You may also be entitled to income-based JSA depending on your income, savings and other circumstances.

2. Occupational pension and early retirement

An occupational pension may be paid to someone under the normal retirement age in their job if the scheme provides for an early pension on grounds of 'incapacity'. The Inland Revenue defines 'incapacity' as 'physical or mental deterioration which makes the individual incapable of his normal employment or which destroys or seriously impairs his earning capacity'. The maximum pension payable under Inland Revenue rules is one based both on the employee's actual service to date and on his or her potential service up to the normal retirement age for that particular firm's pension scheme. There may, or may not, be an actuarial reduction.

Check with your employer, personnel officer or trade union as to what your firm is offering you.

3. State benefits and ill health

You can claim incapacity benefit if you are 'incapable of work', provided you satisfy the contribution conditions. If you have an employer, you should qualify for statutory sick pay – see Chapter 10. If you have been receiving statutory sick pay, your employer will give you a form (SSP1) to claim incapacity benefit. You can continue to receive incapacity benefit until you reach pension age, or your condition improves enough for you to be considered fit enough to work again.

For full details of statutory sick pay and incapacity benefit and the meaning of 'incapacity for work' see Chapters 8, 10 and 11.

43 Benefits in retirement

1. What benefits can you get?

State pension age is 60 for women, and 65 for men (but see Chapter 44 for future changes to equalise pension ages). Once you reach that age, and not before, you can claim the state retirement pension. Retirement pension is dealt with in Chapter 44. This chapter looks at the other benefits you may be able to get at pension age. Sometimes you will need to decide whether to draw your pension or receive another benefit instead. Other benefits such as attendance allowance and income support can be paid in addition to the pension.

European law allows different state pension ages for men and women. However in other situations where standard benefit rules treat men and women of the same ages differently, this may contravene European law. Further information about equal treatment is given in 10 below.

2. What if you go on working?

Since 1.10.89, you can claim retirement pension at pension age whether or not you go on working. Chapter 44 explains more about retirement pension.

If you put off claiming retirement pension, you will:
■ earn extra pension for each week you work between pension age and the age of 65 (women) or 70 (men) as long as you defer your pension for at least 7 weeks and are not receiving certain other benefits – see Chapter 44(4);
■ be able to claim short-term incapacity benefit if you are

aged under 65 (women) or 70 (men) and you fall ill, but only if your 'period of incapacity for work' began before pension age – see 3.

If you work at any time after pension age you will not have to pay National Insurance contributions. Give your employer a certificate of age exception (form CF384). If you haven't got one, or are putting off claiming retirement pension, ask your DSS office for one.

Statutory sick pay

If you are employed and earning £62 pw or more, you should claim statutory sick pay (SSP) from your employer if you are sick for at least 4 days in a row. You are not entitled to SSP once you've reached the age of 65 (men and women). But if you reach 65 while you are getting SSP, your benefit will continue until the end of that period of entitlement.

Unemployment

If you become unemployed after pension age you cannot claim jobseeker's allowance. The rules were different before October 1996 as unemployment benefit could be paid after pension age.

3. Incapacity benefit

Before 13 April 1995 people could choose whether to draw their retirement pension when they reached pension age or continue to receive sickness or invalidity benefit up to the age of 65 (women) or 70 (men). The position is different with incapacity benefit. Whether you can receive incapacity benefit after pension age will depend on whether you were previously receiving invalidity benefit and whether you were over pension age on 13.4.95.

Short-term incapacity benefit

If you became incapable of work before the age of 60 (women) or 65 (men) you can continue to receive short-term incapacity benefit after reaching pension age. The full basic rate of short-term incapacity benefit for people over pension age is £59.90 (the rate does not change after 28 weeks) but you will receive less if you do not have sufficient qualifying years for a full basic pension. You may also receive any additional pension or graduated pension which you would be entitled to with your retirement pension. Short-term incapacity benefit can be paid for up to a year of incapacity. In deciding whether to draw your pension or continue to receive short-term incapacity benefit, you should note that the full basic pension is a little higher than the basic rate of incapacity benefit but while the pension is taxable, short-term incapacity benefit is tax free for the first 28 weeks.

See Chapter 11 for more details on incapacity benefit.

Long-term incapacity benefit

You can only receive long-term incapacity benefit after pension age if you are entitled to a transitional award because you were previously entitled to invalidity benefit and you reached pension age (60 for women, 65 for men) before 13.4.95. If you reach pension age on or after 13.4.95 your incapacity benefit will stop at pension age and you should claim your retirement pension.

If you are entitled to long-term incapacity benefit after pension age, you can continue to receive it until you reach the age of 65 (women) or 70 (men) as long as you remain incapable of work. This is tested under the 'all work' test of incapacity, but you may be exempt from the test – see Chapter 12.

If your contribution record is deficient, you will have got a reduced rate of invalidity benefit (and now incapacity benefit) after you reached pension age – even though you will have got the full rate beforehand. However, if your incapacity is 'industrial', you will have continued to get full-rate incapacity benefit during the 5 years after reaching pension age – see Chapter 12(2). Once you claim retirement pension it will be paid at the appropriate rate given your actual contributions record.

Invalidity allowance or age addition to long-term incapacity benefit is paid before or after retirement at the same rates – but becomes taxable if it is paid with retirement pension, as does the additional earnings-related pension. See Chapter 11 for more details.

Incapacity benefit or retirement pension? – The main advantage of keeping incapacity benefit is that it is tax free (for transitional awards) while retirement pension is taxable. Chapter 51 gives basic details about tax.

A man who has transitional protection which enables him to continue to receive the tapered earnings addition for his wife, will lose this if he switches to the retirement pension.

On the other hand, it might be an advantage to draw the pension if you and/or your partner work. There is no earnings rule with the retirement pension while there is a therapeutic earnings limit of £46.50 with incapacity benefit. For men, if you have a wife you cannot receive an addition for her if she has earnings over a certain level. If she is 60 or over she will be able to claim a pension based on your contributions, regardless of her earnings, if you start to draw the retirement pension (this will only be an advantage if she doesn't have a pension of at least £37.35 based on her own contributions).

In general, if you have enough income to pay tax, it may be best to stay on incapacity benefit unless it is clear there would be advantages for you in drawing the retirement pension.

In some circumstances a woman aged 60 to 64 may be better off claiming severe disablement allowance if she fulfils the conditions.

If you are unsure of your position, you may want to contact an advice agency such as a Citizens Advice Bureau.

Once you draw your retirement pension you can choose to cancel your retirement in order to reclaim long-term incapacity benefit. However, the new date from which you are claiming incapacity benefit must not be more than 8 weeks since the last claim ended. You can only choose to cancel your retirement once.

When can you claim retirement pension?

If you stay on incapacity benefit and then decide you want to draw your retirement pension instead, you just notify your local DSS office that you wish to claim retirement pension. In any event once you reach age 70 (men) or 65 (women) you can no longer get incapacity benefit so you should draw your pension.

4. Invalid care allowance

Both men and women can claim ICA up to the age of 65. You must satisfy the usual conditions of entitlement explained in Chapter 19. Because there is a 3 month time limit on ICA claims, you can actually make your claim up to 3 months after the day before your 65th birthday provided you satisfied the qualifying conditions before you reached 65.

If you were receiving ICA before the age of 65, or would have received it but for the overlapping benefit rules, you can continue to receive it beyond 65. After 65, your ICA continues even if you no longer care for a disabled person, or you start earning over £50 a week.

If you are a woman aged over 65, you may be able to start

getting ICA now. This applies if you were 65 or over before 28.10.94 and would have satisfied the conditions for ICA immediately before your 65th birthday were it not for the UK rules which, at the time, said that a woman must be under 60 when she claimed ICA. This applies even if you did not make a claim at the time. If you did claim before 28.10.94 it is possible to get ICA backdated to 28.10.94 (or earlier in some cases). For more details, see our *Disability Rights Bulletin Summer 1996*. However, in any situation where you start to get ICA after pension age, you should be aware that you may not be better off due to the overlapping benefit rules.

ICA overlaps with retirement pension, so once you reach pension age, if you claim your pension, ICA can only continue to be paid if your pension is less than £37.35 a week. You can be paid ICA on its own, or to top up a retirement pension. You don't have to claim retirement pension.

Carer premium
While you receive ICA, or would receive it but for the overlapping benefit rules, your 'applicable amount' for income support, housing and council tax benefit, includes a carer premium of £13.35 a week.

If your ICA is overlapped, you must have claimed ICA or reclaimed after 1.10.90 in order to get the carer premium.

Once you reach 65, you continue to get ICA even if you are no longer caring for the disabled person. But to keep the carer premium, if your ICA is overlapped, the person you were caring for must continue to receive attendance allowance or DLA care component at the middle or higher rate. However, the carer premium continues for 8 weeks after your ICA ceases, for example, where the disabled person's attendance allowance or DLA is withdrawn after 4 weeks in hospital. If the disabled person regains attendance allowance or DLA care component at the middle or higher rate, your carer premium should resume.

5. Severe disablement allowance
Severe disablement allowance overlaps with retirement pension. But, if you don't qualify for a retirement pension, or it is lower than SDA, your retirement pension can be topped up to your full SDA entitlement, including any age-related addition. On the other hand, you can just put off claiming retirement pension and keep your tax-free SDA.

Entitlement to SDA can continue after you become entitled to retirement pension. This is so even if your retirement pension is equal to or more than your SDA. In this case, you don't count as being 'in receipt' of SDA for the disability premium. However, if you already have a SDA-based disability premium or a higher pensioner premium under income support or housing or council tax benefit, you can continue to get the higher pensioner premium – see Chapter 3(19). See also Chapter 13 for details about SDA.

SDA age additions – These were added to SDA on 3.12.90. The age addition is based on the date you became incapable of work. If you were under 40 when your incapacity arose, your weekly rate of SDA would be £50.90.

After pension age – Both men and women can claim SDA up to the age of 65. You cannot normally be paid SDA for the first time after reaching the age of 65. However pensioners who were receiving the old non-contributory invalidity pension (NCIP) before 29.11.84 were automatically transferred to SDA under Route 1 (see Chapter 13).

To qualify for SDA after 65, you must have been entitled to it (or NCIP) for at least one day before your 65th birthday. So, you must show you met all the necessary qualifying conditions on that day for whichever route to SDA you have to take. You must either be paid SDA for that day, or would be paid SDA but for the overlapping benefit rules (eg your widow's benefit cancels out payment of SDA).

If you are a woman aged over 65, you may also be able to start receiving SDA now if you were 65 or over before 28.10.94 and would have satisfied the conditions for SDA immediately before your 65th birthday were it not for the UK rules which, at the time, said a woman must be under 60 when she claimed SDA. This rule may apply even if you did not make a claim at the time. If you did make a claim before 28.10.94 it is possible to receive payments backdated to 28.10.94 (or earlier in some cases). For more details see our *Disability Rights Bulletin Summer 1996*. However, in any situation if you start to receive SDA after pension age, you should be aware that you may not be better off due to the overlapping benefit rules.

Once you reach 65, you continue to get SDA even if you are no longer incapable of work or 80% disabled, provided you were entitled to SDA immediately before your 65th birthday. You no longer need to send in doctor's statements.

Women claimants – If you are a married woman, there are extra points to consider. Both of them relate to the effect that keeping SDA has on your income tax position.

❑ If you haven't yet reached 60, but your husband is 65 or over and claiming retirement pension, it is sensible for you to claim SDA. The addition for a dependent wife paid with retirement pension is taxable whereas SDA is at least £4.55 higher and all tax free.

❑ If you are over 60 you may be entitled to a Category A retirement pension based on your own contributions and/or a Category B pension on your husband's contributions if he is over 65. If this would be less than your SDA including any age related addition, you can continue to get the difference between your own retirement pension and your SDA. If you decide not to claim retirement pension, the whole of your SDA will be tax free. Note that in some cases it is worth putting off claiming retirement pension, even though you might be entitled to more than SDA in retirement pension. It all depends on the effect on your tax position. You do not have to claim retirement pension if you do not wish to.

6. Attendance allowance
Attendance allowance is only for people aged 65 or older. There is no upper age limit. See Chapter 18 for full details.

Many older people fail to claim attendance allowance. Some people do not realise that it is tax free; that it is not means-tested; and that it can be paid on top of retirement pension or income support (but there are special rules if you are in hospital or residential care – see Chapters 39 and 36). Others put their problems down to 'old age' rather than disability. If you're not sure if you qualify, seek advice.

7. Disability living allowance
If you were getting disability living allowance before you reached 65, you continue to be eligible for DLA, provided you continue to satisfy the other conditions.

You can still claim if you have not yet reached your 66th birthday and missed the opportunity to claim before you reached the age of 65 but only if you claim before 6.10.97. From 6.10.97, the rules are changing. If you claim on or after 6.10.97, you must make your first DLA claim before your 65th birthday. For more information see Chapter 17.

If you are a war pensioner, see Chapter 22 – there is no upper age limit for war pensioners' mobility supplement.

8. Income support

If your savings are not more than £8,000 and your income is not more than about £68.80 for a single person, or £106.80 for a couple, you may be entitled to income support to top up your income. If you are blind, over 75, get a disability benefit, or have certain housing costs you can have more income and still be entitled to income support. See Chapter 3 for full details. If you live permanently in residential care, you may be entitled to income support if your savings are no more than £16,000 – see Chapter 36.

9. Housing and council tax benefit

If you get any income support, you will be entitled to maximum housing and/or council tax benefit. If you do not get income support, you may still be eligible for some housing and/or council tax benefit. In this case claim directly from the local authority, not the DSS. See Chapter 4 for full details.

10. Equal treatment

The principle of equal treatment is that men and women should be treated equally. But the difference in state pension ages for men and women is lawful in so far as that difference relates to state retirement pension and to the overlapping benefit rules where a non-contributory benefit, such as SDA, is reduced by the amount of any retirement pension payable.

A series of court cases suggests that the knock-on effect of the difference in pension ages to other benefits can be discriminatory and in breach of EC Social Security Directive 79/7 on the progressive implementation of equal treatment in statutory social security matters. However in other cases, notably the *Graham* case (see below) the European Court of Justice ruled that unequal treatment is lawful.

The equal treatment directive excludes from its scope the age at which old-age or retirement pensions are granted and also 'the possible consequences thereof for other benefits'. The *Thomas* case related to invalid care allowance and severe disablement allowance (*Secretary of State v Thomas and others*, ECJ case C-328/91, 1993). The judgement stated that discrimination was permitted only if it was *'objectively necessary in order to avoid disrupting the complex financial equilibrium of the social security system or to ensure consistency between retirement pension and other benefits schemes'*. The Court ruled that for ICA and SDA discrimination was not justified and as a consequence UK law was changed to treat men and women equally.

However, in *Graham* (*Secretary of State and Chief Adjudication Officer v Graham and others*, ECJ case C92/94, 1995) the Court ruled that unequal treatment within invalidity benefit was permitted. The judgement found that ending the unequal treatment would undermine the coherence between the retirement pension scheme and the invalidity benefit scheme, (although some legal experts have described the reasoning as inadequate).

'Graham lookalikes'

Many other women were in the same position as Mrs Graham and these are often described as 'Graham lookalikes'. The Social Security Commissioner had ruled in favour of Mrs Graham, and while awaiting the result of the appeal to the European Court, Adjudication Officers followed the decision but payment of benefit was usually suspended under regulation 37A, Social Security (Claims and Payments) Regulations 1987, except in cases of hardship. Now that the *Graham* case has ruled that the unequal treatment is lawful, in most cases it is likely that the suspended benefit will not be paid. However there are still legal arguments being pursued with the DSS, following a case in the Scottish Court of Session (*Mulgrew*, 30.11.95), which held that reg 37A cannot be used where benefit has been awarded on appeal to a tribunal, and a further case, *Sutherland*, QBD, 7.11.96 which held that all reg 37A suspensions are unlawful. We will report on any developments in our *Disability Rights Bulletin*.

Other cases

The *Graham* decision makes it unlikely that a challenge to the unequal age rules within incapacity benefit and other contributory benefits would be successful, while the *Thomas* case has established that for non-contributory benefits discrimination would generally be unlawful.

Industrial injuries benefits, although linked to the contribution system, are not based on a contribution record in the same way as, for example, incapacity benefit. When someone is considered to have given up 'regular employment' and has reached pension age, the industrial injuries benefit, reduced earnings allowance, is replaced by retirement allowance which is paid at a lower rate (see Chapter 21(15)). Women aged 60 to 64 may receive less than a man of the same age and should appeal against the reduction in benefit – and seek advice.

If you do find that you receive less benefit than someone of the opposite sex who is the same age, you may wish to seek advice about your position.

44 Retirement pensions

1. State retirement pensions

There are four categories of state retirement pension. The two main ones are contributory and are known as Category A and B pensions.

Category A pensions are normally based on your own contribution record. Category B pensions are payable only to married women, widows and some widowers and are based on their spouse's contribution record. Category D retirement pensions are non-contributory and are only payable to people aged 80 or more. Category C pensions are for people who were already over pension age in 1948.

All categories of state retirement pension are taxable. For more details see leaflets FB6 *Retiring?* and NP46 *A Guide to Retirement Pensions*.

2. When can you get retirement pension?

You can get a state retirement pension if you've reached the state pension age (60 for women, 65 for men), you meet the contribution conditions and have made a claim. You can claim at any time, from 4 months before pension age. For Category A pensions, you yourself must have met the contribution conditions. You can receive a reduced-rate basic pension, so long as you have met the conditions to give you at least a pension of 25% of the standard rate – see Box M.1. For Category B pensions, your spouse must have met these contribution conditions.

If you do not draw your pension until you reach 65 (women) or 70 (men) you can get extra pension if you have not claimed retirement pension, or give up your pension for a period – see 4. Once you reach the age of 65 (women) or 70 (men) you cannot earn any extra pension.

Changes to state pension age

The Pensions Act 1995 introduces an equal state pension age

of 65 for both men and women. This change will be phased in between 2010 and 2020. Women born before April 1950 will still get their pension at age 60, while those born from April 1955 onwards will not be able to receive a pension until they are 65. Those born between these dates will be able to claim their pension between 60 and 65, depending on their date of birth.

3. Working and the state pension

You can earn what you like without it reducing your pension. If you carry on working during the first 5 years after reaching pension age, you earn extra pension if you put off claiming retirement pension – see 4 below. If you have already claimed retirement pension, you can give up your claim in order to earn extra pension. You can only give up a pension once, and you cannot backdate that choice.

Once you reach 65 (women) or 70 (men), you can no longer earn extra retirement pension.

Note that there is an earnings limit for an addition for a wife or other adult dependant – see 4 below.

4. Contributory pensions

Category A retirement pension

This is normally based on your own personal National Insurance contribution record. But some widows and widowers can get a pension even if they have not met the contribution conditions, so long as they have been getting incapacity benefit just before reaching pension age. Other widows, widowers and divorced people may be able to use the contribution record of their former spouse to help them qualify – see leaflets NP45 and NP46.

If you have met the contribution conditions in full, you can receive a basic pension as follows:

- **for yourself** £62.45
- **for an adult dependant** £37.35
- **for the first dependent child** (tax free) £9.90
- **for each other dependent child** £11.20

An adult dependant can be a wife or someone looking after your dependent child, or in limited circumstances, a husband. The age of an adult dependant makes no difference. If he or she is working, or receiving other NI income maintenance benefits, this affects the £37.35 increase in the same way as for incapacity benefit. The earnings limit for an adult dependant is £49.15; so the increase won't be paid if he or she earns more in any week; occupational and personal pensions count as earnings here.

A woman can only receive an increase for her husband if, immediately before drawing a pension, she was receiving an increase for him with incapacity benefit.

If your partner receives NI income maintenance benefits (eg SDA or incapacity benefit) those benefits will almost always cancel out a dependant's increase to your retirement pension.

Category B pension

This is payable mainly to women over pension age, who are, or have been, married. The Category B pension is based on the contribution record of your spouse or former spouse. If s/he had not fully met the contribution conditions, you will receive a reduced-rate pension.

Married women – If your husband has met the contribution conditions, both of you are over pension age, and he has claimed his own pension, you can get the £37.35 increase paid to you as your own Category B pension. If he has a reduced contribution record, you will receive a proportionally reduced pension. You can earn what you like without it affecting your pension.

Widows and widowers – See DSS leaflet NP45 for details. If you qualify for a full basic Category B pension, you will get £62.45 a week.

Category A and Category B pensions overlap. So if, for example, you are a married woman with a basic pension of £20 on your own contributions, you cannot receive this in addition to £37.35 Category B pension based on your husband's contributions. Instead your pension will be 'topped up' to £37.35 using your husband's contributions.

Extra pension

Your Category A or B pension may also include:

Additional earnings-related pension (SERPS) – This is based on earnings since 1978 on which you paid Class 1 contributions – as long as you were not contracted out of SERPS (see 8 below).

If you reach pension age on or before 6 April 1999, your SERPS pension will be calculated in this way. Your earnings from April 1978 up to the April before you reach pension age are revalued in line with increases in average earnings. From each year's revalued earnings the qualifying level of earnings for the basic state pension is taken away. (For example in 1997-98 the qualifying level of earnings is £3,224.) After this is deducted, all the earnings are added together and divided by 80 to give your yearly amount of SERPS.

The rules are changing if you reach pension age after 6 April 1999. For more details about the calculation for people retiring both before and after 6.4.99 see leaflet NP46.

For additional pension earned up to 5 April 1997, if you were contracted out of SERPS and a member of a company salary-related scheme, all or part of your 'additional' pension will be paid, as a *'guaranteed minimum pension'*, via your employer. In this case, your state pension will include any increases needed to increase your 'guaranteed minimum pension' (GMP) in line with inflation. For GMPs accruing after 6.4.88, the employer pays the first 3% of inflation proofing. If you were contracted out of SERPS and belonged to your company's money purchase scheme or a personal pension scheme, you will receive a pension based on the value of the fund built up (through contributions and the investment return on these). The part of the fund which is intended to replace SERPS is known as your 'protected rights'. There is no GMP as such, but your state additional pension will be reduced by an amount which may be more or less than the pension provided by your scheme. Note that an additional pension can be paid on its own if you aren't entitled to any basic pension. It is also payable with long-term incapacity benefit – but only for people who previously received invalidity benefit and are covered by the transitional rules – and widows' benefits.

Since 6 April 1997 there has no longer been a link between SERPS and contracted-out pension schemes. Instead of providing a GMP, a contracted-out salary-related scheme has to satisfy an overall test of quality. For contributions made from 6 April 1997 the DSS will no longer calculate your pension by making a deduction from your additional pension to take into account the time you have been in a contracted-out scheme. You will either receive an additional pension or, if you are contracted out, an occupational or personal pension based on the scheme's rules.

Graduated retirement benefit – This is based on graduated contributions made between April 1961 and April 1975. However levels of payment are low – for example, average weekly payments in 1995 were about £3.39 for men and £1.36 for

M.1 Retirement pension – the qualifying conditions

Your entitlement to basic retirement pension depends on three factors:
- your National Insurance contributions;
- your qualifying years;
- your working life.

In order to qualify for any retirement pension you must meet two conditions.
- In at least one tax year since April 1975 you must have actually paid contributions on earnings equivalent to 52 times (50 times from 6 April 1975 to 5 April 1978) the lower earnings limit for that year; or 50 flat-rate contributions at any time before 6 April 1975.
- You must also have paid or have been credited with enough contributions to make at least a quarter of the years in your 'working life' count as 'qualifying years'.

National Insurance contributions

From 1948 contributions were paid at a flat rate. From 1961 a system of graduated contributions was introduced which were paid by some people in addition to flat rate contributions. Graduated contributions were paid as a percentage of earnings between specified limits and earned people entitlement to graduated retirement benefit, the predecessor of SERPS.

Since 1975, employees pay Class 1 contributions as a percentage of gross earnings, collected with income tax. You can also be credited with contributions. For example, you will normally be credited with a contribution for any week in which you are signing on as available for work, or in which you are incapable of work. These credits help you pass the contribution condition for retirement pension (but don't help towards a SERPS pension).

You may also be entitled to 'credits', for pension purposes only, for the tax years of your 16th, 17th and 18th birthdays. Class 1 (employee), Class 2 (self-employed) and Class 3 (voluntary) contributions can all count towards your entitlement to retirement pension.

Chapter 9 gives more details about contributions and contribution credits.

Your qualifying years

A 'qualifying year' is a tax year in which you have paid or been credited with enough contributions for a pension.

In the old scheme, qualifying years were worked out by adding up all your stamps and dividing them by 50.

Under the current scheme, a qualifying year is one in which you have paid or been credited with contributions on earnings equivalent to 52 times the lower earnings limit for the year.

The lower earnings limit is the level at which you start paying contributions. This is normally almost the same as the basic rate of retirement pension – £62 a week in 1997-98.

For self-employed people and those paying voluntary contributions, the test is the number of flat-rate contributions, as it was under the old scheme, but divided by 52.

Working life

Your working life is the number of tax years in which you are expected to pay or are credited with contributions. This is normally from the tax year in which you became 16 to the last full tax year before you became 65 for men, or 60 for women. Working life is therefore normally 44 years for a woman and 49 years for a man. But if you were already over 16 (and insured for pension purposes) when the National Insurance scheme started in 1948, your working life is counted from April 1936, or when you last entered insurance, whichever is later, until the April before you reach 65 (for men), 60 (for women). If you weren't insured for pension purposes on 5.7.48, your working life is counted from 6.4.48. In either case you'll get credits for each week from the start of your working life up to 5.7.48.

To get a full basic pension about nine out of every ten years in your working life must be qualifying years. Women with a working life of 44 years need 39 qualifying years for a full basic pension and men with a working life of 49 years need 44 qualifying years.

If you do not have enough qualifying years to get a full pension, you will get a reduced pension as long as you have at least a quarter of the qualifying years you would need for a full pension.

Working out your pension

In most cases, you won't need to work out your entitlement to retirement pension. All your records should be on the computer in Newcastle, so all you have to do is to make sure that you put in a claim.

In a few cases it may be important to work out your pension entitlement. For example, you may have worked for an employer and had full contributions deducted but find that you don't get the full pension. This could be because one of your employers may not have paid over all your contributions – perhaps because of a bankruptcy.

If you think you are entitled to a different pension get in touch with the DSS immediately. They will check your contribution records and investigate any deficiencies. You can also check the calculation yourself. If you reach a different figure and can show that you did not connive with your ex-employer in avoiding paying the contributions, the Secretary of State can accept those contributions you had deducted from your pay, as if they had been paid over at the right time. This power covers all contributory benefits, including SERPS. If you have not kept all your pay slips, or a good proportion of them, you may find that the Inland Revenue will have enough details to satisfy the Secretary of State.

A more normal example of needing to work out your potential entitlement to retirement pension is if you are a married woman deciding whether or not to give up your existing right to pay the reduced-rate married woman's contribution.

Ask the DSS for advice

The easiest, and most accurate, way to do this is to ask your local DSS office for form BR19 to ask for a pension forecast. You can get a pension forecast if you are over 4 months away from your 60th birthday (women) or 65th birthday (men). Send your completed form to the address on form BR19. The forecast will give you your current pension entitlement based on the records held by the DSS. It should allow you (with some help if necessary) to make the right decisions about your future contribution position. The DSS says it takes an average of 17 working days to provide a forecast (40 working days if you are divorced or widowed). Your DSS office, or a Citizens Advice Bureau should be able to translate the forecast for you!

Ask for a pension forecast if you want to work out your entitlement to retirement pension for any other reason.

women. A graduated pension can be paid on its own.

Invalidity addition – This is paid if, within 8 weeks before reaching state retirement age, you were receiving:
- an invalidity allowance with your invalidity benefit; or
- transitional invalidity allowance with incapacity benefit; or
- an age addition with long-term incapacity benefit.

Provided you get some additional (earnings-related) pension, you can get this even if you don't get any basic pension. It is paid at the same rate as your invalidity allowance or age addition but is off-set against an additional pension or GMP.

Increments for deferring retirement – If you put off claiming your retirement pension for at least 7 weeks, your pension (including graduated and additional pension) will be increased by ½p for each £1 of retirement pension that you would have been paid if you had claimed it. Maximum increments are earned by putting off claiming retirement pension for 5 years. If you defer your pension for the full 5 years, it will be increased by about 37.5%.

Note that you cannot clock up extra pension just by keeping another income maintenance benefit such as widow's pension after retirement age. An addition for an adult or child dependant won't be increased if you defer claiming retirement pension. However, a Category B pension may be increased, but not in respect of any period during which a wife receives any pension or graduated retirement benefit (GRB)* based on her own contributions.

After you reach 65 (women), or 70 (men), you can gain no extra increments. However, in some circumstances a married woman can earn extra increments over age 65 – see leaflet NP46.

* *This does not apply in relation to GRB from 19.1.88 to 4.8.92.*

Age addition – 25p for people aged 80 or more.

5. Non-contributory pensions

Category C and D pensions
These are both non-contributory and paid at £37.35 a week. Category C pensions are payable to people who were already over pension age on 5 July 1948 and for the widows, wives and former wives of men in that position. Category D pensions are payable to people currently aged 80 or older and not entitled to another category of pension or entitled to one at a lower rate. To qualify you must satisfy certain residency conditions. Leaflet NI 184 has more about Category D. For Category C pensions, ask the DSS.

6. How do you claim retirement pension?
Normally the DSS will send you a claim form about 4 months before you reach 60 (women) or 65 (men). If you haven't been sent a form, write to the DSS from about 3 months before your 60th/65th birthday and ask for a claim form. Put your National Insurance number on your letter.

If you are a married woman, and haven't worked for some years, the DSS may not have an up-to-date address for you. So, if you don't hear from them and you have at any time paid contributions, write and ask for a claim form. Don't delay. The DSS will let you know if you are entitled to any pension.

If you are working and intend to put off claiming retirement pension in order to gain extra pension, you should complete the form so that the DSS can make the necessary arrangements.

If you have decided that it is sensible for you to keep your incapacity benefit (or ICA or SDA) because of the effect on your own tax or benefits position, complete the form, showing that you don't wish to claim retirement pension yet. (See Chapter 43 for more about benefits and retirement.) You will be sent a notice saying how much your pension will be. You can then work out the effect of retirement pension on your tax and benefits position. You could do this earlier by asking for a pension forecast – see Box M.1.

If you have put off claiming (for whatever reason) and decide that you want to claim your pension, you should claim about 3 months beforehand. Ask for a claim form if you haven't got one. Retirement pensions can be automatically backdated for 12 months if you claim before 4.8.97. For claims made on or after 4.8.97, pensions can only be backdated for 3 months. However, if you want to give up your pension you cannot backdate that choice. You can only give up your pension once.

Note that retirement pension can only start from a pay day, which is normally Monday for people who start to draw their pension now. You cannot receive any pension for days before your first pay day, even if you have reached pension age.

7. How is retirement pension paid?
If your pension is more than £5 a week, you can choose to have it paid at the post office or directly into a bank or building society account. Pensions collected at the post office are paid weekly in advance. At the time of writing, people are sent an order book but over the next two years order books and girocheques will begin to be phased out and replaced by a social security card.

If you prefer to have your pension paid directly into a bank or building society account, this is normally paid in arrears every 4 or 13 weeks. However, if you get income support as well, you can have this and your retirement pension paid weekly into an account. Leaflet NI 105 gives full details and an application form.

If your pension is £5 or less a week, it will normally be paid in a lump sum – along with your £10 Christmas bonus. Before October 1996, the limit to receive a pension weekly was £2 a week.

8. Pension options
This section looks at your pension choices and, in particular, your options regarding contracting out of SERPS. See 4 above for more information about SERPS.

If you are an employee and a member of an occupational pension scheme, you may also be paying into SERPS, or if your scheme satisfies certain requirements, you may be contracted-out of SERPS.

Contracted-out occupational pension schemes provide a pension related to earnings (known as 'salary-related' schemes) or a contribution-based pension (known as 'money purchase' schemes).

Instead of joining a contracted-out occupational scheme, you can choose to opt out of SERPS and enter into an 'appropriate personal pension' (APP) scheme instead. If you opt for an APP it will be a 'money purchase' scheme. That means that there is no guarantee about the level of your final pension (as there is with a 'salary-related' scheme). It may also give you fewer benefits than you could get under a good company scheme (even one which is also a 'money purchase' scheme).

A further choice is to pay additional voluntary contributions (within Inland Revenue limits) into your employer's scheme to top up your occupational pension. Or you can pay contributions into a pension plan which is quite separate from your own occupational scheme. These are known as 'free standing additional voluntary contributions'.

This 'free choice' of additional pension carries with it the major risk of making the wrong choice. If you do nothing, that is the same as making a decision – perhaps the wrong decision. Seek advice from an independent financial adviser, particularly if you are in a borderline age range for the 'better choice'. Always read the small print carefully. Ask for a detailed explanation or answers to your questions in writing if you are unsure about anything. Do not let yourself be hustled into making a decision. If you leave a company pension scheme, your employer does not have to take you back if you find out later that you've made the wrong choice.

If you are under 35 to 40 (for women), or under 40 to 45 (for men), a money purchase scheme may be a better bet than SERPS but do seek professional advice first. If you are 40 (women) or 45 (men) or older, you should probably stay in or switch to SERPS. SERPS, even in its cut-back version, gives a better deal than money purchase schemes for older contributors. At present, the law allows you to switch back and forth. But again, double check to see if there are any penalties for opting out of a company pension or private pension at the age of 40/45. Changes to equalise pension ages for men and women by 2020 may affect your pension options.

If you are getting a personal pension, it may affect your, or your partner's, right to benefits. A personal pension is taken into account on the same basis as an occupational pension – see below.

9. Occupational pensions

Occupational, or company, pensions vary from one firm to another and sometimes between different jobs in the same firm. So it is not possible for us to generalise about the different sorts of benefits available to someone retiring early, or at pension age. For information on what benefits your firm's pension scheme can offer you, ask your employer, personnel department or trade union.

Any pension you get from your firm will count as taxable income but it will not affect your entitlement to incapacity benefit. However, an occupational pension will be taken into account in three ways:
- it counts as earnings if your partner is claiming an increase for you as an adult dependant, or if s/he is claiming an increase for a child dependant. This covers all non-means-tested benefits;
- it counts as income for means-tested benefits such as income support, income-based jobseeker's allowance, housing or council tax benefit;
- if you receive an occupational pension of more than £50 a week, any contribution-based jobseeker's allowance you may be entitled to will be reduced.

45 Home responsibilities protection

1. What is home responsibilities protection?

Home responsibilities protection (HRP) is aimed at protecting your basic retirement pension rights (and widows' benefits) when you are not paying National Insurance contributions because you are looking after someone for a whole tax year at home and are not getting a benefit, such as invalid care allowance, which credits you with contributions. This scheme first

---

M.2 For more information

Occupational and personal pensions
The Pensions Advisory Service (OPAS) may be able to help if you have any problems. If you have tried, but not managed to discover the answer to your problem from the pension scheme trustees or managers, or from the personnel department in your firm it is worth contacting OPAS. OPAS cannot take legal action for you but it does seek to negotiate with the pension scheme authorities on your behalf and can give individual advice on most problems.

Your local Citizens Advice Bureau may be able to answer your query themselves. If not, they can refer you to a local OPAS volunteer adviser. If OPAS cannot solve your problem you may want to ask the Pensions Ombudsman to investigate.

You can write directly to OPAS at: *11 Belgrave Road, London SW1V 1RB*.

Pensions Ombudsman
The Pensions Ombudsman can investigate written complaints if you consider you have suffered injustice because of maladministration in connection with any action, or inaction, of the trustees or managers of an occupational or personal pension scheme; or if you have a dispute with the trustees on a matter of fact or law. The Pensions Ombudsman has wide powers to investigate any dispute within his remit. He has the same powers as the courts to require pension scheme trustees or managers to submit evidence and produce any relevant documentation. His decision is binding on the parties, with a right of appeal on a point of law only to the High Court. Before taking a complaint to the Pensions Ombudsman, you are normally expected to have asked OPAS for assistance. The Pensions Ombudsman is based at: *11 Belgrave Road, London SW1V 1RB*.

Occupational Pensions Regulatory Authority
The Occupational Pensions Regulatory Authority (OPRA) is an independent body established under the Pensions Act 1995 and accountable to Parliament. From April 1997 it has been responsible for the regulation of occupational pension schemes. OPRA can investigate schemes if there appears to be a problem or where a complaint has been made. It has also taken over the responsibility from the Occupational Pensions Board (which closed in April 1997) for the Pensions Registry which provides a tracing service for people who want to contact a scheme in which they have pension rights but do not know the address.

OPRA is based at *Invicta House, Trafalgar Place, Trafalgar Street, Brighton BN1 4DW (01273 627600)*. The Pensions Schemes Registry is at *PO Box 1NN, Newcastle upon Tyne NE99 1NN (0191 255 6437)*.

DSS leaflets
PP 1 *Thinking About a Personal Pension?*
PP 2 *Making the Most of Your Personal Pension*
PP 3 *Personal Pensions for the Self-Employed*
NP 46 *A Guide to Retirement Pensions*
PEC 1 *Information about Pensions (Catalogue)*
PEC 2 *About Pensions*
PEC 3 *The 1995 Pensions Act*
PEC 4 *What Are You Doing After Work?*
These and other leaflets on pensions are available from *DSS Pensions, Freepost BS5555/1, Bristol, BS99 1BL* or by ringing the DSS Pensions Line on 0345 313233.

began in April 1978, so only the tax years after that time can be covered by HRP. HRP is not a contribution credit and does not make up a deficiency in a person's contribution record.

HRP is intended to help you satisfy the second condition for the basic state retirement pension (see Box M.1). This is the condition that nine out of every ten years in your 'working life' must be 'qualifying years'.

The total number of years in which you were awarded HRP will be deducted from the number of qualifying years you normally need for a full basic pension. HRP cannot reduce the required number of qualifying years to less than 20.

2. Do you qualify?
You will qualify for home responsibilities protection if throughout a complete tax year:
- you spend at least 35 hours a week looking after someone who gets attendance allowance, DLA care component at the middle or higher rate, or constant attendance allowance for 48 or more weeks in the year (52 weeks for tax years before 6.4.88); or
- you get income support so that you can stay at home to look after a sick or disabled person; or
- you get child benefit (as the 'main payee') for a child under 16.

3. Does anything affect the provision of HRP?
Work – Makes no practical difference: if you qualify for HRP, you will get it if you have not paid enough contributions for retirement pension in the tax year.

Change of circumstance – If any one of the above conditions covers you for only part of the year but another covers you for the rest of this year, you can apply for HRP. But, if you meet the qualifying conditions for only part of the year, you will lose HRP for the whole of that year.

For example, before 6.4.88, if you were looking after someone who got attendance allowance and s/he went into hospital for 5 weeks, s/he lost the allowance for 1 week (see Chapter 17(9) and Chapter 18), you lost HRP for that year. However, for the tax years from 6.4.88, you would only lose HRP if s/he lost attendance allowance for more than a total of 4 weeks in the tax year because of being in hospital.

Married women and widows – If you are still liable to pay the reduced rate contribution at any time during a tax year, you cannot apply for HRP for that tax year. You can change to paying full NI contributions from the start of the next tax week after you notify the DSS. But this will make no difference to your HRP position until the start of the next tax year after you change to full liability.

Note that after you have spent two consecutive tax years without paying a reduced-rate Class 1 contribution (and were not self-employed), your right to pay reduced contributions will end at the end of the second tax year in any case. If you are likely to have to spend more than two tax years out of the employment field, it may be worth switching to full NI liability.

4. How do you apply?
If you are a man or a woman getting child benefit and your name is the first or only name on the order book or on letters about child benefit, or you are getting income support to look after a sick or disabled person at home, you do not have to apply. Your HRP will be recorded automatically (you can check with your local DSS office that this is happening). If you are the parent whose NI contribution record is affected, it is important that you are the one who is claiming the child benefit. Contact your local DSS office if you wish to change to become the claimant.

If you are looking after someone who is getting DLA care component at the middle or higher rate, attendance allowance or constant attendance allowance, or if you are covered partly by one of the general conditions and partly by another, you will have to apply for each tax year you need HRP. (But note, that if you get ICA (and haven't kept your rights to pay reduced-rate contributions – see 3), you will be credited automatically with NI contributions and so may not need HRP.)

To apply, just complete the form in leaflet CF411. You can get this from your local DSS office.

Other money matters

This section of the Handbook looks at the following:

Widows	Chapter **46**
Christmas bonus	Chapter **47**
Health benefits	Chapter **48**
Housing grants	Chapter **49**
Child support	Chapter **50**
Income tax	Chapter **51**

46 Widows

1. What to do after a death?
To claim widows' benefits, just ask your DSS office for form BW1. The period after a death is really the worst time to have to plough through official leaflets to find out all the mechanical things that have to be done, and all the financial or practical help that could be available. You don't want to have to worry about dealing with bureaucracy as well as coping with bereavement. It is therefore sensible to get hold of the latest editions of DSS leaflets D 49 *What To Do After a Death* and NP 45 *A Guide to Widows' Benefits*. Put them to one side in a safe place so that they will be there if you need them.

You can get practical help and advice from a funeral director, family doctor, solicitor, church, synagogue, mosque or temple, Social Services Department and a Citizens Advice Bureau. A health visitor or district nurse may help if the death was at home, or if it was in hospital, the ward sister or hospital chaplain could help. One of the first things you'll need to do is to transfer any insurance policies into your name (eg for a car, house and belongings).

If you need support and comfort more than practical advice, there are several organisations that are more than willing to help; ranging from national organisations such as Cruse, the organisation for bereavement care, to local branches of national charities such as the Multiple Sclerosis Society.

Chapter 22(8) gives information on help available to war widows.

2. Tax allowances
You are entitled to the widow's bereavement tax allowance during the year of your husband's death, and the next tax year – see Chapter 51.

3. Social fund funeral expenses
If you receive income support, income-based jobseeker's allowance, housing benefit, council tax benefit, family credit or disability working allowance, you may get a payment from the social fund for funeral expenses – see Chapter 6.

4. Income support and jobseeker's allowance
If your available savings are not over £8,000 and you are not working 16 or more hours a week, you may be able to get income support to top up a low income or top up other benefits, or to provide a basic income. Income support can also help with mortgage interest payments. See Chapter 3 for full details. If you are required to sign on as available for work, you may get income-based jobseeker's allowance – see Chapter 14.

Housing benefit and council tax benefit may provide help to pay the rent or council tax if your savings are no more than £16,000 – see Chapter 4.

5. Widow's payment
If your husband died on or after 11.4.88, you may get a lump-sum widow's payment of £1,000. If he died before 11.4.88, see below.

To qualify for the widow's payment, you must have been legally married. If you were in the process of divorcing your husband, you would still qualify for the widow's payment if he died before the divorce was made 'absolute'.

In Scotland, you may also qualify if you were married *'by cohabitation with habit and repute'*. You need to provide substantial evidence of this. If such a marriage is confirmed by a DSS solicitor or through the Court of Session, you may be entitled to a retirement pension based on your husband's contributions.

To get the widow's payment you must be under 60 when your husband dies; or if you are older, your husband was not getting a retirement pension based on his National Insurance contribution record.

Widow's payment depends on your husband's National Insurance contributions. He must have met either of the following two conditions.
- Before 6 April 1975 he must have paid, before age 65, 25 flat-rate contributions. (These can be employee, self-employed, or voluntary contributions, or a combination of them.)
- Since 6 April 1975 Class 1 (employee) contributions have been based on earnings, and he must have paid contributions on earnings in any one tax year equal to 25 times the lower earnings limit for that tax year. He could easily have met this condition in a shorter time than 25 weeks. A Class 2 (self-employed) or Class 3 (voluntary) contribution counts as a Class 1 contribution at the lower earnings limit.

For example, you would qualify for widow's payment if your husband had earned and paid Class 1 contributions on earnings of £437.50 in the 1978/79 tax year. (The lower earnings limit for that year was £17.50 a week. 25 times £17.50 equals £437.50.) If he had only paid Class 1 contributions on earnings of £350 (20 × £17.50) but had also paid five Class 2 or 3 contributions, you would still qualify for the widow's payment.

You have 3 months to claim the widow's payment.

Industrial death benefit – If your husband died before 11.4.88 as a result of an industrial accident or prescribed industrial disease, you will stay on the industrial death benefit scheme. You'll get the same amount of benefit as National Insurance widows. However, if you are also entitled to retirement pension or incapacity benefit, based on your own contributions, you can keep the full amount of that benefit.

If your husband died on or after 11.4.88 as a result of an industrial accident or prescribed industrial disease, you come within the National Insurance widow's benefit scheme. However, your widow's benefit does not depend on your husband having passed the relevant contribution tests.

6. Widows' benefits

See DSS leaflet NP 45 for full details. Widows' benefits are subject to your husband satisfying the contribution conditions. If your husband died on or after 11.4.88, you'll be entitled to the lump-sum widow's payment if he satisfied the contribution conditions.

If you have dependent children, you'll normally be eligible for widowed mother's allowance (WMA). This is payable from the Tuesday pay day on or after the date your husband died. It is based on your husband's contribution record up to his death. The full rate is the same as widow's pension (£62.45 pw). Increases for qualifying dependent children are £9.90 for one child, and £11.20 a week for each other child. If you make a late claim for WMA it may be backdated for up to 3 months. WMA for yourself is taxable. Increases for children are tax free.

If you don't have dependent children and are aged less than 45 on the day your husband died, you won't be eligible for a widow's pension. You'll just get the lump-sum widow's payment – see 5.

If you are aged between 45 and 54 on the day your husband died, or when your widowed mother's allowance ends, you may qualify for an age related widow's pension. If you were aged 55 or older on that day, the full rate pension may be payable. If you re-marry under age 60, it ceases altogether. Widows' benefits are not payable for any period when you are living with a man as his wife. A widow's pension is taxable.

Widowed before 11.4.88?

If you were widowed before 11.4.88 you come under the old rules. If you were between 40 and 49 at the time of your husband's death, or when your widowed mother's allowance ends, you may be entitled to an age related widow's pension. If you were 50 at that time, you may qualify for a full-rate pension.
Widow's allowance – This was payable if your husband died before 11.4.88, for 26 weeks after his death. If you received widow's allowance, you come under the old rules for widowed mother's allowance and widow's pension.

7. What happens to your own incapacity benefit?

Incapacity benefit and widows' benefits overlap. You cannot be paid both benefits in full at the same time. You can, however, choose to continue to receive your incapacity benefit (but not if you get the special long-term incapacity benefit, outlined in 9 below). You must do this in writing.

If your widow's benefit is higher than your incapacity benefit, the DSS will send you a letter to confirm that your widowed mother's allowance or widow's pension includes your incapacity benefit entitlement. Keep this letter safe. You may need to show it to the Inland Revenue or to the Income Support section in your local DSS office, or to the Housing or Council Tax Benefit sections.

If you were required to submit doctor's statements to your local DSS office, you should continue to do so.

If you cannot be paid your widow's benefit because of the overlapping benefit rules, this does not affect any rights as a pre-11.4.88 widow.

Why should you pick this option?

If you choose to have your long-term incapacity benefit continue, with any balance paid as widow's benefit, you will be able to qualify for the disability premium under income support, housing benefit or council tax benefit even if this wasn't included in your IS/HB/CTB assessment before you started to get WMA or widow's pension – see Chapter 3(12).

There may also be a tax advantage for people who transferred to long-term incapacity benefit from invalidity benefit. In this case your incapacity benefit remains tax free whereas widow's benefit is taxable.

It is best to pick this option when you first claim a widow's benefit. Enclose a letter to the DSS with your claim to widow's benefit (form BW1). Say that you would like your incapacity benefit to continue, with any balance coming from widow's benefit.

If you did not do this, you can still improve your future position. You can pick this option at any time. It starts from the widow's benefit payment following the date your letter is received by the DSS. You cannot backdate an option to have your benefit made up of incapacity benefit with the balance coming from your widow's benefit.

8. What about ICA and SDA?

Invalid care allowance of £37.35 a week is taxable and, unless you get a reduced-rate widow's pension, there may be no immediate cash advantage in claiming it. However, it is worth claiming ICA in order to secure Class 1 contribution credits. See Chapters 9 and 19. Entitlement to ICA also qualifies you for the carer premium with income support (or income-based jobseeker's allowance) even if the ICA is completely overlapped by the widow's pension (see Chapter 3(16)).

SDA of £37.75 (plus any age-related addition) cannot be paid along with widows' benefits (unless it is higher) because of the overlapping benefit rules. It is nevertheless worth claiming as it gives you Class 1 contribution credits. It might help you qualify for the disability premium with income support, housing and/or council tax benefit. If a disability premium has been included in your assessment, it won't be withdrawn just because you can no longer be paid SDA – but you must continue to provide evidence that you are incapable of work.

9. Special rules for incapacity benefit

If you are incapable of work but you don't have enough National Insurance contributions to qualify for incapacity benefit, special rules for widows and widowers may help you.

You are entitled to long-term incapacity benefit if:

- you are not entitled to WMA on your husband's death, or entitlement has ended; and
- you are entitled to a reduced rate widow's pension, or you don't get a pension because you were under 45 when your husband died or WMA ended; and
- you are incapable of work on your husband's death or when your WMA ends, (and this was after 5.4.79); and
- you are in the same 'period of incapacity for work' (see Chapter 11(2)) that began before your husband died or WMA ended, and have been incapable of work for 52 weeks. If you are terminally ill, incapacity benefit is payable after 28 weeks of incapacity.

See Chapter 11(3) for the amounts of long-term incapacity benefit. If you get a reduced rate widow's pension, incapacity benefit tops it up to the standard long-term incapacity benefit rate. So if you are getting SDA when your husband dies, you will switch to incapacity benefit when your WMA ends if you are not then entitled to widow's pension, or it is lower than your incapacity benefit entitlement.

Once you reach pension age, your incapacity benefit will stop. You will be entitled to a full retirement pension even if you do not have sufficient NI contributions – see Chapter 44. However, if you received incapacity benefit after 28 weeks of incapacity for work because you are terminally ill, you can choose to stay on incapacity benefit beyond pension age until

you have received 24 weeks of incapacity benefit altogether.
S.40 Social Security Contributions and Benefits Act 1992

A widower can qualify for incapacity benefit on the same basis if he was incapable of work on his wife's death, or within 13 weeks afterwards.
S.41 Social Security Contributions and Benefits Act 1992

47 Christmas bonus

1. What is the Christmas bonus?
It is a tax-free bonus of £10 paid in December with some social security benefits. To get the bonus, you must have been entitled to a payment of one of the qualifying benefits in the week containing the first Monday in December. It is not taken into account as income for any means-tested benefit.

2. How is it paid?
If your benefit is paid by order book, you will find that the extra £10 is included in the payment covering the week from 1 December 1997.

If you don't have an order book, the DSS will pay it by girocheque, payable order, or by an extra credit if you are paid by credit transfer direct to your bank or building society.

If you have not received the bonus by the end of December, contact your local DSS office.

3. Who qualifies for it?
In 1997, you will be entitled to a Christmas bonus if, in the week beginning 1 December 1997:
- you are present or ordinarily resident in the UK, the Channel Islands, the Isle of Man, Gibraltar or in any EEA country; **and**
- you are entitled to a payment of one of the benefits listed below, for a period which includes a day in the week beginning 1.12.97:
- attendance allowance
- constant attendance allowance
- disability living allowance
- income support (claimant over pension age)
- industrial death benefit
- invalid care allowance
- long-term incapacity benefit
- retirement pension
- severe disablement allowance
- unemployability allowance
- unemployability supplement
- war pensioners' mobility supplement
- war widow's pension
- widow's pension
- widowed mother's allowance

A war disablement pensioner, who gets none of the benefits listed above, will also qualify for the Christmas bonus if s/he is over 65.

If each of a couple meet these qualifying conditions, each will be paid the £10 bonus.

If you and your partner are both over pension age but s/he does not receive a bonus in her/his own right, you will get an extra £10 bonus for your partner if you are entitled, or treated as entitled, to an increase of benefit in respect of her/him. Only one Christmas bonus is payable in respect of any person.

48 Health benefits

1. Who qualifies for help?
Some people qualify automatically for help with NHS charges, vouchers for glasses and hospital fares because of their age, or particular personal circumstances. If you qualify automatically, your income and capital makes no difference.

Other people are 'passported' to this help, without going through an additional income test. You, your partner and any dependent children have an automatic right to full help with NHS costs if you get income support, income-based jobseeker's allowance (JSA), family credit, or disability working allowance.

A third group of people can qualify for help with paying all, or part, of NHS charges, hospital travel costs, and vouchers for glasses, on the basis of low income. If you qualify on low-income grounds, your partner and any dependent children also qualify.

NHS leaflets, HC11 and HC13 explain the help available with health costs.

2. Prescription charges
Prescriptions cost £5.65 (in 97/98) for each item, so it is important to take advantage of exemptions from charges if they apply to you, and of prepayment certificates which save money on frequent prescriptions.

Who is automatically exempt?
You can get free prescriptions if:
- you are under 16, or under 19 in full-time education – see below;
- you are aged 60 or over;
- you get income support, income-based JSA, family credit, or disability working allowance – or you are the partner or dependent child of someone who gets one of these benefits.

If you are in any of these groups, you don't need an exemption certificate. Just complete the declaration on the back of the prescription form.

Full-time education – This is defined as receiving qualifying full-time education within the meaning of the NHS Act 77, sch 12, para 7. Para 7 says that this means full-time instruction in a school within the meaning of the Education Act 1944. Unfortunately, the Education Act does not define full-time. It thus depends on whether or not your school considers you to be full-time.

Who can get an exemption certificate?
The following people can get an exemption certificate for free NHS prescriptions:
- expectant mothers – through your doctor, midwife, or health visitor after confirmation of pregnancy;
- women who have had a child during the past year – if you didn't obtain an exemption form during pregnancy, get form FW8 from your doctor, midwife or health visitor;
- people who have a specified condition or who are housebound with a continuing physical disability – see below;
- war/service pensioners – for prescriptions needed for treatment of accepted disabilities;
- people who live in a residential care or nursing home, placed by the local authority, who can't afford the full fees for the home without local authority help – apply on form HC1(RC);
- people who qualify under the low income scheme for an HC2 (full help) certificate – see 5.

Health benefits • 225

What are the specified conditions?
If you have one of the conditions listed below, you can get exemption from prescription charges. Get form FP92A (EC92A in Scotland) from a hospital, chemist, or your doctor. Send the completed form to your local Health Authority, or in Scotland, to your Health Board, who will send you an exemption certificate:

- a continuing physical disability which prevents you from leaving your home except with the help of another person (this does not include a temporary disability, even if it is likely to last a few months);
- permanent fistula, including caecostomy, colostomy, laryngostomy or ileostomy, requiring continuous surgical dressing or an appliance;
- diabetes mellitus (but not if treatment is by diet alone), myxoedema, hypoparathyroidism, diabetes insipidus or other forms of hypopituitarism, forms of hypoadrenalism, including Addison's disease for which specific substitution therapy is essential, or other conditions where supplemental thyroid hormone is necessary, myasthenia gravis;
- epilepsy, requiring continuous anti-convulsive therapy.

What about hospital out-patients?
If you are attending hospital as an out-patient, the exemptions from charges made by the hospital for drugs are the same as those listed above, but the arrangements for claiming are slightly different. If you are covered by any of the following documents, take it with you to the hospital:

- an HC2 exemption certificate – see 5;
- a Health Authority (Health Board in Scotland) exemption certificate or prepayment certificate;
- a DSS war pensioners exemption certificate;
- a DSS award letter or order book.

Who can get the charges refunded?
If you have paid for a prescription, you can claim a refund, within 3 months of paying, if you are:

- assessed by the Health Benefits Division as qualifying on grounds of low income – see 5;
- receiving income support, income-based JSA, family credit, or disability working allowance.

If you are in one of these groups, you can get refunds for your dependants as well.

You can claim a refund within 3 months of paying, if you are an exempt person, ie automatically exempt or covered by an exemption certificate – see above.

But in either case, you cannot claim a refund unless you ask for a receipt on form number FP57 (EC57 in Scotland) when you pay for the prescription. This form tells you how to claim a refund.

The Post Office will refund the cost when you ask for it and present your receipt and proof of exemption.

What is a prepayment certificate?
If none of this applies to you, you may still be able to get your prescription costs reduced by buying a prepayment certificate. A 4-month certificate costs £29.30 and a year's certificate costs £80.50 (in 97/98); it saves money if you need over 14 items a year (or over 5 items in 4 months) on prescription. If your income is too high to get the HC2 (full help) certificate (see 5), you cannot get help with the cost of prescriptions: even if your income is just 1p above the limit. A prepayment certificate is your only option for reducing prescription costs.

You can apply for a prepayment certificate on form FP95 (or EC95 in Scotland). You can get it from a chemist, Health Authority, Health Board, post office, or DSS office. You then use the prepayment certificate like a season ticket whenever you need to collect prescriptions.

3. Vouchers for glasses
You can get a form for applying under the low-income scheme from the DSS or your optician. Eyesight tests are now subject to a charge unless you are an exempt person: eg you are registered as blind or partially sighted; you are aged 40 or over and are the parent, sibling or child of a person who has been diagnosed as having glaucoma; or you have diabetes or glaucoma (if your doctor has referred you for an eye test).

Children under 16, and people aged under 19 who are in full-time education, qualify automatically for vouchers for glasses and free eye tests. So too do people getting income support, income-based JSA, family credit or disability working allowance.

If you need complex lenses, you qualify automatically for lower-rate vouchers (and free eye tests) if you don't qualify for more help under the low income scheme.

You must ask for a voucher when you have your eyes tested. When you buy your glasses, give the supplier your voucher. If the glasses cost more, you'll have to pay the extra yourself.

The value of the voucher depends on the strength of the lenses you need, with additions, eg for clinically necessary prisms or tints.

Low income scheme – See 5 below for details. You must ask for a voucher when you have your eyes tested. Then apply to the Health Benefits Division on form HC1 if you don't have a current HC2 or HC3 certificate (these used to be known as AG2 and AG3). You cannot use your voucher until you get a favourable decision from the unit. If you have an HC2 certificate (full help) your eye tests will also be free.

Refunds – If you've already paid for glasses or a sight test, ask for form HC5 to get a refund of up to the voucher value. Unless prescribed through the Hospital Eye Service, refunds are only available if your sight test was on or after 1.4.97, or you paid for your glasses on or after 1.4.97. You must send in your optical prescription and sight test receipt with the HC5.

4. Free NHS dentures & dental treatment
Children under 16; 16 and 17 year olds; people aged 18 who are in full-time education; pregnant women, and women who have had a child in the past year, all qualify automatically for free NHS dentures and dental treatment. If you are pregnant, you qualify automatically only if you were pregnant when the dentist accepted you for treatment. Similarly, if you start a course of dental treatment on the day before your child's first birthday, that treatment is free.

People getting income support, income-based JSA, family credit or disability working allowance also qualify automatically. You also qualify if you live in a residential care or nursing home and the local authority help with the care home fees – claim on form HC1(RC).

Tell your dentist you qualify automatically, and fill in the declaration on the form s/he gives you. If you've already paid, ask the DSS for form HC5 to get a refund. If you haven't yet claimed under the low income scheme, or don't have a current HC2 or HC3 certificate (or AG1 or AG2), you must also claim on form HC1.

5. Low income scheme
The low income scheme for help with NHS charges and vouchers for glasses is operated by the Health Benefits Division. The assessment is broadly the same as for income support, but with some changes. If your capital is £8,000 or less, you may be eligible for help. The capital limit is £16,000 if you live

permanently in a residential care or nursing home.

If your income is less than or equal to your requirements, you are entitled to full help with any NHS charges and to vouchers for glasses. The Health Benefits Division will send you an HC2 certificate.

If your income is higher than your requirements, you cannot get any help with the cost of NHS prescriptions. However, you may get some help with the cost of other NHS charges and travel expenses to a disablement services centre or to hospital for NHS treatment. You qualify if your income exceeds your requirements by less than a third of the charge, or by less than the travelling expenses. The Health Benefits Division will send you an HC3 certificate to show that you are entitled to partial help with NHS charges and travel expenses.

For travelling expenses to a disablement services centre or to hospital for NHS treatment, you'll get the difference between your excess income and your total fares in any week (Sunday through to Saturday).

For NHS charges, you multiply your excess income by three. If the result is lower than the particular charge, you'll get the difference between the two figures.

For example, if your excess income is £4.65 pw, you would be entitled to have remitted the amount of any weekly travel expenses as an outpatient or patient in excess of £4.65. For other NHS costs, you work out 3 times £4.65 ie £13.95. You'll have to pay this amount towards the cost of NHS dental treatment etc, but if the charge is higher, you'll be entitled to have the balance remitted.

Each HC2 or HC3 certificate lasts, in most cases, for 6 months. Your certificate will last for 12 months if you are aged 60 or over, or you are entitled to a disability premium (as long as you don't have a working partner), or you live in a residential care or nursing home placed by the local authority.

The low income assessment
The assessment of your resources is broadly the same as for income support. However, if you are on strike, your pre-strike income is taken into account. If you are a student, the maximum student loan for your situation is taken into account as income (whether or not you have applied for it). However, the £10 disregard is only available if your assessment includes a premium, or you get a LEA disabled students' allowance because of deafness, or where the claimant is not a student but his or her partner is one.

Your requirements are worked out in almost the same way as the IS applicable amount, including premiums. However a disability premium can be included after 28 weeks of incapacity, rather than 52 weeks; and a higher pensioner premium is included if you or your partner are aged 60 or over (instead of a pensioner or enhanced pensioner premium). For children, the personal allowance at age 11 and 16 is not aligned with the school year as it is with IS, but increases on the child's 11th or 16th birthday. There is no deduction if you could only get IS on an urgent cases basis. Generally, your net weekly housing costs are also taken into account, including: mortgage capital repayments; payments on an endowment policy in connection with buying your home; any repayment of interest and capital on an unsecured loan to adapt your home for the special needs of a disabled person; any rent payments (net of any housing benefit); and any council tax (net of council tax benefit). Amounts for non-dependants are deducted from your housing costs.

How do you claim?
Claim on form HC1 which you can get from the DSS, the Health Benefits Division, an NHS hospital, a family doctor, dentist or an optician. If you are unable to act for yourself, someone else can claim for you. If you haven't claimed before, or don't have a current HC2 or HC3 certificate (or AG2 or AG3 as they were previously known), and have just paid for dental treatment etc, you will also need to claim on form HC5. If your claim doesn't reach a DSS office within 3 months of paying the travel expenses, or dental treatment etc, you cannot get a refund.

After you have claimed on form HC1, the Health Benefits Division will send you a decision. If you are entitled to full help, they will send an HC2 certificate. If you are entitled to partial help, they will send an HC3 certificate. You should make a repeat claim on form HC1 shortly before the end of the period on your certificate. If your circumstances change during the currency of a certificate, you can write to the Health Benefits Division and they will issue a new certificate showing your revised entitlement. There is no right of appeal against a decision made by the Health Benefits Division. However, if you feel they have made a mistake, write and ask them to reconsider, or review, that decision. Write to: *DSS, Health Benefits Division, Sandyford House, Newcastle upon Tyne, NE2 1DB*.

6. Free milk and vitamins
Free liquid or dried milk and vitamins are available as follows. If you get income support or income-based JSA, you will qualify automatically if you, or a dependant:
- are pregnant; or
- are a nursing mother; or
- have one or more children under 5.

Even if you don't get IS, you can get free milk:
- for a disabled child aged over 5 but under 16, who is not registered at school because of physical or mental disability. Claim on Form FW20 which you can get from your local DSS office; or
- for a child under 5 who is looked after by a registered childminder or a registered day nursery (they make the claim – not you).

49 Housing grants

1. The housing renewal grants system
Grants to help repair, improve and/or adapt a property are available from the local housing authority. This chapter describes the main grants available in England and Wales. A similar system is available in Northern Ireland. In Scotland the system is different, see Box N.1.

The current system was introduced in December 1996 under the Housing Grants, Construction and Regeneration Act 1996. If an application for a mandatory renovation grant or minor works assistance was made prior to 17 December 1996 it may be affected by transitional provisions, see Box N.2.

The following types of grant are available:
- renovation grants – for improvement or repair of a dwelling, or for provision of dwellings by conversion of a house or other building;
- disabled facilities grants – for provision of facilities for a disabled person in a dwelling, or a common part of a building, such as a staircase, containing one or more flats;
- home repair assistance – for smaller scale repairs, improvements or adaptations;
- houses in multiple occupation (HMO) grants – for landlords for repairs or improvements to properties in multiple occupation;

- common parts grants – for repairs or improvements to the common parts of a building, such as a roof, containing a number of flats;
- group repair schemes – for external works to a group of properties, such as a block or a terrace.

This chapter describes in more detail the most common grants; renovation grants, disabled facilities grants and home repair assistance. For more information on the other grants contact the local housing authority and see Box N.4.

2. Renovation grants

A renovation grant is a cash grant for larger scale repair and improvement works to a dwelling.

Who is eligible for a grant?

To be eligible for a renovation grant:
- you must be an owner-occupier, including leaseholders with at least 5 years to go on the lease, or a private tenant with an obligation to carry out the repairs to the property; and
- the property must have been built or converted at least 10 years prior to the application; and
- the occupier of the property must have occupied it for at least 3 years prior to the application, unless the property is in a local authority renewal area, the grant is for fire precautions, the grant is to convert a property or the local authority exercise their discretion to accept an application earlier.

What can you get a grant for?

Renovation grants can be awarded to:
- bring a property up to the legal standard of fitness for human habitation – see Box N.3;
- bring a property up to a standard of reasonable repair;
- improve the thermal insulation of a property;
- provide facilities for heating;
- improve the internal arrangements within a property, such as staircases;
- provide a fire escape or other fire precautions;
- improve the provision of services, such as fuel and water, or amenities, such as a bath or toilet, within a property;
- convert an existing property.

All renovation grants are discretionary unless the application was made in the first half of 1996 or earlier – see Box N.2. Each local authority will have its own priorities for renovation grants. Grants to bring a property up to the fitness standard are likely to be high priorities in most local authorities. An application form and details of the local priorities should be available from the local housing authority.

The test of financial resources

All renovation grants are means-tested. The test of resources is similar to housing benefit and council tax benefit. There are, however, a number of important differences.
- The test of resources applies to the grant applicant and anyone else who is both entitled to apply for a grant and lives or intends to live in the property.
- There are no non-dependant deductions in the test of resources.
- There is an extra grant premium, currently £40, in the applicable amount for every grant application.
- If the applicant is in receipt of income support or income-based jobseeker's allowance the applicable amount is automatically £1.00 and all their income and capital is disregarded giving a zero contribution.
- There is no capital cut-off point. The first £5,000 of capital is disregarded. Tariff income is assumed on capital over £5,000.
- There is a system of stepped tapers on 'excess income'.

Working out your contribution

The test of resources is designed to calculate how much, if anything, you can afford to contribute towards the cost of the works. This is done by calculating the value of a notional standard repayment loan you could afford to take out using a proportion of your 'excess income' (see below) to repay the loan. If you have no excess income then your contribution will be zero. Owner-occupiers, including leaseholders, are expected to be able to repay a loan over 10 years; tenants with a repairing obligation, over 5 years. The higher the amount of excess

---

N.1 Grant system in Scotland

Grants for repairs and adaptations to properties in Scotland are available from the local authority. Details of these grants are set out in a booklet, *Improve Your Home With A Grant* produced by the Scottish Office Environment Department, this is available from the local authority or the *Scottish Office, Environment Department, St Andrew's House, Edinburgh, EH1 3DE*.

The legislation governing the grant system is set out in Part XIII of the Housing (Scotland) Act 1987. The system itself is administered by the local authorities. Grants are, in the main, discretionary awards.

There is a *mandatory standard amenity grant* available to disabled people. This improvement grant, at 50% of the total approved expense, is available as of right to a disabled occupant for the provision of an additional standard amenity to meet their particular needs. Standard amenities are:
- a fixed bath or shower with a hot and cold water supply;
- a wash-hand basin with a hot and cold water supply;
- a sink with a hot and cold water supply;
- a toilet.

If your house already has these amenities but they don't meet your needs, you may still get a grant. For example, if you have a toilet upstairs but cannot easily climb up the stairs, you can claim a grant to put in a ground floor toilet.

A *discretionary improvement* grant may also be available for the works and/or adaptations required to make the house suitable for the welfare, accommodation or employment of a disabled person. This grant is available at a rate of up to 75% of a maximum approved expense limit of £12,600. Although under no obligation to do so, many local authorities do treat such applications as a priority. If the cost of the works exceeds the set grant limit and the local authority considers that there are extraordinary reasons for this, they can apply to the Secretary of State for an increase in the grant limit.

All houses are subject to the following three conditions for a period of 5 years from payment of the grant:
- the house must only be used as a private dwelling house (although part can be used for another purpose);
- the house must not be occupied by the owner or a member of the same family, except as their only or main residence (ie it may not be used as a second or holiday home); and
- the house must be kept in a good state of repair.

There is no bar on a person selling a house following the payment of a grant, but the conditions themselves continue to apply to the property for the remainder of the 5 year period. The local authority would only seek repayment of the grant if any of the three conditions were breached during the five years.

income the higher the proportion expected to be used towards repaying the notional loan.

Below we give an outline of how to work out your contribution. This means test takes into account your own resources and your partner's. But, for renovation grants, the means test also applies to other adults who live in or intend to live in the property, and who would be entitled to apply for a grant – see below, under 'Multiple means-testing'.

❑ Work out your capital – Your own capital together with your partner's is taken into account. Certain types of capital are disregarded. The rules are similar to those for income support – see Chapter 3(24) and (31). However the capital value of the dwelling or building to which your grant application relates is disregarded whether or not you live there. The first £5,000 of your capital is ignored. For each £250 you have above £5,000, a 'tariff income' is assumed of £1 a week.

❑ Work out your income – Your average earnings and other income is based on income over the 12 months before your application. The earnings and income disregards are the same as for housing and council tax benefit – see Chapter 4(24).

❑ Work out your 'applicable amount' – This represents your weekly living needs and those of your family – see Chapter 4(25). Add one £40 grant premium.

❑ Work out your 'excess income' – If your income is less than or equal to your applicable amount, you do not have excess income. Your contribution is zero. If your income is greater than your applicable amount, the excess income is the difference between the two figures.

❑ How much is your contribution? – Excess income is apportioned into a maximum of four bands and multiplied by the relevant loan generation factor for that band. For applications made on or after 17.12.96 the bands and multipliers are as follows. The applicable amounts and loan generation factors are usually uprated annually. This uprating does not always coincide with social security April uprating. You may need to check with the local housing authority what the rates are at the time of your application.

Excess income bands	Loan generation factors Owner-occupiers		Tenants
1 The first £47.95	×	18.46	10.77
2 £47.96 to £95.89	×	36.92	21.54
3 £95.90 to £191.78	×	147.68	86.16
4 £191.79 or more	×	369.21	215.40

The aggregate of Bands 1–4 is the value of the notional loan the applicant is expected to contribute towards the cost of the works.

N.2 Transitional provisions

Some applications for mandatory renovation grants made in the first half of 1996 under the previous grant system are preserved as applications for mandatory grants even if they are not approved for some time. Later applications become discretionary applications but are still dealt with under the previous legislation, the Local Government & Housing Act 1989. A briefing paper, *Transitional Provisions for Applications for Mandatory Renovation Grants, Policy Briefing 8/96*, is available from *Care & Repair (England), Castle House, Kirtley Drive, Nottingham, NG7 1LD*.

For example if an applicant who is an owner-occupier has £100 excess income the calculation would be as follows:

1	£47.95	×	18.46	=	£ 885.16
2	£47.94	×	36.92	=	£1,769.94
3	£ 4.11	×	147.68	=	£ 606.96
	£100.00			=	**£3,262.06**

The applicant's contribution would therefore be £3,262.06. If the total cost of the works were £11,000 the grant would be £11,000 – £3,262.06 = £7,737.94.

Multiple means-testing

If there are two or more people, other than a married couple or couple living together as husband and wife, who are subject to the test of resources the calculation is slightly different. For example this might apply to two sisters who are joint owners of a property or same sex partners who jointly own a property. In these cases the combined applicable amounts of the two (or more) people are aggregated with only one grant premium. Their combined income including any tariff income is compared to the applicable amount and any excess income is used to calculate the contribution required for the grant application. The test of resources only calculates the total contribution it does not attempt to apportion the contribution to the two, or more, people. That is entirely a matter for them.

For example, two sisters jointly own a property and both live in it. They are both 73 years old. One of them is on income support, and one gets retirement and private pensions of £130 a week. If the grant application was made on 1.1.97 the calculation would be as follows.

Applicable amount		£
Sister No. 1	(income support)	1.00
Sister No. 2	personal allowance	47.90
	pensioner premium	19.15
	grant premium	40.00
	Total	**108.05**

Income		£
Sister No. 1	(all disregarded)	0.00
Sister No. 2	pensions	130.00
	Total	**130.00**

Excess income is £130.00 – £108.05 = £21.95. This is multiplied by loan generation factor 18.46 giving a joint contribution of £405.20.

Subsequent grants

If an applicant has had to make a contribution to a previous grant, in the last 10 years for owner-occupiers or 5 years for tenants, the value of that contribution is deducted from the assessed contribution on a subsequent grant application. The works under the first grant must have been carried out to the local authority's satisfaction for this offsetting to apply. If the contribution on the earlier grant was more than the cost of the works, leading to a 'nil-grant approval' the value of the works properly carried out can be offset against a subsequent grant contribution.

Applying for a renovation grant

You can get an application form from your local housing authority. An application for a renovation grant must include the details of the property, a list of works for which the grant is required with usually two builders' estimates, details of any other costs such as building regulation fees and all the information required for the test of resources. The application must be accompanied by an owner-occupier's certificate stating that the grant applicant or a member of their family will occupy the property for the next five years, or a tenant's certificate stating that the applicant is a tenant and is liable to carry out the repairs. A tenant's application will normally also require a landlord's certificate.

Approval of the grant – In order to approve an application for a renovation grant for a property which is unfit for human habitation the local housing authority must be satisfied that repairing the property is the most satisfactory course of action for that property and that the property will be fit for human habitation once the repairs have been carried out. The alternatives open to the local authority would be to serve either a deferred action notice or a closing order or a demolition order. See Box N.4 for where to get more information.

The local authority must determine the application not later than six months from the date of formal application. If the application is approved they must specify how much grant is awarded and how it was calculated. If the application is turned down the local authority must specify the reasons why. If approved the building works should usually be completed within one year by one of the contractors who supplied an estimate for the application. A renovation grant may have to be repaid if the property is sold by the grant applicant within five years of completing the works. The grant is not normally repayable if the grant applicant dies after the works have been finished. If the grant applicant dies before the works are finished the local housing authority may still pay for all or part of the works to be completed.

3. Disabled facilities grants

A disabled facilities grant is designed to help meet the cost of adapting a property for the needs of a disabled person.

Who is eligible for a grant?
To be eligible for a disabled facilities grant, you must be:
- an owner-occupier; or
- a private tenant; or
- a landlord with a disabled tenant; or
- a local authority tenant; or
- a housing association tenant.

A person is disabled if:
- his/her sight, hearing or speech is substantially impaired; or
- s/he has a mental disorder or impairment of any kind; or
- s/he is physically substantially disabled by illness, injury, impairment present since birth, or otherwise; or
- s/he is registered or registerable disabled with the Social Services Department.

What can you get a grant for?
There are two types of disabled facilities grants – mandatory and discretionary.

A mandatory grant can be awarded for the following purposes:
- facilitating a disabled occupant's access to and from the dwelling;
- making the dwelling safe for the disabled occupant and others residing with him or her;
- facilitating a disabled occupant's access to a room used or usable as the principal family room;
- facilitating a disabled occupant's access to or providing a room used or usable for sleeping in;
- facilitating a disabled occupant's access to or providing a room in which there is a lavatory, bath or shower, and washhand basin or facilitating the use of any of these;
- facilitating the preparation and cooking of food by the disabled occupant;
- improving the heating system to meet the disabled occupant's needs, or providing a suitable heating system;
- facilitating a disabled occupant's use of a source of power, light or heat;
- facilitating access and movement around the home to enable the disabled occupant to care for someone dependent on them, who also lives there.

Discretionary disabled facilities grants can be awarded for adaptations which make the property more suitable for the accommodation, welfare or employment of the disabled occupant.

The test of financial resources
The test of resources for disabled facilities grants for owner-occupiers and tenants is similar in operation to that for renovation grants above. However, the only person who is subject to the test of resources for a disabled facilities grant is the person with disabilities and their partner if they have one. If the disabled person is less than 18 years old the test of resources is applied to the parent(s) or person who has the primary responsibility for their care. This is the case even if the disabled person is not the applicant for the grant.

For example, if a disabled person lives with his brother who has sole ownership of the property. The brother can apply for a disabled facilities grant to carry out adaptations to his property for the benefit of his brother who has a disability. The test of resources only applies to the brother who has a disability, it will not apply to the brother who made the application.

N.3 The housing fitness standard

Government figures show that there are 1.5 million unfit homes in England alone. Most of these homes are occupied and nearly half are owner-occupied. If a house fails to meet any of the following requirements then it will be considered unfit for human habitation, there is a different fitness standard for flats.

The house must :
- be structurally stable;
- be free from serious disrepair;
- be free from dampness prejudicial to the health of the occupants;
- have adequate provision for lighting, heating and ventilation;
- have adequate piped supply of wholesome water;
- have satisfactory facilities for the preparation and cooking of food, including a sink;
- have a suitable located WC and a suitably located fixed bath or shower and washhand basin for the exclusive use of the occupants;
- have an effective system for the draining of foul waste and surface water;
- have a satisfactory supply of hot and cold water to sinks and baths etc.

The Department of the Environment are currently reviewing the housing fitness standard. A consultation paper is expected to be published towards the end of 1997.

Subsequent grants
A contribution to a previous grant can be offset against a contribution to a subsequent grant as for renovation grants above.

Applying for a disabled facilities grant
Disabled facilities grants are administered by the local housing authority rather than the Social Services Department where these are different local authorities. It is important to ensure an application is made to the local housing authority as the statutory time limit for the application to be determined, of not later than six months, only begins when the formal application has been made. An application form should be available from the local housing authority. An application must be supported by a certificate stating that the disabled occupant will live in the property for at least five years after the works are completed, or a shorter period if there are health or other special reasons.

Approval of a disabled facilities grant – In order to approve an application for a disabled facilities grant the local housing authority must be satisfied that the works in question are both necessary and appropriate for the needs of the disabled person and reasonable and practicable in relation to the property. In determining whether the works are necessary and appropriate the local housing authority must consult with the Social Services Department. This is why some local authorities will direct people to the Social Services Department first for an occupational therapy assessment. But the statutory time limit to determine the application only begins to run when a formal application has been made to the local housing authority.

The maximum grant payable under a mandatory disabled facilities grant is £20,000 in England and £24,000 in Wales. Local authorities have a discretion to pay additional discretionary grant for mandatory items if the cost exceeds the maximum. There is no maximum discretionary grant.

The local authority must determine the application not later than six months from the date of formal application. If the application is approved they must specify how much grant is awarded and how it was calculated. If the application is turned down the local authority must specify the reasons why. If approved, the adaptations should usually be completed within one year by one of the contractors who supplied an estimate for the application. The local housing authority has a discretion to approve a grant but to stipulate that it won't be paid for up to 12 months from the date of application. Government guidance says this discretion should only be used sparingly, but it could delay when the works can be done.

For example, if an application was made on 1 January 1997 and the approval was issued at the end of the statutory time limit on 1 July 1997. The local authority could stipulate that payment will be made in December 1997, within 12 months of the date of application.

If, after the application for a disabled facilities grant has been approved, the disabled person's circumstances change in some way before the works are completed, the local housing authority has a discretion as to whether to proceed with paying for all, part or none of the works. The local housing authority must take into account all the circumstances of the situation before deciding how to proceed in such a situation.

4. Home repair assistance
Home repair assistance is a discretionary grant to help meet the cost of smaller scale repairs, improvements and adaptations.

Who is eligible?
To be eligible for home repair assistance, you must:
- be aged 18 or over;
- live in the dwelling as your only or main residence, or be applying for a grant for the benefit of a person who is 60 years old or more, or disabled or considered to be infirm;
- be an owner-occupier or a private tenant, or have a right of exclusive occupation of the property for at least five years (see below);
- have a power or duty to carry out the works;
- be in receipt of income support, income-based jobseeker's allowance, housing benefit, council tax benefit, family credit or disability working allowance; or be aged 60 or more, or disabled, or infirm; or the application is for adaptations to enable someone who is aged 60 or more or disabled or infirm to be cared for.

The definition of a disabled person is the same as for disabled facilities grants above. There is no statutory definition of 'infirm' in the grants legislation and so this is potentially a wide criteria.

Applicants who are not owner-occupiers or tenants but do have a right of exclusive occupation for at least five years must have lived in the property for at least three years prior to the application unless the works are for:
- fire precautions; or
- to enable an elderly, infirm, or disabled person to be cared for in the property; or
- the property is in a local authority renewal area.

Home repair assistance is also available to some lawful occupiers of house boats and mobile homes, for more information see Box N.4.

N.4 For more information

The main rules for Housing Renewal Grants are set out in the following statutory provisions.
- The Housing Grants, Construction and Regeneration Act 1996, Part 1
- The Housing Grants, Construction and Regeneration Act 1996 (Commencement No. 2 . . .) Order 1996
- The Housing (Fitness Enforcement Procedures) Order 1996
- The Home Repair Assistance Regulations 1996
- The Disabled Facilities Grants and Home Repair Assistance (Maximum Amounts) Order 1996
- The Housing Renewal Grants (Services and Charges) Order 1996
- The Housing Renewal Grants Regulations 1996
- The Housing Renewal Grants (Prescribed Form and Particulars) Regulations 1996

A new Department of the Environment Circular has also been produced which consolidates and updates all previous guidance, Circular 17/96 called *Private Sector Renewal: a Strategic Approach*.

All the statutory provisions and the guidance circular are available from the Stationery Office (formerly HMSO).

In addition to the local authority there may be an independent home improvement agency in your area who can offer advice about grants. Home improvement agencies also help people to apply for grants, obtain other sources of finance to help pay for works, help to find a good builder and ensure the works are properly carried out. To find out if there is a home improvement agency in your area contact the local authority or Care & Repair (England) see our Address List.

For information about VAT relief on building works, see leaflet 701/7/94, *VAT Reliefs for People With Disabilities*, available from your local VAT enquiries office (look in the phone book under 'Customs and Excise').

Home repair assistance is always discretionary. Each local authority will have its own priorities for home repair assistance. An application form and details of the local priorities should be available from the local housing authority.

There is no restriction on the type of repair, improvement or adaptation which can be undertaken. Assistance can be in the form of a cash grant, materials or a mixture of both. The maximum assistance available is £2,000 per application and £4,000 for the same dwelling in any three year period. A previous award of minor works assistance does not count towards the maximum amount of home repair assistance available.

5. Home energy efficiency scheme

The home energy efficiency scheme is administered by the Energy Action Grants Agency, and covers England, Scotland and Wales.

Grants are available to owners and tenants including council tenants.

Who is eligible?

To be eligible for the home energy efficiency scheme, you must be in receipt of any of the following benefits:

- income support
- income-based jobseeker's allowance
- disability living allowance
- attendance allowance
- constant attendance allowance
- family credit
- disability working allowance
- housing benefit
- council tax benefit
- war pension mobility supplement

Under this part of the scheme you will qualify for up to £315 worth of draught-proofing, insulation and energy advice.

If you are not on any of the benefits above but you or your partner are 60 years old or more you will qualify for up to £75 of assistance.

The measures available include draught proofing of doors and windows, loft insulation, cavity wall insulation and better heating system controls. Energy advice can include provision of two low energy light bulbs and a hot water tank jacket. The maximum grant will mean that you may have to choose between draught proofing measures and insulation. Under insulation, loft insulation will take priority.

You can apply for a grant either to a local network installer or to the Energy Action Grants Agency, Freephone 0800 181 667 (Minicom 0191 233 1054) or write to *Energy Action Grants Agency, PO Box 1NG, Newcastle upon Tyne, NE99 2RP*.

50 Child support

A new system to assess and collect child maintenance was introduced in April 1993 which will eventually replace the courts in most aspects of child maintenance. This chapter provides a basic outline of the child support system and the provisions likely to affect parents and children with disabilities.

1. The Child Support Agency

The Child Support Agency was set up to assess, collect and enforce payment of child maintenance. It is located in six Child Support Agency Centres around the UK, with some child support staff based in each Benefits Agency District Office.

The Child Support Agency has phased in the take on of cases as follows.

- Any parent with care of a qualifying child (see below) who makes a new or repeat claim for income support, income-based jobseeker's allowance, family credit or disability working allowance on or after 5.4.93 is required to authorise the Agency to assess and collect child maintenance from the absent parent (see below).
- Parents with care who have been receiving income support since before 5.4.93 who wish to apply to the Agency can do so.
- Anyone else can use the Agency, provided there is no existing court order or written maintenance agreement made before 5.4.93 in force.
- Parents with a court order or written maintenance agreement made before 5.4.93 remain under the jurisdiction of the courts and the take on of these cases has been postponed indefinitely. Parents who have a court order which cannot be enforced or varied through the courts can, however, use the Agency.

2. Duty to maintain

Both parents have a duty to maintain their children, whether they are divorced, separated, remarried, have never been married or never lived together. The parent who does not have the day to day care of the child is required to pay child support to the person caring for the child, unless s/he lives abroad or the child has been adopted.

- A child is a *'qualifying child'* if s/he is under 16, or under 19 and in full-time non-advanced education and one or both of her/his parents are absent. S/he must not be married or entitled to income support in her/his own right.
- A *'person with care'* is the person who provides day to day care (of at least 104 nights a year) for the qualifying child. The person with care may be the child's parent, or someone else who is caring for the child, for example, a grandparent, friend or relative.
- An *'absent parent'* is any parent not living in the same household as the qualifying child and whose child is being looked after by someone else.

3. Requirement to co-operate

A parent with care who claims income support, income-based jobseeker's allowance, family credit or disability working allowance is required to co-operate with the Agency. S/he is required to authorise the Agency to assess and collect maintenance and to provide any information to help trace the absent parent and assess his/her liability.

A parent with care is not required to give authorisation if *'there are reasonable grounds for believing that, if she were to comply, there would be a risk of her, or any child living with her, suffering harm or undue distress'*. The Agency has issued guidelines outlining the circumstances in which parents may be exempt and authorisation may not be required. These include situations where there is a fear of violence or a history of rape or sexual abuse. The list is only guidance and not exhaustive and the individual circumstances of the parent with care should be considered.

If a parent with care refuses to co-operate or give authorisation and s/he is not accepted as being exempt, the Agency may issue a reduced benefit direction. Originally, this reduced the parent with care's weekly benefit for a total of 78 weeks. From 7.10.96 this period was extended to 3 years, with the possibility of renewal for a further 3 years. The parent with care may also be asked to attend a social security fraud interview.

Before issuing a reduced benefit direction, the Child Support Officer must take into account the welfare of any child in the household. From 22.1.96 a reduced benefit direction cannot be made if the parent has the higher pensioner, disability or disabled child premium included in her/his income support applicable amount or, if s/he is not receiving income support, in her/his exempt income calculation. A direction made after this date can be suspended if the parent is having direct payments/deductions made from her/his income support, for example for fuel and rent arrears. The direction will be reimposed 14 days after the direct payments cease.

The parent with care can appeal to a Child Support Appeal Tribunal against the decision to impose a reduced benefit direction and should do so within 28 days.

Paternity disputes
If an absent parent denies he is the father of a qualifying child, both he and the parent with care will be interviewed. If he continues to deny paternity, the parent with care and/or the Agency will have to obtain a court order confirming paternity before a maintenance assessment can be made. In some cases the Agency will offer the alleged father a discounted DNA test, the fee for which will be refunded if he is found not to be the father.

4. The assessment
Both parents are obliged to provide whatever information is necessary for the Agency to assess the amount of maintenance payable. The Agency has considerable powers to obtain information from, for example, employers' records, National Insurance data, Inland Revenue and local authority housing benefit and council tax records.

If the absent parent does not provide the Agency with sufficient information, an interim maintenance assessment can be made, the amount of which will usually be higher than the amount of maintenance the absent parent will eventually be required to pay.

The formula
The Agency uses a standard, complex, formula to assess the amount of maintenance, unless the absent parent is on income support or income-based jobseeker's allowance. In this case, the absent parent will pay the minimum amount of £5 a week maintenance. An absent parent in receipt of income support or income-based jobseeker's allowance will not have this deduction made from her/his benefit if s/he is under 18 years old, has the family premium included in her/his applicable amount (or has day to day care of a child) or receives statutory sick pay, incapacity benefit, severe disablement allowance, attendance allowance, disability living allowance, invalid care allowance, maternity allowance, statutory maternity pay, disability working allowance, industrial disablement benefit, war disablement benefit or payments from the Independent Living Funds.

All absent parents must pay the minimum amount of maintenance, even if they are assessed under the formula as being required to pay less. An absent parent who has been assessed as having to pay less than £5 is exempt from paying anything if s/he:
- or her/his partner, is getting child benefit; or
- is a prisoner; or
- receives one of the benefits listed above; or
- is under 16, or under 19 and in full-time, non-advanced education; or
- has a net income of less than £5.

An absent parent will never have to pay more than an amount equivalent to 30% of her/his net income in maintenance.

The Agency makes numerous mistakes when assessing the amount of maintenance. Parents should check that the Agency has used the correct information and has, for example, included any relevant disability premiums. A parent can request a review if s/he believes the amount of maintenance has been calculated incorrectly.

Liability
If the maintenance enquiry form was sent before 18.4.95, liability to pay maintenance starts from the day the form was sent. If the form was sent on or after 18.4.95 and the absent parent returns it, confirming s/he is the absent parent, within four weeks, the absent parent will be liable to pay maintenance from eight weeks from the date the form was sent.

Absent parents who have an existing maintenance agreement or court orders and whose child support assessment is higher than the previous amount may be able to 'phase in' their payments.

Maintenance can be paid either directly to the person with care or via the Agency.

The new departure system
A new system, allowing 'departure' from the standard formula, came into effect from 2.12.96. This allows a parent with care or absent parent to apply for a departure from the formula after receiving an assessment or after a change of circumstances. The grounds for seeking a departure include: extra costs arising from a disability or long-term illness; the costs of keeping in contact with a child; paying debts incurred for the child's or couple's benefit before separation; a parent appearing to have a lifestyle inconsistent with the income declared or claiming unreasonably high housing costs.

5. Enforcement
If an absent parent fails to make payments and builds up arrears, the Agency has wide powers of enforcement. These include deducting payments from earnings, or obtaining a liability order or debt enforcement order relating to property and bank accounts.

If at least three months of initial arrears have accrued because the Agency has delayed making an assessment, it will write off any arrears over six months, providing the absent parent agrees to pay off any other arrears and continues to make regular weekly payments.

6. Reviews and appeals
All maintenance assessments are reviewed automatically every

N.5 For more information

- *The Child Support Adjudication Guide* (from The Stationery Office) – this sets out all the Chief Child Support Officer's guidance to individual Child Support Officers.
- *Child Support: The Legislation* (£37, published by Sweet & Maxwell) – aimed at advisers.
- *Child Support Handbook* (£9.95 from Child Poverty Action Group, £3.30 for claimants) – this is aimed at parents as well as advisers.

The Child Support Agency produces a range of leaflets and shorter guides. If you want general information, call:
- The Child Support Enquiry Line – 0345 133133.

In Northern Ireland – 0345 139700.

If you just want leaflets, call:
- The Child Support Response Line – 0345 830830.

two years. In addition, all parents can apply for a review if there has been a change of circumstances or against almost any Child Support Officer's decision. Appeals to a Child Support Appeal Tribunal can be made if a parent disagrees with the outcome of the review against a Child Support Officer's decision. An appeal needs to be submitted within 28 days of a decision being issued.

7. Maladministration

The Agency has established a reputation for poor administration and communication. It has a massive backlog of cases to be dealt with and parents will therefore experience delays in the handling of their cases. Complaints should be made to the Customer Services Manager at the relevant Centre, ideally via an MP. If still dissatisfied, a complaint can be made to the Ombudsman. If someone has suffered financial loss as a result of the Agency's maladministration, s/he can apply for compensation. However, these payments are discretionary and, because of the extent of the delays, the Agency is unlikely, in practice, to award compensation in any but the most extreme cases.

8. Role of the courts

The courts will still continue to deal with some issues of child maintenance. They can, for example, make 'top-up' awards for certain additional expenses which are currently not taken into account by the formula, including those arising from a qualifying child's disability. The child must be receiving disability living allowance or *'is blind, deaf, without speech, or is substantially and permanently handicapped by illness, injury, mental disorder or congenital deformity'*.

9. Child maintenance bonus

From April 1997, you can build up entitlement to a new child maintenance bonus of up to £1,000 while you are on income support or income-based jobseeker's allowance. It is payable when you or your partner start work or increase your hours or earnings so that your income support or income-based JSA stops. The bonus builds up by up to £5 a week of the child maintenance payable or the actual amount paid if that is less, up to a maximum of £1,000. Claim within 28 days of your benefit ending, or up to 6 months if you have good cause for the delay.

51 Income tax

1. Introduction

This is a brief outline of some basic income tax facts. For more information, a good tax guide is the *Which? Tax-Saving Guide* published annually by the Consumers' Association (your local library may have a copy). Your local tax office or Tax Enquiry Centre will help with any tax enquiries you might have. Their addresses are in your local phone book under Inland Revenue. For advice, try contacting your local Citizens Advice Bureau, or TaxAid, an independent registered charity based at *Linburn House, 342 Kilburn High Road, London, NW6 2QJ (0171 624 3768, 9 – 11am weekdays)*.

To check if you are paying the right amount of tax you need to know what kinds of income are taxable, which allowances you are entitled to and what the appropriate rate of income tax is. The amounts change from year to year (from 6 April) so find out the amounts for the year you want to check. Here we only give the figures for 6 April 1997 to 5 April 1998.

2. Income

Some income is exempt from tax (eg National Savings Yearly Plan and Bonds) and so is ignored completely when working out your tax; other types of income, such as earnings, are taxable. You are also allowed tax relief on certain outgoings, eg pension contributions and mortgage interest, but this is often deducted at source.

Which benefits are taxable?

The following benefits are the only ones that are taxable:
- higher rate short-term incapacity benefit;
- long-term incapacity benefit (but not if you transferred from invalidity benefit – see Box E.7 in Chapter 11);
- income support if you are directly involved in a trade dispute;
- invalidity allowance when it is paid with a retirement pension;
- industrial death benefit;
- invalid care allowance;
- jobseeker's allowance;
- retirement pension;
- statutory maternity pay;
- statutory sick pay;
- adult dependants' additions paid with these benefits (but not additions for children);
- widowed mother's allowance;
- widow's pension.

For more information on how incapacity benefit is taxed, see Box E.7 in Chapter 11.

3. Tax allowances

You are entitled to a personal allowance. Depending on your circumstances you might also be entitled to other tax allowances. The amount of income you can receive before you pay tax depends on your tax allowances. For a single person this is normally £4,045 (97/98) and for a person with a Married Couple's Allowance this is normally £5,417 (97/98).

From April 1994 some of the tax allowances were restricted to give a reduced amount of tax relief (20% from April 1994 and 15% from April 1995). The allowances which are restricted are the Married Couple's Allowance, Additional Personal Allowance and Widow's Bereavement Allowance; also payments made under maintenance agreements or by order of the Child Support Agency up to a maximum of £1,830 per year.

If you are not getting all the tax allowances due to you, write to your tax office with the details. You can claim for the last six complete tax years and if you have overpaid tax, you will get a refund. In the tax year 97/98 you can claim a refund back to 91/92.

Personal Allowance

Everyone, male or female, married or not, has a Personal Allowance which can be set against all types of income. The amount depends on your age during the tax year:
- aged under 65   £4,045
- aged 65–74   £5,220
- aged 75 or over   £5,400

You can claim the higher allowance for the complete year if your 65th or 75th birthday falls at any time during the tax year. The higher allowances for those aged 65 or over are reduced if your total income is over £15,600 for the 97/98 tax year. £1 is deducted for each £2 extra income over £15,600. But it won't be reduced below the basic Personal Allowance.

A husband and wife each have a separate total income limit.

If you don't use up your full Personal Allowance you cannot transfer it to a partner or carry it forward to future tax years.

Blind Person's Allowance

You will get an allowance of £1,280 if you are registered blind (but not if you are registered partially sighted). A married couple can transfer any surplus allowance from one to the other. If both husband and wife are registered blind, it is therefore possible for one of them to get both his or her own Blind Person's Allowance and the other's surplus allowance. You can receive the allowance for the tax year before the one in which you are registered as blind, provided you had obtained the evidence for registration (eg opthalmologist's certificate) before the end of that tax year.

Married Couple's Allowance

This is an extra allowance for a married couple who live together. It is paid at three rates depending on the age of the older partner:

- aged under 65   £1,830
- aged 65–74   £3,185
- aged 75 or over   £3,225

Tax relief on Married Couple's Allowance is restricted to 15%. The higher Married Couple's Allowance for those aged 65 or over may be reduced if the husband's income is above the £15,600 income limit. It only starts to be affected if his personal allowance has been reduced to the basic personal allowance.

N.6 Check your tax

Example: Ruth gave up work because of ill health. She has earnings for this tax year, as well as statutory sick pay while she was employed and is now on incapacity benefit. She is registered blind and cares for a school-aged child. Her earnings and sick pay were taxed at source by her employers through PAYE. Tax is deducted from her incapacity benefit by the DSS.

Step 1: Add up the taxable income

Gross wages	£5,725
Statutory sick pay	£1,000
Incapacity benefit	£3,000
Total income	**£9,725**

Step 2: Add the personal allowances and deduct from total income

Personal Allowance, aged under 65	£4,045
Blind Person's Allowance	£1,280
Total personal allowances	**£5,325**
Taxable income	**£4,400**

Step 3: Work out the income tax

20% of first	£4,100		£ 820
23% of next	£ 300		£ 69
	£4,400		
Total			**£ 889**

Step 4: Deduct restricted tax allowances

15% of Additional Personal Allowance of £1,830	£ 274.50
Total tax payable	**£ 614.50**

If you get married during the tax year, the allowance is not paid for the months before you marry. It is given in full in the year of death of either spouse or in the year in which separation takes place.

It is claimed in the first instance by the husband, though a couple can elect to transfer the allowance to the wife. Alternatively, the wife can claim half the allowance as of right. This transfer must be done before the start of the tax year (ask your tax office for form 18). If either partner does not use their entitlement to the Married Couple's Allowance, they can transfer the surplus to their spouse up to six years afterwards (ask your tax office for form 575).

Additional Personal Allowance

If you are single or an unmarried couple, you can claim an allowance of £1,830 if you have a qualifying child resident with you for all or part of the tax year, ie a child under 16 living with you, or if your child is still in full-time education or training. Tax relief is restricted to 15%. If there are two or more children and the parents live at separate addresses, and the children spend a good deal of time with each parent, two full amounts of the Additional Personal Allowance can be claimed, one for each parent. If there are two parents claiming for the same child, the allowance must be divided between them.

A married man (but not a woman) can claim this allowance as well as the Married Couple's Allowance if he has a qualifying child living with him, and his wife is totally incapacitated throughout the tax year. Her disability must be such that, in practice, he is in the same position as someone bringing up children on their own.

Widow's Bereavement Allowance

In the year of your husband's death you will receive this allowance of £1,830 to set against income for the whole of the tax year. It is available for the following tax year too provided you have not re-married before the start of it. There is no widower's bereavement allowance. Tax relief is restricted to 15%.

4. Income tax rates

For the tax year 6 April 1997 to 5 April 1998 the rates are:
- 20% (lower rate)   – on first £4,100 taxable income
- 23% (basic rate)   – between £4,101 and £26,100
- 40% (higher rate) – above £26,100.

5. Working out your tax

Step 1 Add up your income from all sources for the year, including any taxable benefits, but don't include any exempt income. The tax year runs from 6 April.

Step 2 Deduct your Personal Allowance (plus the Blind Person's Allowance if you qualify for this) from your total income in Step 1. This gives your taxable income.

Step 3 Work out your tax by adding together:
20% of your taxable income up to £4,100; plus
23% of your taxable income between £4,101 and £26,100; plus
40% of anything above £26,100.

Step 4 Add together the other tax allowances you qualify for which only give restricted tax relief (eg Married Couple's Allowance, Additional Personal Allowance). Work out 15% of this and deduct the result from the tax payable in Step 3. This gives you the total amount of tax you are due to pay.

Before April 1994 none of the tax allowances gave restricted relief, so if you are checking a tax year before April 1994, miss out Step 4 and add all your allowances together at Step 2 to get your taxable income.

See Box N.6 for an example.

6. Notice of coding

If you have earnings or an occupational pension you will generally have tax deducted under PAYE (Pay As You Earn). You should receive a notice of coding which sets out details of the personal allowances, with any necessary adjustments, that are to be set against income.

For example, if you are a single person, registered blind, you would get total allowances of £5,325 (Personal Allowance of £4,045 + Blind Person's Allowance of £1,280). Your code would be 532L – the final digit of your allowance is replaced by the letter L. The letters at the end of tax codes give information about the allowances you get.

- L for a code with basic Personal Allowance
- H for a code with basic Personal Allowance plus the basic Married Couple's Allowance or Additional Personal Allowance
- P for a code with Personal Allowance (age 65–74)
- V for a code with the Personal Allowance for those aged 65–74 plus the Married Couple's Allowance for those aged 65–74
- T in most other cases

There are five special cases which do not have numbers or which have numbers which do not show the amount of allowances.

- BR means that no allowances have been given, tax will be deducted at basic rate (23%) on every pound of income
- D (followed by a number) means that tax is to be deducted at a higher rate (40%)
- K (followed by a number) means that amounts to be taken away from your allowances are more than the total allowances. The negative allowances indicate the amount to be added to your pay or pension on which tax is to be paid
- NT means that no tax is to be deducted
- OT means that no allowances have been given; tax will be deducted at the appropriate rate on every pound of income

7. Tax refunds

If you have paid too much tax you can claim a refund for six years back as well as the current tax year. You should write to your tax office with the necessary details. They will need to know your National Insurance number and any tax reference you might have. If you are unsure what to do, you could telephone your tax office for guidance on how to make a written claim.

Any refund that is due to you if you have to give up work and your income drops can be paid after 4 weeks of leaving work. Send your P45 into the tax office. You will need to estimate your income for the remainder of the tax year. If you have left work and are signing on for jobseeker's allowance, you can't get a tax refund until the end of the tax year.

Savings

Most income from savings is received after deduction of tax by the bank, building society, etc. If you have income, including interest (gross) which amounts to less than your total personal allowances, you are entitled to receive interest from banks, building societies, etc without deduction of tax. Ask your bank or building society for a R85 form.

The rate of income tax deducted from interest credited to depositors, eg by banks and building societies, is 20%. There is no further tax to pay by most depositors even if you are normally liable at the basic rate of 23%.

Before 6 April 1996, tax was deducted at the basic rate. For years up to 95/96, if your income exceeded your personal allowances and you paid tax but only at the 20% level, you could be entitled to a partial refund on any tax deducted at source. In the first instance just write to the tax office for a claim form, R40.

8. Arrears of tax

If you have not paid enough tax, the Inland Revenue can claim it from you. Generally they must do so within six years. If there are special circumstances (eg tax evasion) there is no time limit, and there may be penalties.

In certain circumstances arrears of tax are wholly or partly waived if they have arisen through the failure of the Inland Revenue to take account, within a reasonable length of time, of information you have given them about your income and personal circumstances, so that you could reasonably believe that your affairs were in order. The concession is normally given where you are notified of the arrears after the end of the tax year following that in which the Inland Revenue received information indicating that you had underpaid tax. For example, if in 1995-96 the Inland Revenue received information that you had underpaid tax then you may claim a waiver of liability if the arrears are not notified to you by 5 April 1997.

If you believe this applies to you simply write to your tax office claiming a waiver under extra statutory concession A19.

9. Tax returns and keeping records

You may be asked to complete a tax return, particularly if your circumstances have changed. However, usually only tax payers with more complex tax affairs are asked to do this every year. If in any tax year you have received income or capital gains which should be taxed and which the Inland Revenue do not know about, you should notify them within 6 months of the end of the year, eg for the tax year ending 5 April 1998, the Inland Revenue should be told by 5 October 1998.

You should keep records of your income and capital gains to enable you to complete a tax return, in case it is required. Usually they should be kept for 22 months after the end of the tax year to which they relate. If you are self-employed this period is extended by a further 4 years.

If you regularly complete a tax return, you should be sent it shortly after the end of the tax year, eg for the tax year ended 5.4.97, you should receive your blank tax return by the end of April 1997. If you want the Inland Revenue to calculate your tax, or to collect any arrears through your PAYE code then you should complete and return this by 30.9.97. Alternatively, under the new self assessment scheme, you may calculate your own tax, in which case you have until 31.1.98 to complete your tax return, including your calculation of the amount of tax you should pay or be refunded. If tax is payable, it should be paid by 31.1.98. There is a fixed penalty of £100 if the return is not sent back by 31.1.98.

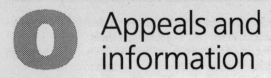

O Appeals and information

This section of the Handbook looks at the following:

Claims and appeals	Chapter **52**
Free legal help	Chapter **53**
Complaining to the Ombudsman	Chapter **54**

52 Claims and appeals

In this chapter we look at:

A. Common questions
Making a claim	see 1
Date of claim	see 2
Interchange of claims	see Box O.1
Time limits for claiming benefit	see Box O.2
Delays in qualifying benefits	see 3
Backdating delayed claims	see 4
Appointees	see 5
Delays in payment – compensation	see 6
Overpayments	see 7

B. Decisions and appeals
Who makes decisions?	see 8
Ways of changing decisions	see 9
Reviews	see 10
Appeals	see 11
How do you ask for an appeal?	see 12
When can you appeal?	see 13
Who can help you?	see Box O.3
Medical Appeal Tribunals	see 14
Medical evidence	see 15
Disability Appeal Tribunals	see 16
Social Security Appeal Tribunals	see 17
What happens when you appeal?	see 18
What can you do before the hearing?	see 19
At the hearing	see 20
The decision	see 21
For more information	see Box O.4
Errors of law	see Box O.5
Commissioners' decisions	see Box O.6

A. COMMON QUESTIONS

1. Making a claim

In order to get any benefit in the first place, you have to claim it. You should claim (or ask the DSS for advice) as soon as you think you might qualify. If you are in any doubt, go ahead and claim. If you cannot make enquiries or claim yourself, get someone else to do so; the DSS will accept a claim made by someone else on your behalf.

If you haven't got the proper claim form and are worried about missing some benefit, note that the Secretary of State has discretion to accept anything written *'as sufficient in the circumstances of any particular case'* to count as a claim.

This discretion also covers cases where you were completely ignorant of your right to a particular benefit. It applies to all benefits except housing or council tax benefit. It only applies to income support and jobseeker's allowance (JSA) until October 1997 when new rules mean that for a claim to be accepted it must be on the right claim form and generally include all the information and evidence requested on the form – see 2.

If the Secretary of State uses his discretion, the date that earlier letter, or other document, was received in a DSS office, counts as your date of claim. Arrears of benefit will be payable from that date (or from the payday following it) even if it was over 3 months ago.

Examples of cases where you could ask the Secretary of State to exercise this discretion include:
- you wrote to the DSS to say you wanted to claim a particular benefit and asked them for the claim form;
- you wrote a general letter to the DSS explaining your situation and asked what help you could get;
- you wrote about your walking difficulties on, eg an income support or social fund claim form;
- your written statement on a medical report for another benefit refers to, eg extreme walking difficulties or your need for constant supervision and personal help.

You cannot appeal to a tribunal if the Secretary of State refuses to exercise this discretion. Your only recourse is to judicial review.

Sometimes making a claim for one benefit can count as a claim for a different benefit – see Box O.1.

2. Date of claim

The date your claim is 'made' is the day it is received in a DSS office. Sometimes your claim can be treated as though it were made on an earlier date.
- For DLA and attendance allowance, your date of claim is the date you requested a claim form from the DSS or their Benefit Enquiry Line so long as you return the completed claim form within 6 weeks – see Chapter 17(25) for more details.
- For income support, JSA, family credit and DWA, your date of claim is the date you notified the DSS (or Jobcentre) of your intention to claim, so long as you return the completed claim form within one month. You can notify the DSS that you wish to claim in any way you like, eg by phone, in person, in writing, or someone else can do it for you. The DSS will send you a claim form. Or you can get one from an advice centre or a post office and simply notify the DSS that you intend to claim.

  For income support and JSA, there are new rules from 6.10.97, requiring the claim form to be returned with all the required information and evidence for it to be accepted – see below.
- If you make a 'defective' claim (not properly completed in accordance with the instructions on the form) or you don't use the correct form, you may have the claim referred back to you or be given the correct form. But this is discretionary. **If** it is referred back to you, then if you return the properly completed claim form within one month of its being sent to you, your claim **must** be treated as

though the original defective claim had been properly made. For income support and JSA, this only applies before 6.10.97, when new rules are introduced – see below. If you don't use the correct form or can't supply full details with the form, explain why this is, including that you don't want to miss out on a week or more of benefit.

Claims for income support or JSA from 6.10.97
From 6.10.97, new rules require that income support and JSA claims must be made on a fully completed claim form and all the information and evidence required on the form provided. Until you do this, you have not made your claim unless you can show that one of the reasons below apply in your case.
If you are unable to complete the form or get all the evidence – Your claim will be accepted only if the difficulty is due to one of the following reasons.
- You have a *'physical, learning, mental or communication difficulty'* and it is not reasonably practicable for you to get help with your claim or get the required information or evidence.
- The information or evidence required:
  - does not exist; or
  - can only be obtained at serious risk of physical or mental harm to you; or
  - can only be obtained from a third party and it's not reasonably practicable for you to get it from them.
- The Secretary of State believes that you've provided enough information to show that you're not entitled to benefit.

Reg 4(1B) SS (Claims & Payments) Regs 1987

If any of these reasons apply, send in your claim form and add a note to explain how the difficulty you have completing your form or getting the required evidence fits into one of these circumstances. The DSS intend to amend the claim forms so that there is space on the form for you to do this. You can also notify the DSS in any other way, eg by phone, or someone else can notify them for you. The decision on whether to accept your reasons is made by the Secretary of State so you can't appeal to a tribunal if you disagree.

If there is other evidence needed to decide your claim but it is not specified in the claim form, it does not affect your date of claim if you can't provide it with your claim.

Date of claim for income support – Your date of claim is the date you first notified the DSS of your intention to claim so long as you return the claim form and all the information and supporting documents required on the form within one month. If you can't supply all the information and evidence, and you tell the DSS within one month, your claim will still be accepted if you can show that your difficulty is for one of the reasons outlined above. If it's over a month since you contacted the DSS

O.1 Interchange of claims

If you make a claim for one benefit, then find you should have claimed a different benefit instead, or you were also entitled to a different benefit, the rules on interchanging benefit claims may help you get arrears of benefit beyond the usual limits. Your original claim may be treated as a claim for another benefit. But not all benefits can count as a claim for any other. Below, in the first column we list the benefit claimed and in the second column the benefit(s) that may be treated as the alternative, or additional benefit(s) claimed.

Benefit claimed	Alternative benefit
incapacity benefit	SDA, maternity allowance
SDA	incapacity benefit, maternity allowance
an increase of incapacity benefit	an increase of SDA
an increase of SDA	an increase of incapacity benefit
maternity allowance	incapacity benefit, SDA
retirement pension of any category	widow's benefit, retirement pension of any category
widow's benefit	retirement pension of any category
attendance allowance	industrial constant attendance allowance, DLA
industrial constant attendance allowance	DLA, attendance allowance
DLA	attendance allowance, industrial constant attendance allowance
income support	invalid care allowance
disability working allowance	family credit
family credit	disability working allowance

SS (Claims & Payments) Regs 1987, Schedule 1

An 'increase' of benefit means an increase for an adult or child dependant.

In addition, a claim for child benefit can be treated as a claim for guardian's allowance, an increase for a child dependant or maternity allowance claimed after confinement, and vice versa.

The decision on whether to treat a claim for one benefit as a claim for another, is made by the Secretary of State and is discretionary (apart from claims made between 6.4.87 and 10.4.88 – for these claims, the decision is made by an Adjudication Officer and you have a right of appeal).

If the Secretary of State uses his discretion, then the date of the original claim counts as the date of claim for the alternative benefit and arrears may be payable from then even if that was more than 3 months ago. However, the overlapping rules could prevent some or all of the arrears being payable.

Claims made before 7.10.96
The regulations governing interchange of benefit claims have been amended several times, most recently on 7.10.96 to remove unemployment benefit. If you made a claim before 7.10.96, the regulations in force at the time you made the claim that you now wish to be treated as a claim for a different benefit generally still apply. See CA/171/93, in which the Commissioner decided that a pre-1987 claim for supplementary benefit could also be treated as a claim for attendant allowance (but note that at the time of writing two decisions on this issue were pending at the Court of Appeal, *Nelson* and *Cullen*).

Pre-7.10.96 claims for unemployment benefit can be treated as claims for invalid care allowance or unemployability supplement. Pre-13.4.95 claims for sickness benefit, invalidity benefit, SDA and maternity allowance are interchangeable with each other (but not with unemployment benefit).

Since 6.4.92 a claim for income support cannot be treated also as a claim for attendance allowance.

For claims (other than supplementary benefit) made before 3.6.85 it may not be possible to use the interchanging claims provisions. If a decision had been made on a pre-3.6.85 claim, you cannot have that claim treated as one for another benefit.

O.2 Time limits for claiming benefit

Benefit	Time Limit
jobseeker's allowance	immediate
incapacity benefit or SDA	3 months
income support	immediate
industrial injuries benefits	3 months (from 15 weeks after date of accident, etc)
family credit	
▪ renewal claim	From 28 days before, up to 14 days after the last day of previous award
▪ post-DWA claims	From 42 days before, up to 14 days after the last day of DWA award
▪ other claims	immediate
social fund	
▪ maternity payment	From 11 weeks before expected week of birth, up to 3 months after date of birth or adoption or parental order
▪ funeral expenses	From the date of death to 3 months from funeral date
DLA, attendance allowance	
▪ initial claim	immediate
▪ renewal claim	6 months (before 1.9.97), immediate (from 1.9.97)
disability working allowance	
▪ renewal claim	From 42 days before, up to 14 days after the last day of previous award
▪ post-FC claim	From 28 days before, up to 14 days after the last day of family credit award
▪ other claims	immediate
retirement pensions	
▪ claim before 4.8.97	12 months
▪ claim on or after 4.8.97	3 months
child benefit, guardian's allowance, ICA, maternity allowance, widows' benefits, dependants' additions (not IS)	3 months

Reg 19 and Schedule 4, SS (Claims & Payments) Regs

The time limits are not cut-off points for claiming benefit, but just limit the extent to which your benefit can be backdated. For example, if you claim ICA it can be automatically backdated for 3 months. However, in the case of disablement benefit for occupational deafness and occupational asthma there is a cut-off point. You must claim within 5 years for occupational deafness, or 10 years for occupational asthma, of working in the prescribed occupation, otherwise you lose entitlement completely – see Chapter 21.

Extending the time limits
For some benefits the time limits can be extended by up to 3 months if you have special reasons for not claiming earlier – see 4 in this chapter.

to start off your claim, your date of claim is the day the fully completed form and required evidence is received at the DSS, or the day you notify the DSS that you are unable to provide all the information and evidence if your reasons are accepted.

If you send in a claim form, rather than notify the DSS in advance that you intend to claim, and you haven't included all the required information and evidence, you have one month to do so.

Date of claim for JSA – If you claim JSA on or after 6.10.97, your date of claim is the date you asked for a claim form, so long as you provide a fully completed claim form and all the required evidence by the time you attend your 'New Jobseeker Interview' (or during the interview). If you can't complete the form or get all the evidence for one of the reasons outlined above, your claim will be accepted. Otherwise, if you haven't got all the evidence or need more time to complete the form, the Secretary of State can extend the time limit by up to a month from the date you first asked for the claim form.

3. Delays in qualifying benefits
Entitlement to some benefits may depend on you getting another qualifying benefit. If you have already claimed the qualifying benefit but there has been no decision on entitlement, and because of this your original claim is refused, a second claim made within three months of the decision on the qualifying benefit can be backdated to the date of your original claim, or to the date from which the qualifying benefit is payable if that is later. But this only applies to:
▪ invalid care allowance – where the person you care for has claimed DLA or attendance allowance (and gets awarded the middle or higher rate care component or attendance allowance);
▪ severe disablement allowance – where you have claimed DLA (and get awarded the higher rate care component);
▪ DWA – where you have claimed any of the DWA qualifying benefits (see Chapter 16(3)): but only if your second claim is made more than 3 months after the decision on your original claim. Within 3 months of the decision, a second claim is treated as a review and benefit is only payable from the date of the second claim;
▪ social fund maternity or funeral payments – where you have claimed any of the qualifying benefits (see Chapter 6).

A similar rule allows a claim for incapacity benefit to be backdated following a decision on a DLA (or constant attendance allowance) claim. This applies if your existing incapacity benefit entitlement ends because you are not 'incapable of work' and you had already claimed DLA. A further incapacity benefit claim, made within 3 months of the decision awarding you higher rate care component, will be backdated to the end of your earlier incapacity benefit entitlement or to the date from which DLA is payable if that is later.

4. Backdating delayed claims
The time limits for claiming benefits are given in Box O.2. They apply to claims made from 7.4.97. If your claim was made before 7.4.97, see below.

For some benefits the time limit can be extended if you have special reasons or for certain administrative reasons. But this only applies to income support, JSA, family credit and DWA. For all other benefits, there is no extension to the time limits for claiming, no matter how good your reasons are for not applying earlier (but see 3 above, and Chapter 4(17)).

Special reasons
For income support, JSA, family credit and DWA the time limits can be extended for up to 3 months if any one or a

combination of the special reasons below apply, as a result of which you could not reasonably have been expected to make the claim earlier.
- ❏ You have difficulty communicating because you are deaf or blind, or have learning, language or literacy difficulties and it was not 'reasonably practicable' for you to get help to make your claim.
- ❏ You are ill or disabled and it was not 'reasonably practicable' for you to get help to make your claim (this is not accepted as a special reason for JSA). There is no definition of 'ill' or 'disabled' in the regulation. Existing case law relating to the previous 'good cause' provisions could be used where this is helpful.
- ❏ You were caring for someone who is ill or disabled and it was not 'reasonably practicable' for you to get help to make your claim. You don't have to live with the person, nor be related to them.
- ❏ You were given information by an official of the DSS or Employment Service which led you to believe that your claim would not succeed.
- ❏ You were given *written* advice by a solicitor or other professional adviser, a medical practitioner, a local authority, or a person working in a Citizens Advice Bureau or similar advice agency, which led you to believe that your claim would not succeed.
- ❏ You or your partner were given *written* information about your income or capital by an employer or ex-employer, or a bank or building society which led you to believe that your claim would not succeed.
- ❏ You were required to deal with a domestic emergency affecting you and it was not reasonably practicable for you to get help to make your claim.
- ❏ You were prevented by bad weather from attending the DSS office or Jobcentre.

Reg 19(4), (5) SS (Claims & Payments) Regs 1987
You should give full details of your reasons for claiming late on your claim form. You can appeal (or for DWA, ask for a review) if you disagree with the decision on backdating.

Administrative reasons
If the Secretary of State considers that it would be consistent with the proper administration of benefits, the time limit for claiming is extended to a maximum of one month if certain circumstances are satisfied. This power applies to JSA, income support, family credit and DWA. This may apply if:
- you couldn't attend the DSS or Jobcentre office to make your claim either because it was closed or because of transport difficulties, and there were no alternative arrangements available; or
- there were adverse postal conditions; or
- you were not sent notice of the end of entitlement to a previous benefit till after it ended; or
- you claim family credit within one month of the end of income support or JSA entitlement; or
- you stopped being part of a couple within one month before claiming (but not for family credit or DWA); or
- your partner, parent, son, daughter, brother or sister died within one month before claiming.

SS (Claims & Payments) Regs 1987, reg 19(6) and (7).

Test cases
If you are claiming following a 'test case' the standard rules on backdating may be modified (under s.68 Social Security Administration Act). In many cases you may only get arrears back to the date the test case decision was given. See 10(f) below for more details.

Claims before 7.4.97
There were major changes in April 1997 to the rules on time limits and backdating of claims. If your claim was made before the rules changed on 7.4.97, the old rules still apply. See the 21st edition of the *Disability Rights Handbook* for full details. Here we give a brief sketch of the old rules.

For invalid care allowance, maternity allowance and widows' benefits, the time limit for claiming was 12 months. For child benefit, guardian's allowance and dependants' additions, the time limit was 6 months. For incapacity benefit and SDA, the time limit was 1 month. For all these benefits, time limits have been aligned at 3 months from 7.4.97.

'Good cause' backdating – Incapacity benefit, SDA, income support, JSA, family credit, DWA, reduced earnings allowance, social fund maternity and funeral expenses could be backdated beyond the time limits for up to 12 months if you could show 'good cause' for the delay. Industrial disablement benefit could be backdated indefinitely if you could show 'good cause'. What counts as 'good cause' was not laid down in the regulations, but there is extensive case law on the issue. From April 1997, there is no provision to backdate claims where you have 'good cause' (except for housing and council tax benefits). Instead, for certain benefits only, the time limit is extended if you have specified special reasons for the delay.

If you want to find out more about good cause and the extensive case law surrounding it, look at *Claim in Time – Time Limits in Social Security Law* by Martin Partington (3rd edition, Legal Action Group, £14.50, 1994).

5. Appointees
If a person is or might be entitled to benefit and cannot act for themselves, the Secretary of State can appoint someone aged 18 or over, the 'appointee', to act on their behalf. An appointee can also be a body of people such as a firm of solicitors or a housing association. An appointment may be appropriate, for example, if the claimant is unable to act for themselves because of a learning disability or mental illness, or is a child or elderly.

If you are the appointee, then it is your responsibility to deal with the claim including for example, notifying changes of circumstances. It is the appointee who is responsible for claiming on time and whose own circumstances will be relevant in deciding whether there are special reasons for backdating a delayed claim, or for not providing all the documentary evidence required for a claim.

If you claimed disability living allowance (DLA) for your child, you will have been appointed by the Secretary of State to act on your child's behalf – but only in relation to DLA. If your child is unable to act for him or herself when s/he reaches 16 and you continue to claim and receive DLA for them, you will have a full appointment covering almost all benefits.

If you are appointed to act for the claimant in relation to one benefit, that appointment covers all non-means-tested benefits as well as income support, family credit, disability working allowance and maternity, cold weather and funeral payments from the social fund. Separate appointments have to be made for housing benefit and for council tax benefit.

If you were appointed before 11.4.88, that appointment does not cover all benefits. It all depended on which benefits you had claimed. You could either have an appointment restricted to an individual benefit: family income supplement, child benefit, social fund maternity and funeral payments, or supplementary benefit. Or you could have an appointment covering all other benefits which came under the Social Security Act 1975 (SSA 75, now consolidated in the SSCBA) – the non-means-tested benefits.

6. Delays in payment – compensation

If you lose money because of delays or mistakes by the DSS in paying your benefit, you can ask them for an ex-gratia payment to cover your actual financial losses (eg the cost of phone calls, stamps and stationery, bank charges, etc). Write, asking for compensation to the Customer Service Manager of the office handling your benefit. The delay or mistake doesn't have to have lasted for any set period of time. It is enough if you have incurred actual financial loss as a result. You may also get compensation if you lose entitlement to a benefit because of wrong or misleading official advice, eg you fail to claim because you were told you were not eligible for benefit.

A separate scheme enables the payment of interest (at fixed rates) on the arrears of benefit. Under this scheme, if the DSS takes longer than their agreed target for clearing the bulk of claims for a benefit, compensation is payable if:
- the arrears of benefit are £100 or more; and
- a significant part of the delay is due to maladministration or administrative error; and
- the compensation would be at least £10; and
- the delay is longer than a set period, which varies according to the type of claim (see below).

Claims and reviews – If you are paid benefit on a claim, or arrears from an underpayment of benefit following a review, compensation is payable if correct payment on that claim has been delayed beyond a set period, called the 'delay indicator' (this is set at about 3 times the official target for processing the benefit). The delay indicators include:
- DLA and AA – 7 months
- income support – 2 months
- JSA – 3 months
- DWA – 1 month
- incapacity benefit – 4 months
- family credit – 6 months
- ICA and SDA – 9 months.

Renewal or current claims – Compensation becomes payable if your benefit payments are interrupted for 3 months.

If you qualify for compensation – Interest is payable on all the benefit owed to you for each complete tax year. It starts to accrue from the end of the set period, but is worked out on all the arrears. Compound interest is only calculated if the delay in payment is over 10 years. Write to the office handling your claim to ask for compensation.

They may however offset any overpayments previously judged to be non-recoverable. They can only do this if there has been an Adjudication Officer's decision that there was an overpayment. You could consider asking for a review or appeal of the AO's decision in order to remove the offset.

Guidance on the various kinds of compensation payable is contained in the DSS manual, *Financial Redress for Maladministration*. This includes details of the 'delay indicators', and the method of calculating interest. You should be able to consult a copy at your local DSS office – contact the Customer Service Manager.

7. Overpayments

There is a common overpayment test for non-means-tested benefits, income support, income-based JSA, disability working allowance (DWA) and family credit. You must show that you did not fail to notify the DSS about a material fact on the relevant date, or as soon as possible afterwards; or that you did not misrepresent a material fact; or that the overpayment arose because of another reason. The AO is responsible for deciding these questions, and for deciding who made the misrepresentation or failed to disclose the material fact, and from whom the overpayment is recoverable. If the overpayment is recoverable from more than one person (eg from the claimant and from his or her appointee), part of the AO's decision will be that the overpayment is recoverable from each person. It is then a matter for the Secretary of State to decide whether to recover that overpayment, how much to recover and from whom.

If the overpayment was made before 6.4.87, a different test applies – see below.

The law on overpayments is found in section 71 of the Social Security Administration Act 1992 (SSAA), and in the Social Security (Payments on Account, Overpayments and Recovery) Regulations 1988, as well as in case law: reg 31 applies these regulations to SB and FIS. Case law on supplementary benefit overpayments also applies to non-means-tested benefit and income support overpayments. For more details about the nature of the overpayment test, read the footnotes to section 71 in *Mesher* or *Bonner* – see Box O.4 – or *Overpayments and Recovery of Social Security Benefits* by Paul Stagg (LAG).

If you have been overpaid any benefit, and the overpayment was *'in consequence of [your] misrepresentation or failure'* to disclose a material fact, the amount of the overpayment is reduced by:
- any amount which has been offset under Part III of the Regulations (generally because of a change in the rate of award of a benefit you had already claimed);
- any extra supplementary benefit or income support which you should have been paid for any period, not necessarily the same period as the overpayment. If the overpayment is of some other benefit, then again the AO must consider offset of income support even if there is no connection between the periods in which the different benefits were payable (reg 13, R(IS)5/92, CSIS/8/95).

If you had not claimed income support, but would have been entitled to it had you not been overpaid another benefit, put in a late claim. If successful, this reduces the amount you have to repay. Since 16.11.92, it is not possible to make a late claim for supplementary benefit. However, the Secretary of State is responsible for taking the final decision on how much, if any, of the overpayment to recover from you. He is only interested in recovering the net loss to public funds: so he should be ready to cut the amount to be recovered by the amount of any other benefit which you would have been paid, had you claimed it at the right time, and had you not been overpaid.

Overpayments made before 6.4.87

The law governing overpayments changed on 6.4.87. Before this, an overpayment of a non-means-tested benefit was recoverable unless you could show that you had used *'due care and diligence'* to avoid being overpaid (s.119 Social Security Act 1975) – see the 12th edition of our Handbook for details. The House of Lords (*Plewa v Chief Adjudication Officer*, 7.7.94) decided that the old rules must still be applied in cases where payments were made before 6.4.87 (no matter when the decision on the overpayment is made). An overpayment which includes periods both before and after 6.4.87 should have both the old and current rules applied separately to each period. If you have had an overpayment recovered under the wrong test after 6.4.87, you can ask for a review of the decision. Note that the rules on limited backdating on review do not apply to overpayments cases.

Diminishing capital

If you have been overpaid because you didn't tell the DSS about all your capital resources, or you misrepresented the nature of your capital, reg 14 may help. At the end of each 13 week period, starting with the first day of the overpayment, your capital is 'treated' as having been reduced by the amount of SB or IS you had been overpaid during that quarter. At the same time, any 'tariff' income would be recalculated.

Your capital cannot be treated as diminished in this way over any shorter period. But obviously, if you actually spent any of that undeclared capital during the overpayment period, the overpayment would end on the day your capital reached the appropriate limit – assuming that the notional capital rules don't apply. The treatment of diminishing capital under reg 14 would also apply to the reduced amount.

The diminishing capital principle applies also to family credit, to DWA, to council tax benefit (under reg 89, CTB Regs), and to housing benefit (under reg 103, HB Regs). Note that this is different from the diminishing notional capital principle – explained in Chapter 3(24).

B. DECISIONS AND APPEALS

8. Who makes decisions?

Decisions on claims for social security benefits are mostly taken by Adjudication Officers (AOs) based at the office where you make your claim.

Decisions on appeal are taken by a Social Security Appeal Tribunal (SSAT) or Disability Appeal Tribunal (DAT) or Medical Appeal Tribunal (MAT). These are run by the Independent Tribunal Service (ITS).

If your claim is for industrial disablement benefit or severe disablement allowance, certain medical or disablement matters are decided by adjudicating medical authorities (AMA). AMAs can consist of:
- a single adjudicating medical practitioner (AMP);
- two or more AMPs sitting as a medical board;

and for certain prescribed industrial diseases:
- a specially qualified AMP;
- a special medical board where at least two members are specially qualified AMPs.

Appeals against AMA decisions are heard by a MAT.

Appeals on decisions of a SSAT, DAT or MAT are made to the Social Security Commissioners.

In addition to the decision makers above, some decisions are taken by the Secretary of State for Social Security, although not in person. He delegates his powers to locally based, authorised DSS officers, who could be the same AO dealing with the claim. The legislation lays down which questions must be decided by the Secretary of State. Many of these are discretionary with no right of appeal. If you disagree, your only recourse is judicial review. An example of a discretionary decision is the suspension of benefit payment pending the outcome of a test case in the courts.

There are separate systems which deal with social fund community care grants and loans (see Chapter 7); housing and council tax benefit (Chapter 4); war disablement pension (Chapter 22); and with vaccine damage payments (Chapter 24). For statutory sick pay and statutory maternity pay, the initial decisions are taken by the employer, with the right to request a formal decision from an Adjudication Officer (Chapters 10 and 26).

9. Ways of changing decisions

Once a decision is made that decision is final. It stands and is binding until or unless one of the specific methods given in the law for changing decisions is set in motion. Even a decision given without legal authority counts as an effective decision until such time as it is challenged.

There are four methods of getting a decision changed:
- correction of an accidental error;
- setting aside the decision;
- review of the decision;
- appeal against the decision.

Each of these methods has specific rules. In general, these rules cover:
- who can apply;
- what types of decisions they can change;
- time limits for applying;
- specific tests for setting the particular method in motion.

If all these are satisfied, then you can look at whether a decision was 'right' or 'wrong'. It is important to remember this because in review cases in particular it is sometimes impossible to have an existing award reviewed, even though everyone agrees the decision was 'wrong'.

We only give a brief outline of the main provisions. Do note that more than one regulation or section of an Act may apply. If in doubt, ask the decision-maker for detailed references to the law which enable the particular procedure to be carried out. You can then ask an adviser with access to the legislation and the *Adjudication Officers' Guide* (see Box O.4) to translate and explain.

(a) Accidental error

An 'accidental' error in any decision, or in the record of a decision, may be corrected by the adjudicating authority who gave the decision, or by an authority of the same status. For example, only an AO can correct an AO's decision; only a SSAT can correct a SSAT's decision. Mathematical or clerical errors can be corrected in this way: eg from the record of a SSAT's decision it is clear that they accidentally gave the wrong starting date for an award of benefit.

There is no time limit, or restriction on who can apply: write to the office that sent you the decision. However, correction is discretionary and there is no appeal against a refusal to correct. A refusal to correct does not start afresh the time limit for applying for leave to appeal to the Commissioner. That time limit starts to run from the date the original decision was sent to you. However, if a decision is corrected it carries the normal rights of appeal.

Regs 9 and 11, Adjudication Regs 1995/1801 cover all the adjudicating authorities except Commissioners. Reg 24, Commissioners Procedure Regs 1987/214 covers the Commissioners.

(b) Setting aside

A decision may be set aside by the adjudicating authority who gave the decision, or by an authority of the same status, if it *'appears just'* to do so because:
- a relevant document wasn't sent or received; or
- a party to the proceedings, or a representative, wasn't present at the hearing – but if you did not opt for an oral hearing (see 18 below), the decision can only be set aside on this ground (unless it is a Commissioner's decision) if *'the interests of justice manifestly so require'*; or
- *'the interests of justice so require'* – this applies to those rules relating to the procedures of the tribunal.

Setting aside a decision means that it is wiped out and the claim, or appeal, can be considered afresh. The process is quicker than, for example, appealing to the Commissioners. You have 3 months to apply for a decision to be set aside (30 days if it is a Commissioner's decision). If your application is refused, there is no right of appeal against that refusal. However, once you get a refusal, the normal time limits for appeal against the original decision start to run.

Any *'party to the proceedings'* can apply in writing to the DSS or to the office which gave the decision to have that decision set aside. This does not include the adjudicating authority which gave the decision. For all types of proceedings it includes the claimant and a person accepted as being 'interested in the proceedings'.

Regs 10, 11, Adjudication Regs cover all the adjudicating authorities except Commissioners. Reg 25, Commissioners Procedure Regs covers the Commissioners. See R(SB)31/85, R(U)3/89 and R(S)3/89.

(c) Review or appeal?

We cover reviews in 10 below, and appeals in 11 onwards. The letter giving you the adjudicating authority's decision will always explain your rights of either review or appeal. If you are in any doubt over which is your best course of action, seek advice.

In some cases you will not have a choice over whether to ask for a review or an appeal. This is true of DLA, attendance allowance and DWA. For these benefits you can only appeal once you've had a decision on a certain type of review, called an 'any grounds' review. If you're within 3 months of the original decision on your claim, you can ask for a review on 'any grounds'. If you're not happy with the review decision, you have the right of appeal. But if it's been longer than 3 months since the original decision, you must first ask for an 'any time' review (on certain grounds). After the decision on this 'any time' review, within 3 months you can ask for an 'any grounds' review of that decision. And only after a decision on this 'any grounds' review, do you then have a right of appeal, within 3 months, to the independent tribunal. The AO may carry out an 'any time' review even though you have not requested one. You can ask for an 'any grounds' review of that decision and again can appeal against that review decision if you still disagree with it. See 10 for more details.

For other benefits, there is a 3 months time limit to appeal. So if it's been more than 3 months since the decision you want to appeal against, although it's not impossible to appeal late, there are strict conditions to meet (see 13(c)). If you are asking for a late appeal, it's worth including a letter asking the AO to treat your appeal request as a request for a review if the late appeal is not admitted. That way you will avoid a delay in the review and thus avoid missing out on backdated benefit.

Where you do have a choice between a review and an appeal, it's usually in your interest to ask for an appeal. Appeals are heard by independent tribunals and you have the right to opt to put your case in person. If the appeal is successful, there is no time limit on the arrears of benefit that can be paid. Note that when you appeal, if an AO reviews the decision in the meantime and considers that a decision on review gives you everything you could have got on a successful appeal, the AO will simply review the decision and your appeal will lapse. If the review would not give you all you could get on appeal, s/he won't implement that review decision, and your appeal will go ahead.

A review is a quicker way of getting a decision changed. But in most cases, you can only get back one month's arrears of benefit if you are successful, although there some situations in which you can get benefit backdated for longer, or without time limit (see 10). If you ask for a review first, you still have a right of appeal against the review decision. But there is an extra hurdle if the AO decided that none of the limited grounds for an 'any time' review were satisfied. Before the tribunal can consider the matter of entitlement that is at issue in the appeal, you must first establish that one of these 'any time' grounds for review were satisfied – see 10(b).

Review of advance awards

Where an advance award has been made, reg 17(4), Social Security (Claims and Payments) Regulations 1987, requires the AO to review the award if you no longer satisfy *'the requirements for entitlement'*. The burden of proof is on the AO who must first establish that one of the specific grounds for review laid down in s.25 or s.30 of the Social Security Administration Act 1992 are satisfied (eg that there has been a change of circumstances or an error of law – see 10(c)). An indefinite award can only be ended by a review. An award for a definite period ends at the end of that period.

If a review is triggered by reg 17(4), that doesn't mean that you automatically lose entitlement to benefit if you are entitled to it for another reason. For example, the AO may decide that you are no longer incapable of work and thus are not eligible for income support. But if you are a carer or a lone parent for example, you may continue to be eligible for income support, albeit on different grounds, so your entitlement should continue. The review would enable the amount of benefit you get to be adjusted to reflect your changed circumstances.

The relationship between reg 17(4) C&P and s.25 and s.30 SSAA was explored in a tribunal of Commissioners' decision, CSIS/137/94.

10. Reviews

A review is the key way of getting a decision changed if you are out of time for appealing against that decision and if it is not possible to get a late appeal – see 13(c). Sometimes you'll have a choice whether to ask for a review or an appeal – see 9(c).

(a) How do you ask for a review?

If you think you have grounds for having a decision changed, write to the office that sent you the decision saying that you would like a review. The AO will look at your application. If it concerns a non-medical question, the AO can deal with it, or, on rare occasions, refer it to a SSAT. However, the AO cannot refer questions on DLA or attendance allowance to a SSAT. The AO must make a decision on the disability questions for DWA, DLA and attendance allowance – there is no power to refer disability questions to a DAT. If your review concerns a medical question, the AO will refer your application to a medical board. Note that the AO and the Secretary of State can initiate a review.

Any grounds reviews – Disability living allowance, attendance allowance and disability working allowance have a special review procedure, under s.30 – s.35 Social Security Administration Act 1992 (SSAA). Within 3 months of any AO decision under s.21, SSAA, you can ask for an 'any grounds' review. In this sort of review, the AO's decision may be reviewed for any reason at all, eg you simply disagree with it. The 3 month time limit cannot be extended unless your letter is delayed in the post due to industrial action.

If you are asking for an 'any grounds' review, you can say what you like. However, this procedure is like an internal appeal, so it is sensible to explain exactly how and why you think the AO's decision is wrong.

Any time reviews – For other social security benefits, reviews are possible at 'any time', but only if one or more of the limited grounds for review are satisfied. These limited grounds are set out in s.25 SSAA and, for DLA, DWA and attendance allowance only, in s.30(2) SSAA. Whoever asks for the review has to show that the grounds for a review are satisfied: showing that the original decision was 'wrong' is not good enough. If the grounds for a review are satisfied, the original decision can be reconsidered or reviewed. The result of the review may be to confirm the original decision or to change it.

(b) DLA, DWA and attendance allowance

For decisions on DWA, DLA and attendance allowance, the review procedure is crucial: you only have the right to appeal to a DAT or SSAT once an AO has made a decision on an 'any grounds' review – under s.30(1) SSAA. If you ask for a review within 3 months of being sent any decision of an AO, you can ask for a review on any grounds: for any reason at all, including that you think the decision wrong – see Chapters 16–18.

Once you are outside the 3 months 'any grounds' time limit, you can ask for an 'any time' review on limited grounds. These are given in s.30(2) SSAA. They are the same as the limited grounds for 'any time' reviews of other social security benefits given in s.25(1), (2) – see (c) below.

Once an AO gives a decision on an 'any time' review, or has refused to review, you can then ask for a further 'any grounds' review of that decision within 3 months. You can only appeal to a DAT or SSAT once you get an 'any grounds' review decision.

Do note that this procedure does not automatically open up the original decision which you (or the AO) were seeking to change. One or more of the limited grounds for an 'any time' review must be satisfied. These are the starting conditions for enabling an 'any time' review at all; they act as a gateway to the original decision.

It is the 'any time' AO's decision which may be reviewed on 'any grounds' (not the original decision you, or the AO, were trying to change). If none of the limited grounds for an 'any time' review are satisfied, the original decision cannot be changed – however 'wrong' or 'right' that decision may be.

Scope of a DLA review

A DLA award consists of one or both DLA components. If you ask for a review of one DLA component or make a top up claim for a component you don't have, the AO could decide to question your entitlement to the other component. But if the other DLA component is a life award, the AO must not disturb it, unless you've asked for your life award to be considered (eg you claim a higher rate) or unless there is information before the AO that gives them 'reasonable grounds' to believe your entitlement should not continue. A change in the law, probably from the beginning of June 1997, will specifically permit the Secretary of State to *'undertake investigations to obtain information and evidence'* and to supply information to the AO reviewing the life award.

From 27.12.93 separate awards of the DLA care and mobility components were combined into one award consisting of two components. But if you had two separate, fixed period (not life) awards set to end at different times, these continued being separate awards until either, on review or renewal, one or both components are awarded for life, or both components are fixed to end on the same day. If you still have two separate awards of DLA, a review of one will not affect the other.

(c) The grounds for a review

Any decision can be reviewed at any time if:
- it was taken in ignorance of any material fact; or if
- it was based on a mistake as to a material fact;
  (if you are asking for a review of a decision on the grounds above, on the assessment of disablement for SDA or industrial injuries you must have *'fresh evidence'* – unless it is an 'unforeseen aggravation' review); or
- there has been a relevant change of circumstances or such a change is anticipated – see below.

A decision by an AO or medical board can also be reviewed if:
- it was based on an error of law – see below.

Change of circumstances

A decision can be reviewed if there has been a material change of circumstances since it was made. A change in the law itself counts as a relevant change of circumstances. However a decision of the Court or a Commissioner's decision does not count as a relevant change of circumstances (but may enable an 'error of law' review – see below). A different medical opinion does not by itself amount to a relevant change of circumstances however the findings of an up to date medical examination and report may be evidence of an actual change of circumstances (see CSIS/137/94).

If the original decision was to refuse benefit completely, that decision cannot be reviewed only because there has been a change of circumstances (see R(A)2/81 and CIS/767/94). The point is that the original decision remains correct. Instead, you make a fresh claim, or your review letter is treated as a fresh claim. DLA is in a special position – see Chapter 17.

A decision may also be reviewed if it is anticipated that a relevant change of circumstances will take place. The decision given on that review would take effect from the appropriate date, depending on the date of the anticipated change of circumstances, and how the rules about altering benefit affect your situation.

Errors of law

A decision by an AO or medical board can be reviewed if it was based on a mistake about the law. Box O.5 explains about errors of law in general. If the original decision-maker was aware of the law and the material facts relevant to your claim, the legal basis for an error of law review can only be satisfied if there has been a changed interpretation of the law (eg by a precedent-setting Commissioner's decision). If the meaning of the law is settled, the fact that the current decision-maker wants to come to a different decision from the original one does not enable an error of law review. The original decision would have to be outlandishly unreasonable to have it reviewed on the basis of an error of law.

A pre-6.4.92 decision of the now defunct Attendance Allowance Board, or one of its delegated medical practitioners, can be reviewed on the basis of an error of law. For review purposes a Board or DMP decision is treated as an AO decision and is subject to review on the same grounds and in the same circumstances as decisions of an AO.

Reg 22(9) SS (Introduction of DLA) Regs

A decision of a DAT, SSAT, MAT, or a Commissioner cannot be reviewed on the basis of an error of law. The best advice if you think a decision is wrong is to challenge that decision on appeal. If you discover that the tribunal (etc) made an error of law when you are outside the time limit for appealing, you can do the following.
- Make a late appeal.
- Apply to have the decision set aside – see 9(b).
- Check to see if a review on the basis of a mistake or ignorance about the facts is possible. Very often what counts as a material fact depends on how one interprets the law and on the understanding of the nature of the tests required by the law. If an error of law has been made, it is likely that the tribunal (etc) won't have explored all the relevant facts. If a review on the basis of mistake or ignorance about the facts is possible then, on review, the whole decision is considered afresh and the current interpretation of the law applied.
- You can, of course, make a fresh claim for the benefit: subject to the normal rules on backdating.
- If you have had a continuing award of benefit, you may find that the current decision on your claim has been taken by

an AO (because the previous decision, including the effect of the tribunal's decision, has been replaced by a fresh decision after being reviewed and revised because of a change of circumstances). If the current decision on your claim has been taken by an AO, that decision is reviewable on the basis of an error of law (even if that error had earlier been confirmed on appeal to a tribunal).
- If a change of circumstances has happened since the original erroneous decision, then on review the AO can also correct the error of law – once you ask for a review, and if the conditions for getting a review are satisfied, then all aspects of the decision can be reviewed.

Appeal rights
If the decision is reviewed but not changed, you have a fresh right of appeal against the new decision. Similarly if the AO refuses to review the old decision, you have the right to appeal against the refusal to review.

If you are trying to show that there are no grounds for review see R(M)5/86, R(S)4/86 and R(I)2/87 – it is irrelevant whether the decision is 'right' or 'wrong', the legal basis for a review must be established before the decision can be reviewed. The main power to review decisions given by AOs, DATs, SSATs and Commissioners is found in s.25, s.30 and s.35 SSAA. S.47 covers reviews of medical questions in disablement benefit and SDA. Reg 24(11), (12), Intro covers mobility allowance reviews. Reg 22(9), Intro enables reviews of Attendance Allowance Board decisions by treating them as AO decisions. Regulations also cover reviews in particular circumstances and the date(s) from which a reviewed award can be revised. Note that if a decision is reviewed because of an error of law, the revised decision cannot be backdated earlier than 23.4.84 – even under reg 57, Adjudication Regs. Note also that a review leading to a reduction in benefit (ie an overpayment) goes back to the start of the period of overpayment. Reviews of s.17 SSAA Secretary of State decisions are covered by s.19 SSAA.

(d) Limited backdating on review
A review of benefit can normally be backdated for no more than one month before the day you asked for a review. If the review is because your circumstances have changed in the month before your review request, benefit cannot be backdated before the date of the change. This time limit cannot be extended (even if you have a good reason for not asking for a review earlier) except in the following cases.
- **Incapacity benefit** – If you become entitled to DLA higher rate care component and as a result your incapacity benefit should have been paid at the long term rate after 28 weeks of incapacity (rather than 52 weeks), the long term rate of incapacity benefit can be fully backdated.
- **Exempt from the all work test** – If, on review, it is decided that you are exempt from the all work test, incapacity benefit and severe disablement allowance can be fully backdated. But this only applies if the review is on the grounds of ignorance or a mistake about a material fact (ie under s.25(1)(a) SSAA). If it is decided that you are exempt because of a change in circumstances, the one month limit on backdating applies.
- **Retirement pension** – If you apply for a review of your retirement pension before 4.8.97, benefit can be backdated automatically for 3 months, or for up to 12 months if you have 'good cause' for your delayed request. For reviews requested on or after 4.8.97, benefit can be backdated for one month only.
- **Contribution conditions** – If the original decision is revised only because of a question relating to NI contribution conditions, benefit can be fully backdated.
- **Income support and JSA** – If you become entitled to another benefit and arrears of that benefit are payable for a period earlier than one month before your review request, then a review of your income support or JSA can be fully backdated. For example, if there is a delay in awarding your DLA, the disability premium can be fully backdated.
- **Full backdating** – In some circumstances there is no time limit on reviews – see (e) below.
- **If you asked for a review before 7.4.97** – The rules described above apply to reviews requested on or after 7.4.97. Before this, for most benefits the limits on backdating were more generous. In addition, a review of most benefits could be backdated for 12 months if you could show 'good cause' for your delayed review request (see 4). If your review request was made before 7.4.97, the old rules still apply. See the 21st edition of the *Disability Rights Handbook*.
- **Housing benefit and council tax benefit** – The changes to the rules from April 1997 on backdating claims and reviews do not apply to housing benefit or council tax benefit. On review, benefit can be backdated for up to 52 weeks.

If you have been underpaid any benefit for over a month, and the special rules for getting full backdating don't apply (see below), you could appeal or try making a late appeal. On a successful appeal, you can receive full arrears. For a late appeal to be heard, you must have exceptional and compelling reasons why you did not appeal in time – see 13(c).

(e) Full backdating
Reg 57 of the Adjudication Regs applies to decisions of all the adjudicating authorities: from AOs to Commissioners. However, it does not apply to a review of a decision by an AO (or SSAT) where the ground for review is that a later decision of the Commissioners or Courts shows that the original decision involved an error of law.

The previous version of reg 57, reg 72, now only applies to reviews which were requested before 31.8.91. For reviews requested from 31.8.91, reg 72 is abolished and replaced by reg 57. Reg 57 provides for the payment of unlimited arrears on review if:
- at the time of making the decision which is now being reviewed the decision maker had before them specific evidence relevant to the claim but failed to take it into account; or someone in the DSS, Employment Service, or DHSS failed to hand over written evidence to the decision maker. In each case the evidence must enable a revision of the decision under review; or
- the original decision is being reviewed as a result of new evidence which has been given to the DSS, etc *'as soon as reasonably practicable after it became available to the claimant'* – so long as that evidence *'did not exist and could not have been obtained'* at the time the original decision was made; or
- the Adjudication Officer, in making the original decision, *'overlooked or misconstrued'* any relevant law or case law which, had it been properly taken into account, would have resulted in an award or a higher award of benefit.

If you cannot get a review of your past benefit entitlement, see if you can put in a late appeal – see 13(c).

(f) Test case backdating
The anti-test case rule limits the extent to which others can benefit from a reinterpretation of the law by the Commissioners or Courts in a test case, by restricting backdating in other cases on review to the date the test case decision was given (or for a maximum of 12 months if the test case is over a year old). The rule is in s.69 Social Security Administration Act 1992. S.68 applies a similar rule to claims. Essentially the rule obliges AOs to ignore the reinterpretation when

considering a related review for any period before the date of the test case. However, the rule does not catch all test cases or all related reviews.

The rule applies to test cases where the AO's decision in the test case is reversed by the Commissioner or Court on the ground that it was wrong in law. It does not apply if the AO's decision is upheld.

If you apply for a review before the date the test case decision is given, the anti-test case rule does not apply (see CDLA/577/94). If your review request is made after the test case then the rule does apply but only if the decision is reviewed on the ground of error of law. A review on any other ground is not caught, nor are appeals or late appeals against a pre-test case decision. Note that if you appeal after the AO has made an error of law review of the earlier decision on your claim, that review decision replaces the earlier decision which ceases to exist.

We only give a sketch of the anti-test case rules here. For more details see the footnotes to s.68 and s.69 SSAA in *Mesher* or *Bonner* (see Box O.4).

In CAO v Bate [1996] 2 All ER 790, the House of Lords ruled that Commissioners and higher courts are also bound by these provisions, as well as AOs and appeal tribunals.

11. Appeals

You have the right to appeal against any decision taken by an Adjudication Officer (AO), unless the sole ground of that AO's decision is a decision already taken by a different type of adjudicating authority. For DLA, disability working allowance and attendance allowance, you have the right to appeal against any decision on an 'any grounds' review, including a refusal to carry out an 'any time' review. You cannot appeal against an AO's initial decision, or 'any time' review decision, on your DLA, disability working allowance or attendance allowance claim – instead you ask for an 'any grounds' review of that decision (see 10).

You also have the right to appeal against any decision taken by an adjudicating medical practitioner (AMP) or medical board. You do not have the right of appeal against a decision taken by the Secretary of State – but see 13(d).

For more information see DSS booklet NI 260 *A Guide to Reviews and Appeals.*

Why appeal?

The law on social security is extensive and detailed. It is not surprising that many people consider that decisions affecting them are cut and dried. In a lot of cases they will be correct, but there are many grey areas where decisions depend on judgement and interpretation. So you should never give up on a claim, or on an appeal, until you understand exactly why a decision was made and you can find no facts and no Commissioners' decisions that support your interpretation of the law. Quite often the people dealing with your claim will not have the time to check all of this thoroughly. As soon as they believe they have enough facts to take a decision they will go ahead.

It is always vital to sort out whether a decision depends on what the law actually says, or whether it depends on a particular interpretation of the law. An understanding of what facts or evidence are relevant, given the legal tests, is also crucial.

Some decisions to refuse people benefits are clearly mistaken. Others are debatable. Appealing means that if you are not satisfied, you can get a second opinion: from the AO or from the independent Social Security Appeal Tribunal (SSAT) or Disability Appeal Tribunal (DAT).

12. How do you ask for an appeal?

You must fill in the form at the back of leaflet NI 246 which you can get from your local DSS office or Jobcentre. If you don't use the correct form, the chair of the tribunal has discretion to accept a written appeal providing you give all the required details.

In your appeal request, you must provide the following details:
- the date of the decision being appealed against;
- the claim or question under appeal;
- a summary of your arguments of why the decision is wrong.

However, if your appeal is detailed and gives as much information as possible about why you think a particular decision should be made (or not made), the decision may well be changed (or 'revised'). If it is wholly revised in your favour, your appeal will not be sent to the SSAT or DAT.

If your appeal is against a decision made over 3 months ago, you must also give 'special reasons' why the appeal is late – see 13(c).

If your appeal request does not contain all the required details, the tribunal chair or clerk may extend the 3 month time limit by up to 14 days. Your appeal is not officially made until the clerk receives all the required details. It is very important to keep to the time limits. If your appeal fails to meet the deadline, there are strict conditions to satisfy before a late appeal will be accepted.

13. When can you appeal?

If you are disallowed a benefit, or are given a review decision on DLA, AA or DWA, the letter the DSS send you will always explain your rights of appeal. If the decision has been taken by an Adjudication Officer, you must appeal within 3 months of the date the decision was sent to you.

If the AO's decision concerns income support, you have the extra right to ask for a written explanation of the AO's decision. You must ask for the explanation within 3 months of the date the decision was sent to you. But any appeal must be made within the 3 month time limit which started with the date that decision was sent to you.

(a) Benefits with one appeal route – to the SSAT

The benefits listed below all follow the same appeal route.

The decision is taken by an Adjudication Officer. You can appeal within 3 months to a Social Security Appeal Tribunal (SSAT). If the SSAT refuses your appeal, or only grants part of your appeal, you can appeal to the Social Security Commissioner – see 21 below.

- child benefit
- child's special allowance
- family credit
- family income supplement
- funeral expenses
- guardian's allowance
- incapacity benefit
- income support
- industrial accident
- industrial death benefit
- invalid care allowance
- invalidity benefit
- jobseeker's allowance
- maternity allowance
- maternity payment
- one parent benefit
- retirement allowance
- retirement pension
- sickness benefit
- statutory maternity pay
- statutory sick pay
- supplementary benefit
- transitional additions
- unemployment benefit
- all widow's benefits

(b) Benefits with two appeal routes

The benefits listed below have two appeal routes. On non-medical questions (including incapacity for work) the right of

appeal is to the SSAT. Where the issue involves or includes a disability question the right of appeal is to the DAT. On medical questions, there is a separate decision and appeal route.
- severe disablement allowance
- attendance allowance
- industrial disablement benefit
- disability living allowance
- reduced earnings allowance
- disability working allowance

Non-medical questions
Non-medical questions are decided by the Adjudication Officer (AO). The right of appeal is the same as in (a) above. These questions include:
- whether you are 'incapable of work' (for SDA);
- whether you meet the residence and presence conditions for SDA, DLA or attendance allowance;
- whether there has been an industrial accident;
- whether your incapacity for work is due to the effects of an industrial accident or disease;
- any question about disability working allowance – except for the 'disadvantage' test.

Disability questions
Disability questions are also decided by the AO, but the right of appeal is to a Disability Appeal Tribunal (DAT). This right arises only if an AO has made a decision on an 'any grounds' review, which includes refusing to carry out an 'any time' review. If a case involves both a disability question and any other question relating to attendance allowance, DLA or DWA, the right of appeal is to a DAT rather than to the SSAT (we call this 'mixed questions'). Appeals against decisions on the equivalent disability questions, and mixed questions, in pre-6.4.92 attendance allowance and mobility allowance are also to a DAT. Disability questions are –
- whether or not you satisfy the disability tests for attendance allowance, DLA care component, or DLA mobility component;
- whether or not you satisfy the relevant qualifying period(s) for the disability tests;
- the period throughout which you are likely to satisfy the disability tests;
- the rate at which attendance allowance, DLA care component, or DLA mobility component is payable; and
- whether you have *'a physical or mental disability which puts [you] at a disadvantage in getting a job'* – for DWA purposes.

O.3 Who can help you?

You are much more likely to succeed with an appeal if someone who is familiar with the procedure can help you. There are a number of people and agencies who can advise you on preparing your appeal and support you at the hearing itself.

The Address List at the back of this Handbook gives addresses of local law centres. Your local Citizens Advice Bureau may be able to help you; they can at least tell you if there is any organisation in your area who could provide a representative. If you are in a union, contact your branch to see if anyone can help. A local DIAL group or other disablement advice centre may be able to offer advice and, in some cases, be willing to represent you. Your local council might have a welfare rights unit that could help, or if not, they are likely to be able to give you a list of local advice centres – contact your town hall for information.

Medical questions
See Chapter 13(8) for how the 80% test under Route 4 for severe disablement allowance is decided.

See Chapter 21 for industrial disablement benefit and reduced earnings allowance.

There is an eventual right of appeal on medical questions to the Medical Appeal Tribunal within 3 months of the date the adjudicating medical practitioner or medical board's decision was sent to you.

(c) Late appeals
If you appeal late, your appeal may still be heard, but there are strict conditions that must be met. The chair of the tribunal must be satisfied that there are reasonable prospects of your appeal succeeding and it is in the interests of justice to allow you to appeal. S/he must also be satisfied that there are special reasons for not appealing in time, that these relate to the facts or history of your case, are wholly exceptional, and have existed from the end of the time limit to the day you asked for an appeal. Your special reasons must clearly amount to a reasonable excuse. The later your appeal, the more convincing must be your reasons. The fact that you or your adviser may have been unaware of or misunderstood the law, will not be taken into account, nor that a Commissioner or court has reinterpreted the law. The time limit cannot be extended for more than 6 years.

These rules make it very difficult to appeal late. But it may still be worth trying if you have special reasons for the delay, for example, due to your ill health or disability. If an appeal is successful you can receive full arrears.

(d) Secretary of State decisions
Decisions made by the Secretary of State fall into two areas: judicial decisions and other decisions. Judicial decisions are made under s.17, SSAA. These judicial decisions carry a right of appeal on a point of law to the High Court, or in Scotland, to the Court of Session.

A Secretary of State's decision is made either when you formally request one (usually once you've received an AO's decision), or where the adjudicating authorities refer the question formally to the Secretary of State under s.37 of the SSAA.

Administrative and other decisions, such as whether to pay attendance allowance on a day other than a Monday, or whether to treat a claim for IS as if it had also been one for invalid care allowance, do not carry any formal rights of appeal. Instead you can use normal methods of negotiation to attempt to change the Secretary of State's mind. If necessary, you can ask your MP to intervene and take up your case with the real Secretary of State. Judicial review of these administrative decisions may be a possibility: but you will need to seek expert advice, from a law centre or solicitor, and to seek that advice really quickly.

14. Medical Appeal Tribunals
If you disagree with an adjudicating medical authority's assessment of the extent of your disablement as a result of an industrial injury or for SDA, you can appeal to a Medical Appeal Tribunal within 3 months of the date the decision was sent to you.

The Medical Appeal Tribunal consists of a lawyer chairperson and two doctors of consultant status. They hear your case completely afresh. They are also concerned with medical facts, so it is essential to get medical evidence to support your case. Try to get a letter from your own consultant, or from an independent specialist, which explains your disabling condition and how it has affected you. Send any medical evidence you collect to the clerk to the tribunal so that copies can be made for the tribunal members. If you can't send them in advance, take them with you to the hearing. The MAT itself can and will direct the DSS to obtain any relevant evidence you have been unable to get – see 15 below.

The procedure for the hearing will be the same as that for SSATs (see 18 to 21), apart from any medical examination which may be required. This usually takes place at the end of the hearing and is carried out by the tribunal doctors in private. You have the right to have a companion of the same sex with you during the examination. See 18 below if you have a problem over access to the MAT. You should discuss any problems with the clerk to the MAT well in advance.

15. Medical evidence

If your appeal concerns a medical question or depends on medical evidence (eg whether or not you are fit for work), you should arrange for medical evidence which you can send in before, or present to, the tribunal.

The Secretary of State, or any adjudicating authority can also direct that the DSS obtain medical evidence to help them come to a decision. This power comes under s.53, SSAA. Although s.53 refers to questions of *'special difficulty'*, the intention is that it should also cover the same type of medical reports that could previously be arranged under reg 8, Adjudication Regs. Although we look at s.53 in the light of AO or SSAT decisions, it does apply across the board. For attendance allowance and DLA, s.54, SSAA also gives wider powers to refer you for a medical examination if a report is needed to help the AO reach a decision on your claim or review. For DATs there is an extra power under reg 30, Adjudication Regs and s.55(1) SSAA.

You can ask the AO to arrange for medical evidence on your appeal form, quoting s.53, (or in your review letter for DLA or AA, quoting s.54), but this is discretionary and you have little control over the questions, or over the doctor you are referred to.

If you are appealing to a DAT, you can also ask the DAT chairperson to use reg 30, Adjudication Regs and s.55(1) to refer you to a medical practitioner for examination and report. S/he must be *'satisfied that [your] appeal ... cannot be properly determined unless'* there is a medical report available to the DAT giving the results of your medical examination. You can do this in your appeal letter, or during a DAT hearing. All that we say below about s.53 applies also to DATs and to the use of reg 30, Adjudication Regs.

If you have been unable to get necessary medical evidence before your SSAT hearing, ask the SSAT to use s.53 to obtain a report. If you have a list of specific questions, ask the SSAT to agree that those questions be put to the doctor, or that you and the AO should agree on the questions. *Stevens v Johnson* [CA, 23.11.84, unreported] says on p.13 of the transcript that, where necessary, the law should be explained to the doctor. The SSAT might want to do this themselves, or pass on the task to you and the AO to agree. Once again this is discretionary, so if the SSAT refuse, ask for an adjournment to allow you to get your own medical evidence.

Unless the medical evidence you need is straightforward, asking the AO or SSAT to use s.53 may be risky. It is best to try and arrange for a report yourself: unless, of course, the rule in *Stevens v Johnson* is followed by the AO, SSAT, DAT, medical board, MAT or Commissioner.

The evidence can come from your GP, or your hospital consultant if you have one. The 'Green Form' scheme may cover the cost of a medical report – see Chapter 53 for details. Under the Green Form scheme a solicitor can arrange for a medical report from an independent consultant or specialist.

When you ask your doctor to give you a letter or statement it is best to ask him or her specific questions, so that you get answers which are directly relevant and not a vague comment about your general condition. Check what the law and case law says about your situation – you will then know what facts you need to prove in order to win your appeal. The relevant chapters in this Handbook should give you some guidance – eg on what counts as being 'incapable of work' or 'virtually unable to walk'.

There is no rule that you must have corroborating medical or other evidence. You can go ahead with your appeal even if you can't get supporting evidence.

O.4 For more information

Statute law
- *The Blue Volumes – The Law Relating to Social Security* (The Stationery Office).

Tribunal members are issued the following books:
- *CPAG's Income Related Benefits: The Legislation*, commentary by Mesher & Wood (Sweet & Maxwell).
- *Non-Means-Tested Benefits: The Legislation*, commentary by Bonner et al (Sweet & Maxwell).
- *Medical and Disability Appeal Tribunals: The Legislation*, commentary by Rowland (Sweet & Maxwell).

The books above have detailed footnotes. Make sure you look at the latest editions.
- *The Law of Social Security*, by Ogus, Barendt & Wikeley (4th ed, Butterworths)
- *SSATs – A Guide to Procedure* (The Stationery Office)
- *MATs – A Guide to Procedure* (The Stationery Office)
- *The Disability Handbook* (The Stationery Office) – see Box G.6.

Case Law
- *Neligan – Social Security Case Law – Digest of Commissioners' Decisions* (The Stationery Office)

This outlines the main reported decisions. In tricky cases it is unlikely to give you enough information and you will need to look up the full reported decisions. You can buy reported decisions from Stationery Office bookshops, or look them up at a local DSS office. You can buy unreported decisions directly from the Commissioners' office – see the Address List at the back of the Handbook.

Interpreting law
- *Industrial Injuries Handbook for Adjudicating Medical Authorities*
- *Income Support Procedure Manual*
- *Social Fund Guide*
- *Adjudication Officers' Guide*
- *Housing Benefit Guidance Manual*

Your local library may have copies of all, or some, of these Stationery Office publications. You can also consult Stationery Office publications and DSS publications at your local DSS office – it is best to phone or write beforehand to make an appointment.

If you are really interested in law and the techniques used in drafting legislation, the best starting point is: *Bennion on Statute Law* (Francis Bennion, Longman, 1990). Borrow a copy through a library.

16. Disability Appeal Tribunals

The Disability Appeal Tribunal (DAT) is independent of the DSS. It is part of the Independent Tribunal Service. The DAT hears appeals against 'any grounds' review decisions of Adjudication Officers on the disability questions (and mixed questions) for attendance allowance, disability living allowance, mobility allowance and disability working allowance. If your appeal does not involve a disability question, it will be heard by a SSAT.

A DAT consists of a lawyer chairperson and two members. A DAT cannot go ahead with consideration of an appeal unless all three are present. One member is a medical practitioner. The other is a person who *'is experienced in dealing with the needs of disabled persons . . . in a professional or voluntary capacity; . . . or because they are themselves disabled'*. This 'disability' member cannot be a medical practitioner – but may well be a paramedic, such as a physiotherapist or a nurse.

If *'practicable'* at least one of the members of the DAT who hears your appeal should be of the same sex as you. However, there won't necessarily be a disabled person serving on the DAT – the Tribunal Service just have to have regard to the desirability of this.

A DAT cannot carry out a physical examination or ask you to undergo a walking test for the mobility component. They will, however, see how you walk into and out of the room, as well as how you cope with what might be a lengthy hearing.

Special needs – If you have any special needs, check with the tribunal clerk beforehand about accessibility, what facilities are available, and how your needs can be met in order to enable you to be present at your hearing and get home within a reasonable time after the hearing. You can and should ask for whatever you need – that is the only way to gain improvements for all people with disabilities. Whether the Tribunal Service can arrange or provide it is a separate matter – if they cannot, seek advice. For example, if it's too far to walk easily to the tribunal room from the nearest point a car can set you down, ask for a wheelchair to be waiting for you. If you need any breaks during a hearing (eg to go to the toilet, to take food, liquids or medication, to stretch your legs, or to change position), ask for them – it helps if the DAT are aware of what might happen beforehand.

Procedures – For details of procedures for the hearing, see 18 to 21 below.

Domiciliary tribunals – If you exercise your right to opt for an oral hearing of your appeal, if necessary, the Tribunal Service can arrange for the DAT to hear your appeal at your home. If you are reluctant to have the DAT visit your home, perhaps because you don't have enough room for a minimum of 5 extra people, a local disability group may know of a suitable and fully accessible venue which could be used instead. Note that the tribunal will normally sit to hear the case to decide whether to adjourn for a domiciliary hearing, but they may go ahead in your absence if they are satisfied there is sufficient evidence before them for a full appeal.

17. Social Security Appeal Tribunals

The Social Security Appeal Tribunal (SSAT) hears all appeals on income support, jobseeker's allowance, family credit, National Insurance benefits, supplementary benefit, and family income supplement. SSATs also hear appeals which only involve non-disability questions on attendance allowance, DLA, DWA and mobility allowance. They should operate in a careful and fair way. You have the right to be present at the hearing of your appeal, but you must request this in writing within the deadline notified to you by the tribunal clerk. The tribunal consists of a lawyer chairperson and two other members representative of people who live or work in the area. They are independent of the DSS, and are under the control of the President of the Independent Tribunal Service.

Where the SSAT are considering a question of whether or not you satisfy the all work test of incapacity, a medical assessor appointed by ITS will sit with the tribunal.

The rules about appealing against a decision of a SSAT (or asking for leave to appeal) to the Social Security Commissioners are in 21 below.

18. What happens when you appeal?

When you appeal to the SSAT or DAT, the Adjudication Officer will check to see whether or not it is possible to revise (or change) the decision.

Sometimes income support decisions get revised in your favour once you have appealed (or asked for a written explanation). This is mainly because the appeals section have more time to go through your case and they tend to be more familiar with the law and case law. It is less common with appeals on National Insurance benefits, but some decisions do get revised in your favour. If you write a detailed appeal letter, the AO clearly has a better chance of seeing if the decision is wrong. If a decision is wholly revised in your favour, you'll get a letter telling you so. In other cases, your appeal just continues.

At all stages of your appeal, make sure you return any forms within the deadlines. If you don't, your appeal could be 'struck out'. You will be sent a warning notice. If your appeal is struck out, it will only be reinstated if you apply within 3 months and only if you did not receive the warning notice even though the tribunal had your address.

If you decide you don't want to go ahead with your appeal, you can withdraw it at any time before the hearing. Just write to the clerk. You don't need the consent of the AO or Secretary of State unless they indicated at the outset that they would oppose this.

Opting for an oral hearing – The tribunal clerk will send you an acknowledgement of your appeal and a form asking whether you want an oral hearing of your appeal, ie whether you want to attend the tribunal hearing in person. Normally you have 14 days to reply. If you don't reply within the deadline given in the letter, the clerk will refer your case to the tribunal to be decided on the papers alone. However, guidance from the Independent Tribunal Service suggests that you will get an oral hearing if you ask for one at any stage right up to the time the hearing is due to start. If a decision is made in your absence despite your late request for an oral hearing, you may be able to get the decision set aside (see 9(b)). The tribunal chair may also require an oral hearing to be held if that is necessary to enable the tribunal to reach a decision.

In most cases, it is better for you to ask for an oral hearing of your case. In some cases, it will be crucial for the success of your appeal. This is particularly true of cases involving any medical or disability questions, eg decisions about incapacity for work or entitlement to DLA. The full extent of your care or mobility needs for example, or your ability to perform the activities in the all work test of incapacity may not become obvious until the tribunal asks you questions at the appeal hearing.

Whether or not you opt for an oral hearing, you will be sent a copy of the appeal papers. If you have requested an oral hearing the clerk will send you details of when and where it will take place. You must be given at least 7 days notice of the time and place of the hearing.

If you need the decision urgently, contact the clerk, giving your reasons. Their address and phone number are on the letter they send you acknowledging the receipt of your appeal.

Asking for a postponement – If the date is inconvenient or it doesn't give you enough time to prepare your case, write to the clerk and ask if the hearing can be postponed. If time is short, you can telephone the tribunal clerk (the number will be at the top of the form AT6) but you should also write to confirm your request. The same applies if you find that you are ill before or on the day. If all the parties have agreed to a postponement, or you have a sudden domestic difficulty, or the case was listed in error, the clerk will generally make the decision on whether to grant a postponement. But in other cases, the tribunal chair will deal with the request. If you are asking for a postponement because of insufficient notice, it is best to go along to the hearing anyway, just in case the postponement is refused.

Access to premises – Check in advance whether the premises are accessible to you, if there is a lift, etc, according to your particular needs. If they are unsuitable, write or telephone the tribunal clerk and ask for the appeal to be heard in premises accessible to you, or at least for help to be made available to you on your arrival and departure.

If the premises aren't accessible to you, the tribunal should adjourn to a time and place where you can be present – quote Commissioner's decision – CI/112/84.

19. What can you do before the hearing?

Tribunals must make decisions in accordance with the law and case law by applying these to the particular facts of your situation. The appeal papers should refer you to the parts of the law relevant to your appeal. You can look these up in the *Blue Volumes* – see Box O.4.

Case law is found in decisions of the Social Security Commissioners and the Courts. The appeal papers should refer you to any relevant decisions. But there may be other Commissioners' decisions that are more helpful for your appeal. It is always worth checking the decisions the AO has quoted. The quickest way is to read *Neligan* (see Box O.4) and look at other decisions in the pages around the decisions that the AO has quoted. If possible you should read the full reported decisions. In really complex cases it is helpful to read, in full, every single reported decision on that topic. Decisions taken by the Social Security Commissioners set precedents. If the principles and facts of a Commissioner's decision are similar to your own situation, the SSAT, DAT or MAT should follow that decision.

Once you have looked at the law and case law, you may have a clearer idea of which facts are important for your appeal and what extra evidence you might need. Almost all appeals concern a dispute about the facts, or a different interpretation of the same facts. So if you feel flummoxed about the law – forget it! Just concentrate on the facts.

You do not have to prove any fact 'beyond all reasonable doubt'. You just have to prove that on a balance of probabilities you are more likely to be telling the truth than not. Your word is just as much 'evidence' as a bit of paper is. But if you get other evidence to back up what you are saying, this helps tip the balance your way.

If you read through the chapter on the benefit you are appealing about, you should get a good idea of what facts could be important. A local advice agency (see Box O.3) may also be able to help – on the law as well as by helping you sort out which facts are important and what other evidence you might need, and might be able to represent you. In some cases you might need to call witnesses – so you'll need to get their agreement and make sure you know what they will be saying and why that backs up your case.

It is best to send in any further evidence and details of your case in advance of the tribunal hearing. Make a copy and take it with you to the hearing.

20. At the hearing

An SSAT can be heard by the chairperson and one member, but only if you or your representative agree. It is usually better not to agree and wait for another hearing – unless of course your need is urgent. A DAT or MAT cannot go ahead unless all members are present.

It is always best to attend the hearing yourself – see 18 above if you have a problem over access.

Besides your partner (if any), you can have one other person with you at the hearing. S/he can represent you. Both of you have the right to speak, and you can also call witnesses if you wish to. You can claim travelling expenses for yourself, and compensation for loss of earnings can be claimed up to a set maximum. You can also claim childminding expenses and subsistence allowance, eg if you are away from home or work for more than 2.5 hours. If you are not sure what you, or

---

O.5 Errors of law

Can you understand the decision?
From reading the full written decision of any tribunal, it must be clear what they decided, and why they decided as they did. If you put forward specific arguments, it must be clear how and why they dealt with your arguments. From the decision it must also be clear that the adjudicating authority understood and applied the law and case law relevant to the decision correctly.

Errors of law are also relevant if you (or the AO or medical board) are seeking to review a previous decision on this ground – see 10(c).

Identifying errors of law
R(A)1/72 lists the tests to be applied in deciding whether a decision is erroneous in law. These have also been considered in later decisions: eg in R(I)14/75. Generally, a decision will be wrong in law if any of the following apply.
- There has been any breach of the rules of natural justice (this is, loosely, incorrect or unfair procedures).
- The adjudicating authority has failed to make sufficient findings of fact on the key questions at issue so as to enable it properly to come to a decision.
- The adjudicating authority has failed to give adequate reasons for the decision. (Listing a string of Commissioners' decisions and/or legal references, or repeating the question at issue in the appeal, is not good enough.)
- The decision contains a misdirection or misunderstanding of the relevant law. (For example, if a DAT's decision shows they thought that 'required' meant only medically required, rather than reasonably required, they would have erred in law. They would have made the decision on the basis of a wrong construction, or understanding, of the law, and the meaning of the words used in the law.)
- The decision is supported by no evidence. (Seek advice.)
- The facts found were such that no person acting judicially and properly instructed about the relevant law could have come to the decision. (Seek advice. To succeed on this ground, the decision must be way out of line.)

O.6 Commissioners' decisions

We quote a number of Social Security Commissioners' decisions in the Handbook. These decisions are part of case law, setting precedents which must be followed in similar cases. In general, decisions of the courts are binding on Commissioners, tribunals and AOs. The legal position is that Commissioners speak with equal authority R(I)12/75, p.19–22. However, a decision of a Tribunal of Commissioners should be followed in preference to a decision of a single Commissioner. A reported decision of a single Commissioner may be given more weight than an unreported one, but AOs and tribunals are free to follow whichever decision they consider correct. There is no obligation on tribunals to prefer an earlier decision to a later one, or vice versa.

The most important decisions are published, or reported by the Stationery Office (formerly HMSO). Decisions which are of general significance are starred; while the vast majority of decisions are unreported, or not published by the Stationery Office.

Reported decisions

These are referred to as: for example, R(M)2/78. Where: R = reported; (M) = the series initial, in this case standing for mobility allowance; '2/78' = the second decision in that series reported in 1978. Some decisions were made by a Tribunal of Commissioners, rather than by a single Commissioner; this would be noted by the suffix (T) eg R(M)3/86(T). Until 1.2.50 reported decisions were referred to in the same way as unpublished decisions eg CS/371/49(KL).

Unreported decisions

Since 1982, unreported decisions of more general significance are starred; some may well be reported at a later stage. Unreported decisions are referred to as, for example, CM/60/86. Where: C = Commissioner; M = the series initial; 60 = the number of the file; 86 = the year in which the file was opened by the Commissioner.

Until 28.10.82 there were three types of decisions – unreported, numbered, and reported decisions. Numbered decisions were referred to as, for example, CS/7/82; where the first numeral refers to its order in the sequence of numbered decisions, rather than to the sequence in which the files were opened.

Series initials

- (A) = attendance allowance
- (CR) = compensation recovery
- (DLA) = disability living allowance
- (DWA) = disability working allowance
- (F) = child benefit, formerly family allowance
- (FC) = family credit
- (G) = general: child's special allowance, death grant, guardian's allowance, invalid care allowance, maternity allowance, maternity grant, statutory maternity pay, widow's benefits
- (I) = industrial injuries benefits
- (IB) = incapacity benefit
- (IS) = income support
- (M) = mobility allowance
- (P) = retirement pensions
- (S) = sickness and invalidity benefit and SDA
- (SB) = supplementary benefit
- (SMP) = statutory maternity pay
- (SSP) = statutory sick pay
- (U) = unemployment benefit

someone with you, can claim, ask the tribunal clerk: phone the number on the AT6 form.

If everyone agrees, any other person can be present during the hearing (including another friend) but they cannot take part in the proceedings. You can request a private hearing or the tribunal chair can, in any case, decide that the hearing should be in private. In practice, the only members of the public who are likely to be present are other claimants (so that they can see what happens before their own appeal is heard) or advisers (to help them in their work). If you ask for a private hearing, the chairperson must grant your request. But note that some people, such as a trainee AO, have the right to be present at a private hearing, even though they are not allowed to take part in the proceedings.

The hearing itself should be fairly informal but this may vary. Apart from the three tribunal members, there will be a presenting officer (who is an Adjudication Officer, but not necessarily the one who took the decision) to put the AO's case. The presenting officer should also identify any points in your favour. This is because the procedure is inquisitorial, and not adversarial (with you against the AO). There will also be a clerk who will deal with any administrative matters that arise during the hearing such as photocopying documents.

Where the hearing concerns the all work test of incapacity, a medical assessor appointed by ITS will also be present. The Government has indicated that the role of the medical assessor is to comment on and explain the medical evidence and advise the tribunal on the weight to be given to it. They have been described as a 'talking medical dictionary'. The advice should be given openly. The assessor should not give an opinion on capacity for work nor take part in the tribunal's questioning or deliberations. The assessor should enter and leave the tribunal room at the same time as you and the presenting officer.

The usual procedure is for the chairperson to ask the presenting officer to read the tribunal papers and to put the AO's case first, but this can vary. You will then be asked to explain your case, and you should try to put your main points without interruption. It is useful to put them in writing so that you don't forget anything at the hearing. If you are interrupted, ask tactfully if you can make all your points before answering questions. Wherever possible back up your statement with documentary evidence, eg bills, doctor's letter, etc. At the end of your statement repeat the decision you want the tribunal to make. You can question the presenting officer and any witnesses. Listen carefully to what s/he has to say, and be prepared to ask questions if you think the facts are being misrepresented.

21. The decision

You normally get a verbal decision at the end of the hearing. Normally you will also be given a handwritten summary decision on the day, which, if your appeal is successful, will speed up the payment of the tribunal award. The tribunal chair may decide to send you a full written decision, including all the things that the tribunal have found as 'facts' and explaining how and why they made their decision. Otherwise, you will be told that this full decision is available to you if you request it within 21 days of the summary decision being given or sent to you. Unless the appeal is successful, it is best to ask for a full written decision, ideally on the day of the tribunal. If you want to appeal to the Commissioners, you **must** have this full decision, so make sure to ask for it within 21 days. If you have been unsuccessful, you should always be able to understand how and why you have been unsuccessful. If you cannot, or are left guessing in any way, this is an error of law and it may be possible to appeal further – to the Social Security Commissioners.

Seeking leave to appeal to the Commissioners
It is only possible to appeal to the Social Security Commissioners on a point of law – see Box O.5. You cannot appeal about the facts. But it is sometimes hard to separate the law from the facts – so it is worth asking an experienced adviser to check the decision.

If you want to appeal to the Commissioner, you must first apply to the chair of the SSAT, DAT or MAT for leave to appeal. You must have the tribunal's full decision before you can appeal. You can ask the tribunal clerk for a special form, OSSC1, or just write a letter setting out all the reasons why you think the decision was legally wrong. Head it *'Application for leave to appeal to the Commissioner'*. Send your OSSC1 form or letter to the office of the clerk to the tribunal and include a copy of the full decision. You must do this within 3 months of being sent the full decision.

If you miss this time limit, apply directly to the Commissioner for leave to appeal, s/he can consider your late application if there are *'special reasons'*. The Commissioner has complete discretion to hear your appeal. The strict rules that apply to late appeals to a tribunal do not apply to the Commissioners. You use form OSSC1 to apply for leave to appeal. But you can just write a letter headed *'Application for leave to appeal to the Commissioner'*. Enclose a copy of the tribunal's full decision. Send the form or letter and the tribunal's decision to the Commissioners' office – see the Address List at the back of this Handbook.

If the chairperson refuses leave to appeal, you have another 42 days in which to apply directly to the Commissioner for leave to appeal. The 42 days start to run from the date the chairperson's decision refusing leave to appeal is sent to you. Your application should go to the Commissioners' office.

If the chairperson grants leave to appeal, you must appeal to the Commissioner within 42 days of the date the decision granting leave to appeal is sent to you. Once again, you send your appeal to the Commissioners' office.

The AO has the same rights of appeal as yourself.

Attendance Allowance Board – You can still apply for leave to appeal to the Commissioners if the Board's written reasons for a decision on review are erroneous in law*. The time limits are the same as for DATs, so this is now only possible if the Commissioner extends the time limit for special reasons. See the 16th edition of this Handbook for more details.

* *Reg 23(1), (1A), Intro (as amended by SI 1992/728).*

The Commissioner's decision
If the Commissioner finds that a SSAT or DAT decision is wrong in law (see Box O.5) s/he can:
- give the decision which s/he considers the tribunal should have given, if s/he can do so without making any other findings of fact; or
- if s/he considers it *'expedient'* the Commissioner can make findings of fact, including calling for more evidence to enable this; or
- if there aren't enough findings of fact, and the Commissioner doesn't think it *'expedient'* to look at the evidence afresh, the case must be referred back to a tribunal. The Commissioner should give the tribunal directions so that they can make a fresh decision along the right lines.

In MAT cases involving medical questions, the Commissioner cannot make findings of fact as s/he is not an adjudicating medical authority. So, if the Commissioner grants the appeal, the case must be referred back, with directions, for a fresh decision. Another MAT will completely re-hear your appeal.

In pre-6.4.92 attendance allowance and mobility allowance cases, the Commissioner will refer back the case to an 'any grounds' Adjudication Officer, rather than to a DAT. However, the Commissioner may make a decision awarding or refusing benefit.

53 Free legal help

1. What help is available?

If you live or work in the catchment area of a law centre, contact the law centre first to see if they can help. Otherwise, many Citizens Advice Bureaux have volunteer lawyers and can refer you to one at a special advice session. Other agencies also organise free legal advice sessions. You can check whether there are any in your area by asking your local CAB. Many trade unions also offer free legal advice to their members.

Even if there are no free legal advice sessions in your area, you may still be able to get free legal advice and initial assistance from any legal aid solicitor. Your local CAB or other advice centre may be able to refer you to a solicitor for a low cost or free first interview through a local referral scheme. If you have been injured in an accident, you can arrange for a free legal consultation with a local solicitor specialising in injury claims, by phoning The Accident Line on Freephone 0500 192939. However, if you qualify for help under the government's Legal Advice and Assistance Scheme you can get help from any legal aid solicitor. This scheme is usually called the 'Green Form' scheme, as the form you have to sign before the solicitor can advise you, is coloured green. In Scotland, it is called the 'Pink Form' scheme. This chapter will only deal with the Green (or Pink) Form scheme. This is different from the Legal Aid and the Criminal Legal Aid Schemes. A solicitor or your local CAB can give you more details about these other types of legal aid.

The Legal Aid Board has overall responsibility for legal aid and advice, acting under the guidance of the Lord Chancellor.

The Green Form scheme does not cover conveyancing (except in very limited circumstances) or making a will (other than for specific categories of clients). Most people with disabilities can continue to get Green Form help with making a will. Others who can get that help are people aged 70 or over; a parent of a disabled person who wants to provide for that person in the will; and a lone parent wishing to appoint a testamentary guardian. Note that the Green Form still covers advice on intestacy, on probate etc of an existing will.

2. Who qualifies for help?

Anyone who receives income support, income-based jobseeker's allowance, disability working allowance, or family credit automatically qualifies for free legal advice under the Green Form scheme, if their savings are not over the set limits.

Other people, in or out of work, may also qualify if their savings and income are not over the set limits for the size of their family.

There is no means test for assistance by way of representation for proceedings before a mental health review tribunal; so you will get assistance at no cost, no matter what your income or capital.

3. The capital limits

The capital limits for the Green Form scheme from 7.4.97 are given below:
- £1,000 for the client;

- plus £335 for a first dependant: husband, wife, child, or other relative if you wholly or mainly support them;
- plus £200 for a second dependant;
- plus £100 for each other dependant.

The capital value of your home, furniture, household effects, tools of your trade and your clothing is ignored. The value of the thing you want advice about is also ignored. For applications made on or after 1.6.96, the market value of your home will be taken into account above £100,000.

If you are one of a couple, both partners' capital and income are added together. However, if you have a contrary interest to your partner, only your own capital and income is taken into account and any housekeeping money you are given will be ignored.

The capital limit for assistance by way of representation is £3,000 for the client (with additions for dependants as above). If you get IS or income-based JSA, you qualify automatically for assistance by way of representation on capital grounds.

4. Disposable income

If your disposable income is no more than £77 a week (£69 in Scotland), you can get free legal advice.

To work out your disposable income, add up your own (and your partner's) total weekly income from all sources. This does not include attendance allowance or DLA care component, or mobility component, or any social fund payment, or any payment under the Community Care Direct Payment scheme.

Once you have added up your total weekly income, deduct any income tax and NI contributions. Then deduct:

- £28.00 (for your partner. NB if you are separated and are paying maintenance, deduct your actual maintenance payment)
- £16.90 (for each child aged 0–11)
- £24.75 (for each child aged 11–16)
- £29.60 (for each child aged 16–18)

The deduction for a child goes up to the next age band from the first Monday in September following the child's 11th or 16th birthday. These age bands changed in April 1997. If your child is already aged 11 before 7.4.97, deduct £24.75; £29.60 if already aged 16; £38.90 if already aged 18.

Once you have deducted the appropriate amounts, you are left with your disposable income. If this is £77 or less, you qualify for free legal advice and assistance from any legal aid solicitor.

In Scotland, if your disposable income is no more than £69, you can get free legal advice. If your income is over £69, you will pay a one-off contribution. The contribution goes up in steps of £7 for each £7 you have over £69; the maximum payable is £95. If your income is over £166, you cannot get help under the Pink Form scheme.

For assistance by way of representation, you can get help if your income is no more than £166. However, you have to pay a weekly contribution of one-third of your income above £69.

5. What work can the solicitor do?

A solicitor can normally do 2 hours' worth of work for you (expenses have to be met within this limit, but not VAT). However, s/he can do more work if an extension to the Green Form limit is granted. An extension to cover the cost of a medical report for use at an appeal tribunal or mental health review tribunal should normally be fairly easy to get if the solicitor needs it in order to advise you properly. The Green Form can cover the cost of preparing for a tribunal eg writing letters, advising you on the law, preparing a written submission for you to hand to the tribunal. However it does not cover actual representation at the tribunal hearing except at mental health review tribunals. It can also cover separate representation for a parent involved in child care proceedings.

In matrimonial cases involving the preparation of a petition, 3 hours' worth of work can be done.

The Green Form cannot be used for help in making a will or with conveyancing – unless you are an exempt person, or in certain circumstances (ask your CAB for advice). Nor can it be used for advice about foreign law, other than EC law.

6. Which solicitor?

You may already have a solicitor who normally deals with your family's legal matters. If s/he does legal aid work, s/he might also be able to advise you, under the Green Form scheme, on other matters.

Your local CAB or the local Law Society will have a full list of legal aid solicitors' firms in your area. However, beyond telling you whether or not a particular firm deals with the topic you need advice on, they cannot recommend a particular firm.

If you have had an accident at work and want to make a claim against your employers it is always best to go to a solicitor. Do not go to Claims Assessors – you are likely to have to wait longer and get less at the end of the day than if you had gone to a solicitor in the first place. Your union may be able to arrange a solicitor for you. Or you can get a free first interview about your compensation rights following any type of accident with a solicitor specialising in injury claims, by contacting The Accident Line on Freephone 0500 192939.

Most solicitors will not be familiar with the intricacies of the social security system. So your first step should normally be to see what advice or help your local CAB, or other advice agency, can give you. If there is a problem the CAB cannot readily answer, they can at least help you express the issue clearly. This will save time if you later seek advice from a solicitor. It is also sensible to write down all the facts about the particular problem facing you.

54 Complaining to the Ombudsman

1. Introduction

Many people have the chance of complaining to an Ombudsman, but do not realise how effective this can be. There are two main kinds of Ombudsmen.

Government Ombudsmen – These are individuals appointed by the Government to investigate complaints that there has been injustice caused by the maladministration of central or local government, or part of the National Health Service. They also investigate complaints about refusal of access to official information.

Other Ombudsmen – There are now a large number of other Ombudsmen, including the Banking Ombudsman, Housing Associations Ombudsman, Insurance Ombudsman and the Investment Ombudsman. This chapter does not give information about these, but your Citizens Advice Bureau can give you their addresses and advise you whether one of them may be able to assist you. Box M.2 in Chapter 44 gives information about the Pensions Ombudsman.

In the remainder of this chapter when we use the word 'Ombudsman' we are referring only to Government Ombudsmen.

2. What can Ombudsmen investigate?

Complaining to an Ombudsman is not an alternative to the normal appeals process, nor is it an extension of that process. You would normally complain to an Ombudsman about the way a decision was taken, or the way you were treated, rather than about the actual decision that was taken. But an Ombudsman would expect you to have complained first to the relevant department or authority: the Ombudsman is not your first line of complaint.

An Ombudsman investigates whether maladministration has caused injustice. The Health Service Ombudsman can also investigate cases where maladministration has caused hardship. Ombudsmen do not investigate personnel matters, except in some cases the Northern Ireland Ombudsman.

Maladministration – This includes such things as bias, muddle, unreasonable delay, failure to follow (or have) proper procedures and rules.

Injustice – This does not only cover financial and other material or tangible loss. It also includes anxiety or stress, even a sense of outrage about the way in which something has been done.

Time limits

Each Ombudsman has a time limit of some kind. Most Ombudsmen would not normally investigate complaints from people about something they knew of more than one year before they complained. However, the Northern Ireland Ombudsman has a two month time limit in some cases.

3. How to complain to an Ombudsman

Before you can complain to an Ombudsman, you should first use the normal complaints procedure. You should be able to get help from a Citizens Advice Bureau, or in health cases, your Community Health Council (in England and Wales), Local Health Council (in Scotland) or Health and Social Services Council (in Northern Ireland).

It is best to keep a copy of your letter of complaint and of anything connected with it. If you are not satisfied, you must put your complaint to the Ombudsman in writing. You do not have to pay a fee to make a complaint.

Which Ombudsman?

In Great Britain, you need to complain to the correct Ombudsman – there is only one Ombudsman for Northern Ireland. In Britain you complain to:
- Parliamentary Ombudsman about central government
- Local Government Ombudsman about local government
- Health Service Ombudsman about health authorities and trusts, doctors, dentists, opticians, etc.

You can ask your CAB to check with the Ombudsman first if you want to make sure whether an Ombudsman can investigate a complaint against a particular government body, such as a quango.

Direct and indirect

You can complain directly to any of the Ombudsmen except the Parliamentary Ombudsman and, in cases concerning central government, the Northern Ireland Ombudsman.

Only an MP (not even a member of the House of Lords) can refer a complaint to the Parliamentary Ombudsman. If you wish to complain to the Parliamentary Ombudsman, you should normally approach your own MP and only approach another MP if yours has refused to refer your complaint. If you do approach an MP for another constituency, they will usually contact your own MP before they decide whether to refer your complaint.

4. What can an Ombudsman do?

An Ombudsman can investigate thoroughly any complaint you make. The Ombudsmen have similar powers to the High Court (Court of Session in Scotland) for obtaining evidence.

If an Ombudsman upholds your complaint, they will expect the body against which you have complained to provide you with some remedy. This may be an apology, a change in procedures, financial compensation, or any combination of these or similar measures.

5. Further information

Each Ombudsman publishes a leaflet or booklet about their services. See Box O.7 for their addresses. Most Ombudsmen now publish their material in ethnic minority languages.

Complaint form – You do not need a special form to complain to an Ombudsman, but most Ombudsmen now include a simple complaint form in their information booklet.

O.7 Contacting the Ombudsmen

Parliamentary Ombudsman
Church House, Great Smith Street, London, SW1P 3BW (0171 276 2130)

Health Service Ombudsman
- England: *Millbank Tower, Millbank, London, SW1P 4QP (0171 217 4051)*
- Scotland: *28 Thistle Street, Edinburgh, EH2 1EN (0131 225 7465)*
- Wales: *4th Floor, Pearl Assurance House, Greyfriars Road, Cardiff, CF1 3AG (01222 394621)*

Local Government Ombudsman
- London and South East: *21 Queen Anne's Gate, London, SW1H 9BU (0171 915 3210)*
- East Anglia, South, South-West, West and West Midlands: *The Oaks No.2, Westwood Way, Westwood Business Park, Coventry, CV4 8JB (01203 695999)*
- East Midlands, North, North-West: *Beverley House, 17 Shipton Road, York, YO3 6FZ (01904 663200)*
- Scotland: *FREEPOST, Edinburgh, EH3 0EE (0131 225 5300)*
- Wales: *Derwen House, Court Road, Bridgend, Mid Glam, CF31 1BN (01656 661325)*

Northern Ireland
There is one Ombudsman service which combines the three roles of Parliamentary, Health Service and Local Government Ombudsmen: *FREEPOST, Belfast, BT1 6BR (0800 343424)*.

Useful Publications

Listed below are a number of publications produced by other organisations which give further information on social security benefits and other rights.

After Age 16 What Next?
£4.00 (free to young disabled people)
Services and benefits for young disabled people.
Published by the Family Fund, PO Box 50, York, England YO1 2ZX

Benefits for People with HIV
£7.00
A handbook for advisors.
Published by The Terrence Higgins Trust, 52–54 Grays Inn Road, London WC1X 8JU

The Care Maze
£15
The law and your rights to community care in Scotland.
Published by ENABLE/The Scottish Association for Mental Health, 6th Floor, 7 Buchanan Street, Glasgow G1 3HL

CHAR's Guide To Means-Tested Benefits For Single People Without a Permanent Home
£9.50
Looks at benefits for boarders, hostel dwellers and single homeless people.
Published by CHAR, 5–15 Cromer Street, London WC1H 8LS

Child Support Handbook
£9.95 (£3.30 for individual claimants)
Published by Child Poverty Action Group (CPAG), 1–5 Bath Street, London EC1V 9PY

Community Care and the Law
£25
Published by Legal Action Group, 242 Pentonville Road, London, N1 9UN

Council Tax Handbook
£9.95
Published by Child Poverty Action Group

Fuel Rights Handbook
£9.95
Published by Child Poverty Action Group

Guide to Housing Benefit and Council Tax Benefit
£14.95
Published by the Chartered Institute of Housing/Shelter, 88 Old Street, London EC1V 9HU

Jobseeker's Allowance Handbook
£6.95 (£2.50 for individual claimants)
Published by Child Poverty Action Group

Migration & Social Security Handbook
£10.95
Published by Child Poverty Action Group

National Welfare Benefits Handbook
£8.95 (£3 for individual claimants)
Published by Child Poverty Action Group

Rights Guide To Non-Means-Tested Benefits
£8.95 (£3 for individual claimants)
Published by Child Poverty Action Group

Unemployment and Training Rights Handbook
£9.95
Published by the Unemployment Unit, 322 St John's Street, London EC1V 4NJ

Your Rights 1997–98
A guide to money benefits for older people.
£3.99
Published by Age Concern England, 1268 London Road, London SW16 4ER

Youthaid's Guide to Training & Benefits for Young People
£6.95
Available from Child Poverty Action Group

Leaflets

You can get all the DSS leaflets mentioned in this handbook from your local DSS office. If you want more than five leaflets, you can order them from:
The Stationery Office
The Causeway
Oldham Broadway Business Park
Chadderton
Oldham
OL9 9XD

Disability alliance
educational & research association

Publications list

	Price	No. Copies	Total £
Rights Publications			
❏ **Disability Rights Handbook 22nd Edition (April 1997–April 1998)** ■ Concessionary price for customers on any social security benefit *A fully comprehensive guide to all social security benefits for disabled people. Contains information on other services – community care, home renovation grants – and an extensive directory of disability organisations in Great Britain and Northern Ireland.* Note: prices may increase from 23rd edition – please phone for details.	£10.50 £6.50		
❏ **Disability Rights Bulletins – Summer, Winter and Spring.** *Update the Handbook and carry feature articles on topical issues in the disability field.*	£3.75 each		
❏ **Rights subscription** A package which includes both the Handbook and Bulletins. ■ Individuals ■ Voluntary organisations/trade unions ■ Statutory organisations/others	£15.50 £17.50 £21.50		
Research & Policy Publications			
❏ *NEW* **Endurance Test – Older people's experience of claiming Attendance Allowance (1996)** *A research report produced jointly with Help the Aged which examines how well the self-assessment process for claiming AA is working.*	£10.00		
❏ **Coalition on Charging campaign guide (1996)** *A guide for individuals and local groups covering the legal position on charges for domiciliary (non-residential) community care services, plus how to use complaints systems and ideas for lobbying.* **Please note you must order at least 5 copies.**	£1.00 each		
❏ **There May be Trouble Ahead – why occupational pensions and permanent health insurance are no substitute for a state disability income scheme (1995)** *A research report produced jointly by Disability Alliance and the Disablement Income Group which looks at the adequacy of private insurance provision.*	£6.75		
❏ **Too Young to Count – the extra mobility-related costs of disabled children under five (1994)** *A report of a nationwide survey of 84 families with disabled children under five with detailed evidence of the extra costs incurred as a result of their child's disability.*	£3.50		
❏ **Too little – too late (1992)** *A joint report from Disability Alliance and RADAR based on a national survey of claimants' and advisers' experiences of Disability Living Allowance and Disability Working Allowance.*	£3.50		

Disability Alliance Educational and Research Association. Charity No. 273128

TOTAL ORDER VALUE

Organisations can join us as members and get a free copy of all our current publications.
Tick if you would like to be sent details ❏

I/we are pleased to add a donation of

I/we enclose a cheque/postal order for

Payment must be sent with your order
If you need a pro-forma invoice please send us your official order and one will be supplied. All publications are sold post free.

Organisation (if any):

Name:

Address:

Postcode:

Send your cheque or postal order to: Disability Alliance ERA, Universal House, 88–94 Wentworth Street, London E1 7SA.
Please allow 28 days for delivery.

Address list

This section of the Handbook contains useful addresses:

1	Government Departments and Benefits Agency	Page **257**
2	A to Z of UK-wide and England organisations	Page **258**
3	A to Z of organisations in Northern Ireland	Page **266**
4	A to Z of organisations in Scotland	Page **267**
5	A to Z of organisations in Wales	Page **268**
6	DIAL UK member groups	Page **268**
7	London-wide organisations	Page **269**
8	Law Centres	Page **269**

Using the address list

Below is a list of names and addresses of a number of general and specialist organisations, all dealing in some way with disability issues. The main A-Z listing contains organisations which cover England, or have a broader eg UK-wide, remit. There are separate lists for organisations based in Northern Ireland, Scotland and Wales. We do not have sufficient space to list locally based organisations and instead provide a list of DIAL UK local groups as a first point of contact.

Each list is organised alphabetically, with entries beginning with the words National, British etc listed by the disability or community which they serve, eg 'Schizophrenia Fellowship, National' or 'Black Mental Health Association, National'.

Acronyms such as RNIB (Royal National Institute for the Blind) are listed by disability (Blind) or remit of work (CHAR – see Housing).

Government Departments and Benefits Agency

Benefits Agency, Chief Executive's Office, Room 4C06, Quarry House, Quarry Hill, Leeds LS2 7UA (0113 232 4000)
Department for Education and Employment, Disability Services, Rockingham House, 123 West Street, Sheffield S1 4ER (0114 275 3275)
Department of Social Security, The Adelphi, 1–11 John Adam Street, London WC2N 6HT (0171 962 8000)
Department of Transport, Mobility Unit, 1/11 Great Minster House, 76 Marsham Street, London SW1P 4DR (Voice and Minicom 0171 271 5252)

Disability Benefits Centres

Olympic House, Olympic Way, Wembley, Middlesex HA9 0DL (0181 795 8400)
Deals with claims from London postal districts EC1–EC4, E1–E18, N1–N27, NW1–NW11, W2–W5, W7, W9–W13, Buckinghamshire, Bedfordshire, Cambridgeshire, Essex, Hertfordshire, Middlesex (except Hounslow and Twickenham), Oxfordshire, Suffolk, Norfolk.

Five Ways Complex, Frederick Road, Edgbaston, Birmingham B15 1SL (0121 626 2000)
Deals with claims from West Midlands, Shropshire, Hereford and Worcester, Staffordshire, Leicestershire, Warwickshire, Northamptonshire, Derbyshire, Nottinghamshire, Lincolnshire.
Government Buildings, Otley Road, Lawnswood, Leeds LS16 5PU (0113 230 9000)
Deals with claims from North Lincolnshire, Yorkshire, Humberside.
Regent Centre, Arden House, Regent Centre, Gosforth, Newcastle upon Tyne NE3 3JN (0191 223 3000)
Deals with claims from Tyne and Wear, Durham, Northumberland, Cleveland.
St Martin's House, Stanley Precinct, Bootle, Merseyside L69 9BN (0151 934 6000)
Deals with claims from Merseyside, Central and North-West Lancashire, Cumbria, North, South and West Cheshire.
Albert Bridge House, Bridge Street, Manchester M60 9DA (0161 831 2000)
Deals with claims from Greater Manchester, East Lancashire, Derbyshire (High Peak), East Cheshire.
Sutherland House, 29–37 Brighton Road, Sutton, Surrey SM2 5AN (0181 652 6000)
Deals with claims from London postal districts WC1 and WC2, SE1–SE28, SW1–SW20, W1, W6, W8 and W14, Hounslow, Twickenham, Berkshire, Hampshire, Surrey, Kent, East Sussex, West Sussex, Isle of Wight.

Government Buildings, Flowers Hill, Bristol BS4 5LA (0117 971 8311)
Deals with claims from Cornwall, Devon, Avon, Gloucestershire, Wiltshire, Somerset, Dorset.
Northern Ireland Disability Benefits Administration Centre, Castlecourt, Royal Avenue, Belfast BT1 1DF (01232 336556)
Deals with claims from all over Northern Ireland.
Edinburgh Disability Benefits Centre, Argyle House, 3 Lady Lawson Street, Edinburgh EH3 0XY (0131 229 9191; Minicom 0131 222 5494)
Deals with claims from all over Scotland except Strathclyde.
Glasgow Disability Benefits Centre, 29 Cadogan Street, Glasgow G2 7BN (0141 249 3500)
Deals with claims from Strathclyde (Postal districts G, KA, ML, PA)
Wales Disability Benefits Centre, Government Buildings, St Agnes Road, Gabalfa, Cardiff CF4 4YJ (01222 586002)
Deals with claims from all over Wales.

Central Units

Child Benefit Centre, (Washington), Newcastle upon Tyne NE88 1BR (0541 555501)
Disability Appeal Tribunals Central Office, PO Box 168, Nottingham NG1 5JX (0345 247246)

Disability Benefits Unit, Warbreck House, Warbreck Hill Road, Blackpool, Lancashire FY2 0YE (0345 123456; Textphone 0345 224433)
Handles all disability living allowance and attendance allowance claims (except initial claim which is processed by Disability Benefits Centres listed above).

Disability Working Allowance Unit, Freepost PR1211, Preston, Lancashire PR2 2TF (01772 883300)
Processes all disability working allowance claims.

Family Credit Unit, Government Buildings, 1 Cop Lane, Penwortham, Preston, Lancashire PR1 0SA (01253 500050; Textphone 01253 500504)
Deals with all family credit claims.

Independent Review Service for the Social Fund, 4th Floor, Centre City Podium, 5 Hill Street, Birmingham B5 4UB (0121 606 2100)

Independent Tribunal Service, Office of the, Whittington House, 19–30 Alfred Place, London WC1E 9LW (0171 957 9200)
Deals with Disability Appeal Tribunals, Social Security Appeal Tribunals, Medical Appeal Tribunals, Child Support Appeal Tribunals and Vaccine Damage Tribunals.

Independent Tribunal Service, Northern Ireland, President: Mr CG MacLynn, 6th Floor, Cleaver House, 3 Donegal Square North, Belfast BT1 5GA (01232 539900)

Invalid Care Allowance Unit, Palatine House, Lancaster Road, Preston, Lancashire PR1 1NS (01253 856123)
Deals with all invalid care allowance claims.

Medical Service, Benefits Agency (BAMS), Dr C Hudson, Director of Medical Services, Room 124, Albert Edward House, 3 The Pavilions, Ashton-on-Ribble, Preston PR2 2PA (01772 898052)

Overseas Benefits Directorate, Tyneview Park, Whitley Road, Benton, Newcastle upon Tyne NE98 1BA (0191 218 7878; Textphone 0191 218 2160)

Social Security and Child Support Commissioners England and Wales, Office of the, Harp House, 83 Farringdon Street, London EC4A 4DH (0171 353 5145)

Social Security and Child Support Commissioners Northern Ireland, Office of the, Lancashire House, 5 Linenhall Street, Belfast BT2 8AA (01232 332344)

Social Security and Child Support Commissioners Scotland, Office of the, 23 Melville Street, Edinburgh EH3 7PW (0131 225 2201)

Phone Lines

Disability Living Allowance Central Telephone Answering Unit 0345 123456
For claimants with an enquiry on their disability living allowance claim or for general enquiries on disability benefits.

Disability Working Allowance Central Telephone Answering Unit 01772 883300
For claimants with an enquiry on their disability working allowance claim.

Family Credit Helpline 01253 500050
Advice and information on family credit.

Benefit Enquiry Line (BEL) 0800 882200; Textphone 0800 243355 (in Northern Ireland 0800 220674; Textphone 0800 243787)
BEL specialises in benefits for people with disabilities their carers and representatives. BEL has no access to personal records and so provides general advice only.

Disability Working Allowance Response Line 0800 444000
Information and leaflets but not advice.

Forms Completion Service 0800 441144
Help over the telephone to fill in disability related benefit claim packs. This service can also be provided in Braille and Large Print.

Incapacity Benefit Line 0800 868868
Provides information and leaflets but cannot give advice.

Senior Line 0800 650065
General benefit advice and information for older people, run by Help the Aged.

England and UK-wide organisations

A

Access Committee for England, 12 City Forum, 250 City Road, London EC1V 8AF (0171 250 0008; Minicom 0171 250 4119)
National focal point on access issues.

Achondroplasia Group – see Child Growth Foundation

Across Trust, Bridge House, 70–72 Bridge Road, East Molesey, Surrey KT8 9HF (0181 783 1355)
Provides accompanied holidays for disabled people. Also provides accessible transport.

Acupuncture Council, The British, Park House, 206 Latimer Road, London W10 6RE (0181 964 0222)
Handbook with directory of practitioners in UK and abroad, £3.50.

AFASIC, Overcoming Speech Impairments, 347 Central Markets, London EC1A 9NH (0171 236 3632)
Information and advice.

African-Caribbean Mental Health Association, 35–37 Electric Avenue, London SW9 8JP (0171 737 3603)
Counselling, group work, legal, advocacy and befriending.

African-Caribbeans, Organisation of Blind, 1st Floor, Gloucester House, 8 Camberwell New Road, London SE5 0RZ (0171 735 3400)

Age Concern England, Astral House, 1268 London Road, London SW16 4ER (0181 679 8000)

AIDS Ahead, c/o British Deaf Association, Health Promotion Unit, 17 Macon Court, Herald Drive, Crewe, Cheshire CW1 6EE (01270 250736; Minicom 01270 250743)
Information and counselling for deaf people on health issues (particularly HIV and AIDS).

AIDS Helpline, National 0800 567123; Minicom 0800 521 361
Confidential advice by trained advisers. Ethnic minority language lines
    Welsh 0800 371131 10am–2pm Monday – Friday
    Cantonese 0800 282446 6–10pm Mondays
    Bengali 0800 371132 6–10pm Tuesdays
    Punjabi 0800 371133, Hindi 0800 371136, Urdu 0800 371134, Gujarati 0800 371134 all 6–10pm Wednesdays
    Arabic 0800 282447 6–10pm Thursdays

AIDS Trust, National, New City Cloisters, 188–196 Old Street, London EC1V 9FR (0171 814 6767)

Al-Anon Family Groups, 61 Great Dover Street, London SE1 4YF (Helpline 0171 403 0888)
Self-help groups for relatives and friends of problem drinkers.

Alateen, 61 Great Dover Street, London SE1 4YF (Helpline 0171 403 0888)
Part of Al-Anon, for young people aged 12–20 affected by a problem drinker.

Alcohol Concern, Waterbridge House, 32–36 Loman Street, London SE1 0EE (0171 928 7377)

Alcoholics Anonymous, PO Box 1, Stonebow House, Stonebow, York YO1 2NJ (01904 644026; Helpline 10am – 10pm 0171 352 3001)

Alzheimer's Disease Society, Gordon House, 10 Greencoat Place, London SW1P 1PH (0171 306 0606)
Advice and support for those coping with dementia.

Amnesia – see Headway

Ankylosing Spondylitis Society, National, 3 Grosvenor Crescent, London SW1X 7ER (0171 235 9585)

Ann's Neurological Trust Society (ANTS), 1 Abbey Drive, Little Heywood, Stafford ST18 0QQ
Self-help groups UK wide.

ARISE (The Scoliosis Research Trust), Graham Hill Building, Royal National Orthopaedic Trust, Brockley Hill, Stanmore HA7 4LP (0181 954 8939)
Information available for patients and professionals.
Army Benevolent Fund, 41 Queen's Gate, London SW7 5HR (0171 584 5235)
Arthritic Association, 1st Floor Suite, 2 Hyde Gardens, Eastbourne BN21 4PN
Promotes natural methods of treating arthritis.
Arthritis, Horder Centre for, St John's Road, Crowborough, East Sussex TN6 1XP (01892 665577)
Rehabilitation, long- and short-term nursing and orthopaedic surgery.
Arthritis and Rheumatism Council, Copeman House, St Mary's Court, St Mary's Gate, Chesterfield, Derbyshire S41 7TD (01246 558033)
Range of information leaflets available, please send sae.
Arthritis Care, 18 Stephenson Way, London NW1 2HD (0171 916 1500; Freephone Helpline 0800 289170)
Action by and for people with arthritis.
Arthritis Care, Young, 18 Stephenson Way, London NW1 2HD (0171 916 1500)
Information and self-help.
Arthrogryposis Group (TAG), Mrs D Piercy, 1 The Oaks, Gillingham, Dorset SP8 4SW (01747 822655)
Contacts, support and information for parents, affected adults and professionals.
ASBAH (Association for Spina Bifida and Hydrocephalus), ASBAH House, 42 Park Road, Peterborough PE1 2UQ (01733 555988)
Asian Peoples with Disabilities Alliance (APDA), The Disability Alliance Centre, The Old Refectory, Central Middlesex Hospital, Acton Lane, London NW10 7NS (0181 961 6773)
Respite care, advice and advocacy, daycare for elderly Asians and disabled people.
Asian Women and Stress Project, Shanti, Health Promotion Services, Coventry Health Authority, Ground Floor Annexe, Christchurch House, Greyfriars Lane, Coventry CV1 2GA (01203 633066)
Produces videos in five Asian languages on helping Asian women deal with stress.
Asians, Association of Blind, 322 Upper Street, London N1 2XQ (0171 226 1950)
Organisation of blind and partially sighted Asian people.
Asthma Campaign, National, Providence House, Providence Place, London N1 0NT (0171 226 2260; Helpline 0345 010203)
Ataxia, The Stable, Wiggins Yard, Bridge Street, Godalming, Surrey GU7 1HW (01483 417111)
Friedreich's, Cerebellar and others. Information, advice and support.

Autistic Society, National, 276 Willesden Lane, London NW2 5RB (0181 451 1114)

B

Back Pain Association, National, 16 Elmtree Road, Teddington, Middlesex TW11 8ST (0181 977 5474)
Information service and local branch support.
Barnardo's, Tanners Lane, Barkingside, Essex IG6 1QG (0181 550 8822)
BHAN (Black HIV, AIDS Network), 1st Floor, St Stephen House, 41 Uxbridge Road, London W12 8LH (0181 749 2828)
Black Mental Health Association, National, c/o Roachford Trust, 70 Grand Parade, Green Lanes, London N4 1DU (0181 800 2039)
Blackliners, Unit 46, Eurolink Business Centre, 49 Effra Road, London SW2 1BZ (0171 738 5274)
AIDS and HIV advice, counselling and support for black people.
Blind, General Welfare of the, 37–55 Ashburton Grove, London N7 7DW (0171 609 0206)
Blind, Guide Dogs for the, Hillfields, Burghfield, Reading RG7 3YG (01734 835555)
Blind, National Federation of the, Unity House, Smyth Street, Wakefield, West Yorkshire WF1 1ER (01924 291313)
Pressure and campaigning group.
Blind, National Library for the, Cromwell Road, Bredbury, Stockport, Cheshire SK6 2SG (0161 494 0217)
Free lending service in Braille, Moon and large print.
Blind, Royal National Institute for the (RNIB), 224 Great Portland Street, London W1N 6AA (0171 388 1266; Tape, Braille and equipment service 0345 023153)
Blind and Disabled, National League of the, 2 Tenterden Road, London N17 8BE (0181 808 6030)
Registered trade union of blind and disabled people.
Blind People, Action for, 14–16 Verney Road, London SE16 3DZ (0171 732 8771)
Employment, grants, information and benefits advice.
Bliss – Baby Life Support Systems, 17–21 Emerald Street, London WC1N 3QL (0171 831 9393; Freephone Helpline for parents 0500 151617)
Supports families of a 'special care' baby.
Body Positive, 51b Philbeach Gardens, London SW5 9EB (0171 835 1045; Helpline 0171 373 9124)
Drop-in centre and nightly Helpline for people living with and affected by HIV and AIDS.
Bone Dysplasia – see Child Growth Foundation

Break, 20 Hooks Hill Road, Sheringham, Norfolk NR26 8NL (01263 823170)
Holidays for people with physical and mental learning difficulties.
Breakthrough, Deaf-Hearing Integration, Birmingham Centre, Charles W Gillett Centre, 998 Bristol Road, Birmingham B29 6LE (0121 472 6447; Minicom 0121 471 1001)
Promotes the integration of deaf people into society. Outreach and information service for deafened people of all ages.
Breast Cancer Care, Kiln House, 210 New Kings Road, London SW6 4NZ (0171 384 2984; Helpline Freephone 0500 245345)
Information, practical and emotional support.
British Legion, Royal, 48 Pall Mall, London SW1Y 5JY (0171 973 7200)
Brittle Bone Society, 30 Guthrie Street, Dundee, DD2 2PW (01382 204446/7)

C

Calibre, Aylesbury, Bucks HP22 5XQ (01296 432339/81211)
Free cassette library for blind or disabled children & adults.
Camping for the Disabled, 20 Burton Close, Dawley, Telford, Shropshire TF4 2BX (evenings 01952 507653; day 01743 761889)
Gives details of campsites abroad.
Cancer, Association for New Approaches to, 5 Larksfield, Egham, Surrey TW20 0RB (01784 433610)
Information on therapies.
Cancer Care, Marie Curie, 28 Belgrave Square, London SW1X 8QG (0171 235 3325)
Provides nursing care at home and in centres.
Cancer Care Society, 21 Zetland Road, Redland, Bristol BS6 7AH (0117 942 7419)
Emotional support to those who have been affected by cancer.
Cancerlink, 11–21 Northdown Street, London N1 9BN (Freephone Helplines 0800 132905; Asian – Bengali, Hindi, Punjabi, Urdu 0800 590415; MAC Helpline for young people affected by cancer 0800 591028)
Support for anyone affected by cancer. List of local groups available.
Cancer Prevention Advice, Clinic for, 6 New Road, Brighton, East Sussex BN1 1UF (01273 727213)
Check-up including cholesterol, mammography, ultrasound osteoporosis assessment, health counselling etc.
Cancer Relief, Macmillan, 15–19 Britten Street, London SW3 3TZ (0171 351 7811)
Information and financial help offered.
Cancer Research Campaign, 10 Cambridge Terrace, London NW1 4JL (0171 224 1333)

Cancer United Patients, British Association of (BACUP), 3 Bath Place, London EC2A 3JR (0171 696 9003; Freephone information 0800 181199; One-to-one counselling 0171 696 9000; Glasgow 0141 553 1553)
Information, counselling and support to anyone affected by cancer.
Car Purchase, Disabled, 114 Commonwealth Road, Caterham, Surrey CR3 6LS (01883 345298)
Specialist vehicle supply.
Care and Repair, Castle House, Kirtley Drive, Nottingham NG7 1LD (0115 979 9091)
Carers National Association, 20–25 Glasshouse Yard, London EC1A 4JS (0171 490 8818; Advice 0171 490 8898)
Informs and supports carers. Brings needs of carers to the attention of government.
Catholic Housing Aid Society, 209 Old Marylebone Road, London NW1 5QT (0171 723 7273; Advice 0171 723 5928)
Cerebral Palsy – see Scope
CHAR – see Housing Campaign for Single People
Child Growth Foundation, 2 Mayfield Avenue, London W4 1PW (0181 994 7625)
Supports families and patients who have conditions which affect growth.
Child Poverty Action Group (CPAG), 1–5 Bath Street, London EC1V 9PY (0171 253 3406)
Childcare Campaign, National, The Daycare Trust, 4 Wild Court, London WC2B 4AU (Helpline 0171 405 5617)
Advice on child care services.
Children, NCH Action for, 85 Highbury Park, London N5 1UD (0171 226 2033)
Community and residential projects for children with disabilities.
Children, Council for Disabled, 8 Wakley Street, London EC1V 7QE (0171 843 6058)
Children, Lady Hoare Trust for Physically Disabled, 44–46 Fleet Street, London EC4Y 1BN
Practical and financial support to children with arthritic conditions and limb deficiencies.
Children in Hospital – Action for Sick Children, Argyle House, 29–31 Euston Road, London NW1 2SD (0171 833 2041)
Children with Heart Disorders, The Association for, Mrs G Hitchen, 26 Elizabeth Drive, Helmshore, Rossendale, Lancashire BB4 4JB (01706 213632)
Children with Tracheostomies, Aid for (ACT), 215a Perry Street, Billericay, Essex CM12 0NZ (01277 654425)
Children's Legal Centre, University of Essex, Wivenhoe Park, Colchester, Essex CO4 3SQ

Children's Liver Disease Foundation, 138 Digbeth, Birmingham B5 6DR (0121 643 7282)
Funds research, provides education and gives emotional support.
Children's Society, The (registered as Church of England Children's Society), Edward Rudolf House, 69–85 Margery Street, London WC1X 0JL (0171 837 4299)
Chinese Mental Health Association, c/o Ginny Lee, Oxford House, Derbyshire Street, London E2 6HG (0171 613 1008)
Citizen Advocacy Information and Training (CAIT), Unit 2K, Leroy House, 436 Essex Road, London N1 3QP (0171 359 8289)
Citizens Advice Bureaux, National Association of (NACAB), Myddelton House, 115–123 Pentonville Road, London N1 9LZ (0171 833 2181)
Will provide details of your local Citizens Advice Bureau.
Colitis and Crohn's Disease, National Association for, 4 Beaumont House, Sutton Road, St Albans, Hertfordshire AL1 5HH (Answerphone 01727 844296)
Colostomy Association, British, 15 Station Road, Reading, Berkshire RG11LG (0118 9391537)
Advice on having a colostomy and rehabilitation.
Combat Stress (Ex-Services Mental Welfare Society), Broadway House, The Broadway, London SW19 1RL (0181 543 6333)
Communication for the Disabled, Foundation for, Beacon House, Pyrford Road, West Byfleet, Surrey KT14 6LD (01932 336512)
Supplies computer systems designed for disabled people.
Community Health Councils for England and Wales, Association of, Earlsmead House, 30 Drayton Park, London N5 1PB (0171 609 8405)
Community Service Volunteers, 237 Pentonville Road, London N1 9NJ (0171 278 6601)
Full-time volunteers involved in independent living, home care etc.
Compassionate Friends, 53 North Street, Bedminster, Bristol BS3 1EN (Helpline 0117 953 9639)
Support for bereaved parents.
Computability Centre, The, PO Box 94, Warwick CV34 5WS (Voice and Minicom 01926 312847)
Helps disabled people through the use of computers at work, at home, in education.
Contact a Family, 170 Tottenham Court Road, London W1 0HA (0171 383 3555)
Advice and help for families caring for disabled children.

Contact the Elderly, 15 Henrietta Street, London WC2E 8QH (0171 240 0630)
Friendship and regular monthly outings for elderly people who live alone without family support.
Continence Foundation, 2 Doughty Street, London WC1N 2PH (Helpline 0191 213 0050 Mon–Fri 9am–6pm)
Counselling, British Association for, 1 Regent Place, Rugby, Warwickshire CV21 2PJ (01788 578328)
Directory of counselling agencies, local agencies also available on receipt of A4 sae.
Cranio Facial Support Group, c/o Steve Moody, 44 Helmsdale Road, Leamington Spa, Warwickshire CV32 7DW (01926 334629)
Crossroads Care, 10 Regent Place, Rugby, Warwickshire CV21 2PN (01788 573653)
Professional support to carers and people with care needs. Services in England, Wales and N. Ireland.
Cruse Bereavement Care, 126 Sheen Road, London TW9 1UR (0181 940 4818; Bereavement Care Line 0181 332 7227)
Counselling and advice to all bereaved people.
Crypt (Creative Young People Together), Forum Workspace, Stirling Road, Chichester, West Sussex PO19 2EN (01243 786064)
Opportunities for disabled young people to live in small group homes.
Cued Speech, National Centre for, 29–30 Watling Street, Canterbury, Kent CT1 2UD (01227 450757)
Cystic Fibrosis Trust, Alexandra House, 5 Blyth Road, Bromley, Kent BR1 3RS (0181 464 7211)
Cystic Hygroma and Lymphangioma Support Group, Villa Fontane, Church Road, Worth, Crawley, West Sussex RH10 4RS (01293 883901)
Contact between parents to share experiences, information, problems.

D

Deaf People, Friends for Young (FYD), East Court Mansion, College Lane, East Grinstead RH19 3LT (01342 323444; Minicom 01342 312639)
Deaf Association, The British, 1–3 Worship Street, London EC2A 2AB (0171 588 3520; Minicom 0171 588 3529)
Deaf Children's Society, National, 15 Dufferin Street, London EC1Y 8PD (Voice and Minicom 0171 250 0123; Freephone 0800 252380)
Deaf People, Royal Association in Aid of, 27 Old Oak Road, London W3 7HN (0181 743 6187; Minicom 0181 749 7561)

Deaf People, Royal National Institute for (RNID), 19–23 Featherstone Street, London EC1Y 8SL (0171 296 8000; Text 0171 296 8001; Tinnitus Helpline 0345 090210)
Local information service via regional offices (list available).
Also: John Wood House, Glacier Building, Harrington Road, Brunswick Business Park, Liverpool L3 4DF (0151 709 9494; Text 0800 500888 (CCITT))
Text users' help scheme, Typetalk national telephone relay service, text rebate scheme.
Deafblind UK, 100 Bridge Street, Peterborough, Cambs PE1 1DY (01733 358100)
Deafblind and Rubella Association, The National (SENSE), 11–13 Clifton Terrace, London N4 3SR (0171 272 7774; Minicom 0171 272 9648)
Deafened People – Link, The British Centre for, 19 Hartfield Road, Eastbourne, East Sussex BN21 2AR (Voice and Minicom 01323 638230)
Residential courses for deafened adults and their families.
DEBRA – see Dystrophic Epidermolysis Bullosa Research Association
Demonstration Centre, National, Pinderfields Hospitals NHS Trust, Aberford Road, Wakefield, West Yorkshire WF1 4DG (01924 814856)
Information on disability aids.
Depression Alliance, PO Box 1022, London SE1 7QB (Answerphone 0171 721 7672)
Self-help for depressives and their families. Send sae for details.
Diabetic Association, British, 10 Queen Anne Street, London W1M 0BD (0171 323 1531)
Information and advice on diabetes.
DIAL UK, St Catherine's Hospital, Park Lodge, Tickhill Road, Balby, Doncaster DN4 8QN (01302 310123)
Supports UK-wide disability information and advice services. See DIAL groups listing.
Disability Equipment Register, 4 Chatterton Road, Yate, Bristol BS17 4BJ (01454 318818)
Nationwide service to buy and sell used disabled equipment.
Disability Law Service – see Law Centres section
Disabled Access to Technology Association, Broomfield House, Bolling Road, Bradford BD4 7BG (01274 370019)
Provides training in computing, CAD, Internet & Email and DTP for people with physical and/or sensory disabilities.
Disabled Christians' Fellowship, 213 Wick Road, Brislington, Bristol BS4 4HP (0117 983 0388)
Fellowship by correspondence, cassettes, local branches, holidays, youth section.

Disabled Drivers' Association, The, National Headquarters, Ashwellthorpe, Norwich NR16 1EX (01508 489449)
Self-help association aiming for independence through mobility.
Disabled Drivers' Motor Club, Cottingham Way, Thrapston, Northamptonshire NN14 4PL (01832 734724)
Offers advice on all problems for the disabled motorist and family.
Disabled Housing Trust, First Floor, Market Place, Burgess Hill, West Sussex RH15 9NP (01444 239123)
Disabled Living Centres Council, 1st Floor, Winchester House, 11 Cranmer Road, London SW9 6EJ (Voice and Text 0171 820 0567)
Co-ordinates work of Disabled Living Centres UK wide. List of centres available.
Disabled Motorists Federation, National Mobility Centre, Unit 2a, Atcham Estate, Shrewsbury SY4 4UG (01743 761181)
Disabled People, British Council of Organisations of (BCODP), Litchurch Plaza, Litchurch Lane, Derby DE24 8AA (01332 295551; Minicom 01332 295581)
Disabled People, Queen Elizabeth's Foundation for, Leatherhead, Surrey KT22 0BN (01372 842204)
Works with disabled people to increase abilities and independence.
Disabled Professionals, Association of, Chair: Sue Maynard Campbell, 170 Benton Hill, Wakefield Road, Horbury, West Yorkshire WF4 5HW (01924 283253; Minicom 01924 270335)
Disablement Income Group, The (DIG), Unit 5, Archway Business Centre, 19–23 Wedmore Street, London N19 4RZ (0171 263 3981)
Works to improve the financial circumstances of disabled people through advice, advocacy, information and research.
DISCERN (Disability Information Service for Sexuality Counselling, Education and Research Nottingham), Suite 6, Clarendon Chambers, Clarendon Street, Nottingham NG1 5LN (0115 947 4147)
Disfigurement Guidance Centre – Laserfair, PO Box 7, Cupar, Fife KY15 4PF, Scotland (01334 839084)
Information, help, publications. Stamped addressed envelope essential for reply.
Down's Heart Group, Mrs M Clayton, 17 Hall Hill, Bollington, Macclesfield, Cheshire SK10 5ED (01625 572417)
Down's Syndrome Association, 155 Mitcham Road, London SW17 9PG (0181 682 4001)
Drug Abuse, Standing Conference on (SCODA), Waterbridge House, 32–36 Loman Street, London SE1 0EE (0171 928 9500)

Dyslexia Association, British, 98 London Road, Reading, Berkshire RG1 5AU (0118 966 2677; Helpline 01189 66 8271)
Dyslexia Institute, 133 Gresham Road, Staines, Middlesex TW18 2AJ (01784 463851)
Educational assessment, teaching, training and advice.
Dyslexia Organisation, Adult, c/o 336 Brixton Road, London SW9 7AA (0171 737 7646; Advice 0171 924 9559)
Dysphasic Adults, Action for, 1 Royal Street, London SE1 7LL (0171 261 9572)
Advice and help for those with a language impairment following a stroke, head injury or other neurological conditions.
Dystonia Society, Weddel House, 13–14 West Smithfield, London EC1A 9HY (0171 329 0797)
Dystrophic Epidermolysis Bullosa Research Association (DEBRA), Debra House, 13 Wellington Business Park, Dukes Ride, Crowthorne, Berkshire RG45 6LS (01344 771961)

E

Eating Disorders Association, National Information Centre, 44–48 Magdalen Street, Norwich NR3 1JU (Helpline 01603 621414; Youth helpline 01603 675050)
Eczema Society, National, 163 Eversholt Street, London NW1 1BU (0171 388 4097)
Education, The Alliance for Inclusive, Unit 2, 70 South Lambeth Road, London SW8 1RL (0171 735 5277)
Campaigns for a national policy to achieve an inclusive education system.
Endometriosis Society, The National, 50 Westminster Palace Gardens, 1–7 Artillery Row, London SW1P 1RL (0171 222 2781; for current helpline numbers ring 0171 222 2776)
Environmental Therapy, Society for, Mrs H Davidson, 521 Foxhall Road, Ipswich, Suffolk IP3 8LW (01473 723552)
Works to discover the environmental causes of disease. Advises on low technology medicine.
Environments, Centre for Accessible, 60 Gainsford Street, London SE1 2NY (Voice and Minicom 0171 357 8182)
Information, training and consultancy on the design of accessible buildings.
Epilepsy, National Society for, Chalfont St Peter, Gerrards Cross, Buckinghamshire SL9 0RJ (01494 601300)
Assessment, rehabilitation, long-term care, advice and local groups.

Epilepsy Association, British, Anstey House, 40 Hanover Square, Leeds LS3 1BE (0113 243 9393; Freephone Helpline 0800 309030)
Equal Opportunities Commission, Overseas House, Quay Street, Manchester M3 3HN (0161 833 9244)

F

Family Fund Trust, The, PO Box 50, York YO1 2ZX (01904 621115)
Financial help and information for families with severely disabled children.
Family Rights Group, The Print House, 18 Ashwin Street, London E8 3DL (Advice 0171 249 0008)
Family Service Units, 207 Old Marylebone Road, London NW1 5QP (0171 402 5175)
Projects providing help to families under pressure.
Family Welfare Association, 501–505 Kingsland Road, London E8 4AU (0171 254 6251)
Services and grants for families in need.
Far East (Prisoners of War and Internees) Fund, 30 Copsewood Way, Bearsted, Maidstone, Kent ME15 8PL (01622 737124)
Foster Care Association, National, Leonard House, 5–7 Marshalsea Road, London SE1 1EP (0171 828 6266)
Free Representation Unit, Room 140, 49–51 Bedford Row, London WC1R 4LR (0171 831 0692)
Claimants requiring representation must contact the Free Representation Unit via a Citizens Advice Bureau or Law Centre. FRU is exclusively a representation service.

G

Gemma, BM Box 5700, London WC1N 3XX
National friendship network of lesbian and bisexual women.
Gingerbread, 16–17 Clerkenwell Close, London EC1R 0AA (0171 336 8183; Advice 0171 336 8184)
Support network for lone parent families.
GLAD – Greater London Association of Disabled People – see London-wide section
Growth Hormone Insufficiency – see Child Growth Foundation
Guideposts Trust, Two Rivers, Witney, Oxfordshire OX8 6BH (01993 772886)
Guillain-Barre Syndrome Support Group, c/o Lincolnshire County Council, Council Offices, Sleaford, Lincolnshire NG34 7EB (01529 304615)

H

Haemophilia Society, 123 Westminster Bridge Road, London SE1 7HR (0171 928 2020)

Handicapped Children's Aid Committee, Mrs Emden, 11 Fairholme Gardens, London N3 3ED (0181 349 2829)
Handihols, 12 Ormonde Avenue, Rochford, Essex SS4 1QW (01702 548257)
House exchange or hospitality scheme for disabled people.
HAPA, Pryor's Bank, Bishop's Park, London SW6 3LA (0171 731 1435; Text minicom 0171 384 2596)
Adventure play for disabled children.
Headway, National Head Injuries Association Ltd, 7 King Edward Court, King Edward Street, Nottingham NG1 1EW (0115 924 0800)
Help, information and support to people with problems created by head injuries.
Hearing Concern, 7–11 Armstrong Road, London W3 7JL (Voice and Minicom 0181 743 1110)
Self-help clubs, advisory and information service for deaf and hard of hearing people.
Heart Foundation, British, 14 Fitzhardinge Street, London W1H 4DH (0171 935 0185)
Help for Health Trust, Highcroft, Romsey Road, Winchester SO22 5DH (Freephone 0800 665544)
Information service on health and self-help groups.
Help the Aged, St James's Walk, London EC1R 0BE (0171 253 0253; Freephone Advice 0800 650065)
Range of free advice leaflets available.
Holiday Care Service, 2nd Floor, Imperial Buildings, Victoria Road, Horley, Surrey RH6 7PZ (01293 774535)
Holiday information and support.
Holiday Homes Trust, Scouts, Baden Powell House, Queen's Gate, London SW7 5JS (0171 584 7030)
Source of holiday and travel information for disabled and disadvantaged people (no scouting connection necessary).
Holidays, Help the Handicapped (3H Fund), 147a Camden Road, Tunbridge Wells, Kent TN1 2RA (01892 547474)
Contact Peggie King (holiday organiser).
Home Farm Trust Ltd, Merchants House, Wapping Road, Bristol BS1 4RW (0117 927 3746)
Individual care service for people with learning disabilities.
Homeopathic Association, British, 27a Devonshire Street, London W1N 1RJ (0171 935 2163)
Send sae for information.
Horticultural Therapy, Society for, Goulds Ground, Vallis Way, Frome, Somerset BA11 3DW (01373 464782)
Advice service to disabled gardeners.
Housing Campaign for Single People (CHAR), 5–15 Cromer Street, London WC1H 8LS (0171 833 2071)

Housing Service, National Disabled Person's, Brunswick House, Deighton Close, Wetherby, West Yorkshire LS22 7GZ (01937 588 580)
Promoting and supporting the creation of local disabled person's housing services.
Huntington's Disease Association, 108 Battersea High Street, London SW11 3HP (0171 223 7000)
Hyperactive Children's Support Group, 71 Whyke Lane, Chichester, West Sussex PO19 2LD (01903 725182)

I

Ileostomy and Internal Pouch Support Group (IA), Amblehurst House, PO Box 23, Mansfield, Nottinghamshire NG18 4TT (01623 28099)
Helps people return to active lives following surgery for removal of the colon. Local groups UK wide.
Immigrants, Joint Council for the Welfare of, 115 Old Street, London EC1V 9JR (0171 251 8708; Adviceline 0171 251 8706 Mon/Tues/Thurs 2–5pm)
In Touch Trust, 10 Norman Road, Sale, Cheshire M33 3DF (0161 905 2440)
For parents of children with special needs.
Incapacity Action, 65 Casimir Road, Clapton, London E5 9NU
Campaigning group working for rights for long-term sick and disabled people.
Independent Living Alternatives, Trafalgar House, Grenville Place, London NW7 3SA (0181 906 9265)
Independent Living Fund, PO Box 183, Nottingham NG8 3RD (0115 942 8191)
Independent Living, National Centre for, 250 Kennington Lane, London SE11 5RD (0171 587 1663)
Provides information, consultancy and training on personal assistance and direct payments.
Invalid Children's Aid Nationwide (ICAN), Barbican Citygate, 1–3 Dufferin Street, London EC1Y 8NA (0171 374 4422)
Irritable Bowel Syndrome Network, St John's House, Hither Green Hospital, Hither Green Lane, London SE13 6RU (0181 698 4611 ext 8194; 10.30am–1.30pm Mon/Wed/Fri.)
Send A4 or A5 sae for information.

J

JCWI – see Immigrants, Joint Council for the Welfare of
Jewish Association for the Mentally Ill (JAMI), 707 High Road, London N12 0BT (0181 343 1111)
Jewish Blind and Physically Handicapped Society, 164 East End Road, London N2 0RR (0181 883 1000)
Sheltered housing and welfare services.

Jewish Care, 17 Highfield Road, London NW11 9LS (0181 381 4816)
Services to people with a visual impairment or a physical disability.
Jewish Deaf Association, Resource Centre, 90 Cazenove Road, London N16 (0181 806 2028), also at 21a Accommodation Road, London NW11 (0181 455 1557)
Jewish Society for the Mentally Handicapped – see Norwood Ravenswood
John Grooms Association for Disabled People, 50 Scrutton Street, London EC2A 4PH (0171 452 2000)
Provides residential care, housing, holidays and work.

K

Kidney Patient Association, British, Bordon, Hampshire GU35 9JZ (01420 472021)
Financial help, advice and counselling. One holiday dialysis centre available.
Kidney Research Fund, National, 3 Archers Court, Stukeley Road, Huntingdon, Cambridgeshire PE18 6XG (01480 454828)
Funds research, trains doctors, provides equipment and supports kidney patients.
Kurdish Disability Organisation, Manor Gardens Centre, 6–9 Manor Gardens, London N7 6LA (0171 727 4231 ext 211)

L

LAGER (Lesbian and Gay Employment Rights), Unit 1G, Leroy House, 436 Essex Road, London N1 3QP (Voice and minicom Lesbians 0171 704 8066; Gay men 0171 704 6066)
Laryngectomy Clubs, National Association of, Ground Floor, 6 Rickett Street, London SW6 1RU (0171 381 9993)
Law Centres Federation, Duchess House, 18–19 Warren Street, London W1P 5DB (0171 387 8570)
Also: 3rd Floor, Arundel Court, 177 Arundel Street, Sheffield S1 2NU (0114 278 7088)
Information on your nearest Law Centre.
Law Society, 114 Chancery Lane, London WC2A 1PL (0171 320 5793)
Group for solicitors with disabilities. Contact Judith McDermott.
Learning Difficulties – Values into Action, Oxford House, Derbyshire Street, London E2 6HG (0171 729 5436)
Campaigns for the right of people with learning difficulties to live in the community.
Learning Disabilities, British Institute of (formerly British Institute of Mental Handicap), Wolverhampton Road, Kidderminster DY10 3PP (01562 850251)

Leonard Cheshire Foundation, 26–29 Maunsel Street, London SW1P 2QN (0171 828 1822)
Provides services to people with mental and physical disabilities and their carers.
Leukaemia Research Fund, 43 Great Ormond Street, London WC1N 3JJ (0171 405 0101)
Booklets on leukaemia and related blood cancers.
Liberty (The National Council for Civil Liberties), 21 Tabard Street, London SE1 4LA (0171 403 3888)
Library, The Listening, 12 Lant Street, London SE1 1QH (0171 407 9417)
A talking book library for disabled people (other than visually impaired) & hospital patients.
Limbless Association, The Rehabilitation Centre, Roehampton Lane, London SW15 5BL (0181 788 1777)
Limbless Ex–Service Men's Association, British, Frankland Moore House, 185–187 High Road, Chadwell Heath, Romford, Essex RM6 6NA (0181 590 1124)
London Lighthouse, 111–117 Lancaster Road, London W11 1QT (0171 792 1200; Minicom 0171 792 2979)
Residential and support centre for people affected by HIV and AIDS.
Long-Term Medical Conditions Alliance (LMCA), c/o Unit 212, 16 Baldwin's Gardens, London EC1N 7RJ (0171 813 3637)
Aims to improve the quality of life of people with long-term medical conditions.
Low Pay Unit, 27–29 Amwell Street, London EC1R 1UN (Employment Rights Helpline 0171 713 7583)
Lupus UK, 1 Eastern Road, Romford, Essex RM1 3NH (01708 731251)
Self-help and fund-raising charity.

M

Macfarlane Trust, PO Box 627, London SW1H 0QG (0171 233 0342)
Grants to people infected with HIV through treatment for haemophilia.
Maternity Alliance, 45 Beech Street, London EC2P 2LX (Office & Minicom 0171 588 8583; Advice 0171 588 8582)
Pressure group on maternity rights.
ME – see Myalgic Encephalomyelitis
Medic Alert Foundation, 1 Bridge Wharf, 156 Caledonian Road, London N1 9UU (0171 833 3034)
Provides internationally recognised medical identification emblems in the form of bracelets or necklets for people with hidden medical conditions.
Medical Accidents, Action for Victims of, Bank Chambers, 1 London Road, London SE23 3TP (0181 291 2793)
Advisory service for victims of medical negligence.

Mencap (Royal Society for Mentally Handicapped Children and Adults), 123 Golden Lane, London EC1Y 0RT (0171 454 0454)
Mencare, 37 Sunningdale Park, Queen Victoria Road, New Tupton, Chesterfield S42 6DZ (01246 865069)
Database of services for people with mental health problems.
Meningitis Trust, The National, Fern House, Bath Road, Stroud, Gloucestershire GL5 3TJ (01453 751738; Support line 0345 538118)
Mental After Care Association (MACA), 25 Bedford Square, London WC1B 3HW (0171 436 6194)
Provides services for people with mental health needs and their carers.
Mental Health Act Commission, Maid Marian House, 56 Houndsgate, Nottingham NG1 6BG (0115 943 7100)
Statutory body to protect the rights of people with mental health problems.
Mental Health, National Association for – see Mind (The Mental Health Charity)
Mental Health Foundation, 37 Mortimer Street, London W1N 8JU (0171 580 0145)
Mental Welfare Society, Ex-Services – see Combat Stress
Metabolic Diseases in Children, Research Trust for, Golden Gates Lodge, Weston Road, Crewe CW2 5XN (01270 250221)
Migraine Association, British, 178a High Road, Byfleet, West Byfleet, Surrey KT14 7ED (01932 352468)
Research, newsletter, leaflets, free information service. Membership £3 per year.
Migraine Trust, 45 Great Ormond Street, London WC1N 3HZ (0171 831 4818)
Full sufferer service, literature, newsletter, helpline, clinic, educational service and research.
Mind (The Mental Health Charity), Granta House, 15–19 Broadway, London E15 4BQ (0181 519 2122; London info line 0181 522 1728; Outside London 0345 660163)
Mobility Centre, Banstead, Damson Way, Orchard Hill, Queen Mary's Avenue, Carshalton, Surrey SM5 4NR (0181 770 1151)
Free information service, assessments for car drivers, passengers & wheelchair users. Driving tuition & residential accommodation.
Mobility for Disabled People, Joint Committee on, 14 Birch Way, Warlingham, Surrey CR6 9DA
Liaising and campaigning body on mobility, access and transport.
Mobility Information Service, National Mobility Centre, Unit 2a, Atcham Estate, Shrewsbury SY4 4UG (01743 761889)
Information on mobility. Driving assessment for disabled drivers.

Moebius Syndrome Contact Group, Mrs L Anderson, 21 Shields Road, Whitley Bay, Tyne and Wear NE25 8UJ (0191 253 2090)
Provides contact between parents for sharing problems and information.
Motability, Goodman House, Station Approach, Harlow, Essex CM20 2ET (01279 635666)
Motor Neurone Disease Association, PO Box 246, Northampton NN1 2PR (01604 250505; Helpline 0345 626262)
Mucopolysaccharide Diseases, The Society for, 55 Hill Avenue, Amersham, Buckinghamshire HP6 5BX (01494 434156)
Support, advocacy and help for families.
Multiple Sclerosis Resource Centre, 4a Chapel Hill, Stansted, Essex CM24 8AG (01279 817101)
Information, educational literature, advice and support counselling by phone.
Multiple Sclerosis Society of Great Britain and Northern Ireland, 25 Effie Road, London SW6 1EE (0171 610 7171; Helpline 0171 371 8000 10am–4pm Mon–Fri)
Muscular Dystrophy Group, 7–11 Prescott Place, London SW4 6BS (0171 720 8055)
Myalgic Encephalomyelitis, Action for, PO Box 1302, Wells, Somerset BA5 2WE (01749 670577; Helpline 0891 122976; Counselling line 01749 670402)
Myalgic Encephalomyelitis Association, Stanhope House, High Street, Stanford-le-Hope, Essex SS17 0HA (01375 642466; Helpline 01375 361013 1.30pm–4pm Mon–Fri)
Myasthenia Gravis Association, Central Office, Keynes House, Chester Park, Alfreton Road, Derby DE21 4AS (01332 290219)

N

Narcolepsy Association UK, 1 Brook Street, Stoke on Trent ST4 1JN (01782 416417)
Support to sufferers and their families, information and advice.
National Association of Citizens Advice Bureaux (NACAB) – see Citizens Advice Bureaux, National Association of (NACAB)
NCVO – see Voluntary Organisations, National Council of
Neurodisability Service, Wolfson Centre, Great Ormond Street Hospital, Mecklenburgh Square, London WC1N 2AP (0171 837 7618)
Assessment and advice on children who have complex neurodevelopmental problems.
Neurofibromatosis Association, The (formerly Link), 82 London Road, Kingston upon Thames KT2 6PX (Voice and Minicom 0181 547 1636)

Noonan Syndrome Society, The, Chelsea House, Westgate, London W5 1DR (0181 991 2536)
Promotes awareness and offers support.
Norwood Ravenswood, Broadway House, 80–82 The Broadway, Stanmore, Middlesex HA7 4HR (0181 954 4555)
Services for children and adults with learning disabilities.
Not Forgotten Association, 158 Buckingham Palace Road, London SW1W 9TR (0171 730 2400)
Services for disabled ex-service people.
NSPCC (National Society for the Prevention of Cruelty to Children), 42 Curtain Road, London EC2A 3NH (0171 825 2500; Freephone Helpline 0800 800500)
Runs network of child protection teams.

O

Occupational and Environmental Diseases Association (ODEA), Mitre House, 66 Abbey Road, Bush Hill Park, Enfield EN1 2QH (0181 360 8490)
Advice and information.
One Parent Families, National Council for, 255 Kentish Town Road, London NW5 2LX (0171 267 1361)
Opportunities for People with Disabilities, 1 Bank Buildings, Prince's Street, London EC2R 8EU (0171 726 4961; Minicom 0171 726 4963)
Employment service (13 regional centres and 2 job clubs).
Orange Badge Network, 52 High Street, Blackheath, Rowley Regis, W. Midlands B65 0EH (0121 561 3265)
Represents the rights and needs of the Orange Badge Holder. Information, membership and newsletter available.
Organic Acidaemias UK, Mrs E Priddy, 5 Saxon Road, Ashford, Middlesex TW15 1QL (01784 245989)
Arranges contacts between families of children with organic acidaemias.
Outset, Drake House, 18 Creekside, London SE8 3DZ (0181 692 7141)
Promotes employment and training for all people with disabilities.

P

Paget's Disease, National Association for the Relief of, 207 Eccles Old Road, Salford, Manchester M6 8HA (0161 707 9225)
Pain Society, The, 9 Bedford Square, London WC1B 3RA (0171 636 2750)
Parentability (National Childbirth Trust), Alexandra House, Oldham Terrace, London W3 6NH (0181 992 2616)
National network of disabled parents. Newsletter, childcare equipment helpline, resource list.

Parkinsonians Partners and Relatives, Young Alert (YAPP&RS), Emma Bennion, Church Farm, Bircham Newton, Kings Lynn, Norfolk PE31 6QZ (01485 578592)
Information group for young people with Parkinson's disease.
Parkinson's Disease Society of the UK, 22 Upper Woburn Place, London WC1H 0RA (0171 383 3513)
Partially Sighted Society, PO Box 322, Doncaster DN1 2XA (01302 323132; London Office 0171 372 1551)
Patients' Association, The, 8 Guilford Street, London WC1N 1DT (0171 242 1524)
Help and advice for patients. Leaflets and self-help directory available.
Pensions Advisory Service (OPAS), 11 Belgrave Road, London SW1V 1RB (0171 233 8080)
Free help to people with pension problems.
People First, Instrument House, 207–215 King's Cross Road, London WC1X 9DB (0171 713 6400)
Independent self-advocacy organisation run by and for people with learning difficulties. Send sae for details.
Perthes Association, 42 Woodland Road, Guildford, Surrey GU1 1RW (01483 306637)
Support on Perthes disease and other forms of osteochondritis.
PHAB England, Summit House, Wandle Road, Croydon CR0 1DF (0181 667 9443)
Clubs and holidays to bring disabled and able-bodied people together.
Phenylketonuria UK Limited, National Society for, 7 Southfield Close, Willen, Milton Keynes MK15 9LL (01908 691653)
Polio Fellowship, British, Unit A, Eagle Office Centre, The Runway, South Ruislip, Middlesex HA4 6SE (0181 842 4999)
Prader Willi Syndrome Association UK, Rosemary Johnson, 2 Wheatsheaf Close, Horsell, Woking, Surrey GU21 4BP (01483 724784)
Premature Sexual Maturation – see Child Growth Foundation
Premenstrual Syndrome, National Association for (NAPS), PO Box 72, Sevenoaks, Kent TN13 1XQ (01732 459378; info line 01732 741709)
Primary Immunodeficiency Association, Alliance House, 12 Caxton Street, London SW1H 0QS (0171 976 7640)
Information on treatment and care, and advice on benefits.
Psoriasis Association, 7 Milton Street, Northampton NN2 7JG (01604 711129)
Psychiatric Rehabilitation Association, Bayford Mews, Bayford Street, London E8 3SF (0181 985 3570)
Provides a range of services to people undergoing psychiatric rehabilitation.

Q

QUIT, Victory House, 170 Tottenham Court Road, London W1P 0HA (0171 388 5775; Quitline 0800 002200)
Offers help to those wanting to quit smoking.

R

Racial Equality, Commission for, Elliott House, 10–12 Allington Street, London SW1E 5EH (0171 828 7022)
RADAR (Royal Association for Disability and Rehabilitation), 12 City Forum, 250 City Road, London EC1V 8AF (0171 250 3222; Minicom 0171 250 4119)
National disability campaigning and information service.
Rathbone Community Industry, 1st Floor, Excalibur Building, 77 Whitworth Street, Manchester M1 6EZ (0161 236 5358; Advice 0161 236 1877)
Ravenswood Foundation – see Norwood Ravenswood
Raynaud's and Scleroderma Association Trust, 112 Crewe Road, Alsager, Cheshire ST7 2JA (01270 872776)
Support, advice, newsletters, publications.
Reach, National Co-ordinator, 12 Wilson Way, Earls Barton, Northamptonshire NN6 0NZ (01604 811041)
Advice and information for children with hand or arm deficiency.
Real Life Options, Tayson House, Methley Road, Castleford, West Yorkshire WF10 1PA (01977 556917)
Services for people with learning disabilities.
Refugee Action, The Offices, The Cedars, Oakwood, Derby DE21 4FY (01332 833310)
Refugee Legal Centre, Sussex House, 39–45 Bermondsey Street, London SE1 3XF (0171 827 9090; Advice line 0171 378 6242; Detention phone line 0171 378 6243)
Refugee Legal Group, c/o NILC, 161 Hornsey Road, London N7 6DU (0171 607 2461)
Co-ordinates activities of lawyers dealing with cases of asylum seekers. Does not give advice to individuals.
REMAP, JJ Wright, National Organiser, Hazeldene, Ightham, Sevenoaks, Kent TN15 9AD (01732 883818)
Makes or adapts aids for disabled people when not commercially available, at no charge to the disabled person.
Remploy Ltd, 415 Edgware Road, London NW2 6LR (0181 235 0500)
Restricted Growth Association, Mrs Honor Rawlings, PO Box 8, Countesthorpe, Leicester LE8 5ZS (0116 2478 913)
Information and support for those affected by restricted growth.

Retinitis Pigmentosa Society, British, PO Box 350, Buckingham MK18 5EL (01280 860363)
Retirement Pensions Associations, National Federation of, (Pensioners Voice), Thwaites House, Railway Road, Blackburn, Lancashire BB1 5AX (01254 52606)
Rett Syndrome Association, UK, c/o A Matthews, 113 Friern Barnet Road, London N11 3EU (0181 361 5161)
Rheumatism, British League Against, 41 Eagle Street, London WC1R 4AR (0171 242 3313)
Riding for the Disabled Association, Avenue 'R', National Agricultural Centre, Kenilworth, Warwickshire CV8 2LY (01203 696510)
Provides the opportunity of riding and driving to disabled people.
Rights Now Campaign, c/o RADAR, 12 City Forum, 250 City Road, London EC1V 8AF (0171 250 3222)
Pressure group for civil rights for disabled people.
Road Peace, PO Box 2579, London NW10 3PW (0181 964 9353; Advice 0181 964 1021)
Emotional and practical support to bereaved and injured road traffic victims.
Royal Air Forces Association, 43 Grove Park Road, London W4 3RX (0181 994 8504)
Regional offices UK wide.
Royal National Institute for Deaf People (RNID) – see Deaf People, Royal National Institute for
Royal National Institute for the Blind (RNIB) – see Blind, Royal National Institute for the
RSI (Repetitive Strain Injury) Association, Chapel House, 152 High Street, Yiewsley, West Drayton, Middlesex UB7 7BE (01895 431134)
Advice and information on RSI.

S

SANE, 199 Old Marylebone Road, London NW1 5QP (0171 724 6520; Saneline 0345 67 8000 2pm–midnight)
Provides information and support for anyone coping with mental illness.
St Dunstan's, PO Box 4XB, 12–14 Harcourt Street, London W1A 4XB (0171 723 5021)
Care for men and women blinded in the services.
St Loyes College for Training Disabled People for Employment, Fairfield House, Topsham Road, Exeter, Devon EX2 6EP (01392 55428)
Residential vocational training for disabled people.
St Vincent de Paul Society, Damascus House, The Ridgeway, London NW7 1EL (0181 906 1339)
Catholic charity helping the needy and poor.

Sarcoidosis and Interstitial Lung Association (SILA), Chest Clinic Office, Dulwich Hospital, London SE22 8PT
Self-help group for people with sarcoidosis and related illnesses.
Sarcoidosis Association, c/o Mrs A Cook, 19 Ashurst Close, Blackbrook, St Helens, Merseyside WA11 9DN (01744 28020)
Schizophrenia Association of Great Britain, Bryn Hyfryd, The Crescent, Bangor, Gwynedd LL57 2AG, Wales (01248 354048)
Helpline and information packs available.
Schizophrenia Fellowship, National, 28 Castle Street, Kingston upon Thames, Surrey KT1 1SS (0181 547 3937; Advice Line 0181 974 6814 Mon–Fri 10am–3pm)
Scleroderma Treatment Unit, Bretforton Hall Clinic, Bretforton, Hereford and Worcester WR11 5JH (01386 830537)
Research, treatment, enquiries.
Scope (formerly The Spastics Society), 12 Park Crescent, London W1N 4EQ (0171 636 5020; Helpline 0800 626216)
Sense – see Deafblind and Rubella Association, The National
Sequal Trust, The (formerly Possum Users' Association), Ddol Hir, Glyn Ceiriog, Llangollen, Clwyd LL20 7NP, Wales (01691 718331)
Assessment and provision of communication aids.
Sex Education Team, Horizon Trust, Harperbury Hospital, Harper Lane, Radlett, Hertfordshire (01923 427420)
Direct work with people with learning disabilities. Advice and training available.
Shaftesbury Society, 16 Kingston Road, London SW19 1JZ (0181 542 5550)
Residential centres, schools, colleges and holiday centres for disabled people.
Shelter (National Campaign for Homeless People), 88 Old Street, London EC1V 9HU (0171 505 2000)
Has regional offices.
SIA, The National Development Agency for the Black Voluntary Sector, Winchester House, 9 Cranmer Road, Kennington Park, London SW9 6EJ (0171 735 9010)
Sickle Cell and Thalassaemia Association of Counsellors, George Marsh Sickle Cell and Thalassaemia Centre, St Ann's Hospital, St Ann's Road, London N15 3TH (0181 442 6230)
Sickle Cell Society, 54 Station Road, London NW10 4UA (0181 961 7795)
Silver-Russell Syndrome – see Child Growth Foundation
Skill – see Students with Disabilities, National Bureau for
Skin Foundation, British, 19 Fitzroy Square, London W1P 5HQ (0171 383 0266)

Snowdon Award Scheme, The, 22 Horsham Court, 6 Brighton Road, Horsham, West Sussex RH13 5BA (01403 211252)
Bursaries to help physically disabled students with the additional costs of further education or training.
Social Workers, British Association of (BASW), 16 Kent Street, Birmingham B5 6RD (0121 622 3911)
Soldiers', Sailors' and Airmen's Families Association – Forces Help (SSAFA), 19 Queen Elizabeth Street, London SE1 2LP (0171 403 8783; 0171 962 9696)
Sotos' Syndrome Society – see Child Growth Foundation
Spastics Society – see Scope
Special Education Advice, Independent Panel for, 4 Ancient House Mews, Woodbridge, Suffolk IP12 1DH (01394 382814)
Speech Impaired Children, Association For All – see AFASIC
Spina Bifida – see ASBAH
Spinal Injuries Association, 76 St James's Lane, London N10 3DF (0181 444 2121; Counselling line 0181 883 4296)
Spod (The Association to Aid the Sexual and Personal Relationships of People with a Disability), 286 Camden Road, London N7 0BJ (0171 607 8851)
Sports Association for the Disabled, British, Mary Glen Haig Suite, Solecast House, 13–27 Brunswick Place, London N1 6DX (0171 490 1919; Minicom 0171 336 8721)
Stammering Association, The British, 15 Old Ford Road, London E2 9PJ (0181 983 1003)
Stroke Association, The, CHSA House, Whitecross Street, London EC1Y 8JJ (0171 490 7999)
Advice, publications, welfare grants. List of local stroke clubs. Visiting services in some areas.
Students, National Union of, Nelson Mandela House, 461 Holloway Road, London N7 6LJ (0171 272 8900)
Students with Disabilities, National Bureau for (Skill), 336 Brixton Road, London SW9 7AA (Voice and Minicom 0171 274 0565; Information line 0171 978 9890 Mon–Fri 1.30pm–4.30pm)
Information on post-16 education for disabled people.
Sue Ryder Foundation, Cavendish, Sudbury, Suffolk CO10 8AY (01787 280252)
Swimming Clubs for the Handicapped, National Association of, The Willows, Mayles Lane, Wickham, Hampshire PO17 5ND (01329 833689)

T

Terrence Higgins Trust, The, 52–54 Gray's Inn Road, London WC1X 8JU (0171 831 0330; Helpline 0171 242 1010; Legal 0171 405 2381)
Thalassaemia Society, UK, 107 Nightingale Lane, London N8 7QY (0181 348 0437)
Education, information, counselling. Publicity available in Greek, Italian, Chinese, Turkish, Arabic, Hebrew, Portuguese and Asian languages.
Thalidomide Society UK, 19 Central Avenue, Pinner, Middlesex HA5 5BT (0181 868 5309)
Tinnitus Association, British, 4th Floor, White Building, Fitzalan Square, Sheffield S1 2AZ (0114 279 6600)
Information, self-help groups.
Tracheo-Oesophageal Fistula Support, St George's Centre, 91 Victoria Road, Netherfield, Nottingham NG4 2NN (0115 940 0694)
Support for families of babies unable to swallow.
Tuberous Sclerosis Association, Mrs Janet Medcalf, Little Barnsley Farm, Catshill, Bromsgrove B61 0NQ (01527 871898)
Provides support and information and promotes research.
Turner's Syndrome Society – see Child Growth Foundation
Turning Point, New Loom House, 101 Backchurch Lane, London E1 1LU (0171 702 2300)
Help with drink, drugs, mental health & learning disabilities.

U

Urostomy Association, Buckland, Beaumont Park, Danbury, Essex CM3 4DE (01245 224294)
Support for people who have had surgery for urinary diversion.

V

Vaccine-Damaged Children, Association of Parents of, 2 Church Street, Shipston on Stour, Warwickshire CV36 4AP (01608 661595)
Values into Action – see Learning Difficulties
Vision Homes Association, 153 Warstone Lane, Hockley B18 6NZ (0121 233 2290)
Provides homes for people with visual impairments and additional disabilities.
Voluntary Organisations, National Council of (NCVO), Regent's Wharf, 8 All Saints' Street, London N1 9RL (0171 713 6161)

W

Widows – see Cruse Bereavement Care
Williams Syndrome Foundation (incorporating Infantile Hypercalcaemia), The Little Ruin, Edge Road, Edge, Stroud GL6 6NE (01452 812277)
Winged Fellowship Trust, Angel House, 20–32 Pentonville Road, London N1 9XD (0171 833 2594)
Respite care and holidays for severely physically disabled people.
Wireless for the Blind Fund, British, Gabriel House, 34 New Road, Chatham, Kent ME4 4QR (01634 832501)
Women, Rights of, 52–54 Featherstone Street, London EC1Y 8RT (Advice 0171 251 6577)
Women's Aid Federation, England, P O Box 391, Bristol BS99 7WS (0117 963 3494; Advice 0345 023 468)
Advice and information or referral to a refuge.
Women's Alcohol Centre, 66a Drayton Park, London N5 1ND (0171 226 4581)
Counselling, group work, residential rehabilitation, children and young people's service.
Women's Health, 52–54 Featherstone Street, London EC1Y 8RT (0171 251 6580)
Information and support on women's health matters.
Women's Royal Voluntary Service (WRVS), 234–244 Stockwell Road, London SW9 9SP (0171 416 0146)
Provides care and practical help for disabled people.
Women's Therapy Centre, 6–9 Manor Gardens, London N7 6LA (0171 263 6200)
Provides individual and group therapy.
Writers, National Association of Disabled, 18 Spring Grove, Harrogate, North Yorkshire HG1 2HS (01423 563103)
Researches political repression of writers.

Y

Youth Exchange Centre, The British Council, 10 Spring Gardens, London SW1A 2BN (0171 389 4030)
Administers grant aid for exchanges of groups of young people aged between 15 and 25.

Northern Ireland

Age Concern, Northern Ireland, 3 Lower Crescent, Belfast BT7 1NR (01232 245729)
Alzheimer's Disease Society, 403 Lisburn Road, Belfast BT9 7EW (01232 664100)

ANTS (Syringomyelia) Self-Help Group, c/o F Somers, 166 Battleford Road, Armagh BT61 8BX (01861 548382)
Arthritis Care, R Douglas, 31 New Forge Lane, Belfast BT9 5NW (01232 669882)
Blind, Royal National Institute for the, 40 Linenhall Street, Belfast BT2 8BG (01232 329373).
Carers National Association, Northern Ireland, Regional Office, 113 University Street, Belfast BT7 1HP (01232 439843)
Chest, Heart and Stroke Association Northern Ireland, Mrs M Beggs, 21 Dublin Road, Belfast BT2 7FJ (0345 697299)
Disability Action, 2 Annadale Avenue, Belfast BT7 3JH (01232 491011) *also at 174 North Street, Belfast BT1 1NE (01232 322504; Textphone 01232 324338)*
Aims to ensure disabled people attain their rights.
Down's Syndrome Association Northern Ireland, J McMaster, 2nd Floor, 28 Bedford Street, Belfast BT2 7FE (01232 243266)
Epilepsy Association, British, Helen Hood, Graham House, Knockbracken Healthcare Park, Saintfield Road, Belfast BT8 8BH (01232 799355)
Extra Care for Elderly People, 11 Wellington Park, Belfast BT9 6DJ (01232 683273)
Domiciliary care for carers in most of Northern Ireland.
Families in Contact, 175 Orby Drive, Belfast BT5 6BB (01232 705097)
Support for parent carers and families with any type of disability.
Fermanagh Voluntary Association of the Disabled, Mill Street, Enniskillen, County Fermanagh (01365 325522)
Haemophilia Society (N. Ireland Group), Society House, 6 Kilcoole Park, Belfast BT14 8LB (Phone/Fax 01232 729559)
ME Association, Northern Ireland, 28 Bedford Street, Belfast BT2 7FE (01232 439831)
Mencap in Northern Ireland, 4 Annadale Avenue, Belfast BT7 3JH (01232 691351)
Mental Health, Northern Ireland Association for, 80 University Street, Belfast BT7 1HE (01232 328474)
Multiple Sclerosis Society, 34 Annadale Avenue, Belfast BT7 3JJ (01232 644914)
Law Centre (NI), 7 University Road, Belfast BT7 1NA (01232 321307)
NICOD Disability Organisation, Malcolm Sinclair House, 31 Ulsterville Avenue, Belfast BT9 7AS (01232 666188)
Training, accommodation and support for people with physical disabilities.

PHAB (NI), Mourne Villa, Knockbracken Healthcare Park, Saintfield Road, Belfast BT8 8BH (01232 796565; North-West Office 01504 371030; Independent Living Centres – Belfast 01232 439703 & Londonderry 01504 372757)
Polio Fellowship, Northern Ireland, J Thompson, 198 Belvoir Drive, Belvoir Park, Belfast BT8 4PJ (01232 643367)
Riding for the Disabled, G Shillington, Altafort, Skeagh Road, Dromore, County Down BT25 2QB (01846 692236)
Shelter, Old Market Place, Omagh, County Tyrone BT78 1DW (01662 244985).
Also at 165 University Street, Belfast BT7 1HR (01232 247752), and 39 Bowling Green, Strabane BT82 8BW
Spina Bifida and Hydrocephalus, The Association for (ASBAH), 73 New Row, Coleraine BT52 1EJ (01265 51522)

Scotland

Age Concern Scotland, 113 Rose Street, Edinburgh EH2 3DT (0131 220 3345)
Alcohol, Scottish Council on, 2nd Floor, 166 Buchanan Street, Glasgow G1 2NH (0141 333 9677)
Alzheimer Scotland – Action on Dementia, 22 Drumsheugh Gardens, Edinburgh EH3 7RN (0131 225 1453; Advice 0131 220 6155; 24 hr Freephone 0800 317 817)
Information and support for people with dementia and their carers.
Autistic Children, The Scottish Society for, Hilton House, Alloa Business Park, Whins Road, Alloa FK10 3SA (01259 720044)
Promotes the welfare and care of children with autism.
British Legion Scotland, New Haig House, Logie Green Road, Edinburgh EH7 4HR (0131 557 2782)
Cancerlink, 9 Castle Terrace, Edinburgh EH1 2DP (0131 228 5557; Macline 0800 591028; Freephone 0800 132905; Asian language line 0171 713 7867; Admin line 0131 228 5567)
Support and information about cancer.
Capability Scotland, 22 Corstorphine Road, Edinburgh EH12 6HP (0131 337 9876)
Chest, Heart and Stroke Scotland, 65 North Castle Street, Edinburgh EH2 3LT (0131 225 6963).
Regional offices: Glasgow (0141 633 1666); Inverness (01463 713433; Adviceline 0345 720720)
Crossroads (Scotland) Care Attendant Schemes, 24 George Square, Glasgow G2 1EG (0141 226 3793)
Charity providing respite relief for carers in their own homes.

Cystic Fibrosis Research Trust, Princes House, 5 Shandwick Place, Edinburgh EH2 4RG (0131 221 1110)
Deaf, Scottish Association for the, Moray House Institute of Education, Holyrood Road, Edinburgh EH8 8AQ (0131 557 0591)
DIAL Scotland, Braid House, Labrador Avenue, Howden, Lothian EH54 6BU (01506 433468)
DIAL local groups and members:
    Carluke (01555 770123)
    Dumfries (01387 247580)
    East Kilbride (01355 222955)
    Falkirk (01324 611567)
    Fife (01383 313333)
    Glasgow (0141 248 1899)
    Glasgow (0141 420 6480)
    Glasgow (0141 882 5632)
    Glasgow (0141 945 3522)
    Grangemouth (01324 504304)
    Johnstone (01505 324120)
    Kirkintilloch (0141 776 0068)
    Knightswood (0141 954 8432)
    Lothian (0131 555 4200)
    Lothian (0131 662 1962)
    Maryhill (0141 946 5011)
    Renfrewshire (0141 848 1123)
    Scotland (0141 550 4455)
    Stirling (01786 462178)
Disability Information Service, Freepost, Grangemouth FK3 9BR (01324 504304)
Disability Resource Centre, 130 Langton Road, Pollok, Glasgow (0141 883 2997)
Disability Scotland, 5 Shandwick Place, Edinburgh EH2 4RG (Voice and Minicom 0131 229 8632)
Disablement Income Group Scotland, 5 Quayside Street, Edinburgh EH6 6EJ (0131 555 2811)
Down's Syndrome Association, Scottish, 158–160 Balgreen Road, Edinburgh EH11 3AU (0131 313 4225)
ENABLE (formerly The Scottish Society for the Mentally Handicapped), 6th Floor, 7 Buchanan Street, Glasgow G1 3HL (0141 226 4541)
Energy Action, Scotland, 21 West Nile Street, Glasgow G1 2PS (0141 226 3064)
Promotes energy efficiency, energy conservation and affordable warmth.
Epilepsy Association of Scotland, 48 Govan Road, Glasgow G51 1JL (0141 427 4911)
Huntington's Association, Scottish, Thistle House, 61 Main Road, Elderslie, Johnstone PA5 9BA (01505 322245)
Law Society of Scotland, 26 Drumsheugh Gardens, Edinburgh EH3 7YR (0131 226 7411)
Provides details of Scottish solicitors.
LEAD (Linking Education and Disability) Scotland, Queen Margaret College, Clerwood Terrace, Edinburgh EH12 8TS (0131 317 3439)
Educational information for physically disabled and/or sensorily impaired adults.

Mental Health, Scottish Association for, Atlantic House, 38 Gardners Crescent, Edinburgh EH3 8DQ (0131 229 9687)
Mental Health Foundation Scotland, 24 George Square, Glasgow G2 1EG (0141 221 2092)
Grant-making charity in the areas of mental health and learning disabilities.
Mental Welfare Commission for Scotland, 25 Drumsheugh Gardens, Edinburgh EH3 7RN (0131 225 7034)
Statutory body to protect the rights of people with mental health problems.
Mental Welfare Society, Ex-Services and Merchant Navy, Hollybush House, Hollybush KA6 7EA (01292 560214)
Motor Neurone Disease Association, Scottish, 76 Firhill Road, Glasgow G20 7BA
Multiple Sclerosis Society in Scotland, 2a North Charlotte Street, Edinburgh EH2 4HR (0131 225 3600; Helpline 0131 226 6573)
PHAB Scotland, 5a Warriston Road, Edinburgh EH3 5LQ (0131 558 9912)
Physically Disabled, Scottish Trust for the, Craigievar House, 77 Craigmount Brae, Edinburgh EH12 8YL (0131 317 7227)
Grant applications considered in relation to housing and transport only.
Red Cross Society, British (Scottish Branch), 204 Bath Street, Glasgow G2 4HL (0141 332 9591)
Limited equipment loan, escort and transport services.
Sense Scotland, 5/2, 8 Elliot Place, Glasgow G3 8EP (0141 221 7577; Text 0141 204 2778)
Shelter Scotland, 8 Hampton Terrace, Edinburgh EH12 5JD (0131 313 1550)
Sign Language Interpreters, Scottish Association of, 31 York Place, Edinburgh EH1 3HP (Voice and Minicom 0131 557 6370)
Holds register of interpreters for Scotland. Also provides training.
Spina Bifida Association, Scottish, 190 Queensferry Road, Edinburgh EH4 2BW (0131 332 0743)
Spinal Injuries Scotland, Festival Business Centre, 150 Brand Street, Glasgow GS1 1DH (0141 314 0056; Helpline 0141 314 0057)
Sports Association for Disabled People, Scottish, The Fife Sports Institute, Viewfield Road, Glenrothes KY6 2RB (01592 415700)
Thistle Foundation, Niddrie Mains Road, Edinburgh EH16 4EA (0131 661 9970)
Accommodation for physically disabled people. Also has a respite care unit.
War Blinded, Scottish National Institution for the, Gillespie Crescent, Edinburgh EH10 4HZ (0131 229 1456)
Women's Aid, Scottish, 12 Torphichen Street, Edinburgh EH3 8JQ (0131 221 0401)

Women and HIV/AIDS Network, The, 13a Great King Street, Edinburgh EH3 6QW (0131 557 5199)
Women's Royal Voluntary Service (WRVS), 19 Grosvenor Crescent, Edinburgh EH12 5EL (0131 337 2261)

Wales

Action Aid for the Disabled, 3 Griffin Street, Newport, Gwent NP9 1GL (01633 258212)
Information, advice, tribunal representation, counselling service.
Agoriad Cyf, Porth Penrhyn, Bangor, Gwynedd LL57 4HN (01248 361392)
Employment agency supporting disabled people into work.
AIDS Helpline and Clinic Newport (01633 841901)
Arts Disability Wales, Chapter Arts Centre, Market Road, Canton, Cardiff CF5 1QE (01222 377885)
Cardiff Law Centre, 15 Splott Road, Splott, Cardiff CF2 2BU (01222 498117)
Cardiff Women's Aid, 20 Moira Terrace, Adamsdown, Cardiff CF2 1EJ (01222 460566)
Computer Workshop, Coleg Glan Hafren, Trowbridge Road, Cardiff CF3 8XZ (01222 250284)
Employment initiative for people with learning disabilities.
Cystic Fibrosis Research Trust, c/o WCVA, Llys Ifor, Crescent Road, Caerphilly, Mid Glamorgan CF83 1XL (01222 852751)
DIAL groups
  Llan Harry (01443 237937)
  Swansea (01792 588322)
Disability Wales, Llys Ifor, Crescent Road, Caerphilly, Mid Glamorgan CF83 1XL (01222 887325)
Information and campaigning body.
Disablement Welfare Rights, 2 Glanrafon, Bangor, Gwynedd LL57 1LH (01248 352227)
Drugaid (SWAPA Ltd), 64–66 Cardiff Road, Caerphilly CF83 1JQ (01222 881000)
Drop-in and group counselling.
Mind, Cymru/Wales (National Association for Mental Health), 23 St Mary Street, Cardiff CF1 2AA (01222 395123; Info Line 0345 660163 9.15am–4.45pm Mon–Fri)
Service offers information on a wide range of mental health issues.
Scope (formerly the Spastics Society), 3 Links Court, Links Business Park, St Mellons, Cardiff CF3 0SP (01222 797706)
Shelter Cymru, 25 Walter Road, Swansea SA1 5NN (01792 469400)
Wales Council for the Blind, Shand House, 20 Newport Road, Cardiff CF2 1DB
Wales Council for the Deaf, Glenview House, Courthouse Street, Pontypridd CF37 1JW (01443 485686; Text 01443 485686)

DIAL UK member groups

There are a huge number of locally based disability groups and it is impossible for us to list them all. We give below a list of DIAL local groups and suggest you contact the one nearest you for details of other organisations or services in your area. Alternatively, we keep a directory of local disability organisations in our office and you can ring us for more information. This is a list of groups in England. For Scotland and Wales, see separate sections.

Amersham (01494 434460)
Ashington (01670 522070)
Basildon (01268 294401)
Barnsley (01226 240273)
Blackpool (01253 699722)
Blyth (01670 364657)
Bradford (01274 594173)
Brigg (01652 650585)
Brighton (01273 778266)
Bristol (0117 983 2828)
Calderdale (01422 346040)
Cambridge (01223 313600)
Carlisle (01222 818555)
Chester (01244 345655)
Coventry (01203 226747)
Devon (01392 464205)
Dewsbury (01484 559513)
Doncaster (01302 327800)
Dorset (01202 716363)
Dunstable (01582 470999)
Ellesmere Port (0151 356 8253)
Folkestone (01303 226464)
Gillingham (01634 262321)
Gravesend (01474 537666)
Great Yarmouth (01493 337650)
Hampshire (01705 824853)
Havering (01708 730226)
Haywards Heath (01444 416619)
Hertfordshire (0800 181067)
High Wycombe (01494 442601)
Hereford (01432 277770)
Hull (01482 226234)
Huntingdon (01480 830833)
Isle of Wight (01983 522823)
Kendal (01539 740508)
Leeds (0113 268 2689)
Leicestershire (0116 251 5565)
London – see under London-wide section
Lowestoft (01502 511333)
Maidstone (01622 692256)
Mansfield (01623 25891)
Margate (01843 230515)
Mid Suffolk (01449 672781)
Middlesbrough (01642 827471)
Milton Keynes (01908 231344)
Northamptonshire, Corby (01536 204742)
Northamptonshire, Daventry (01327 704223)
North Staffordshire (01782 269744)
North Worcester (01562 68248)
Northwich (01606 350611)
Norwich (01603 623543)
Nuneaton and Bedworth (01203 349954)
Oldham (0161 628 2271)

Oxford (01865 791818)
Peterborough (01733 265551)
Rotherham (01709 373658)
Rugby (01788 568368)
Runcorn (01928 590361)
St Helens (01744 453053)
Sandwell (0121 558 7003)
Selby and District (01757 210495)
Sheffield (0114 272 7996)
Shropshire (01743 240404)
Skelmersdale (0800 220676)
Solihull (0121 770 0333)
Stretford (0161 865 5021)
Surrey (01883 744255)
Tameside (0161 320 8333)
Tamworth (01827 66393)
Tendring (01255 435566)
Tunbridge Wells (01892 526368)
Wakefield (01924 379181)
Warrington (01925 240064)
Weston-super-Mare (01934 419426)
Whitstable (01227 771155)
Wigton (016973 45775)
Wiltshire (01380 871003)
Worcester City (01905 27790)
Workington (01900 65555)

London-wide organisations

Artsline, 54 Chalton Street, London NW1 1HS (0171 388 2227)
London information and advice service for disabled people on arts and entertainment.
Black Disabled People's Association, PO Box 7610, London NW6 5BN (0181 933 3826)
London-wide group of and for Black disabled people.
Blind, Metropolitan Society for the, Duke House, 4th Floor, 6–12 Tabard Street, London SE1 4JU (0171 403 6184)
Small grants available.
Chinese Health and Resource Centre, London, 1 Leicester Place, Leicester Square, London WC2H 7BP (0171 287 0904)
Counsel and Care for the Elderly, Twyman House, 16 Bonny Street, London NW1 9PG (0171 485 1566 Mon–Fri 10.30am–4pm)
Advice service on care at home, residential care and financial help.
Cypriot Advisory Service, 26 Crowndale Road, London NW1 1TT (0171 387 6617)
DART, Unit 11, Spectrum House, 32–34 Gordon House Road, London NW5 1LP
Campaign group for accessible transport.
Disability Resource Team, Bedford House, 125–133 Camden High Street, London NW1 7JR (Voice and Minicom 0171 482 5299)
Disabled Living Foundation, 380–384 Harrow Road, London W9 2HU (0171 289 6111)
Disabled Living Centre for London area.

Greater London Association of Disabled People (GLAD), 336 Brixton Road, London SW9 7AA (0171 346 5800; Minicom 0171 346 5811; Info Line 0171 346 5813)
Information, publications, newsletter and training.
Immunity Legal Centre, 1st Floor, 32–38 Osnaburgh Street, London NW1 3ND (0171 388 6776)
Free legal service for people living in London, affected by HIV or AIDS.
Kenté, 356 Holloway Road, London N7 6PA (0171 700 8148)
The London organisational development agency for the black voluntary sector.
Kith and Kids, c/o Haringey Irish Centre, Pretoria Road, London N17 8DX (0181 801 7432)
Parent self-support group with London and Home Counties remit.
Naz Project London, Palingswick House, 241 King Street, London W6 9LP (0181 741 1879)
HIV, AIDS and sexual health agency for South Asian, Middle Eastern and North African communities.
Parents for Children, 41 Southgate Road, London N1 3JP (0171 359 7530)
Specialist fostering and adoption agency, placing children with exceptional needs.
Refugee Action, 240a Clapham Road, London SW9 OPZ (0171 735 5361)
Shape, LVS Resource Centre, 356 Holloway Road, London N7 6PA (0171 700 8139)
Disability arts agency. Workshops, training, festivals, ticket scheme, deaf arts.
London DIAL local groups and members
   Barking and Dagenham (0181 595 8181)
   Catford (0181 698 3775)
   Tower Hamlets (0181 980 2200)
   Twickenham (0181 898 4225)
   Waltham Forest (0181 520 4111)
   Wandsworth (0181 333 6949)
   Westminster (0171 289 2360)

Law Centres

Law centres provide free legal advice. However, they are usually restricted to providing services in a specific catchment area and are unlikely to be able to help you if you do not live or work in their area. You are best advised to ring them first to check if they are able to assist you. This is a list of law centres in England, with centres in the London area listed at the end. For centres in Northern Ireland, Scotland and Wales see separate sections.

Avon and Bristol Community Law Centre
2 Moon Street, Bristol BS2 8QE (0117 924 8662)
Bradford Law Centre
31 Manor Row, Bradford BD1 4PS (01274 306617)
Carlisle Law Centre
43 Cecil Street, Carlisle, Cumbria CA1 1NS (01228 515129)
Chesterfield Law Centre
44 Park Road, Chesterfield S40 1XZ (01246 550674; Minicom 01246 204570)
Coventry Law Centre
The Bridge, Broadgate, Coventry CV1 1NG (01203 223051/3)
Same location includes Coventry Disability Rights Service (01203 555567)
Disability Law Service
Room 241, 49–51 Bedford Row, London WC1R 4LR (0171 831 8031)
Free legal advice and information for disabled people.
Gateshead Law Centre
Swinburne House, Swinburne Street, Gateshead NE8 1AX (0191 477 1109)
Gloucester Law Centre
Widden Old School, Widden Street, Gloucester GL1 4AQ (01452 423492)
Wheelchair accessible.
Harehills and Chapeltown Law Centre
263 Roundhay Road, Leeds LS8 4HS (0113 249 1100)
Highfields and Belgrave Law Centre
Seymour House, 6 Seymour Street, Highfields, Leicester LE2 0LB (0116 2532 928)
Humberside Law Centre
95 Alfred Gelder Street, Hull HU1 1EP (01482 211180)
Kirklees Community Law Centre
Unit 5, Lion Chambers, John William Street, Huddersfield HD1 1EU (01484 518525)
Liverpool 8 Law Centre
34–36 Princes Road, Liverpool L8 1TH (0151 709 7222)
London – see list at end
Luton Law Centre, 28 Clarendon Road, Luton, Bedfordshire LU2 7PQ (01582 481000)
Middlesbrough Law Centre
St Mary's Centre, 82–90 Corporation Road, Cleveland TS1 2RW (01642 223813)
Newcastle Law Centre
51 Westgate Road, Newcastle upon Tyne NE1 1SG (0191 230 4777)
North Manchester Law Centre
Community Services Centre, Paget Street, Manchester M40 7UU (0161 205 5040)
Nottingham Law Centre
119 Radford Road, Nottingham NG7 5DU (0115 9787 813)
Oldham Law Centre
Prudential Assurance Buildings (2nd Floor), 79 Union Street, Oldham OL1 1HL (0161 627 0925)
Rochdale Law Centre
Smith Street, Rochdale OL16 1HE (01706 57766)
Salford Law Centre
498 Liverpool Street, Salford, Manchester M6 5QZ (Voice and Minicom 0161 736 3116)

Saltley Action Centre
2 Alum Rock Road, Saltley, Birmingham B8 1JB (0121 328 2307)

South Manchester Law Centre
584 Stockport Road, Manchester M13 0RQ (0161 225 5111)

Vauxhall Law Centre
Multi-Services Centre, Silvester Street, Liverpool L5 8SE (0151 207 2004/3502)

Warrington Law Centre
64–66 Bewsey Street, Warrington, Cheshire WA2 7JQ (01925 651104)

Wiltshire Law Centre
26 Victoria Road, Swindon, Wiltshire SN1 3AW (01793 486926/7)

Wythenshawe Law Centre
260 Brownley Road, Manchester M22 5EB (0161 498 0905/6)
List of other advice agencies within the Manchester area available.

London Law Centres

Brent Community Law Centre
Advice by telephone only (0181 451 1122)

Brixton Law Centre
506–508 Brixton Road, London SW9 8EN (0171 737 0440)

Cambridge House Legal Centre
137 Camberwell Road, London SE5 0HF (0171 701 9499)

Camden Community Law Centre
2 Prince of Wales Road, London NW5 3LG (0171 485 6672)

Central London Law Centre
47 Charing Cross Road, London WC2H 0AN (0171 437 5854)

Ealing Borough Law Centre
11b King Street, Southall, Middlesex UB2 4DF (0181 574 2434)

Greenwich Law Centre
187 Trafalgar Road, London SE10 9EQ (0181 853 2550)

Hackney Law Centre
236–238 Mare Street, London E8 1HE (0181 985 8364)

Hammersmith and Fulham Law Centre
142–144 King Street, London W6 0QU (0181 741 4021)

Hillingdon Legal Resource Centre
12 Harold Avenue, Hayes, Middlesex UB3 4QW (0181 561 9400)

Hounslow Law Centre
51 Lampton Road, Hounslow, Middlesex (0181 570 9505)

Mary Ward Legal Advice Centre
26–27 Boswell Street, London WC1N 3JZ (0171 831 7079)

Newham Rights Centre
285 Romford Road, London E7 9HJ (0181 555 3331)

North Islington Law Centre
161 Hornsey Road, London N7 6DU (0171 607 2461)

North Kensington Law Centre
74 Golborne Road, London W10 5PS (0181 969 7473)

North Lambeth Law Centre
14 Bowden Street, London SE11 5DS (0171 582 4373)

North Lewisham Law Centre
28 Deptford High Street, London SE8 3NU (0181 692 5355)

Paddington Law Centre
439 Harrow Road, London W10 4RE (0181 960 3155)

Plumstead Law Centre
105 Plumstead High Street, London SE18 1SB (0181 855 9817)

Southwark Law Centre
Hanover Park House, 14–16 Hanover Park, Peckham, London SE15 5HS (0171 732 2008)

Springfield Law Centre Ltd
Springfield Hospital, Glenburnie Road, London SW17 7DJ (0181 767 6884)

Stockwell and Clapham Law Centre
57–59 Old Town, Clapham, London SW4 0JQ (0171 720 6231)

Tottenham Legal Advice Centre
754–758 High Road, London N17 (0181 808 5354; Advice line 0181 801 6064)

Tower Hamlets Law Centre
341 Commercial Road, London E1 2PS (0171 791 0741)

Wandsworth & Merton Law Centre
248 Lavender Hill, London SW11 1LJ (0171 228 9462/2566)

Index

A

abroad, benefits payable 209–212
see also – person from abroad
absence from home 40, 101, 102, 143
Access Funds 173
Access to Work 108
Accident Line 154, 251
accidents at work – *see industrial injuries scheme*
actively seeking work 101–102
adaptations
    help from social services 182–184
    housing benefit 41
    housing grants 226–231
    income support for mortgages and loans 26
additional earnings-related pension (SERPS)
    incapacity benefit 89
    retirement pensions 217, 218, 219
adjudicating medical authority 9, 97, 151, 241
adjudicating medical practitioner 94, 95, 151, 241
adjudication officer 9, 241
age
    discriminatory age limits 216
    pension age 216
    retirement 155, 213, 216–220
    tax allowance 233, 234
agent – *see appointees*
all work test 70–76
    appeals 16, 75, 76
    exemptions, standard 70
    exemptions, transitional 91
    medical examination 74
    mental disabilities, descriptors 74
    mental health assessment 70, 74–75
    physical disabilities, descriptors 72–73
    questionnaire 71
allowance for lowered standard of occupation 157
alternative claims 237
appeals
    appeal or review 242
    appeals to Commissioners 251
    attendance allowance 119, 141–142, 242, 245–246, 248
    council tax benefit 49
    disability living allowance 139, 242, 245–246, 248
    disability working allowance 117, 242, 245–246, 248
    housing benefit 49
    incapacity for work 16, 75, 76, 103
    income support 38, 245, 248
    Independent Living Funds 186
    industrial injuries scheme 153, 245–247
    late appeals 246
    Secretary of State decisions 241, 246
    social services 181–182
    supplementary benefit 37
    time limits 245
    war disablement pension 158–159
see also – Disability Appeal Tribunals
    – Medical Appeal Tribunals
    – Social Security Appeal Tribunals
applicable amounts
    council tax benefit 52–53
    disability working allowance 115
    family credit 168
    housing benefit 52–53
    income-based jobseeker's allowance 108
    income support 18
    residential care 192–193, 200–201
appointees 140, 171, 239
arrears of benefit
    and review of income support 244
    ignored as capital 36
    invalid care allowance 21, 144
see also – backdating
asbestos related diseases 148, 149
asthma, occupational 149
asylum seekers 17, 18
attendance allowance 140–142
    abroad 211
    age limits 140, 142
    amount 141
    appeals 141–142, 245–246, 248
    attention 128–129, 132–133, 140
    backdating 138, 139, 141, 238, 244
    claims 141
    daily rate 205
    dialysis 133, 140
    hospital 123–125, 141, 204
    other benefits 141
    residential care/nursing home 125–126, 141, 191, 199
    respite care 124, 196–197
    reviews 141–142, 242–244
    supervision 129, 132, 140
    tax 140
    terminal illness 130–131, 141
    watching over 130–132, 140
see also – disability living allowance
    – disability living allowance care component
available for work
    jobseeker's allowance 100–101
    part-time students 175

B

back to work bonus 105
backdating
    claims 48, 238–239
    reviews 244–245

Banstead Mobility Centre 146
benefit penalty 76, 103–105, 231–232
benefit week 34, 47
benefit year 78
benefits, checklist 4–5
see also – under name of benefit
Benefits Agency 8
Benefits Agency Medical Services (BAMS) 10, 74, 151
blind
   all work test
     – descriptors 73
     – exemption 70
   care services 180
   child support 233
   disability living allowance
     – care component 128, 171
     – mobility component 134, 137
   disability premium 20
   disability working allowance 114
   disabled child allowance 115
   disabled child premium 23
   disablement, percentage assessments 94, 96, 152
   equipment for work 108
   exemption from signing on 16
   non-dependant deduction 51
   pensioner in residential care 201
   reader service 108
   severe disability premium 21, 22
   severe disablement allowance 94, 172
   sight tests 225
   students 173, 176
   tax allowance 234
boarders 34, 42, 88, 168
bridging allowance 110
budgeting loans 60–66
byssinosis 148, 149

C

capital or savings
   council tax benefit 51
   dependent child 28
   deprivation of capital 29–30, 194
   diminishing capital 30, 240–241
   disability working allowance 113
   family credit 167
   housing benefit 51
   income-based jobseeker's allowance 107
   income support 28–30, 34–36
   notional capital 29–30, 195
   residential care
     – income support 192, 200
     – local authority charging assessment 188, 189, 193, 194–195, 197
   social fund 59, 60, 61, 62
   tariff income 34, 51
   trust fund 36
care component – see disability living allowance care component
care services 177–182
   help with the cost of care 184–186
careers 176
carer premium 23, 53, 144, 215
carers
   absence from home 41, 143
   council tax 57
   council tax benefit 41, 53
   credits 78
   help for 178–179, 180
   hospital 145, 204, 206
   housing benefit 41, 53
   income support
     – carer premium 23
     – housing costs waiting period 27, 28
     – not signing on 17
     – remunerative work 15–16
   jobseeker's allowance 100
see also – invalid care allowance
Carers (Recognition and Services) Act 1995 178, 180
cars 146, 147
charging
   for local authority care services 179–181
   for residential care 193–198
charitable payments 32–33
child benefit 165–167
   abroad 211
   extension period 165
   in hospital 205
   lone parent 166
   residence test 166
child maintenance bonus 233
child support 231–233
childcare costs 52, 88, 115, 168
children 164–165, 169–171
see also – young people
Christmas bonus 224
chronic bronchitis, miners 151
Chronically Sick & Disabled Persons Act (1970) 179, 180
claims
   alternative 237
   backdating 238–239
   date of claim 236–237
   delays 238–239, 240
   information and evidence 237
   late claims 48, 238–239
   reviews 242–245
   time limits 238
see also – under name of benefit
close relative
   claimant in residential care 197, 199
   housing benefit 39
   severe disability premium 22
   social fund funeral payment 59
clothing
   clothing allowance 157
   community care grant 63
   help from the Family Fund 169
   school clothing grant 165
cold weather payments 60
comforts allowance 157
Commissioners' decisions 241, 250, 251
see also – appeals
communication aids 183, 184
Community Care 177–182
   charging 179–181
   complaints 181–182
   direct payments 186, 191
   equipment 182–184
   local authority assessments 177–178, 180
   services 178–179
community care grants 60–66

Community Health Council 253
compensation
    criminal injuries compensation 159–161
    delays in benefit payment 48, 240
    industrial injury 148–149
    maladministration 253
    recovery of benefit from compensation 160, 162
Compensation Recovery Unit 162
complaints 10, 182, 252–253
constant attendance allowance 154, 156
    abroad 212
    in hospital 204
contracting out of SERPS 219
contribution-based jobseeker's allowance 98, 106
see also – jobseeker's allowance
contributions – see National Insurance
contributory benefits 8
council tax 55–58
    disability reduction scheme 58
    discount scheme 58
    exempt dwellings 55, 56
    liability 56
    severe mental impairment 57
council tax benefit 45
    second adult rebate 53–54
see also – housing benefit
councillors 16, 68–69
credits 77–78
criminal injuries compensation 159–161
crisis loans 60–66
customer service manager 10

D

date of claim 236–238
day centres 179
deaf
    care component 128, 132
    children's care component 165, 171
    incapacity for work 73
    mobility component 134, 137
    occupational deafness 149
    students 172, 174
death 5, 59, 160, 222
decisions 241, 250
see also – reviews
       – appeals
delays
    in claiming 48, 238–239
    in payment 48, 240
delegated medical practitioner 243
dental treatment 225
diabetes 97, 225
dialysis – see kidney dialysis
direct payments for care 186, 191
direct payments from benefit 37–38
Disability Appeal Tribunals (DAT) 9, 139, 142, 242–243, 246, 248
    members' duties for incapacity benefit 68
Disability Discrimination Act 1995 10–13, 109
Disability Employment Adviser 108
disability living allowance 119–140
    abroad 211
    age limits 120, 121, 142

appeals 139, 242–243, 246, 248
appointees 140, 171, 239
awards 138–139, 140
blind 128, 134, 137, 171
care component 126–133
children
    – age rules 121
    – extra disability test 126–127, 133, 170–171
    – hospital and special accommodation 124–125
    – presence test for babies 122
claims 137–138
    – administration 138
    – backdating 138
    – help with claiming 137
    – interchangeable 237
    – late claims 138
    – linked claims 122
    – renewal 120–122, 138
    – terminal illness 130–131
    – time limits 138, 238
compensation for delays 138, 240
deaf 128, 132, 134, 137, 171
decisions 138, 241
disability tests 126–133, 133–137
hospital 123–125, 204, 205, 209
medical examinations 123, 137, 138, 248
non-disability tests 120–122
other benefits 123
payment 140
payment at daily rate 205
prison 123
qualifying periods 122, 133
residence and presence tests 122
residential care 125–126, 191, 199
reviews 139, 140, 242–244
    – backdating 139, 244
    – change of circumstances 139, 140, 243
    – grounds for review 139, 242–243
    – life awards 139, 243
    – terminal illness 131
self-assessment 137
tax 123
terminal illness 130–131
see also – disability living allowance care component
       – disability living allowance mobility component
disability living allowance care component 126–133
amount 122
attention 128–129
    – bodily function 128
    – frequent 128–129
    – night attention 129
    – overlap with supervision 132–133
    – prolonged 129
    – reasonably required 128
    – repeated 129
    – significant portion 129
    – simpler methods 132
children
    – disability tests 126–127, 170–171
    – hospital and special accommodation 124–125
cooking test 127–128
dialysis 133
disability tests 126
intermittent disability 127
night 126, 129, 130–132
residential care/nursing home 125–126, 191, 196–197, 199

– independent care homes 191
– local authority homes 191
– local authority not funding 126, 191
– preserved rights 199
respite care 124
students 176
supervision 129–130, 132
terminal illness 130–131
watching over 130–132
work 122–123
see also – disability living allowance
disability living allowance mobility component 133–137
amount 122
amputations 133, 134
artificial aids 135, 136
behavioural problems 133, 136–137
children 133
coma 134
deaf/blind 134
disability tests 133
exemption from road tax 147
exertion 133–134
guidance or supervision 137
higher rate 133–137
hospital 123–125, 204, 205, 209
ignored as income for benefits/services 123
intermittent abilities 136
learning disabilities 134–135, 137
lower rate 133, 137
Motability 125, 146
severe discomfort 135–136
severe mental impairment 136–137
terminal illness 135
virtually unable to walk 135–136
walking tests 135, 248
see also – disability living allowance
disability premium 20–21, 53
disability reduction scheme 58
disability working allowance 111–118
age limit 112
appeals 117, 242–243, 246, 248
applicable amounts 115
assessment, disability 113, 114
assessment, means-test 115–116
backdating 116–117, 238–239
'better off' 112
change of circumstances 117
claims 116–117
contribution credits 78
decisions 117
disability questions 117, 246
disability test 113, 114
family credit 116
linking rules
– for qualifying benefits 113, 116
– for training courses 113
– linked spells of sickness 117
– two year rule 117–118
off-sick
– effect on hours 112
– effect on other benefits 117
qualifying benefits 113
reviews 117, 242–243
therapeutic work 112
disabled child allowance 115
disabled child premium 23, 53

disabled facilities grant 229–230
Disabled Living Centres 183
Disabled Living Foundation 183
Disabled Persons Act (1986) 180
disabled students' allowance 173
disablement benefit 149–154
discount scheme 58
discrimination
disability 10–13, 109
sex 216
dismissal
disabled 11, 109
jobseeker's allowance 104
draughtproofing 231
DSS structure 8–10

E

EC 210
EEA 210
early retirement 213
earnings
adult dependant limit 88, 90, 97
child dependant limit 88, 97
councillors 69
earnings disregards, income support 31
invalid care allowance 144
jobseeker's allowance 106, 107
occupational pension 32, 87, 88, 106, 195, 200, 213
retirement pension 217
therapeutic 68
education
credits 78
full-time education
– child benefit 165
– income support 15, 17, 172, 174
– severe disablement allowance 92, 171–172, 176
grants 172–173, 175
part-time education 174, 175
special educational needs 164, 165
Eileen Trust 32–33, 36, 51
employed earner, status 110
employment rehabilitation course 109, 111
Employment Service 108
equal treatment 216
equipment 108, 173, 182–184
errors of law 243, 249
European Community 210
European Economic Area 210
exceptionally severe disablement allowance 154, 157
exemption from all work test 70, 91
exemption from road tax 147
ex-gratia payments 32, 36, 48, 240
eye tests 225

F

family credit 167–169
Family Fund 169
family premium 22–23, 53
fares
to Disablement Services Centres 226
to hospital 203, 226

to school 165
to tribunal 249
to work, Access to Work 108
foster parents 16, 125, 166
fresh evidence 153, 243
full-time education – see education
full-time work 15–16, 102–103, 112–113, 167
funeral payment 59–60

G

gay partner 63, 86, 198
glasses 225
good cause for late claim 48, 239
graduated retirement benefit 217
grants
    community care grants 60–66
    housing grants 226–230
grants for students 172–173
green form scheme 251–252
guaranteed minimum pension 217
guide dogs 102, 135, 137

H

habitual residence test 17
Health Authorities 183, 187
health benefits 224–226
health care 177, 183–184
Health Service Ombudsman 253
health visitors 178
higher pensioner premium 24, 53
Home Energy Efficiency Scheme 231
home helps 178
Home Responsibilities Protection 220–221
home visits 178
hospices 123, 188
hospital 203–209
    after one year 207, 208–209
    attendance allowance 123–124, 141, 204
    children 124–125, 205
    daily rate 205
    disability living allowance 123–125, 204, 205, 209
    fares 203
    linking rule 204, 206
    temporary absence 205, 209
    treatment allowance 157
housing benefit 39–55
    absence from home 40–41
    appeals 49
    applicable amount 52–53
    assessment 49–50
    backdating 48
    benefit period 47
    benefit week 47
    capital 51–52
    change of circumstances 47
    childcare costs 52
    claims 45–47
    complaints 49
    counselling and support services 42
    eligible rent 41
    ex-gratia payments 48
    extended payments 47
    extra benefit in exceptional circumstances 48
    fuel charges 42
    hospital 41, 206–207
    income 52
    joint occupiers 40
    meal deductions 42
    moving home 41
    non-dependant deductions 50–51
    payments 47
    premiums 53
    rent restrictions 42–45
    residential care/nursing homes 40, 41, 191–192, 199–200
    reviews 49
    service charges 42
    students 39, 174–175
    water charges 42
housing costs, income support 24–28
housing for disabled people 182
housing grants 226–231
    disabled facilities grants 229–230
    home energy efficiency scheme 231
    home repair assistance 230
    improvement grants 227
    renovation grants 227–229

I

improvement grants 227
incapacity benefit 85–89
    abroad 210
    additional pension (SERPS) 89
    age addition 86, 90
    amount 86, 88, 89–90
    appeals 75, 76, 89, 245, 248–250
    backdating 89, 238, 244
    claims 88–89
    contribution conditions 79, 85
    credits 77
    dependants' additions 86, 88, 90
    disability living allowance 70, 87, 89
    disability working allowance 87, 90, 113, 117–118
    disqualification 69, 87
    earnings 68, 87, 88
    equal treatment 216
    hospital 87, 204
    industrial incapacity 89, 90
    maternity allowance 164
    over pension age 88, 89, 90, 214, 216, 219
    period of incapacity for work 78–79, 85–86
    statutory maternity pay 164
    statutory sick pay 83, 84
    tax 87
    terminal illness 70, 86, 87
    training 87, 90, 111
    transferring from invalidity benefit 89–90
    transferring from sickness benefit 89
    widows 85, 223
see also – all work test
        – incapacity for work
incapacity for work 67–76
    all work test 69, 70–75
    appeals 16, 75, 76
    credits 77

councillors 68–69
descriptors 72–73, 74
disability premium 20–21, 91
disqualification 69
exceptional circumstances 76
exempt from all work test 70, 91
income support
 – claiming while appealing 16, 76, 103
 – exemption from signing on 16
jobseeker's allowance 103
medical certificates 70, 75, 89, 91
medical examinations 74–75
mental health assessment 70, 74–75
own occupation test 69–70
pregnancy 68, 164
questionnaire 71–74
severe mental illness 70
tests of incapacity 69
therapeutic work 68, 90
treated as incapable of work 68
tribunal members 68
variable conditions 71
voluntary work 68
see also – *statutory sick pay*
 – *incapacity benefit*

income support 14–38
abroad 210–211
appeals 38, 245, 248–250
applicable amounts 18
appointee 37, 239
assessment 18
asylum seekers 17, 18
backdating claims 37, 238–239
backdating on review 38, 244
benefit week and paydays 34–35
capital 28–30, 34–36
carers 15–16, 17, 23
claims 36–37, 237–238
direct payment 37–38
eligibility 16–17
'gateway' to other benefits 14
habitual residence test 17
hospital 206–207
housing costs 24–28
incapacity appeals 16
income 28–34
interest on mortgages and loans 26
liable relatives 28, 193, 201–202
maintenance 28, 193, 201–202, 231
people from abroad 16–18
personal allowances 19
premiums 20–24
remunerative work 15–16
residential care/nursing homes 19, 192–193, 195, 199, 200–202
students 15, 17, 173–174
tax 233
income tax 87, 233–235
income-based jobseeker's allowance 98, 106–108
see also – *jobseeker's allowance*
incontinence 129, 137, 183
Independent Living Funds 184–186
industrial accident or disease 148–155
industrial death benefit 149, 222
industrial injuries scheme 148–155
accidents at work 148, 150

aggregating assessments 152–153, 153–154
appeals 153, 246–247
assessment of disablement 95, 96, 152
backdating 149, 239, 244
constant attendance allowance 154
disablement benefit 149–153
exceptionally severe disablement allowance 154
prescribed diseases 148, 151
reduced earnings allowance 154–155
retirement allowance 155
reviews 153–154, 242–245
unforeseen aggravation 153
Industrial Tribunals 11, 13, 109
invalid care allowance 142–145
abroad 211
amount 144
backdating 144, 238
carer premium 23, 144, 215
claiming jobseeker's allowance 79, 100, 145
credits 78, 144
dependants' additions 144
earnings 144
entitlement 143–144
hospital 145, 204, 205
income support 15–16, 17, 144
over pension age 214–215
overlapping benefits 21, 144
residence and presence 143
severe disability premium 21
tax 142, 233
time off caring 144
invalid trike 146
invalidity benefit
additional pension (SERPS) 89, 90, 214
age allowance (invalidity allowance) 90, 214, 219
dependants' additions 90
disability working allowance 90, 118
industrial incapacity 90
over pension age 90, 214, 219
therapeutic work 90
training 90, 111
transferring to incapacity benefit 89–91

J

Job Introduction Scheme 108
Jobcentres 108
jobseeker's allowance 98–108
abroad 211
actively seeking work 101–102
age 16 or 17 107–108
amounts 106, 108
available for work 100–101
back to work bonus 105
capable of work 103
claiming 98–100, 237–238
contribution-based jobseeker's allowance 106
 – contribution conditions 79
hardship payments 105–106
hospital 204
incapacity cut-offs 103
income-based jobseeker's allowance 106–108
jobseeker's agreement 102
jobseeker's direction 100

jobseeking period 79
just cause for voluntarily leaving work 104
over pension age 98, 214
permitted period 100
sanctions 103–105
students 98, 100, 175
transferring from income support 99
transferring from unemployment benefit 99
trial period 104
judicial review 246
jury service 17, 78, 79

K

kidney dialysis 68, 85, 122, 133, 140

L

late appeals 246
late claims 238–239
laundry
    disability living allowance 128
    Family Fund 169
    incontinence services 183
    social fund 63
learning disabilities
    all work test 70, 74, 91
    appointees 37, 140, 171, 239
    backdating benefit 239
    disability living allowance 134–135, 137, 171
    severe disablement allowance 172
leaving hospital 187–188, 205, 209
legal aid 251–252
lesbian partner 63, 86, 198
liable relatives 28, 189, 193, 195, 201–202
linking rules
    attendance allowance 123–124, 141
    disability living allowance 122, 123–124
    disability premium 20
    disability working allowance 117–118
    higher pensioner premium 24
    hospital 123–124, 204, 206
    invalid care allowance 145
    jobseeker's allowance 79
    training 111
see also – period of incapacity for work
        – period of interruption of employment
loans for repairs 26, 65
loans, social fund 60–66
loans, students 173
local authority accommodation – see residential care homes
local authority, help for disabled people 177–179
Local Government Ombudsman 253
Local Health Council 253
lone parent
    child benefit 166
    child support 231–233
    earnings disregard 31, 52
    family premium 22–23
    hospital 207
    residential care 193
lone parent premium 22

M

MacFarlane Trusts 32–33, 36, 51, 178
maintenance payments 28, 193, 195, 201
    Child Support Agency 231
    disregard 52, 115, 168
maternity 163–165
maternity allowance 163–164
maternity payment, social fund 59
meals allowance, residential care 202
Meals on Wheels 178, 179
means-tested benefits 8
Medical Appeal Tribunals 241, 246–247
    access to 249
    appeals from 251
    evidence 247
medical assessor 250
medical evidence, backdating 21, 89, 92
medical examinations 74–75, 94, 141, 151, 247
milk and vitamins 165, 226
mobility checklist 146
mobility component – see disability living allowance mobility component
mobility housing 182
Mobility Information Service 146
mobility supplement 156
mortgage interest 24–28
Motability Scheme 125, 146
Motor Insurers' Bureau 160

N

National Assistance Act (1948) 177, 180, 187, 190
National Disability Council 12–13
National Health Service Act (1977) 181, 190
National Health Service and Community Care Act (1990) 180, 187, 190
National Insurance
    benefit year and contribution year 78–79
    contributions, amounts 76–77
    contributions and benefits 76
    contribution conditions 79–80, 218
    contribution credits 77–78
    contributions deducted but not recorded 218
NHS benefits 224–226
non-contributory benefits 8
non-contributory invalidity pension 92–93
non-dependants 21–22, 50–51
non-means-tested benefits 8
notional capital 29–30, 194–195
notional income, residential care home 202
nursing homes
    benefit entitlement 125–126, 187, 190–193, 198–202
    choice of home 187–190
    continuing nursing care 187–188
    local authority charging 193–198
    maintenance 193, 195, 201
    preserved rights 198–202
    registration with health authority 187
see also – residential care homes

O

OPAS (Pensions Advisory Service) 220
occupational pensions 213, 217, 220
    dependants' additions 87, 88, 97
    income support 32
    invalid care allowance 144
    jobseeker's allowance 106
    residential care 32, 195, 200
Occupational Pensions Regulatory Authority 220
occupational sick pay 81–82
occupational therapists 178, 183
Ombudsman 252–253
one parent benefit 166
orange badge scheme 145
overpayments of benefits 48, 240
own occupation test 69–70

P

PIW – *see period of incapacity for work*
parking concessions 145
Parliamentary Ombudsman 253
Part III accommodation – *see residential care homes*
partner 18, 53, 87
part-time student 174, 175
part-time work
    disability working allowance 112–113
    family credit 167
    income support 15–16, 105
    jobseeker's allowance 102–103, 105
    therapeutic work 68
'passport' or gateway to other benefits 14, 112, 120
pay day for benefits 34–35, 47, 205
pension – *see retirement pension*
pensioner premium 23, 53
Pensions Ombudsman 13, 220
period of incapacity for work (PIW)
    contribution conditions 78–79
    day of incapacity 85
    linking
    – incapacity benefit 78–79, 85–86
    – unemployment benefit 79
    maternity allowance 85
    statutory sick pay 80
period of interruption of employment (PIE) 79
person from abroad
    attendance allowance 122
    disability living allowance 122
    disability working allowance 112
    family credit 167
    housing benefit/council tax benefit 39
    income support 16–18
    invalid care allowance 143
    jobseeker's allowance 107
    severe disablement allowance 92
personal allowance 19, 53
personal injury
    compensation recovery 160, 162
    legal advice 148, 154, 251–252
    trust funds 36
personal pensions 219
see also – *occupational pensions*
personal reader service for blind people 108
physiotherapists 179, 183

Placement, Assessment and Counselling Teams 108, 109
plasmapheresis 68, 85
pneumoconiosis 148, 149, 151
pre-1976 vehicle scheme 146
pregnancy 17, 59, 68, 80, 106, 163–165
premiums 20–24, 53
prescribed industrial diseases 148, 151, 246
prescription charges 224–225
preserved rights, residential care 198–202
prison 17, 41, 51, 62, 80, 81, 100, 101, 123
public transport concessions 146

R

RADAR (Royal Association for Disability and Rehabilitation) 183
RNIB (Royal National Institute for the Blind), students 176
radiotherapy 68, 80, 85
Railcard 146
rate rebate, Northern Ireland 54–55
reduced earnings allowance 154–155, 216
refugees – *see person from abroad*
register of disabled people 7, 11, 108, 178
relative – *see close relative*
remunerative work 15–16, 51, 102–103, 107
renovation grants 227–229
rent – *see housing benefit*
resettlement benefit 32
residential allowance 19, 192
residential care homes 187–202
    benefit entitlement 125–126, 190–193, 198–202
    benefits and charges 196–197
    charging assessment 193–198
    choice of home 189
    complaints 181–182, 190
    couples and maintenance 193, 195, 201–202
    eviction 201, 202
    hospices 123, 188
    hospital 123–125, 206, 207
    local authority needs assessment 177–178, 180, 188–189
    personal expenses allowance 196–197, 200
    preserved rights 198–202
    residential allowance 19, 192
    respite care 40, 124, 192, 193, 196, 197, 198
    treatment of former home 35, 191, 194–195, 197–198
    trial period in residential care 41, 192, 193
    types of residential care 187–188
retirement 213–220
    early retirement 213
    equal treatment 216
    increments towards pension 219
    pension age 216–217
retirement allowance 155, 216
retirement pension 216–220
    abroad 212
    deferring claims 213–214, 219
    extra pension 217–219
    hospital 204–205
    incapacity benefit 214
    invalid care allowance 214–215
    severe disablement allowance 215
reviews
    appeal or review 242
    backdating on 244

change of circumstances 243
grounds for 242–243
life awards, disability living allowance 139, 243
terminal illness 131

S

savings – *see capital or savings*
Secretary of State 9, 241, 246
self-certification
   incapacity benefit 88
   statutory sick pay 80
SERPS – *see additional earnings-related pension*
service charges 25, 42
services checklist 178–179
setting aside decisions 241
severe disability premium
   housing benefit/council tax benefit 53
   income support 21–22
   residential care 192
severe disablement allowance 91–97
   16–18 year olds 171–172, 176
   abroad 210
   age additions 97
   backdating 93, 97, 238, 239, 244
   disability working allowance 94, 117–118
   disablement assessment 94–96
   employment rehabilitation course 109, 111
   in hospital 204–205
   incapacity for work 70, 90, 91, 92
   interchangeable claims 237
   over pension age 215
   passporting benefits 94
   residence and presence 92
   routes to qualification 92
   students 92, 171–172, 176
   therapeutic work 68, 97
   training allowance 111
   volunteers 68
   work trial concession 93–94
severe disablement occupational allowance 157
sheltered employment – *see supported employment*
sheltered housing 182
sick notes 21, 69, 83, 88–89, 92, 203
sickness benefit 89, 111, 118
see also – incapacity benefit
signing on 16, 76, 77, 98–100
social fund, discretionary 60–66
   budgeting loans 61–62, 63–64
   claims 64–65
   community care grants 61, 62–63
   crisis loans 62, 63–64
   decisions 66
   exclusions 64–65
   repayment of loans 66
   repeat applications 61
   reviews 66
social fund, regulated 59–60
   cold weather payment 60
   funeral payment 59–60
   maternity payment 59
social fund inspector 66
Social Security Administration Act 8
Social Security Appeal Tribunals 9, 245, 248

Social Security Contributions and Benefits Act 8
social services, personal 177–182
Social Work (Scotland) Act (1968) 201
special educational needs 164, 165, 176
special hardship allowance 149
statutory maternity pay 163
statutory sick pay 80–85
   abroad 212
   age rules 81, 214
   evidence of sickness 83
   in hospital 204
   leaver's statement 84
   period of incapacity for work 80
   pregnancy 80, 164
   qualifying conditions 80
   transfers to incapacity benefit or SDA 83
see also – incapacity benefit
strikers 17, 33, 35, 52, 64, 77, 81, 233
students 172–176
   access funds 173
   benefits 173–176
   blind 176
   career development loans 173, 174
   deaf 174
   disabled students' allowance 173
   equipment 173
   grants 172–173
   loans 173
   part-time study 174, 175
supplementary benefit 37
supported employment 109

T

tax – *see income tax*
telephone 179
terminal illness 21, 70, 87, 130–131
test case backdating 244–245
therapeutic work 68, 90
time limits
   appeals 245, 246, 250, 251
   claims 238–239
   reviews 242–244
traffic accidents 160
training allowance 110, 111
Training and Enterprise Councils 109
training credits 78, 110
Training for Work 110–111
training schemes 103, 109
transport schemes 146, 179
see also – fares
treatment allowance 157

U

unemployability supplement 154, 156–157
unemployment benefit 99
see also – jobseeker's allowance
unfit for human habitation 229
unforeseen aggravation 153, 243

V

VAT 230
vaccine damage payments 161–162
vehicle excise duty, exemption from 147
vitamins 163, 165, 226
voluntary early retirement 213
voluntary work, effect on benefits 16, 29, 68, 101, 102
vouchers for glasses 225

W

War Pensioners' Welfare Service 157
war pensions scheme 156–159
    appeals 158
    constant attendance allowance 156
    in hospital 157, 204, 205
    mobility supplement 156
    war disablement pension 156
    war widows 158
water charges 25, 42, 65
wheelchair housing 182
Wheelchair Service Centre 184
wheelchairs, provision of 184

widowed mother's allowance 223
widows 222–224
    benefits abroad 212
    bereavement tax allowance 234
    contribution credits 78
    funeral expenses 59–60, 158
    incapacity benefit 223
    invalid care allowance 223
    severe disablement allowance 223
widows' allowance 223
widows' payment 222
work – see *full-time work, part-time work*

Y

young people 171–172
    education grants 172–173
    income support 15, 172
    jobseeker's allowance 107–108
    'normal' schooling 171–172
    training 109–110
Youth Training 109–110